CURRENT THERAPY IN OBSTETRICS AND GYNECOLOGY

CURRENT THERAPY IN OBSTETRICS AND GYNECOLOGY

5TH EDITION

Edited by

EDWARD J. QUILLIGAN, M.D.

Professor Emeritus
Department of Obstetrics and Gynecology
University of California, Irvine, Medical Center
Orange, California

and

FREDERICK P. ZUSPAN, M.D.

Professor Emeritus
Department of Obstetrics and Gynecology
Ohio State University
Columbus, Ohio

W.B. SAUNDERS COMPANY
A Division of Harcourt Brace & Company
Philadelphia   London   Toronto   Montreal   Sydney   Tokyo

W.B. SAUNDERS COMPANY
A Division of Harcourt Brace & Company

The Curtis Center
Independence Square West
Philadelphia, Pennsylvania 19106

Library of Congress Cataloging-in-Publication Data

Current therapy in obstetrics and gynecology / [edited by] Edward J. Quilligan,
Frederick P. Zuspan.—5th ed.

   p.   cm.

Includes index.

   ISBN 0–7216–7579–4

1. Generative organs, Female—Diseases—Treatment.   2. Pregnancy—
Complications—Treatment.   I. Quilligan, Edward J.   II. Zuspan, Frederick P.

[DNLM: 1. Genital Diseases, Female—therapy.   2. Fetal
Diseases—therapy.   3. Infant, Newborn, Diseases—therapy.   4. Pregnancy
Complications—therapy.   WP 650 C976 2000]

RG125.C87   2000

618′.046—dc21

DNLM/DLC   99-16181

CURRENT THERAPY IN OBSTETRICS AND GYNECOLOGY   ISBN 0–7216–7579–4

Printed in the United States of America.

Last digit is the print number: 9   8   7   6   5   4   3   2   1

To Betty and Jane, our wives,
for over 50 years of unwavering support.

CONTRIBUTORS

W. Allen Addison, MD

Walter L. Thoma Professor of Obstetrics and Gynecology, Division of Gynecological Specialities, Duke University Medical Center, Durham, North Carolina

Androgen Insensitivity Syndrome

Paula Amato, MD

Assistant Adjunct Professor, University of California, San Diego, LaJolla, California

Polycystic Ovarian Syndrome

Janice Andreyko, MD

Co-Medical Director, Northern California Fertility Medical Center, Roseville, California

Hypopituitarism

Fernando Arias, MD, PhD

Division of Maternal-Fetal Medicine, The Toledo Hospital, Toledo, Ohio

Third Trimester Bleeding

Edward R. Ashwood, MD

Professor, Department of Pathology, University of Utah Health Sciences Center, Salt Lake City, Utah

Lung Maturity Testing

Tamerou Asrat, MD

Associate Clinical Professor, University of California, Irvine, Department of Obstetrics/Gynecology, Division of Maternal-Fetal Medicine, University of California, Irvine, Medical Center, Orange; Medical Director, Perinatal Services at Hoag Memorial Hospital, Newport Beach, California

Breech Delivery; Post-term Pregnancy

Ricardo Azziz, MD, MPH

Professor of Medicine and Obstetrics/Gynecology, University of Alabama at Birmingham, Birmingham, Alabama

Androgen Excess of Adrenal Origin

David A. Baker, MD

Professor, Department of Obstetrics, Gynecology, and Reproductive Medicine; Director, Division of Infectious Diseases, Health Sciences Center, State University of New York at Stony Brook, Stony Brook, New York

Herpes Genitalis

Marina Ball, MD

Associate Clinical Professor, University of California, Irvine, College of Medicine and Medical Center, Irvine, California

Acne Vulgaris

David A. Baram, MD

New York, New York

Premenstrual Dysphoric Disorder (PDD)

Marie H. Beall, MD

Associate Professor of Clinical Obstetrics/Gynecology, University of California, Los Angeles, School of Medicine, Los Angeles; Chief, Division of Obstetrics, Harbor-UCLA Medical Center, Torrance, California

Chorionic Villus Sampling for Prenatal Diagnosis

Fritz K. Beller, MD, DrSci, FACOG, FACS

Professor Emeritus, Westfaelische Wilhelms University, Muenster, Germany; University of Iowa, Iowa City, Iowa

Breast Cancer: Principles for Therapy

Andrew Berchuck, MD

Professor of Obstetrics and Gynecology and Gynecologic Oncology, Duke University, Durham, North Carolina

Endometrial Carcinoma

Ross S. Berkowitz, MD

William A. Baker Professor of Gynecology, Harvard Medical School; Chief, Division of Gynecologic Oncology; Co-Director, New England Trophoblastic Disease Center, Brigham and Women's Hospital, Boston, Massachusetts

Gestational Trophoblastic Disease; Hydatidiform Mole

Michael J. Birrer, MD, PhD

Senior Investigator, Division of Clinical Sciences, National Cancer Institute, Rockville, Maryland

Ovarian Cancer

Jorge D. Blanco, MD

Professor and Associate Chairman, Department of Obstetrics and Gynecology, University of Florida College of Medicine; Medical Director, Women's Hospital, Pensacola, Florida

Chorioamnionitis

Adam F. Borgida, MD

Assistant Professor of Obstetrics and Gynecology, Division of Maternal-Fetal Medicine, University of Connecticut School of Medicine, Farmington, Connecticut

Twin Pregnancy

Michel Boulvain, MD, PhD

Chef de Clinique, Unité de developpement en obstétrique, Université de Genève and Hôpitaux Universitaires de Genève, Geneva, Switzerland

Dysfunctional Labor

Diane Blake Brashear, PhD

Clinical Associate Professor of Obstetrics/ Gynecology and Psychiatry, Indiana University School of Medicine, Indianapolis, Indiana

Sexual Abuse and Rape

Robert F. Burrows, MD, FRCS, FRACOG

Professor and Chair, Maternal-Fetal Medicine, Monash University and Medical Centre, Department of Obstetrics and Gynaecology, Clayton, Victoria, Australia

Idiopathic Thrombocytopenic Purpura

Nancy A. Callan, MD

Director, Division of Maternal Fetal Medicine, Department of Obstetrics and Gynecology, Boston University Medical Center, Boston, Massachusetts

Intrauterine Growth Retardation

Bruce R. Carr, MD

Paul C. MacDonald Professor of Obstetrics and Gynecology and Director, Division of Reproductive Endocrinology, The University of Texas Southwestern Medical Center at Dallas;

Attending Staff Physician, Zale Lipshy University Hospital, Dallas, Texas

Evaluation and Treatment of the Infertile Couple

Linda F. Carson, MD

Associate Professor, Obstetrics, Gynecology, and Women's Health, and Director, Division of Gynecologic Oncology, University of Minnesota, Minneapolis, Minnesota

Vulvar Neoplasms

Denis Cavanagh, MD

Professor of Obstetrics and Gynecology, University of South Florida; Director of Division of Gynecologic Oncology, University of South Florida Health Sciences Center/Tampa General Hospital, Tampa, Florida

Septic Shock in the Gynecologic Patient

Douglas A. Cesario, BS

Resident, University of California, San Diego, California

Pneumonia: Viral and Bacterial

Thomas C. Cesario, MD

Dean, College of Medicine, University of California, Irvine, Irvine, California

Pneumonia: Viral and Bacterial

R. Jeffrey Chang, MD

Professor, University of California San Diego School of Medicine, La Jolla, California

Polycystic Ovarian Syndrome

Samuel J. Chantilis, MD

Assistant Professor and Director, In Vitro Fertilization Program, The University of Texas Southwestern Medical Center at Dallas, Dallas, Texas

Evaluation and Treatment of the Infertile Couple

Patricia S. Choban, MD

Adjunct Professor, Human Nutrition, Ohio State University, Columbus; Bariatric Specialist of Ohio—Surgeon, Bariatric Treatment Centers, Grove City, Ohio

Ileus

Steven L. Clark, MD

Professor of Obstetrics-Gynecology, University of Utah School of Medicine; Director, Women's and Newborns' Services, Intermountain Health Care, Salt Lake City, Utah

Amniotic Fluid Embolism

Daniel L. Clarke-Pearson, MD

James Ingram Professor of Gynecologic Oncology, Department of Obstetrics and Gynecology, Duke University School of Medicine, Durham, North Carolina

Venous Thromboembolic Disease in Pregnancy

Elizabeth B. Connell, MD

Professor Emeritus, Department of Gynecology/Obstetrics, Emory University School of Medicine, Atlanta, Georgia

Barrier Contraception: The Reality Female Condom

Leandro Cordero, MD

Professor, Pediatrics and Obstetrics, The Ohio State University College of Medicine; Director, Newborn Services, The Ohio State University Medical Center, Columbus, Ohio

Glucose Metabolism, Hypocalcemia and Hypomagnesemia in the Newborn; Seizures in the Neonatal Period

Jonathan A. Cosin, MD

Assistant Professor, Obstetrics, Gynecology, and Women's Health, University of Minnesota School of Medicine, Minneapolis, Minnesota

Vulvar Neoplasms

Carolyn B. Coulam, MD

Clinical Professor, University of Illinois School of Medicine; Director, Reproductive Immunology, and Vice President, Medical Affairs, The Center for Human Reproduction, Chicago, Illinois

Recurrent Spontaneous Abortion

Daniel L. Coury, MD

Professor of Clinical Pediatrics, The Ohio State University College of Medicine and Public Health; Chief, Section of Behavioral-Developmental Pediatrics, Children's Hospital, Columbus, Ohio

Congenital Anomalies of the Neonate

Stephanie Marie Culver, MD, MS

Department of Obstetrics and Gynecology, University of Minnesota School of Medicine and Hennepin County Medical Center, Minneapolis, Minnesota

Pelvic Inflammatory Disease

F. Gary Cunningham, MD

Professor, Obstetrics and Gynecology, and Chairman, Obstetrics and Gynecology, The University of Texas Southwestern Medical Center at Dallas; Attending Physician, Parkland Health and Hospital System, Dallas, Texas

Group B Streptococcus in Pregnancy

Douglas C. Daly, MD

Clinical Associate Professor of Obstetrics-Gynecology, Michigan State University College of Human Medicine, East Lansing; Director of Reproductive Endocrinology, Spectrum Health East and Grand Rapids Fertility, Grand Rapids, Michigan

Induction of Ovulation

Vicki C. Darrow, MD

Obstetrician/Gynecologist, Kaiser Permanente Hospital, Novato, California

Annual Examination

John M. Davison, MD

Professor of Obstetric Medicine, University of Newcastle upon Tyne Medical School; Consultant Obstetrician and Gynaecologist, Newcastle upon Tyne Hospitals NHS Trust, Royal Victoria Infirmary, Newcastle upon Tyne, United Kingdom

Renal Disease in Pregnancy (Chronic)

M. Yusoff Dawood, MB, ChB, MD, MMed

The Berel Held Professor of Obstetrics, Gynecology, and Reproductive Sciences and Director, Division of Reproductive Endocrinology, University of Texas Medical School; Attending Obstetrician and Gynecologist, Hermann Hospital and Lyndon Baines Johnson Hospital, Houston, Texas

Dysmenorrhea

John O. L. DeLancey, MD

Normal F. Miller Professor of Gynecology and Associate Chair, Division of Gynecology, University of Michigan, Ann Arbor, Michigan

Genital Prolapse

Lawrence D. Devoe, MD

Professor and Chairman, Department of Obstetrics/Gynecology, and Director of Maternal-Fetal Medicine, Medical College of Georgia; Director, Obstetric Services, Medical College of Georgia Hospitals and Clinics, Augusta, Georgia

Antepartum Fetal Surveillance

Michael P. Diamond, MD

Kamran S. Moghissi Professor of Obstetrics and Gynecology and Director, Division of Reproductive Endocrinology and Infertility, Wayne State University, Detroit, Michigan

Endoscopic Surgery

Philip J. DiSaia, MD

Professor, Department of Obstetrics and Gynecology, The Dorothy Marsh Chair in Reproductive Biology, University of California, Irvine; Attending Staff, University of California Irvine Medical Center, Orange, California

Cervical Carcinoma

James O. Donaldson, MD

Professor of Neurology, University of Connecticut School of Medicine, Farmington, Connecticut

Seizure Disorder in Pregnancy

Arie Drugan, MD

Vice Chairman, Department of Obstetrics and Gynecology, and Director, Labor and Delivery, Rambam Medical Center, Haifa, Israel; Associate Professor, Department of Obstetrics and Gynecology, Wayne State University, Detroit, Michigan

Amniocentesis and Other Tests for Antenatal Diagnosis of Genetic Disorders

Patrick Duff, MD

Professor and Residency Program Director, Department of Obstetrics and Gynecology, University of Florida, Gainesville, Florida

HIV in Pregnancy

Daniel A. Dumesic, MD

Associate Professor, Division of Reproductive Endocrinology, Department of Obstetrics and Gynecology, Mayo Clinic, Rochester, Minnesota

Menopause

E. Christopher Ellison, MD

Zollinger Professor and Chief of General Surgery, Ohio State University, Columbus, Ohio

Pancreatitis in Pregnancy; Hemorrhoids and Anal Fissure

David A. Eschenbach, MD

Professor, Department of Obstetrics and Gynecology, and Chief, Division of Gynecology, University of Washington, Seattle, Washington

Vaginosis (Bacterial)

Mark I. Evans, MD

Charlotte B. Failing Professor, Acting Chairman and Chief of Obstetrics and Gynecology, Professor of Molecular Medicine and Genetics, and Professor of Pathology, Wayne State University; Director, Division of Reproductive Genetics, Center for Fetal Diagnosis and Therapy, and Human Genetics Program, Hutzel Hospital/The Detroit Medical Center, Detroit, Michigan

Amniocentesis and Other Tests for Antenatal Diagnosis of Genetic Disorders

Mary P. Evans, MD

Staff Obstetrician/Gynecologist, Olmsted Medical Group, Rochester, Minnesota

Menopause

Mark J. Fallen, MD

Partner in Urologic Physicians, P.A.; Chief of Urology, Abbott Northwestern Hospital, Minneapolis, Minnesota

Male Sterilization

Lisa J. Farkouh, MD

Clinical Assistant Professor, Maternal-Fetal Medicine, University of Colorado Health Sciences Center, Denver, Colorado

Percutaneous Umbilical Blood Sampling

Sebastian Faro, MD, PhD

John M. Simpson Professor, Department of Obstetrics and Gynecology, Rush Medical College; Chairman, Department of Obstetrics and Gynecology, Rush-Presbyterian-St. Luke's Medical Center, Chicago, Illinois

Sexually Transmitted Diseases; Urinary Tract Infections

Louis Flancbaum, MD

Adjunct Professor, Human Nutrition, Ohio State University College of Medicine, Columbus, Ohio

Ileus

Michael R. Foley, MD

Clinical Associate Professor, Department of Obstetrics/Gynecology, University of Arizona Medical Center, Tucson; Medical Director, Phoenix Perinatal Associates, and Director of Obstetric Intensive Care, Good Samaritan Regional Medical Center, Phoenix, Arizona

Fetal Surgical Management of Congenital Hydronephrosis

William D. Fraser, MD, MSc, FRCSC (Can)

Professor and Chairman, Laval University; Chief of Obstetrics and Gynecology, Pavillon St. François d'Assise (CHUQ), Quebec City, Quebec, Canada

Dysfunctional Labor

Andrew J. Friedman, MD

Private Practice, Wellesley, Massachusetts

Leiomyomata Uteri

Steven G. Gabbe, MD

Professor and Chair, Department of Obstetrics and Gynecology, University of Washington School of Medicine and University of Washington Medical Center, Seattle, Washington

Diabetes Mellitus in Pregnancy

Thomas J. Garite, MD

Professor and Chairman, Department of Obstetrics and Gynecology, University of California, Irvine, Irvine, California

Fetal Fibronectin: Its Role in Obstetrics; Premature Rupture of Membranes

Margaret Graf Garrisi, MD

Associate Professor of Obstetrics and Gynecology, Cornell University Medical College; Associate Attending, Department of Obstetrics and Gynecology, New York Presbyterian Hospital, New York, New York

Adnexal Masses

Donald P. Goldstein, MD

Clinical Professor of Obstetrics, Gynecology, and Reproductive Biology, Harvard Medical School; Co-Director, New England Trophoblastic Disease Center, Brigham and Women's Hospital, Boston, Massachusetts

Gestational Trophoblastic Disease; Hydatidiform Mole

Mary Jane Gray, MD, DMedSci

Professor Emeritus, Obstetrics-Gynecology, University of North Carolina Medical School, Chapel Hill, North Carolina

Oral Contraceptives

Nancy B. Hansen, MD

Attending Neonatologist, Children's Hospital, Columbus, Ohio

Congenital Anomalies of the Neonate

Robert L. Harris, MD

Assistant Professor of Obstetrics/Gynecology and Director, Section of Urogynecology and Reconstructive Pelvic Surgery, University of Mississippi School of Medicine, Jackson, Mississippi

Androgen Insensitivity Syndrome

John C. Hauth, MD

Professor and Director, Center for Research in Women's Health, and Vice Chairman for Research, University of Alabama at Birmingham, Birmingham, Alabama

Postpartum Hemorrhage

Perry A. Henderson, MD

Professor, Obstetrics and Gynecology, University of Wisconsin—Madison; Attending Physician, Meriter Hospital, Madison, Wisconsin

Fetal Death Syndrome

Geri D. Hewitt, MD

Assistant Clinical Professor, Departments of Obstetrics/Gynecology and Pediatrics, Ohio State University College of Medicine and School of Public Health; Physician, Ohio State University Medical Center and Columbus Children's Hospital, Columbus, Ohio

Pediatric Gynecology; Pelvic Pain (Chronic)

William H. Hindle, MD

Professor, Clinical Obstetrics and Gynecology, University of Southern California School of Medicine; Director, Breast Diagnostic Center, Women's and Children's Hospital, LAC&USC Medical Center, Los Angeles, California

Mastalgia and Fibrocystic Changes in the Breast

Endrika L. Hinton, MD

Co-Director, Assisted Reproductive Technologies Program, The Johns Hopkins Medical Institutions, Department of Gynecology and Obstetrics, Baltimore, Maryland

Galactorrhea and Hyperprolactinemia

John C. Hobbins, MD

Professor of Obstetrics and Gynecology and Chief of Obstetrics, University of Colorado Health Sciences Center, Denver, Colorado

Percutaneous Umbilical Blood Sampling

Daniel Hollander, MD

Professor of Medicine, University of California, Los Angeles, School of Medicine; President/CEO, Harbor-UCLA Research and Education Institute, Torrance, California

Gastrointestinal Disorders in Pregnancy

Walter B. Hull, MD

Assistant Professor, Department of Obstetrics and Gynecology, Ohio State University College of Medicine, Columbus, Ohio; Former Staff Physician, Christian Medical Institute of Kasai, Kanaga, Democratic Republic of Congo, Africa

Vesicovaginal Fistulas

W. Glenn Hurt, MD

Professor, Department of Obstetrics and Gynecology, Medical College of Virginia, Virginia Commonwealth University, Richmond, Virginia

Urinary Incontinence

Jay D. Iams, MD

Frederick P. Zuspan Professor and Director, Division of Maternal-Fetal Medicine, Department of Obstetrics and Gynecology, The Ohio State University College of Medicine, Columbus, Ohio

Obstetrical Care of Preterm Births

Robert Israel, MD

Professor, Department of Obstetrics/Gynecology, University of Southern California School of Medicine, Los Angeles, California

Intrauterine Adhesions

David Jackson, MD

Associate Professor, Seattle University, Department of Sonography, Seattle; Clinical Staff, Sacred Heart Medical Center, Eugene, Oregon

Fetal Distress in the Intrapartum Period

Mark P. Johnson, MD

Associate Professor, Departments of Obstetrics and Gynecology, Molecular Medicine and Genetics, and Pathology, Wayne State University School of Medicine; Associate Director, Division of Reproductive Genetics and Center for Fetal Diagnosis and Therapy, Hutzel Hospital/The Detroit Medical Center, Detroit, Michigan

Amniocentesis and Other Tests for Antenatal Diagnosis of Genetic Disorders

Georgeanna S. Jones, MD

Professor Emeritus, Johns Hopkins University School of Medicine, Department of Gynecology and Obstetrics, Baltimore, Maryland; Professor Emeritus, Eastern Virginia Medical School, Norfolk, Virginia

Luteal Phase Defect

John B. Josimovich, MD

Retired; 43 Royal Ave., Cambridge, Massachusetts

Systemic Lupus Erythematosus in Pregnancy

Vern L. Katz, MD

Associate Director, Center for Genetics and Maternal-Fetal Medicine, Eugene, Oregon

Nonimmune Hydrops

Raymond H. Kaufman, MD

Professor, Department of Obstetrics-Gynecology and Pathology, Baylor College of Medicine, Houston, Texas

Non-neoplastic Epithelial Disorders of the Vulva; Vulvar Vestibulitis

William M. Kaylor, Jr., MD

Urologist, Abbott Northwestern Hospital, Minneapolis, Minnesota

Male Sterilization

Thomas F. Kelly, MD

Associate Professor of Reproductive Medicine, Division of Perinatal Medicine, University of California, San Diego, School of Medicine, La Jolla; Chief of Maternity Services, UCSD Medical Center; Consultant, Mercy Hospital, San Diego; Consultant, Scripps La Jolla Medical Center, La Jolla, California

Rheumatic Heart Disease: Safe Conduct in Pregnancy

Elizabeth Kennard, MD

Assistant Professor, Ohio State University College of Medicine, Columbus, Ohio

Precocious Puberty

Omid Khorram, MD, PhD

Assistant Professor of Obstetrics/Gynecology, University of Wisconsin, Division of Reproductive Endocrinology, Madison, Wisconsin

GIFT Procedure

Dirk G. Kieback, MD, PhD

Professor and Chairman, Department of Obstetrics and Gynecology, Freiburg University Medical Center, Freiburg, Germany; Adjunct Associate Professor, Departments of Obstetrics and Gynecology and of Cell Biology, Baylor College of Medicine; Adjunct Associate Professor, Department of Gynecologic Oncology, The University of Texas M.D. Anderson Cancer Center, Houston, Texas

Breast Cancer: Principles for Therapy

Moon H. Kim, MD

Professor and Director, Division of Reproductive Endocrinology, Department of Obstetrics and Gynecology, University of California, Irvine, School of Medicine, Orange, California

Secondary Amenorrhea

David Z. Kitay, MD

Ormond Beach, Florida

Iron Deficiency

Matthew F. Kohler, MD

Associate Professor, Division of Gynecologic Oncology, Department of Obstetrics and Gynecology, Medical University of South Carolina, Charleston, South Carolina

Cervical Carcinoma

Mark B. Landon, MD

Associate Professor and Vice Chairman, Department of Obstetrics and Gynecology, The Ohio State University College of Medicine and Public Health, Columbus, Ohio

Diabetes Mellitus in Pregnancy

Janet D. Larson, MD

Clinical Instructor, Department of Obstetrics and Gynecology, Section of Maternal-Fetal Medicine, The University of Oklahoma College of Medicine, Oklahoma City, Oklahoma

Hyperemesis Gravidarum

Roger R. Lenke, MD

Director, Indiana Center for Prenatal Diagnosis, Indianapolis, Indiana

Lung Maturity Testing

Luanna Lettieri, MD

Director of Maternal-Fetal Medicine, John Peter Smith Hospital, Fort Worth, Texas

Biophysical Profile

Michael P. Levine, PhD

Professor of Psychology, Kenyon College, Gambier, Ohio; Member, Academy for Eating Disorders; Board Member, Eating Disorders Awareness and Prevention, Inc.

Bulimia Nervosa

Frank W. Ling, MD

Professor and Chairman, Department of Obstetrics and Gynecology, University of Tennessee, Memphis, Tennessee

Ectopic Pregnancy

Gary H. Lipscomb, MD

Associate Professor and Director, Division of Gynecology, Department Obstetrics and Gynecology, University of Tennessee, Memphis, Tennessee

Ectopic Pregnancy

A. Brian Little, MD

Clinical Professor, Obstetrics, Gynecology, and Women's Health; University of Medicine and Dentistry of New Jersey, New Jersey Medical School, Newark, New Jersey; Professor, Obstetrics and Gynecology, McGill University Faculty of Medicine, Montreal, Canada

Dysfunctional Uterine Bleeding

Lauren Lynch, MD

Associate Professor and Director of Maternal-Fetal Medicine, University of Puerto Rico School of Medicine, San Juan, Puerto Rico

Multifetal Pregnancy Reduction

Everett F. Magann, MD

Associate Professor of Obstetrics and Gynecology, Division of Maternal-Fetal Medicine, University of Mississippi Medical Center, Jackson, Mississippi

HELLP Syndrome

Alberto Manetta, MD

Professor and Senior Associate Dean, University of California, Irvine, School of Medicine, Irvine, California

Endometrial Hyperplasia

Douglas J. Marchant, MD

Emeritus Professor of Surgery and of Obstetrics/Gynecology, Tufts University School of Medicine, Boston, Massachusetts; Adjunct Professor, Brown University; Director Emeritus, Breast Health Center, Women and Infants Hospital, Providence, Rhode Island

Breast Mass and Nipple Discharge

Stanley C. Marinoff, MD, MPH

Clinical Professor, Obstetrics/Gynecology, George Washington University School of Medicine and Health Sciences; Attending Physician, George Washington University Hospital and Columbia Hospital for Women, Washington, DC

Vulvodynia and Pruritus

Mark G. Martens, MD

Professor and Vice Chairman, Department of Obstetrics and Gynecology, University of Minnesota School of Medicine; Chairman, Department of Obstetrics and Gynecology, Hennepin County Medical Center, Minneapolis, Minnesota

Pelvic Inflammatory Disease

James N. Martin, Jr., MD

Professor of Obstetrics-Gynecology and Director of Maternal-Fetal Medicine and Obstetrics; Director, Maternal-Fetal Medicine Fellowship Program, University of Mississippi Medical Center, Jackson, Mississippi

HELLP Syndrome

Dev Maulik, MD, PhD

Professor of Obstetrics and Gynecology, State University of New York at Stony Brook, Stony Brook; Chairman, Department of Obstetrics and Gynecology, Winthrop-University Hospital, Mineola, New York

Doppler Velocimetry in Fetal Surveillance

Ernest L. Mazzaferri, MD, FACP

Professor and Chairman, Department of Internal Medicine, and Professor of Physiology, The Ohio State University College of Medicine and Medical Center, Columbus, Ohio

Thyrotoxicosis

Paul G. McDonough, MD

Professor of Obstetrics-Gynecology, Medical College of Georgia, Augusta, Georgia

Gonadal Dysgenesis

Peter G. McGovern, MD

Assistant Professor, Department of Obstetrics, Gynecology, and Women's Health, University of Medicine and Dentistry of New Jersey, New Jersey Medical School, Newark; Associate Director, Center for Reproductive Medicine, Hackensack University Medical Center, Hasbrouck Heights, New Jersey

Dysfunctional Uterine Bleeding

W. Scott Melvin, MD

Assistant Professor of Surgery, Ohio State University College of Medicine, Columbus, Ohio

Pancreatitis in Pregnancy

Lance Jay Mercer, MD

Professor of Obstetrics and Gynecology, Northwestern University Medical School, Chicago, Illinois

Chlamydial Infections

Jorge H. Mestman, MD

Professor of Medicine and Obstetrics and Gynecology, University of Southern California School of Medicine; Director, USC Center for Diabetes and Metabolic Diseases, University of Southern California Department of Medicine, Los Angeles, California

Hypothyroidism

Frank C. Miller, MD

Professor and Chair, Department of Obstetrics/Gynecology, University of Kentucky Medical School, Lexington, Kentucky

Fetal Scalp Stimulation

Randy R. Miller, MD

Associate Professor of Clinical Pediatrics and Director, Apnea Program, Children's Hospital, Columbus, Ohio

Seizures in the Neonatal Period

Jane E. C. Milne, MBChB

Research Associate, University of Newcastle upon Tyne, The Medical School, Newcastle upon Tyne; Specialist Registrar, Queen Elizabeth Hospital, Tyne and Wear, United Kingdom

Renal Disease in Pregnancy (Chronic)

Edward R. Newton, MD

Professor and Chairman, East Carolina University School of Medicine; Chief of Service, Department of Obstetrics and Gynecology, Greenville, North Carolina

Genital Tract Trauma

David H. Nichols, MD*

Former Chairman, Department of Obstetrics and Gynecology, Brown University, Providence; Head, Women and Infants' Hospital, Providence, Rhode Island
*Deceased

Disorders of Pelvic Support

David J. Nochimson, MD

Professor and Vice Chairman, Obstetrics and Gynecology and Reproductive Sciences; Associate Dean, Hospital Affiliation, Robert Wood Johnson Medical School, University of ﹒edicine and Dentistry of New Jersey; Physician, St. Peter's Hospital, New Brunswick, New Jersey

Biophysical Profile

Kenneth L. Noller, MD

Professor and Chair, Department of Obstetrics/ Gynecology, University of Massachusetts Medical School; Chair, Department of Obstetrics/Gynecology, University of Massachusetts Memorial Health Care, Worcester, Massachusetts

Colposcopy

James A. O'Leary, MD

Professor of Obstetrics and Gynecology, University of South Florida, Tampa, Florida

Hydrocephalus: Diagnosis and Treatment

James L. O'Leary, II, JD

Tampa, Florida

Hydrocephalus: Diagnosis and Treatment

James W. Orr, Jr., MD, FACOG, FACS

Clinical Professor, University of South Florida, Tampa, Florida; Director, Gynecologic Oncology, Gynecologic Oncology Research and Cancer Care, Fort Myers, Florida; Lee Cancer Care, Fort Myers, Florida

Nutritional Support

Pamela Jo Orr, RN, OCN

Data Manager, Florida Gynecologic Oncology, Fort Myers, Florida

Nutritional Support

Pasquale Patrizio, MD

Assistant Professor of Obstetrics/Gynecology, Division of Human Reproduction, and Director, Male Infertility Program, Hospital of the University of Pennsylvania, Philadelphia, Pennsylvania

GIFT Procedure; Male Infertility: Intrauterine Insemination; Microsurgical Epididymal Sperm Aspiration

George Paulson, MD

Kurtz Professor of Neurology, The Ohio State University College of Medicine and Medical Center, Columbus, Ohio

Headache

Jordan H. Perlow, MD

Associate Director, Maternal-Fetal Medicine, Good Samaritan Regional Medical Center, Phoenix, Arizona

Asthma Management During Pregnancy

Donald E. Pittaway, MD, PhD

Brookview Women's Center, Winston-Salem, North Carolina

Laboratory Diagnosis of Pregnancy

John T. Queenan, MD

Professor of Obstetrics and Gynecology, Georgetown University School of Medicine, Washington, DC

Rh Factor in Pregnancy

Edward J. Quilligan, MD

Professor Emeritus, Department of Obstetrics and Gynecology, University of California, Irvine, Medical Center, Orange, California

Breech Delivery: Post-term Pregnancy; Fetal Surgical Management of Congenital Hydronephrosis

Papineni S. Rao, PhD

Professor of Obstetrics and Gynecology, University of South Florida, Tampa, Florida

Septic Shock

William F. Rayburn, MD

Professor and Chairman, Department of Obstetrics and Gynecology, The University of New Mexico School of Medicine, Albuquerque, New Mexico

Hyperemesis Gravidarum; Prostaglandin E₂ for Cervical Ripening; Fetal Movement Charting

Thomas E. Reilley, DO

Associate Professor, The Ohio State University College of Medicine, Columbus, Ohio

Atelectasis in the Postoperative Period

Eli Reshef, MD

Clinical Associate Professor, University of Oklahoma Health Sciences Center, Department of Obstetrics/Gynecology; Medical Director, Integris Baptist Bennett Fertility Institute, Oklahoma City, Oklahoma

Hysteroscopic Evaluation and Therapy of Müllerian Anomalies

Robert Resnik, MD

Professor of Reproductive Medicine and Associate Dean of Admissions, University of California, San Diego, School of Medicine; Faculty, Reproductive Medicine Department of UCSD, Mercy Hospital—Consultant Service, San Diego, and Scripps La Jolla Medical Center—Consultant, La Jolla, California

Rheumatic Heart Disease: Safe Conduct in Pregnancy

Daniel H. Riddick, MD, PhD

Professor, Department of Obstetrics and Gynecology, University of Vermont College of Medicine; Attending, Women's Health Care Service, Fletcher Allen Health Care, Burlington, Vermont

Primary Amenorrhea

John W. Riggs, MD

Associate Professor, University of Texas; Health Science Center, Department of Obstetrics, Gynecology, and Reproductive Sciences, Lyndon B. Johnson General Hospital, Houston, Texas

Chorioamnionitis

John F. Rodis, MD

Associate Professor of Obstetrics and Gynecology, Division of Maternal-Fetal Medicine, University of Connecticut School of Medicine, Farmington, Connecticut

Twin Pregnancy

Robert E. Rogers, MD

Emeritus Professor, Obstetrics and Gynecology, Indiana University School of Medicine, Indianapolis, Indiana

Cancer Screening

Joseph S. Sanfilippo, MD

Professor of Obstetrics and Gynecology, MCP Hahnemann, School of Medicine; Chairman, Department of Obstetrics and Gynecology, Allegheny General Hospital, Pittsburgh, Pennsylvania

Hysteroscopic Evaluation and Therapy of Müllerian Anomalies

George Schaeffer, MD*

Former Emeritus Professor of Clinical Obstetrics and Gynecology, Cornell University Medical College, New York, New York
*Deceased

Female Genital Tuberculosis

Cynthia S. Shellhaas, MD

Assistant Professor, Department of Obstetrics/ Gynecology, Division of Maternal-Fetal Medicine, The Ohio State University College of Medicine, Columbus, Ohio

Drug Abuse in Pregnancy

Rebecca Shiffman, MD

Clinical Assistant Professor of Obstetrics/ Gynecology, SUNY Health Center, Brooklyn, New York; Assistant Professor of Obstetrics/ Gynecology, Cornell University Medical College, New York, New York; Director of Obstetrics, Vice Chairman, Department of Obstetrics and Gynecology, New York Methodist Hospital, Brooklyn, New York

Systemic Lupus Erythematosus in Pregnancy

Baha M. Sibai, MD

Professor and Chief, Division of Maternal Fetal Medicine/Department of Obstetrics/Gynecology, University of Tennessee, Memphis, Memphis, Tennessee

Chronic Hypertension in Pregnancy; Prediction and Prevention of Preeclampsia: The Role of Low-Dose Aspirin and Calcium in Hypertensive Diseases in Pregnancy

Robert M. Silver, MD

Associate Professor, Department of Obstetrics and Gynecology, Division of Maternal-Fetal Medicine, University of Utah School of Medicine, Salt Lake City, Utah

Antiphospholipid Antibodies in Reproductive Loss

John F. Steege, MD

Professor, Department of Obstetrics and Gynecology, University of North Carolina, Chapel Hill, North Carolina

Dyspareunia

Phillip G. Stubblefield, MD

Professor and Chairman, Obstetrics and Gynecology, Boston University School of Medicine; Director of Obstetrics and Gynecology, Boston Medical Center, Boston, Massachusetts

Intrauterine Devices

Eric S. Surrey, MD

Associate Clinical Professor, Department of Obstetrics-Gynecology, University of California, Los Angeles, School of Medicine, Los Angeles; Medical Director, Reproductive Medicine and Surgery Associates, Beverly Hills, California

Endometriosis and Adenomyosis

Robert R. Taylor, MD

Associate Director, Gynecologic Oncology and Pelvic Reconstructive Surgery, Saint Barnabas Medical Center, Department of Obstetrics and Gynecology, Livingston, New Jersey

Ovarian Cancer

William Benbow Thompson, Jr., MD

Professor Emeritus, Gynecology, University of California, Irvine, College of Medicine; Attending Physician, University of California, Irvine, Medical Center, Orange, California

Bartholin's Cyst and Abscess; Therapeutic Abortion

Julianne S. Toohey, MD

Assistant Clinical Professor, University of California, Irvine, School of Medicine and Medical Center, Orange, California

Battered Woman

Stanley van den Noort, MD

Professor of Neurology, University of California, Irvine, School of Medicine, Department of Neurology, Irvine, California

Multiple Sclerosis; Myasthenia Gravis

Donald G. Vidt, MD

Professor of Medicine, The Ohio State University College of Medicine, Columbus; Consultant, Department of Nephrology and Hypertension, Cleveland Clinic Foundation, Cleveland, Ohio

Hypertension in the Nonpregnant Patient

Anthony M. Vintzileos, MD

Professor, Obstetrics and Gynecology and Reproductive Sciences, Director, Maternal-Fetal Medicine and Obstetrics, Robert Wood Johnson Medical School, University of Medicine and Dentistry of New Jersey; Physician, St. Peter's Medical Center, New Brunswick, New Jersey

Biophysical Profile

Gerald Weinstein, MD

Chairman, Department of Dermatology, University of California, Irvine, Irvine, California

Acne Vulgaris

George D. Wendel, Jr., MD

Professor, Obstetrics and Gynecology, The University of Texas Southwestern Medical Center at Dallas; Physician, Parkland Health and Hospital System, Dallas, Texas

Group B Streptococcus in Pregnancy

David A. Wininger, MD

Assistant Professor, Clinical Internal Medicine, Ohio State University College of Medicine and Public Health, Columbus, Ohio

AIDS and HIV Infection

William E. Wise, Jr., MD

Clinical Associate Professor, Ohio State University School of Medicine; President-Elect, Medical Staff, Riverside Methodist Hospitals, Columbus, Ohio

Hemorrhoids and Anal Fissure

Andrea G. Witlin, DO

Assistant Professor, The University of Texas Medical Branch at Galveston, Galveston, Texas

Prediction and Prevention of Preeclampsia: The Role of Low-Dose Aspirin and Calcium in Hypertensive Diseases in Pregnancy

Russell P. Woda, DO

Assistant Professor, The Ohio State University College of Medicine, Columbus, Ohio

Atelectasis in the Postoperative Period

Howard A. Zacur, MD, PhD

Theodore and Ingrid Baramki Professor and Director of the Division of Reproductive Endocrinology and Infertility, The Johns Hopkins Medical Institutions, Department of Gynecology and Obstetrics, Baltimore, Maryland

Galactorrhea and Hyperprolactinemia

Gerald I. Zatuchni, MD, MSc

Professor Emeritus, Obstetrics and Gynecology, Northwestern University, Chicago, Illinois

Female Sterilization

Frederick P. Zuspan, MD

Professor and Chairman Emeritus, Department of Obstetrics and Gynecology, The Ohio State University College of Medicine and Public Health, Columbus, Ohio

Preeclampsia

Kathryn Zuspan, MD

Clinical Assistant Professor, Department of Anesthesia, University of Minnesota; Anesthesiologist, Hennepin County Medical Center and Fairview Southdale Hospital, Minneapolis, Minnesota

Anesthesia for Obstetrics; Control of Postpartum Pain

PREFACE

This is the fifth edition of *Current Therapy in Obstetrics and Gynecology*. There have been many significant changes in obstetrics and gynecology since the first edition of this book was published in 1980. There have been remarkable advances in intrauterine fetal diagnosis as a result of marked improvements in ultrasonography and chemical and chromosomal abnormality detection. The entire field of reproductive technology has exploded, permitting patients who had little or no chance of becoming pregnant to have a child or in some cases many children. The therapy of gynecologic cancer involves new chemotherapeutic agents, with increased survival occurring in such deadly diseases as ovarian cancer.

Accompanying these and many other signficant changes in diagnostic and therapeutic modalities is a major shift in the way care is given. The care giver is shifting from a he to a she; 70% of today's obstetrics and gynecology residents are female. Also, we have gone from solo practitioners to groups, bringing both advantages and disadvantages to the patient. The physician may be less sleep-deprived when she or he sees the patients but may not know them as well. Many of the procedures requiring hospitalization are now done on an outpatient basis, and when patients are admitted to the hospital, the stay is significantly shorter than before. Obstetrics and gynecology is becoming an ambulatory care and an enlarging specialty in that we are emphasizing primary care.

The format of this book has not changed. It is still oriented toward a short description of the modern therapy of a variety of obstetric and gynecologic disorders. It now includes primary care problems that the obstetrician and gynecologist has always encountered but in some cases in the past were referred to the internist or family physician. In most chapters, we have new authors giving you their insight into the problem; however, in some chapters the therapy has not changed and therefore we have elected to repeat the chapter from the last edition. As in the past, the book is written for all health care givers, whether they are physicians, nurses, medical students, or nursing students. We sincerely hope there will be many nuggets in this book that will help you to help your patient. That is what we are really here for, isn't it?

Enjoy having more than a hundred consultants at your fingertips for modern health care.

EDWARD J. QUILLIGAN, M.D.
FREDERICK P. ZUSPAN, M.D.

CONTENTS

Gynecology

Adnexal Masses

Margaret Graf Garrisi, MD

Adnexal masses may originate from the ovary, the fallopian tube, or the uterus. Ovarian adnexal masses may be physiologic in women of reproductive age (follicular or corpus luteum cysts). These cysts may be numerous and result in very large ovaries in women undergoing induction of ovulation for insemination or in vitro fertilization. Benign pathologic ovarian masses commonly include endometriomas, or are the result of pregnancy (luteoma) or infection; less common are benign neoplastic ovarian masses such as hyperthecosis (polycystic ovary disease) or fibromas. Malignant ovarian masses include germ cell tumors and, more commonly, epithelial carcinomas. Fallopian tube masses are rarely malignant and most commonly include ectopic pregnancy and infection-related hydrosalpinges or pyosalpinges; endometriosis may also lead to a hydrosalpinx. Paratubal structures such as hydatid cysts of Morgagni (wolffian duct remnants) are very common. Pedunculated subserous leiomyomas of the uterus may also present as adnexal masses.

Adnexal masses may be symptomatic, causing acute or chronic pain of moderate to severe intensity. Adnexal torsion usually results in sudden colic-like pain and is more frequently seen with ovaries enlarged through stimulation with fertility medications for ovulation induction than with those in natural cycles. Pain from an ectopic pregnancy may be more acute than pain developing slowly from an infectious or endometriotic etiology. Often, however, asymptomatic adnexal masses may be palpated on routine examination or found incidentally on abdominal or pelvic imaging studies.

The differential diagnosis of adnexal masses begins with a history from the patient and an examination. Age and menstrual history may make certain masses more or less likely, such as functional cysts in women of reproductive years versus neoplasias in postmenopausal women. Sexual history and contraceptive use may reveal pregnancy or infectious etiologies of adnexal masses. A past history of salpingitis, endometriosis, or prior surgery may be very pertinent. Current symptoms of pain, bleeding, and gastrointestinal or genitourinary symptoms are also important. Physical examination of the patient includes vital signs and abdominal, pelvic, and rectal examination. Tenderness as well as size and location of the adnexal mass may be appreciated.

The patient's history and physical examination will suggest the appropriate laboratory tests to perform, such as cervical cytology, cultures, blood counts, pregnancy test, sedimentation rates, ^{125}Ca levels, and hormone levels. Office vaginal pelvic ultrasonograms are very helpful to evaluate uterine and adnexal pathology, especially with early pregnancy problems such as a corpus luteum cyst versus ectopic pregnancy. Once the presence of an adnexal mass has been established, further imaging with computed tomographic scan, magnetic resonance imaging, or Doppler flow studies may provide more accurate estimation of size, consistency, and malignant potential.

Current therapies of adnexal masses include observation and surgery and medical management. Expectant follow-up of suspected physiologic adnexal masses with repeat examination or ultrasonogram, or both, in a subsequent menstrual cycle will usually confirm the diagnosis of the follicular or corpus luteum cyst, which would be absent or significantly smaller. Laparoscopy or laparotomy may be necessary to remove a mass, drain a cyst or abscess, or treat an ectopic pregnancy. Ectopic pregnancies are also frequently treated with methotrexate, either primarily or after surgical failure. Patients with endometriosis who have suspected recurrent disease may be treated medically (gonadotropin-releasing hormone agonists) for recurrent adnexal masses; sometimes they may have large endometriomas drained transvaginally with ultrasonographic guidance. Depending on the pathology and the desires of the patient, efforts to preserve adnexal structures are generally advocated; preoperative consultation should inform the patient of the possibility of salpingectomy or oophorectomy, however, and consent must be obtained.

Androgen Excess of Adrenal Origins

Ricardo Azziz, MD, MPH

Androgen excess affects between 2% and 10% of all women. Although the majority of patients demonstrate excessive ovarian androgen secretion, many of these patients also have excess adrenocortical secretion of androgens. Furthermore, others will demonstrate androgen excess that is almost exclusively of adrenal origin, including nonclassic adrenal hyperplasia (NCAH), adrenocortical neoplasias, Cushing's disease, and functional adrenal androgen excess. In this article, we review these disorders and their diagnosis and treatment.

Clinical and Hormonal Markers of Adrenal Androgen Excess

The zona fasciculata and reticularis of the adrenal cortex secrete both C-21 (eg, cortisol) and C-19 steroids (ie, adrenal androgens). The adrenal androgens primarily measured in the circulation include dehydroepiandrosterone (DHA) and its sulfate (DHS), Δ^5-androstene-3β,17β-diol or androstenediol (ADIOL), and 11β-hydroxyandrostenedione (11-OHA4). The vast majority of these steroids are produced by the adrenal cortex. While androstenedione can also be considered an adrenal androgen, it is significantly less specific, since in adult women approximately 50% of this steroid is secreted by the ovary.

The direct measurement of circulating levels (in serum) by radioimmunoassay has replaced the measurement of 17-ketosteroids in 24-hour urine collections. Nonetheless, it should be noted that some of these androgens vary significantly with the time of the day, although minimally with the menstrual cycle. Circulating levels of DHA, ADIOL, and 11-OHA4 exhibit a circadian rhythm similar to that of cortisol, with peak serum concentrations in early morning and a nadir in late evening. In contrast, circulating DHS levels change minimally or not at all throughout the day, reflecting its longer half-life. Although some investigators have noted that androstenedione levels follow the adrenocortical circadian cycle, we were unable to demonstrate a significant difference in mean androstenedione levels obtained between 0700 and 0900 hours and 1500 and 1700 hours in healthy control women. DHA, DHS, ADIOL, and 11-OHA4 do not vary with

the menstrual cycle. In contrast, androstenedione increases in the late follicular and luteal phase, presumably secondary to variations in ovarian secretion, although in normal premenopausal women these values generally remain within normal limits.

Clinically, the measurement of circulating DHS is used as the marker for adrenal androgen excess, since this hormone is (1) 97% to 99% of adrenocortical origin; (2) the second most abundant steroid; (3) relatively stable throughout the day and the menstrual cycle; and (4) easily measured. Although various investigators have proposed the use of 11-OHA4 as a marker of adrenal androgen excess, it should be noted that the radioimmunoassay for this steroid is difficult to perform and standardize. Since adrenal androgens are generally less potent than testosterone or dihydrotestosterone, the signs and symptoms directly attributable to their excess are also usually mild. In fact, adrenal androgens appear to have a greater effect on sebum secretion and are more frequently related to the development of persistent acne in both males and females than with hirsutism and oligo-ovulation (see later).

Adrenal Androgen Excess in the Polycystic Ovary Syndrome

Serum levels of DHS and 11-OHA4 are elevated in 20% to 60% of patients with the functional ovarian hyperandrogenism or the polycystic ovary syndrome (PCOS). Alternatively, there is less agreement regarding abnormalities of circulating DHA. Some investigators observed that the mean circulating DHA level at 0800 hours, or its 24-hour integrated concentration, was normal or only minimally elevated in these women. Alternatively, other investigators noted that over 50% of hyperandrogenic women demonstrated elevated DHA levels, including free DHA. In general, the circulating level (or 24-hour integrated concentration) of ADIOL is normal in PCOS patients, although the production rate of ADIOL may be increased in these patients. Further confirming the increased adrenocortical secretion of these androgens in PCOS, the uptake of iodocholesterol by the adrenal cortex exceeds normal in approximately 50% of these women.

All of these data serve to support the concept that, in addition to ovarian androgen excess, over one half of patients with PCOS also demonstrate adrenocortical oversecretion of androgens. Thus, the clinician should not be misled into excluding PCOS just because the circulating DHS level is elevated. In fact, a high DHS level is more common in PCOS than it is among patients with NCAH (see later). Therapeutically, the presence of an elevated DHS level may indicate the need for glucocorticoid suppression, either to enhance the success of clomiphene ovulation induction or to improve acne. Specifically, PCOS patients who do not respond to standard clomiphene citrate doses (ie, 50–100 mg/day × 5 days) and demonstrate a circulating DHS level above the mean (although not necessarily above the upper normal limit for the laboratory) may benefit from the addition of dexamethasone 0.5 mg daily, taken through conception. Alternatively, we have noted that the sole administration of dexamethasone to hyperandrogenic oligo-ovulatory patients does not result in a significant improvement in ovulatory function, regardless of circulating DHS levels.

Adrenal Androgen Excess in Nonresponsive, Persistent, or Adult Acne

Acne that is nonresponsive to standard therapy (whether in adolescence or otherwise) persists into adulthood, or appears postpubertally (adult) is a common and distressing problem affecting both males and females. While excessive circulating levels of many different androgens have been noted in 30% to 50% of patients with this condition, it appears that the adrenal steroids are most directly related to the development of this problem.

In these patients we have found that the administration of dexamethasone (0.5 mg/day × 30 days, then 0.5 mg qod) results in a dramatic improvement in skin quality in a significant fraction of these patients. Therapeutic benefit, if it is to occur, is evident within 4 to 8 weeks. Thus, if acneic patients have not demonstrated a beneficial result after 3 months of glucocorticoid therapy, it is unlikely that they will do so, and other therapeutic options should be considered.

Nonclassic Adrenal Hyperplasia

Adrenal enzyme deficiencies that lead to the appearance of hyperandrogenic symptoms some time after birth have been called postpubertal, attenuated, mild, acquired, or late-onset, although NCAH is the preferred term. By definition, NCAH is an autosomal recessive disorder that causes symptomatic hyperandrogenism (eg, hirsutism, acne, androgenic alopecia, ovulatory dysfunction, premature pubarche) peripubertally

or postpubertally in the presence of normal female external genitalia. If a girl presenting with evidence of an adrenal enzyme deficiency also demonstrates virilization of the genitalia, however minor, the disorder should be classified as congenital or classic adrenal hyperplasia (CAH), because the hyperandrogenism was present in utero during genital development.

21-Hydroxylase (21-OH)-deficient CAH and NCAH are among the most common genetic disorders known. Although 21-OH deficiency accounts for the vast majority of NCAH, defects in 11β-hydroxylase (11-OH) and 3β-hydroxysteroid dehydrogenase (3β-HSD) function may rarely result in the disorder.

21-Hydroxylase Deficient Nonclassic Adrenal Hyperplasia

Endocrinologically evident 21-OH deficient NCAH appears to affect between 1% and 10% of women with androgen excess, depending on the population studied. Surveys in the United States generally note a lower prevalence than studies in Europe or Canada, and the prevalence appears highest among Ashkenazi Jewish and Middle Eastern populations.

Clinically, these NCAH patients cannot be differentiated from those suffering from PCOS. In fact, androgenic signs and symptoms are often mild, with severe hirsutism or virilization being an infrequent finding. Patients tend to be shorter than would be expected from the midparental height, although their mean final height is greater than for individuals with CAH.

Biochemically it is difficult to distinguish NCAH women from other hyperandrogenic patients. Mean circulating testosterone and DHS levels are not different from those observed in patients with PCOS. In fact, DHS levels are often normal. In contrast to CAH, patients with NCAH do not demonstrate a decrease in cortisol production, nor elevated circulating adrenocorticotropic hormone (ACTH) levels.

Measurement of the immediate 17-hydroxylated steroid precursor to 21-OH, 17-hydroxyprogesterone (17-HP), in the morning and in the follicular phase of the menstrual cycle can be used to screen for 21-OH-deficient NCAH. The majority of untreated NCAH women demonstrate basal 17-HP levels above 200 ng/dL (2 ng/mL or 6 nmol/L). Alternatively, a basal follicular phase 17-HP level of less than 200 ng/mL almost completely rules out the disorder. It is important that the screening basal 17-HP be obtained in the follicular phase of the menstrual cycle, since the levels of this steroid increase luteally. Furthermore, if 17-HP is sampled in the afternoon (when the adrenocortical secretion is at its nadir) or following dexamethasone administration, the diagnosis of NCAH may be masked. Hyperandrogenic women who demonstrate a basal follicular phase 17-HP level above 200 ng/dL merit an acute ACTH stimulation test to rule out the disorder. If the 17-HP level 30 or 60 minutes following the intravenous administration of 0.25 mg ACTH-(1-24) (one vial of Cortrosyn, Organon, Inc.) is above 1000 to 1500 ng/dL (10–15 ng/mL or 30–45 nmol/L), the diagnosis is established.

Little information regarding the treatment and outcome of NCAH patients is available. In general, glucocorticoid suppression (eg, dexamethasone 0.5 mg qod) improves acne in all patients. Ovulatory function and hirsutism improve, but less readily in older patients with the disorder. It is possible that long-standing adrenal hyperandrogenism alters the hypothalamic-pituitary-ovarian axis, such that the suppression of adrenal androgens is not sufficient to induce normal ovulation. Furthermore, once hair follicles that normally yield vellus have been stimulated by androgens to produce terminal hairs (ie, hirsutism), glucocorticoid suppression alone is of little value. We highly encourage the use of antiandrogens (eg, spironolactone) in the treatment of hirsutism of any origin, including that associated with NCAH.

To monitor the adequacy of treatment, we measure the circulating androstenedione and free testosterone (and/or sex hormone-binding globulin) levels at 3 and 6 months of therapy, and yearly thereafter, aiming to normalize these values. Alternatively, physicians should not try to normalize the 17-HP levels, since adrenal androgens are more sensitive to the suppressive effects of glucocorticoid administration than are C-21 steroids (including 17-HP). It is extremely important to keep in mind that these measures simply serve as a guideline and that clinical response is of greater value in determining the adequacy of therapy. In fact, androgen measures are primarily useful when clinical improvement is *not* evident, suggesting the possibility of persistent hyperandrogenemia.

Although many patients with NCAH benefit from glucocorticoid suppression, it is also true that many do not tolerate or simply dislike the side effects of these medications (see later). In those women complaining of acne, hirsutism, or oligomenorrhea, we recommend the usual treatment for hyperandrogenism, including oral contraceptives and androgen blockers (eg, spirono-

lactone). Not surprisingly, most of these women will demonstrate a significant improvement in symptomatology.

In some patients, achieving fertility may be the primary issue. The principal cause of the reduced fertility in patients with NCAH is probably ovulatory dysfunction, secondary to hyperandrogenism. Furthermore, chronic elevations in circulating progesterone and 17-HP levels may result in an inadequate cervical mucus or an atrophic endometrium, or both. Nonetheless, while NCAH patients may be subfertile, it should be stressed that many of these women become pregnant without requiring treatment, and often prior to diagnosis. Assuming that other infertility factors have been ruled out, we first initiate glucocorticoid therapy to improve ovulatory function. If the patient fails to demonstrate adequate or satisfactory ovulation after 4 months of adrenocortical suppression, we then proceed to ovulation induction with clomiphene citrate, and human menopausal gonadotropin therapy if necessary. As noted previously, it is possible that long-term chronic hyperandrogenemia results in the disruption of the hypothalamic-pituitary-ovarian axis and the development of a PCOS-like phenotype. Overall prognosis for fertility in oligoovulatory NCAH patients is good and should not be any different from that of other hyperandrogenic women seeking ovulation induction.

It is a matter of debate whether patients with NCAH are at risk for adrenal insufficiency. Although we have never observed acute or chronic hypocortisolism in our NCAH patients, with many of them having undergone surgery or obstetric deliveries without glucocorticoid supplementation, this possibility cannot be discounted. Therefore, we inform patients of this theoretical risk and counsel them and their families regarding the presenting symptoms of adrenal insufficiency, particularly in the event of trauma, accidents, or surgery. Glucocorticoid supplementation during these events may also be considered.

Children of patients with NCAH are at risk for inheriting 21-OH deficiency. Affected children may suffer from either CAH or NCAH, since many NCAH patients are actually compound heterozygotes; that is, they carry one mutation encoding for a severe defect and the other for a mild defect. Most efforts at preconceptual and prenatal therapy will be directed at preventing CAH in a female infant. The actual risk of giving birth to an affected infant depends on (1) the genotype of the mother, and (2) the probability that the father is a carrier (heterozygote). In the absence of molecular analysis of the

*CYP*21 genes of both parents, the theoretical risk of a patient with NCAH delivering a child with CAH is between 1.7 and 2.3 per 1000.

11-Hydroxylase Deficient Nonclassic Adrenal Hyperplasia

Patients with 11-OH deficient NCAH are extremely rare. As in the 21-OH variant, they appear to be clinically indistinguishable from other hyperandrogenic women. The blood pressure in 11-OH deficient NCAH patients ranges from normal to moderately elevated. The diagnostic criteria for 11-OH deficient NCAH are unclear. In the absence of a reliable genetic marker, the diagnosis of 11-OH deficient NCAH may be presumed when the 11-deoxycortisol level following ACTH stimulation exceeds a pre-established arbitrary value, generally sixfold the upper 95th percentile of normal.

3β-Hydroxysteroid Dehydrogenase Deficient Nonclassic Adrenal Hyperplasia

The diagnosis of 3β-HSD deficient NCAH is based on an abnormally elevated 17-hydroxypregnenolone (17-HPREG) or DHA response, or both, to ACTH stimulation. Various reports have documented the existence of a 3β-HSD deficient form of NCAH. However, the diagnostic criteria for this disorder are unclear and have been recently revised, based on genetic data. If we include only those individuals with confirmed mutations of the 3β-HSD-II gene, we can presume that these patients will demonstrate a 17-HPREG sixfold to 10-fold the upper 95th percentile of control subjects. In fact, when genotyping is used to confirm the diagnosis, 3β-HSD deficient NCAH also appears to be extremely rare.

Androgen-Producing Tumors of the Adrenal

Androgen-producing tumors of the adrenal are relatively rare and include adenomas and carcinomas. These neoplasms can be suspected when the circulating DHS is greater than 7000 ng/mL, although the clinical presentation is the most sensitive indicator. The vast majority of patients demonstrate cushingoid features or virilization or both. Furthermore, most demonstrate a time course of less than 2 years. The diagnosis is usually established by a computed tomographic (CT) scan of the adrenal, with images obtained at 0.5 cm intervals. The presence of oligo-ovulation or hirsutism depends on tumor histopathology. More differentiated neoplasms tend to produce higher levels of androgens, while less differentiated tumors do not. Overall, adrenocortical neoplasias demonstrate less efficient steroidogenesis than normal adrenocortical tissue. However, because these tumors are frequently very large, the overall steroid secretion by these neoplasms can be significant.

Unfortunately, most functioning adrenocortical neoplasms are carcinomas and demonstrate a very poor prognosis. They are generally large (greater than 6 cm) and can be easily identified on CT scan by their irregular outline. Alternatively, an isolated adenoma of the adrenal cortex, solely secreting DHA, DHS, androstenedione, or testosterone, may be present but is extremely rare. It should be remembered that patients with NCAH frequently demonstrate silent adenomas of their adrenal cortex, presumably secondary to chronic, if not measurable, ACTH hyperstimulation. Thus, NCAH (especially 21-OH deficient) should be first excluded in those patients presumed to have an androgen-secreting adenoma. Furthermore, in patients with rapid or severe virilization, particularly children, liberal use of adrenal CT scanning is justified.

Cushing's Disease

Excessive ACTH-dependent adrenocortical function, due to either an ectopic ACTH-producing tumor or a pituitary tumor (Cushing's disease), can lead to excessive adrenal androgen secretion and hyperandrogenism. Ectopic tumors that produce ACTH and corticotropin-releasing hormone are infrequently associated with virilization, since they are rare tumors in females. Hirsutism is present in 60% to 70% of women with Cushing's disease and is generally diffuse, mild, and accompanied by varying degrees of hypertrichosis. Hirsutism, with or without menstrual irregularity, is among the presenting symptoms in one third of such women, and the only presenting complaint in approximately 20%. Overall menstrual irregularities are seen in 80% to 100% of women with Cushing's disease.

Circulating testosterone levels are often elevated in women with pituitary Cushing's disease. An adrenal origin is ascribed to the increased androgen levels, since dexamethasone causes a parallel decrease in cortisol and testosterone, while ACTH stimulation induces an increase in testosterone that is more profound in women with Cushing's disease than in normal women. Furthermore, bilateral adrenalectomy dramatically decreases circulating testosterone, correcting the oligomenorrhea and hirsutism. Nonetheless, an increase in the adrenal secretion of androgens may not be the only factor accounting for the androgenic symptoms in Cushing's disease. It is possible that an increase in ovarian androgen secretion may, in part, account for the hyperandrogenism. The role that the increased insulin resistance and gonadotropin abnormalities noted in Cushing's disease play in promoting ovarian hyperandrogenemia is unknown. Finally, a direct effect of long-term hypercortisolemia on hair growth, particularly that of vellus hairs, cannot be ruled out.

In spite of the high frequency of hirsutism reported among women with Cushing's disease, hirsute women are rarely diagnosed as having the disorder. As illustration, among approximately 1000 hyperandrogenic women with whose care the author has been involved, only one patient has been diagnosed as suffering from Cushing's disease. Thus, screening for glucocorticoid excess (ie, Cushing's syndrome) in hyperandrogenism probably should be restricted to individuals with obvious cushingoid features, particularly those with recent weight gain, easy bruisability and generalized weakness, and centripetal obesity. In general, the diagnosis of excessive cortisol production can best be established by a 24-hour urine free cortisol test. Although a more simple screening method is the measurement of morning fasting serum cortisol level following the administration of 1 mg of dexamethasone the evening before, the false-positive rate can be significant, particularly among patients with endogenous depression or obesity or those on diphenylhydantoin (Dilantin) therapy.

Functional Adrenal Androgen Excess

Most patients who demonstrate excess circulating levels of adrenal androgens, principally DHS, have PCOS. Nonetheless, we and others have also postulated that some of these patients may actually demonstrate "functional adrenal androgen excess" (FAE), that is, the presence of adrenal androgen excess in the absence of adrenal hyperplasia, adrenal tumors, or PCOS. Presumably these patients have oversecretion of androgens by the adrenal cortex, independent of any abnormality of ovarian function. Tentatively, the diagnosis of FAE can be established by an elevated DHS level, generally greater than 4000 ng/

mL (400 μg/dL), in the presence of normal total testosterone and in the absence of ovulatory disturbances. Nonetheless this definition is flawed, because many patients with PCOS may not demonstrate overt ovulatory dysfunction and may have a "normal" total testosterone level.

We have noted that patients with presumed FAE generally are younger and less obese than those with PCOS. This suggests that the normal peak in adrenal androgens seen between the ages of 18 and 25 years may be exaggerated in these patients. Furthermore, many of these women demonstrate acne with minimal hirsutism and regular ovulation, consistent with the preferential stimulation of sebum secretion by adrenal androgens. These patients may benefit solely from glucocorticoid suppression. Nonetheless, it remains to be demonstrated that patients with presumed FAE actually represent a distinct group of patients, separate from those with PCOS.

Glucocorticoid Suppression: Considerations and Risks

In considering adrenocortical suppression for the improvement of androgenic symptoms, various factors must be considered. The metabolism of dexamethasone, a frequently used fluorinated steroid with almost exclusive glucocorticoid activity, varies significantly among patients. The concomitant use of antiseizure medications, or other drugs stimulating hepatic metabolism, may decrease the half-life and thus the efficacy of dexamethasone. Alternatively, in other patients dexamethasone demonstrates an excessively long half-life, with the development of cushingoid features. In fact, many patients will demonstrate weight gain of between 3 and 15 lbs, which usually is lost following discontinuation of therapy. Side effects may be reduced by using a shorter-acting glucocorticoid, such as prednisone or even hydrocortisone, and by administering the drug every other day.

Other common side effects include gastritis, jitteriness and irritability, anxiety, and insomnia. Although we generally recommend that glucocorticoids be taken orally at bedtime to suppress the morning surge in adrenocortical function, it should be noted that this becomes irrelevant after a few days of therapy. Thus, if patients are experiencing significant insomnia we suggest taking the medications in the morning. Some hyperandrogenic patients, particularly those with obesity or insulin resistance, may develop frank glucose intolerance during glucocorticoid treatment.

Two more serious complications of chronic glucocorticoid therapy to consider are adrenocortical suppression and osteoporosis. In general, significant adrenocortical hypofunction is uncommon with doses of less than 0.5 mg of dexamethasone, 5.0 to 7.5 mg of prednisone, or 15 to 20 mg hydrocortisone daily. Nonetheless, it is recommended that these patients, when undergoing surgery or experiencing serious illness, receive hydrocortisone supplementation intravenously (eg, 100–300 mg q 6–8 hours). Bone loss has been reported with even the lowest doses of glucocorticoids. Thus, if patients are receiving long-term therapy, consideration should be given to obtaining a bone density measurement every 2 years.

Androgen Insensitivity Syndrome

Robert L. Harris, MD
W. Allen Addison, MD

Androgen insensitivity syndrome (AIS) is the preferred designation for the condition that Morris first referred to as testicular feminization in his 1953 report. His patients were genetic males with cryptorchid testes and female phenotype. These patients would now be recognized as having complete AIS. It is now known that there are two mechanisms for the failure of androgen expression in such patients. The more common cause is unresponsiveness due to androgen receptor mutations, now referred to as Type I AIS. An additional cause, referred to as Type II AIS, is less common and is the result of a deficiency of 5α-reductase, which is necessary for the production of dihydrotestosterone, requisite for the expression of the biologic effects of androgen. Type I AIS is genetically transmitted as an X-linked recessive disorder, whereas Type II AIS is genetically transmitted as an autosomal recessive disorder. Both defects can result in complete absence of androgen expression peripherally and the unblemished female phenotype of complete AIS. Both defects, can, however, also result in incomplete AIS, producing varying degrees of androgenization ranging from almost complete lack of virilization to almost normal phenotypic expression of androgen influence. Any phenotypic expression of end organ response to androgen qualifies for the designation of incomplete AIS.

Diagnosis

The most common presentation of AIS likely to be encountered by the practicing gynecologist is a phenotypically normal female with primary amenorrhea or difficulty consummating coitus. These individuals generally have normal growth and development and are usually tall. Their hands and feet tend to be large. Their secondary sexual characteristics are strikingly feminine, with female habitus, large breasts, and normal-appearing external genitalia. Pubic and axillary hair is usually scant. Their nipples tend to be lightly pigmented and the labia minora may appear hypoplastic. Inguinal testes may be palpable and there may be evidence of inguinal hernias, extant or repaired. Vaginal depth varies from a dimple to a blind pouch that is usually foreshortened. Müllerian structures are absent on rectal examination.

The differential diagnosis of the well-feminized patient with vaginal agenesis primarily involves distinguishing AIS from müllerian dysgenesis, the former being much less common. In müllerian dysgenesis, unlike in AIS, patients may report cyclic molimina from normal cyclic ovarian function. In contrast to patients with AIS, genital and axillary hair growth is normal in patients with müllerian dysgenesis. There is a greater variation in vaginal development in patients with müllerian dysgenesis and müllerian structures may be palpable on rectal examination or may be imaged ultrasonographically.

Patients with AIS have a chromatin-negative buccal smear (normal male pattern), estrogen levels in the normal male range, and testosterone levels in the normal male range (300–1000 ng/dL). In contrast, patients with müllerian dysgenesis have chromatin-positive buccal smears (normal female pattern), serum estrogen levels in the normal female range, and serum testosterone levels in the normal female range (20–70 ng/dL). For practical purposes, these studies can distinguish effectively between AIS and müllerian dysgenesis. Karyotyping is the definitive diagnostic study and should be performed in all patients. Patients with AIS have a normal 46XY male karyotype, in contrast to patients with müllerian dysgenesis who have a normal female 46XX karyotype. In both complete and incomplete forms of AIS, patients have similar levels of estrogen and testosterone. Patients with incomplete forms of AIS may have varying degrees of virilization or masculinization, determined by the androgen expression permitted by the severity of their defect. It is possible to differentiate the two types of AIS with serum testosterone and dihydrotestosterone levels, fibroblast cultures for 5α-reductase activity, and dihydrotestosterone to testosterone ratios after gonadotropin stimulation. This is, however, of little clinical utility.

Management

Primary goals of management of the patient with AIS include removing the testes because of their neoplastic potential, providing effective estrogen replacement therapy, and establishing a coitally functional vagina. The incidence of neoplasia in testes left in situ after puberty has been reported to be as high as 52%, and the incidence of malignant neoplasia as high as 22%. It was traditional to allow complete pubertal development prior to testicular removal because of a belief that endogenous hormones provided a smoother transition through puberty than did exogenous estrogen replacement. There are, however, no data to support this, and there have been reports of malignant change in the testes prior to puberty in patients with AIS. Additionally, some patients with apparent complete AIS have exhibited unexpected virilization during puberty. The current trend is for earlier gonadectomy followed by institution of estrogen replacement therapy at the expected age of pubescence. The feasibility of providing hormone replacement therapy with androgens has been investigated but seems to provide no clear advantage over estrogen. Effective estrogen replacement therapy can be delivered by any of the available routes, oral, transdermal, or parenteral. It has been reported that patients with AIS do not experience significant vasomotor symptoms after gonadectomy. Other investigators have observed, however, that some of these patients exhibit intense vasomotor symptomatology and require greater than usual doses of estrogen to control these symptoms. The most common recommendation for estrogen replacement is 1.25 mg of conjugated equine estrogens or their equivalent, but doses of 2.5 mg or greater may be required. A coitally functional vagina can be established in some patients by progressive dilatation employing the Frank technique, the bicycle seat technique described by Ingram, or, on occasion, by coital thrusting. A high degree of motivation is required for success. A number of surgical techniques have been described for neovaginal creation, the most important being the McIndoe operation. With this operation, perineal cavitation is followed by a split thickness skin graft held over the surfaces of the cavity by a stent. Dilatation should be attempted prior to any surgical intervention and surgery definitely should not be performed until the patient is highly motivated to comply with the demanding instructions necessary to maintain patency of the neovaginal lumen during the critical 6-month period after cavitation and grafting.

Appropriate psychological management of these patients is of paramount importance and may require the involvement of mental health care professionals. The patient, whose female gender identity is fully established by rearing, orientation, and appearance, should be told that her gonads must be removed because of neoplastic potential and that, except for procreation, she can function in all ways as a normal female after a neovagina has been established. The family should be told nothing different and any reference to testes or genetic maleness should be avoided. Involvement in the management of a patient with AIS should direct the physician toward the screening of other phenotypic females in the family, as this may afford earlier diagnosis and more timely intervention for affected individuals.

Antiphospholipid Antibodies in Reproductive Loss

Robert M. Silver, MD

Antiphospholipid antibodies (aPL) are a heterogeneous group of autoantibodies that bind to negatively charged phospholipids. Although several have been characterized, two aPL, lupus anticoagulant (LA) and anticardiolipin antibodies (aCL), are generally accepted as having clinical relevance. Circulating levels of these antibodies are associated with several medical problems including pregnancy loss, arterial and venous thrombosis, and autoimmune thrombocytopenia. In addition to fetal loss, several obstetric disorders have been associated with aPL. Successful pregnancies are often complicated by preeclampsia, intrauterine growth retardation, abnormal fetal heart rate tracings, and preterm delivery.

Antiphospholipid Syndrome

When characteristic clinical features occur in a patient with specified levels of aPL, the patient is considered to have antiphospholipid syndrome (APS).

Clinical criteria for APS include the following:

1. Fetal loss:
   Three or more spontaneous abortions with no more than one live birth.
   Unexplained second- or third-trimester fetal death.
2. Unexplained thrombosis, including stroke.
3. Autoimmune thrombocytopenia.
4. Unexplained transient ischemic attacks, amaurosis fugax, livedo reticularis, Coomb's positive hemolytic anemia, chorea, and chorea gravidarum.

Laboratory criteria include the following (see subsequent text for details):

1. Lupus anticoagulant
2. Anticardiolipin antibodies
   Immunoglobulin (Ig) G isotype greater than 15 to 20 GPL (Ig G binding) units (medium- to high-positive) detected in standardized assay using standard serum calibrators.

Connective tissue diseases, especially systemic lupus erythematosus (SLE), have also been associated with APS. Patients meeting criteria for APS who also have underlying autoimmune disease are considered to have secondary APS. Primary APS is diagnosed when individuals do not have another multisystem autoimmune disorder.

Pregnancy Loss and Antiphospholipid Antibodies

A relationship between circulating aPL and pregnancy loss has been recognized since the 1950s, and numerous studies have confirmed the association. Indeed, the rate of pregnancy loss in untreated patients with APS has been reported as high as 90%. A relatively large proportion of aPL-related pregnancy losses are second or early third trimester fetal deaths. Fifty percent of pregnancy losses in women with APS at the University of Utah were fetal deaths and over 80% of women with APS suffered at least one fetal death. Thus, clinicians should be suspicious of APS in women with unexplained fetal death. aPL also account for some cases of recurrent spontaneous abortion. Positive test results for aPL have been detected in up to 20% of women with recurrent pregnancy loss; however, many of these positive results are for low levels of aPL or aPL other than LA or aCL. We have found low positive levels of aPL and aPL other than LA and

aCL (see later) to be of questionable clinical relevance. At the University of Utah, we found APS to be the cause in 4% to 5% of couples with recurrent spontaneous abortion.

As opposed to recurrent pregnancy loss or fetal death, aPL have not been associated with sporadic spontaneous abortions. This is not surprising given the myriad causes of individual pregnancy loss and the infrequency of APS.

Obstetric Features of Antiphospholipid Syndrome

Successful pregnancies in women with APS are often complicated by obstetric disorders associated with abnormal placentation. Very high rates of pre-eclampsia have been reported in women with well-characterized APS. At the University of Utah, one half of women with APS developed pre-eclampsia and one quarter had severe pre-eclampsia. APS is also an important cause of *very severe pre-eclampsia*. Several studies have noted aPL in approximately 15% of women with early onset (<34 weeks') severe preeclampsia. Testing for aPL is recommended for women developing severe pre-eclampsia prior to 34 weeks' gestation but not for those with mild disease or pre-eclampsia at term.

Intrauterine growth retardation (IUGR) is also common. IUGR has been reported in one third of APS pregnancies. However, aPL have not been demonstrated to be a common cause of idiopathic growth impairment. Similarly, abnormal fetal heart rate tracings requiring delivery occur in one half of pregnancies complicated by APS. As with IUGR, aPL are rarely found in idiopathic cases of abnormal fetal heart rate tracings. Thus, idiopathic IUGR and "fetal distress" are not indications for testing for aPL in the absence of other features of APS.

These obstetric disorders all dramatically increase the risk of preterm delivery in women with APS. Patients should be counseled regarding an approximately 40% chance of delivering prior to 34 weeks' gestation if they are fortunate enough to achieve a live birth.

Medical Features of Antiphospholipid Syndrome

One of the most worrisome complications of APS is thrombosis. A majority of thrombotic events (65–70%) are venous, but arterial thromboses and stroke are also common. The most common site of venous thrombosis is the lower extremity, and up to one third of patients will have at least one pulmonary embolus. Thromboses in unusual locations have been reported in association with APS, however, and should cause the clinician to contemplate the diagnosis. Unexplained venous thrombosis should be considered an indication for testing for aPL, which is present in approximately 2% of cases.

Similarly, unexplained arterial thrombosis is also an indication for aPL testing. APS may explain up to 40% of cerebrovascular accidents in otherwise healthy individuals under the age of 50 years. Arterial thromboses can also occur in unusual locations such as the retinal artery.

Both pregnancy and oral contraceptive use appear to increase the risk of thromboembolism in women with APS. In fact, the prospective risk of thrombosis has been reported as 5% to 12% during pregnancy and the puerperium. Thus, prophylactic anticoagulant therapy should be considered during pregnancy and the postpartum period (see later). In addition, women with APS should not be treated with estrogen-containing oral contraceptives.

Autoimmune thrombocytopenia is also strongly associated with aPL. Although APS-related thrombocytopenia is difficult to distinguish from idiopathic thrombocytopenic purpura, the two disorders are treated similarly. Numerous other medical disorders associated with APS include autoimmune hemolytic anemia, livedo reticularis, chorea gravidarum, pyoderma-like leg ulcers, and transverse myelitis.

Laboratory Testing for Antiphospholipid Antibodies

Laboratory testing for aPL is a relatively new science that is still evolving. Problems have included nonstandardized assays, interlaboratory variation of assays, and confusion as to which aPL to test. Many of these issues are being resolved through international workshops, but the clinician is best served by using a laboratory with a special interest and expertise in aPL testing.

The two aPL that are best characterized and recommended for clinical use are LA and aCL. The antibody causing a false-positive serologic result for syphilis is an aPL often present in individuals with LA and aCL. It is not recommended for routine testing, however, because the relationship between it and clinical disorders is less clear. Similarly, other aPL such as antiphosphatidylserine antibodies are sometimes present in patients with APS, but most individuals with aPS also have LA or aCL. Also, assays for aPL other than LA and aCL have not been subjected to any standardization. Thus, although assays for additional aPL may prove useful, they cannot be recommended for routine clinical use at present.

Lupus anticoagulant is a classic misnomer and an unusual name for an autoantibody. Recall that many individuals with LA do not have SLE, and that LA is associated with thrombosis, not anticoagulation. LA is detected in plasma using any of several phospholipid-dependent clotting assays. Examples include the activated partial thromboplastin time (APTT), dilute Russel viper venom time, and kaolin clotting time. If LA is present, it will bind to the phospholipid used in the assays, thus interfering with the assay and resulting in an apparent prolongation of the clotting time. This observation prompted use of the term *anticoagulant*. The sensitivity of these tests for LA is greatly affected by the reagents used and varies among laboratories.

Factors other than LA, for example improperly processed specimens, clotting factor deficiencies, or anticoagulant medications, can also result in an apparent prolongation of clotting time. Thus, plasmas suspected of containing LA should undergo confirmatory testing. First, a mixing study is done wherein the patient's plasma is "mixed" with normal plasma. If an inhibitory antibody such as LA is present, the clotting time will remain abnormal. However, if the patient has a clotting factor deficiency, adding normal plasma will correct the clotting time. A second confirmatory test involves the addition or removal of phospholipid to the plasma. For example, if pretreatment with phospholipid normalizes the clotting time (by binding LA and removing it from the reaction), the patient is considered to have LA.

The clinician should order an "LA screen," which includes some combination of phospholipid-dependent clotting assays and confirmatory tests. Regardless of the assay used, LA cannot be quantified and is reported as present or absent.

Anticardiolipin antibodies are detected by immunoassays. Interlaboratory variation in these assays prompted the development of standard sera, which can be obtained from the Antiphospholipid Standardization Laboratory in Atlanta, Georgia. Assays using standard sera are reliable and allow for the semiquantitation of antibody levels, reported as GPL for IgG aCL, MPL for IgM aCL, and APL for IgA aCL. Results are reported as negative, or low-, medium-, or high-positive. Medium- or high-positive IgG aCL correlate well with clinical disorders and are considered to be laboratory criteria for APS. Low-positive results and isolated IgM or IgA antibodies are common, nonspecific, and of questionable clinical relevance. They should not be considered diagnostic of APS.

There is substantial overlap between LA and aCL, but the correlation is imperfect. Since both LA and aCL independently correlate with clinical disorders, testing for both LA and aCL is recommended.

Indications for Antiphospholipid Antibody Testing

1. Three or more first trimester pregnancy losses.
2. Unexplained second or third trimester fetal death.
3. Severe pre-eclampsia at less than 34 weeks' gestation.
4. Unexplained arterial or venous thrombosis.
5. Autoimmune thrombocytopenia.
6. Stroke, transient ischemic attacks, or amaurosis fugax, especially in patients less than 50 years old.
7. Autoimmune hemolytic anemia.
8. Systemic lupus erythematosus.
9. False-positive serologic test result for syphilis.
10. Unexplained severe fetal growth impairment or uteroplacental insufficiency (?; testing of questionable benefit in the absence of other clinical features of APS).

Obstetric Management of Antiphospholipid Syndrome

Extremely high rates of pregnancy loss and obstetric complications prompted clinicians to seek treatments during pregnancy to improve fetal outcome. Although still unproven in optimally designed clinical trials, accumulating evidence indicates that fetal survival is dramatically improved in treated pregnancies.

Medical treatments are based on proposed mechanisms of fetal loss in women with APS. Strategies intended to suppress the immune system include steroids and intravenous immune globulin. Heparin and other anticoagulants are intended to prevent thrombosis in the uteroplacental circulation, and low-dose aspirin can increase the prostacyclin-to-thromboxane ratio by suppressing platelet production of thromboxane.

Considerable success has been reported after treatment with either high-dose prednisone (40 mg per day) and low-dose aspirin (81 mg per day) or prophylactic doses of heparin (e.g. 5000 to 10,000 units per day) and low-dose aspirin. At the University of Utah, both regimens have resulted in a 70% success rate in a cohort of women with only a 10% live-birth rate in previous pregnancies. In a small randomized trial by Cowchock and colleagues,* both prednisone and heparin were equally efficacious, but prednisone had more side effects. Since heparin has fewer side effects and may also provide prophylaxis against thrombosis, heparin and low-dose aspirin are recommended as primary therapy. Low molecular weight heparin has been used safely during pregnancy and may eventually replace unfractionated heparin.

Heparin use has several adverse effects, including bleeding, thrombocytopenia, and osteopenia, which can lead to vertebral compression fractures. Since the risks of osteoporosis and bleeding increase with increasing doses of heparin, and "anticoagulant" doses of heparin are not superior to "prophylactic" doses with regard to fetal outcome, prophylactic doses should be used in the absence of acute thrombosis. Also, weight-bearing exercise and calcium and vitamin D supplementation should be encouraged to diminish the risk of osteoporosis. Heparin and high-dose prednisone should not be used simultaneously, since they both predispose women to osteopenic fractures and combination therapy is no better than either drug alone.

Therapy should be initiated after confirmation of a viable embryo with cardiac activity. Any theoretical (and unproven) benefit of preconception treatment is offset by the side effects of prolonged therapy. Thromboprophylaxis should be continued during the postpartum period because of the risk of thromboembolism. Coumarin can be used postpartum to limit the risk of heparin-induced osteoporosis.

Intravenous immune globulin has been extremely promising in a small number of cases that were refractory to heparin or prednisone. However, it is extremely expensive and cannot be recommended as primary therapy without further proof of efficacy.

Ideally, women with APS should receive preconceptional counseling regarding their risk for fetal loss, preterm birth, pre-eclampsia, fetal growth impairment, cesarean delivery, and

---

*Cowchock FS, Reece EA, et al: Repeated fetal losses associated with antiphospholipid antibodies: a collaborative randomized trial comparing prednisone with low-dose heparin treatments. Am J Obstet Gynecol 166:1318–1323, 1992.

thromboembolism. They should also have confirmation of relevant levels of aPL. Once the diagnosis of APS is made, however, serial antibody determinations are unnecessary. Intensive surveillance (weekly clinic visits and biweekly nonstress tests) for pre-eclampsia, fetal growth impairment, and uteroplacental insufficiency should be instituted at 30 to 32 weeks' gestation. Earlier (24–25 weeks' gestation) and more frequent ultrasonograms and fetal testing are indicated in selected cases, such as for women with poor obstetric histories, fetal growth retardation, or pre-eclampsia. My group and others have noted spontaneous decelerations in the second trimester in APS pregnancies. Intervention with preterm delivery may improve fetal outcome in severe cases. Finally, women with SLE, autoimmune thrombocytopenia, or other related diseases should receive specialized care as appropriate.

Medical Management of Antiphospholipid Syndrome

Women with APS are at substantial risk for developing nonobstetric medical problems associated with aPL. Individuals with previous thromboses and APS should receive lifelong anticoagulation with coumarin to achieve an international normalized ratio of 2.5 to 3.0. Acute thromboses require anticoagulation with heparin to elevate the APTT to 1.5 to 2 times normal. Phospholipid-dependent clotting assays such as the APTT cannot be used to assess anticoagulation in women with LA. Anticoagulation is considered adequate when the thrombin time is elevated to 100 seconds or greater. It is unclear whether patients with APS and no previous thromboses require treatment.

Barrier Contraception: The Reality Female Condom

Elizabeth B. Connell, MD

A new contraceptive device, the polyurethane vaginal pouch, or Reality Female Condom, is approved for sale in the United States. It is currently available in Switzerland, Austria, Norway, Portugal, the Netherlands, and the United Kingdom.

As the occurrence of unplanned pregnancies and sexually transmitted diseases (STDs) reached epidemic proportions, the need for products like the pouch, designed to address both of these issues, was ever more evident. With this in mind, the Obstetrics and Gynecology Devices Panel of the US Food and Drug Administration (FDA) drew up a new set of preclinical and clinical guidelines for an expedited "fast-track" review procedure for products that fall into this category. The vaginal pouch is the first product to be studied and approved under the new guidelines.

The pouch is a sheath, 17 cm in length, made of soft, thin polyurethane and closed at one end. It has a flexible ring at both ends. The inner closed ring covers the cervix like a diaphragm; the outer open ring is placed externally, covering the central portion of the perineum. Since the entire vagina, cervix, and part of the perineum are covered, the device offers a women maximum protection against contact with the penis and the ejaculate. It also prevents contact with the base of the penis. The pouch is made in only one size and is sold over-the-counter. It is prelubricated with silicone and packaged with a water-soluble lubricant. It may be inserted immediately before or up to several hours prior to sexual intercourse, but is to be used only once.

When the FDA's Devices Panel met on January 31, 1992, it reviewed preliminary data on the pouch supplied by the Wisconsin Pharmacal Company. It was reported that the polyurethane film, approximately twice as thick as latex rubber condoms for men, had been tested in the laboratory and found to be less permeable to viruses and dyes than latex. In addition, tests on the film using gases such as helium and nitrogen showed no permeability. It was suggested that, in view of these data, it was unlikely that the much larger STD organisms could leak through the walls of the pouch. Studies also showed that the pouch was impermeable to *Trichomonas*.

Data gathered on 81 women in clinical studies conducted in the United States and Latin America showed a failure rate of 15.1 per 100 women during the first 6 months of use. Twenty-five pregnancies were reported, about three quarters of which were classified as user failures. This rate is comparable to results obtained with other barrier methods.

After the presentation, the panel decided that the preliminary clinical data that were submitted were inadequate for final evaluation. It therefore recommended that the studies, originally planned to provide 12-month data on 200 women, be concluded. Second, the panel stated that the failure rate must continue to be equal to or better than the preliminary rate of 15% if final approval is to be recommended. It also indicated that the polyurethane film should be further tested to obtain more conclusive data on its ability to withstand ripping and breaking.

There are two key advantages to the vaginal pouch. First of all, it provides maximum physical protection to both partners. Second, and of equal or greater importance, this barrier method is female-controlled. There is ample evidence in the medical and lay literature that, for various personal, cultural, and psychological reasons, the male condom is not always used in high-risk situations. This is particularly disturbing as STD rates, especially human immunodeficiency virus and acquired immunodeficiency syndrome, are rising dramatically in women. Furthermore, it is now well established that male-to-female transmission of HIV infections is 12 to 17 times greater than female-to-male. Therefore, there is a great impetus to find a barrier method that allows a woman to protect herself against STD transmission as well as pregnancy.

Even with excellent data on safety and efficacy, there are a number of unanswered questions about the ultimate acceptability of this device. Individuals who are at high risk for pregnancy and STDs may, in all likelihood, be highly motivated to use the vaginal pouch. However, its size and aesthetic qualities may make it less attractive than other currently available options, particularly to low-risk women.

On the issue of consumer labeling for the pouch, the panel took the position that the company's claims for protection against specific STDs were unproven, except in the case of trichomoniasis. It was suggested that its labeling be similar to that allowed by the FDA for the male condom, which is nonspecific as regards possible protection against particular STDs. In addition, it was recommended that accurate and clear information be made available to potential users about the degree of protection against unwanted pregnancy that proper use of the pouch provides.

Despite their reservations, the panel concluded that the preliminary data on the contraceptive vaginal pouch looked quite encouraging. It recommended that the various laboratory and clinical studies that were discussed be completed and that the information from them be gathered, collated, and submitted to the FDA. On December 10, 1992, the panel again reviewed the data. Although there were still concerns about the pregnancy rate and the limited data on STD transmission, the panel felt that the pouch should be approved. The FDA gave final approval on April 26, 1993, pending agreement on the specific labeling.

The following day the FDA issued a press release, announcing the approval "with restrictive labeling." It stated that the product was "the first barrier contraceptive for women that also offers limited protection against sexually transmitted diseases." However, it continued to recommend the male latex condom as "the best shield against AIDS and other sexually transmitted diseases."

The press release also listed two conditions: first, the label must compare the pregnancy rate—26% per year—to rates associated with other female barriers, which are lower; second, the manufacturer must take part in further effectiveness studies. On November 27, 1994, it was announced that $5.5 million had been awarded by the National Institute of Child Health and Human Development and the Center for Disease Control and Prevention to the University of Alabama in Birmingham. The grant was an extension of a 1991 study looking for methods to help control STD transmission in high-risk populations.

Continuing interest in the female condom has stimulated new programs and studies. In early 1995, programs for safer, smarter sex were started in many major university student health services. Focus groups of African-American women in New Orleans indicated strong support for a method that gave them control. Finally, a review published in 1994 concluded that the efficacy and continuation rates were similar to those of other female barrier methods.

Bartholin's Cyst and Abscess

William Benbow Thompson, Jr, MD

Cysts and tumors of the vulva and probably of Bartholin's duct have been known for all time. Aëtius of Amida referred to vulvovaginal cysts as "hernia aquosa" of the labia and described them as early as the sixth century AD. Numerous observers and anatomists referred to drainage through the duct into the vestibule. The anatomist Duverney probably was the first to actually find the glands—in the cow. He later was able to dissect them in a human and demonstrated them to Bartholin, whose first accurate description in 1676 gave him the eponymic rights to this structure.

The Bartholin glands are the homologues of the greater vestibular glands of mammals. They lie deep beneath the fascia and underlie the lower margin of the bulbocavernosus muscle directly beneath the vestibular bulb. The duct penetrates the superficial fascia and enters the vestibule in its posterior aspect, about 2 cm from the central tendon of the perineum. The gland is a lobulated, racemose structure with multiple acini that secrete mucin; secretion is increased during excitatory sexual stimulation and is an important function of this gland in lower animals. Cysts and abscesses of this structure involve primarily the duct, whereas neoplastic alterations of the structure involve the gland itself.

It is important to keep the basic anatomy in mind when attempting operative procedures for correction of abnormalities of the Bartholin gland and duct. For practical purposes, it is best to divide disorders or diseases of this structure into (1) inflammatory conditions—acute and chronic, (2) conditions that obstruct the duct, and (3) neoplastic disease.

Carcinoma of the Bartholin gland is an extremely rare tumor. It is usually diagnosed after the spread has reached surface epithelium, and at that point it is obvious that something is happening. Prespread diagnosis may be made by palpation of a hard 1 to 1.5 cm nodule in the deep structures of the vulva in the location of the Bartholin gland. Unfortunately, this is usually mistaken for Bartholin's adenitis, and long periods of delay are the rule, even in those patients in whom the gland has been palpated. The association between inflammatory changes in the duct and gland and carcinoma is incidental at best. Neoplastic changes in Bartholin's gland will be discussed under carcinoma of the vulva.

Noninflammatory ductal obstruction, although relatively uncommon, may account for 25% or more of cystic tumors of Bartholin's duct. These are usually traumatic in origin and may occur following repair of straddle injuries in young children but may not become evident until the postpubertal period. They also occur following obstetric laceration or mediolateral episiotomy, and, for this reason, they are most frequently encountered in the left Bartholin duct region. These tumors seldom become larger than 2 to 3 cm in diameter and are easily palpable, are usually nontender, and may be treated by either excision or marsupialization. From the fifth decade and beyond, it is advisable to undertake excision, although, as previously mentioned, the association between cystic change in the duct and carcinoma of the gland is not established.

The most common Bartholin's tumor encountered is acute inflammatory change secondary to infection and obstruction of the duct from adhesions and distortion. Patients with such tumors need immediate treatment. One cannot easily temporize when a patient is in severe pain and relief is so easily accomplished. The traditional approach of incision and drainage is still a logical method of treatment. Unfortunately, the recurrence rate from simple incision and drainage is quite high. The use of a Word catheter has a somewhat more beneficial long-term effect and, like incision and drainage, can be done under topical local anesthesia in the office. The balloon should be inflated so as to occupy approximately one-half to two-thirds of the preinsertion dimensions. Drainage should always be accomplished through the mucous surface of the vestibule in the lower one third and not through the skin, even though this may be the area of greatest distention. In chronic inflammatory changes, the condition is generally relatively asymptomatic, and the patient is seen because of difficulties with intercourse. These patients are ideal candidates for primary marsupialization and have a better success rate than with incision and drainage. A reasonable number of these patients with chronic cystic change have had an incision and drainage in the past, and after the inflammation has gone from their abscess, they have a residual cyst.

Treatment

Before commencing treatment, it is important to review the patient's past history. These are "clean contaminated" cases at best. One must think of possible antibiotic therapy in conjunction with surgical approach. All patients with prosthetic replacements, as well as patients with valvular cardiac disease, should receive intraoperative antibiotics. The choice should cover the common contaminants—*Escherichia coli* and the gram-negative flora associated with the genital tract.

The treatment of the acute Bartholin's duct abscess is best accomplished immediately. It is easiest to perform this procedure if an assistant is available to hold the tissues. The labia are rolled inferiorly and laterally, presenting the mucous surface of the vestibule. This surface should be painted with a topical anesthetic (benzocaine [Hurricaine] spray or gel provides a good topical anesthesia). The mucosa may then be further anesthetized using 1% lidocaine in a 25-gauge needle. The point of introduction of the scalpel for drainage or of the Word catheter via the trocar should be along the lower third of the vestibule near the anatomic orifice of the duct. Cultures should be obtained from the drainage material for both predominant organisms and gonococcus. Although gonococcus used to be the primary infecting organism, it now occupies a secondary position to enteric and anaerobic organisms. Once drainage has been accomplished, the patient immediately feels better. If a Word catheter is used, she may begin taking sitz baths in about 48 hours. If no Word catheter is used, this process can begin earlier. Since most patients do not have the hospital type of equipment for sitz baths, an easy method is to put 4 inches of warm water (approximately 100 to 120°F) along with 2 cups of ordinary Epsom salts in the bathtub. The patient may then sit in this for a period of 20 minutes, two or three times daily. Other adjunctive agents to put in the sitz bath include table salt, povidone-iodine (Betadine), and chlorine bleach (it is unnecessary to use more than one agent at a time). If a Word catheter is used, the preparatory maneuvers are the same. When the balloon is inflated, the patient has almost immediate relief of her symptoms. She should be seen in 3 or 4 days for removal of the Word catheter, although many of these catheters deflate and are expelled in this period of time. It is unnecessary to attempt packing of an incised and drained abscess in the office. The increased success rate is marginal, and the discomfort to the patient is maximal.

Attempted marsupialization of an acute abscess is an expensive exercise in futility. The probability of having a clear stoma at the end of this procedure is very small, and the expense for the patient of undergoing a general or regional anesthetic and going through an operating room procedure seems unwarranted when the success rate using a Word catheter is almost the same. In general, marsupialization of the Bartholin's cyst should be done in the hospital or out-patient surgery center. Regional or general anesthesia is preferred. I prefer to remove a segment of mucosa, although there are others who believe that this affords no decrease in recurrence rate following marsupialization. Generally, I remove a circular segment of the mucosa of the vestibule of 1 to 1.5 cm. When the cyst wall is encountered, it is simply incised in a linear fashion from top to bottom. The contents of the cyst should be cultured and examined for cellular material, and then the cyst wall is sutured to the mucosa using fine, interrupted sutures. Our preference is 4–0 Vicryl or Dexon, but 4–0 chromic catgut certainly has been used for generations with reasonable success. As noted previously, packing does not seem to increase the likelihood of suc-

cess; however, I still pack the cyst with a small segment of iodoform gauze. This can be sewed into the cyst simply by pushing a needle through the top of the cyst and out of the mucosa superiorly, then rethreading the needle and doing the same with the opposite end. Thus, the tie is external and removal can be accomplished simply by cutting the suture and pulling the drain loose.

There are occasional indications for removal of Bartholin's gland. These include recurrence following marsupialization and presence of an asymptomatic cyst in women over 40 years of age. Although the association between cystic change and neoplastic change is not established, it is still believed to be advisable to remove tissue in this instance. This procedure tends to be difficult and is fraught with problems (the usual one is perforation of the cystic tumor during the procedure). It is important to palpate and find the pea-sized Bartholin gland, since excision of a Bartholin duct cyst without the glandular material often leads to a recurrent, deep cyst that is more difficult to remove. The other hazard encountered is related to the vasculature of the bulb, which may produce considerable intraoperative and postoperative bleeding and may cause wound disruption postoperatively.

In attempting an enucleation of the Bartholin duct cyst, the labia are stretched laterally so as to expose the mucous surface of the vestibule. The incision is linear and should be ample for the size of the cyst. This is not a simple enucleation as with an inclusion cyst but, rather, is a tedious dissection with numerous adhesions between the cyst wall and the adjacent structures. Small Metzenbaum scissors are best, in my opinion, for accomplishing this dissection. The initial incision must go to the area of the cyst wall; otherwise, too much of the intervening blood supply to the mucosa is destroyed, which is a detriment to healing. The cysts usually have their largest component above the area of the anatomic duct and above the base of the Bartholin gland itself. It is advisable, however, to do a careful rectal examination, palpating to discover whether the cyst extends inferiorly into the perirectal space. Such an extension is another danger signal in removal, and one must be extremely careful in dissecting the deep structures from such a cyst. If the gland is inadvertently opened, which occurs in 25% to 75% of attempts, the contents should be cultured. (Sending a specimen for cytologic evaluation seems unnecessary, since a pathologic specimen will be forthcoming.) In some respects, this simplifies the removal, since one can see both sides of the cyst as the dissection is continued, and one often can then trace the origin of the gland area itself, facilitating the removal of the deep Bartholin gland. Drainage should be instituted. A ¼ to ½ inch Penrose drain sutured in the manner previously described is usually sufficient. The layers are closed from the base toward the mucosa, and 3–0 catgut or 4–0 Dexon is appropriate suture material.

Immediately after surgery, icebags to the perineal area will reduce edema. After approximately the third day, sitz baths may be instituted. Drains can usually be removed after the third to fourth day unless there seems to be excessive drainage on the dressing. The presence of a drain in these wounds usually prevents the development of a labial hematoma, even in instances in which the bulb of the vestibule has been damaged. The recovery period after removal of the cyst and gland is relatively prolonged (2 to 3 weeks of home care is usual).

Chlamydial Infections

Lane Jay Mercer, MD

Chlamydia is an obligate intracellular parasite that has a tropism for specific tissue types, commonly columnar and cuboidal epithelium. It has a complex life cycle characterized by both bacterial and viral elements. This two-part life cycle starts with an elementary stage during which a metabolically inert but infectious form attaches to a susceptible host cell and facilitates its ingestion via phagocytosis. This elementary body has a cell wall structure similar to that of gram-negative bacteria. Once inside the cell, it combines with a host phagosome to form a reticulate body, so named because of its characteristic microscopic appearance. This metabolically active form uses energy "stolen" from the host much in the manner of a virus to divide by binary fission every 8 to 24 hours to form new elementary bodies to infect nearby cells. This life cycle takes approximately 36 to 48 hours to complete. Therefore, short-term prophylactic antibiotic therapies are not effective against this organism.

Epidemiology

There are an estimated 3 to 5 million new cases of *Chlamydia trachomatis* infection every year in the United States, with a reported incidence of 198 cases per 100,000 population in 1991, which was more than double that found in 1987. Unprotected sexual contact is the only identified mode of transmission of *Chlamydia trachomatis*. A transmission rate per sexual contact with an infected partner of 30% is estimated. Race has been identified as a significant risk factor for chlamydial infection, with African-Americans having a higher incidence than whites. However, reanalysis of this data suggests that socioeconomic status rather than race appears to be the important risk factor. Among adolescents, perhaps the greatest reservoir of this organism, race, socioeconomic status, and geography do not appear to be significant risk factors. There appears to be a seasonal variation in the reported rates of detection of chlamydiosis, with highest rates reported in August and September. This may reflect the increased sexual activity identified during that time of year or the increased utilization of Student Health Services at the beginning of the school year.

Risk Factors

A number of risk factors have been identified to facilitate screening for chlamydial infections. Objectively, age less than 24 years, a new sexual partner in the preceding 2 months, use of non-barrier contraception or no contraception, cervical cytologic atypia, and a history of sexually transmitted diseases have all been correlated with infection. Subjectively, mucopurulent cervical discharge, bleeding upon swabbing of the cervix, and cervical ectopy have indicated an increased risk for *Chlamydia trachomatis* infection.

Screening

The use of selective screening for chlamydia has been shown to be both effacious in the identification of the asymptotic carrier and cost-effective in the prevention of subsequent pelvic inflammatory disease. Screening women with two or more of the following risk factors identified approximately 90% of infections: new sex partner in the preceding 2 months, age less than or equal to 24 years, purulent cervical discharge, endocervical bleeding with swabbing, and the use of no or nonbarrier contraceptive methods. The application of these selective screening techniques has been successful in large-scale family planning clinics, where, when combined with education and aggressive therapy of the patient and partner, reduced prevalence rates in both high- and low-risk patients by half.

Tests

Two considerations must be taken into account when utilizing any test for the detection of chlamydial infections. First, asymptomatic patients carry quantitatively fewer chlamydia in their cervices than do symptomatic patients. The reported accuracy of most tests was ascertained in high-risk or high-prevalence populations. The accuracy of the test may be lower when used in a screening population. Second, regardless of the outcome of a confirmatory test, if there is high suspicion that a patient may have a chlamydial infection, that patient should be treated. The consequences of a false-negative result could have such a great effect on future reproduction that the benefit of such treatment may outweigh the cost or potential side effects.

Cell culture, once considered the standard against which all other tests are compared, is now recognized as having sensitivity of 75% to 100%, when compared with two independent nonculture tests. Handling of the specimen, cleansing of the cervix, the type of swab used, type of cells cultured, passaging, and staining methods are all variables that can affect the accuracy of this technique. Once a specimen for culture is obtained, it should be plated within 24 hours. Cultures left at room temperature for 24 hours have shown a decreased yield of 65%. Specimens held for 24 to 48 hours can be refrigerated at 4°C with only a 5% decrease in yield. Those held longer should be frozen at −70°C for optimal results. Other limitations of this test are the relatively high expense, labor intensive nature, and the long turnaround time of 3 to 7 days.

Enzyme immunoassay utilizes polyclonal antibodies to lipopolysaccharides and membrane proteins to achieve a sensitivity of 73% to 95% and a specificity of 97% to 99%. The advantages of this test include rapid turnover time, no need for viable organisms, and its low cost. Although largely eliminated through the use of blocking antibodies, false-positive reactions can occur with specific strains of *Escherichia coli* and other bacteria.

Direct immunofluorescent antibodies utilize chlamydial antibodies conjugated to a fluorescent molecule that can be detected with a fluorescent microscope. Sensitivities of 86% to 100% and specificities of 95% have been reported. The advantages of this technique is that

fixed slides can be kept at room temperature for days before being read, allowing for batch processing and a relatively short turnaround time. The main disadvantage is the reliance on the skill of the microscopist in the interpretation of the slides. One study demonstrated as much as 30% intermicroscopist variance in the identification of positive slides.

DNA probes are directed against *Chlamydia*-specific nucleic acids. Early studies were highly specific in high-prevalence populations but much less so in low-prevalence screening populations. The use of polymerase chain reaction has increased the specificity of these tests to equal to that of the enzyme immunoassay, with specificities and sensitivities of 99% and 78%, respectively.

Dealing with the false-positive test result is particularly problematic when screening a low-risk population, particularly in light of the social implications such a result may engender. As false-positives are inherent to any test, the test should be applied to a population with known risk factors. False-positives may occur due to cross-reactivity to other bacteria such as *E. coli*, *Acinetobacter*, and *Citrobacter*, misinterpretation such as with the use of direct immunofluorescent antibodies, and contamination with foreign DNA with the DNA probe. A positive test result occurring in an unlikely situation should be confirmed using a culture technique or a dissimilar nonculture technique. Persistently positive test results in spite of adequate therapy and appropriate compliance should be confirmed with an alternative test.

Clinical Manifestations of Infection

Cervicitis is the most common manifestation of a chlamydial infection. Mucopurulence, friability with swabbing, and ectropion are common findings, with two of these three findings demonstrated in 60% of patients with chlamydial infection. However, in a general population with mucopurulent cervicitis alone (yellow-green cervical discharge and greater than 10 polymorphonuclear leukocytes per high-power field), *Chlamydia* was isolated in only 7% to 22% of patients.

Chlamydia trachomatis is associated with 20% to 30% of cases of pelvic inflammatory disease (PID) in the United States. Chlamydia may play two distinct roles in the pathophysiology of this disease. First, it may manifest as pure chlamydial PID characterized by lower abdominal pain, irregular uterine bleeding, and pelvic tenderness during bimanual examination. Fever, rebound tenderness, and adnexal masses are rarely found. Laboratory findings include elevated erythrocyte sedimentation rates and C-reactive protein, but white blood cell counts are not usually markedly elevated. As these findings are nondescript, suspicion for this "out-patient PID" is the most useful diagnostic tool. Therapy consists of appropriate oral anti-chlamydial agents and re-examination in 24 to 48 hours to ensure an adequate response to therapy. Second, *Chlamydia* plays an important role in the pathogenesis of acute bacterial PID characterized by high fever, elevated white blood cell counts, diffuse abdominal tenderness, and extremely tender pelvic organs. Although frequently isolated from the endocervices of patients with PID, it is much less commonly isolated from the fallopian tubes. The multibacterial nature of this disease is well recognized, and broad-spectrum parenteral therapy remains the standard care. An indication for parental therapy is any one of the following: temperature over 38°C, white blood cell count over 12,000, four-quadrant tenderness, rebound tenderness, and the finding of an adnexal mass.

Urethritis and **urethral syndrome** are commonly caused by *Chlamydia trachomatis*. As many as 65% of afebrile women presenting with urinary frequency or urgency, or both, and negative urine cultures had chlamydial infections. Again, patient populations must be taken into account and other common causes of dysuria such as estrogen deficiency should be sought. Although simultaneous culturing of the endocervix and urethra may increase the yield of positive cultures by as much as 20%, the technique can be uncomfortable. Therefore, a patient with a negative urine culture and urinary symptoms may be empirically treated with an antibiotic such as trimethoprim/sulfamethoxazole or ofloxacin, which are active against both *Chlamydia* and common urinary pathogens.

Perihepatitis, characterized by right upper quadrant pain, tenderness upon palpation of the liver, and mildly elevated liver function tests, occurs in 4% to 25% of patients with PID. Although PID was once thought to be exclusively caused by *Neisseria gonorrhoeae*, *Chlamydia* is now recognized as a significant etiologic pathogen. *Chlamydia trachomatis* has been isolated from liver biopsies and has been cultured from the cervix of half of women with gonorrhea-negative PID and laparoscopically proven perihepatitis. The diagnosis of perihepatitis does not alter the treatment of PID but sequelae such as chronic right upper quadrant pain may occur.

Infertility is the most serious consequence of chlamydial infection. Fifty percent of women with infertility due to tubal occlusion but no history of PID had serologic evidence of past infection with *Chlamydia*. Following a single episode of acute PID, 15% of women develop tubal occlusion and infertility, with the incidence of infertility doubling with each subsequent infection.

An increased rate of **ectopic pregnancy** has been associated with chlamydial infection. Patients with a history of PID had a five- to sevenfold increase. Women with antichlamydial antibodies had two- to sixfold increased risk of developing an ectopic pregnancy.

Therapy

Although some beta-lactam antibiotics have been shown to be inhibitory to the development of the cell wall of the *Chlamydia* within the reticulate body, this is a bacteriostatic event, and after withdrawal of the antibiotic reproduction continues. Therefore, this class of antibiotics is not considered an adequate therapy. Indeed, some concerns have been raised as to the effect of these drugs on the function of other antibiotics when administered simultaneously.

Most antibiotics for the treatment of chlamydial infection are effective and retesting to ascertain eradication of chlamydia is unnecessary. However, patient compliance is an important factor in the success of this therapy. It is difficult for patients, particularly adolescents, to complete a course of therapy that has considerable side effects to treat an asymptomatic infection. Therefore, the choice of antibiotic should include patient acceptability as well as efficacy. Recommended antibiotics are as follows:

> Doxycycline 100 mg PO bid for 7 days
> Azithromycin 1 g PO as a single dose
> Erythromycin 500 mg PO qid or equivalent
> for 7 days
> Ofloxacin 300 mg PO bid for 7 days

Other antibiotics have been shown to be effective therapeutic agents but are not generally considered first-line therapies.

Chlamydial Infections During Pregnancy

Some studies have indicated that infection with *Chlamydia trachomatis* in pregnant women may result in premature labor, premature rupture of membranes, and chorioamnionitis. An association between the presence of antichlamydial antibodies and low birth weight infants has been made.

Furthermore, it has been suggested that recently infected women are more likely to deliver preterm infants than chronically infected women.

Infection in the first trimester is associated with a 20% incidence of postabortal endometritis, with appropriate screening and treatment successful in preventing this complication. Postpartum endometritis occurs in 20% to 25% of women with evidence of chlamydial infection. This late-onset endometritis presents 3 to 6 weeks after delivery and manifests as fever, vaginal discharge, lower abdominal pain, and postpartum hemorrhage.

Some practitioners have suggested screening all parturient patients at initial presentation for chlamydia; however, this has not been proven cost-effective. Using similar criteria to those used for nonpregnant women, *Chlamydia* has been identified in 10% of pregnant women in middle-class practices in one study. No test has been proven superior to another during pregnancy. As with the nonpregnant patient, a suspicion of infection should constitute an indication for the initiation of therapy.

Recommended therapy in pregnancy is erythromycin base or equivalent, 500 mg PO qid for 7 days. Alternative regimens include clindamycin, azithromycin, and trimethroprim/sulfamethoxazole.

Perinatal Infections

Transmission from the mother to the neonate during the birthing process is 30% to 60%. Neonatal manifestations include conjunctivitis, respiratory tract infection, and vaginitis. Conjunctivitis presents 1 to 3 weeks after delivery with mucopurulent discharge and possible pseudomembrane formation. Symptoms are usually self-limited but may lead to corneal ulceration with severe consequences for vision. Pneumonitis is characterized by a staccato cough, bulging eardrums, and a protracted course. Children with chlamydial pneumonia are at a higher risk for developing asthma or chronic obstructive pulmonary disease in the future. Neonatal vaginitis is characterized by a mucopurulent vaginal discharge due to infection of the endocervical cells which extend onto the upper vagina. Sequelae of vaginal synnechiae have been reported.

Treatment of the infant consists of erythromycin liquid 50 mg/kg in four divided doses for 10 days. Topical therapy for chlamydial conjunctivitis is inadequate, as the infant may harbor the organism in the nasopharynx. Other therapies in the infant have been reported as successful, but

limited use and experience make them second line.

Lymphogranuloma Venereum

Lymphogranuloma venereum (LGV) is an unusual disease in the United States caused by a different serovar of *Chlamydia trachomatis* than is found in the more common infections. The most frequent clinical manifestation of LGV is enlarged, painful inguinal lymph nodes. These lymph nodes, which are exquisitely tender, may be bilateral but are usually unilateral. In one third of the cases they are found above and below the inguinal ligament, presenting as the "groove sign," which is strongly suggestive, but not pathognomonic, of LGV. Systemic symptoms are common and include chills, myalgias, fever, and lassitude. Diffuse systemic symptoms may be found in some patients. If left untreated, the inguinal lymph nodes may form buboes, which break down and form chronically draining sinus tracts.

The primary site of infection is rarely identified in most patients, but appropriate testing of common infection sites is warranted. *Chlamydia* can seldom be cultured from the inguinal lesions. Secondary infection with other organisms, including anaerobics, is common. Therapy should be initiated to cover not only the *Chlamydia* but also these secondary organisms. Failure to treat adequately can result in scarring, fibrosis, and lymphedema with subsequent disfigurement.

Colposcopy

Kenneth L. Noller, MD
Jeffrey O. Riley, MD

Colposcopy is a diagnostic procedure originally introduced into the United States in the 1960s. It allows early detection and diagnosis of premalignant cervical lesions, which can be effectively treated by simple office-based procedures. Additionally, colposcopy has been found to be useful for detecting premalignant changes of the vagina and vulva.

Colposcopy is an office-based procedure that utilizes a low power binocular microscope to examine the lower genital tract. No special patient preparation is required (eg, prophylactic antibiotics, analgesia). An experienced colposcopist can recognize specific patterns that are associated with premalignant and early invasive disease of the lower genital tract. Directed biopsies of suspicious areas can be performed, which are evaluated by standard histologic techniques to establish a definitive diagnosis. Because of the sensitivity of colposcopy in detecting lower genital tract disease, it has emerged as the primary method for evaluating women with abnormal Pap smears in the United States. Appropriate use of colposcopy requires proper patient selection, an understanding of normal and abnormal cytoarchitecture, good technique, and ongoing experience.

Patient Selection

Although colposcopy is sensitive in detecting premalignant lesions, it is neither necessary nor cost effective to screen all women with annual colposcopic examinations. It is a diagnostic technique to evaluate prescreened women who are at high risk for lower genital tract disease. Usually, screening is accomplished by a Pap smear. Since its introduction in 1988, the Bethesda System (TBS) has become the dominant reporting system used by U.S. cytology laboratories. Various diagnostic categories are reported with the TBS system. The presence of cytologic abnormalities suggestive of a high grade squamous intraepithelial lesion or squamous carcinoma represent clear, unequivocal indications for colposcopic examination. However, the immediate use of colposcopy with less severe cytologic changes is controversial (Fig. 1).

Cytologic abnormalities diagnosed as low grade squamous intraepithelial lesions (LGSIL) can be indicative of underlying early preneoplastic changes. However, most women with LGSIL cytologic abnormalities will be found, after evaluation, to have only subclinical human papilloma virus (HPV) infections. Most HPV infections are thought to be completely reversible. Additionally, if colposcopic examination of a woman with LGSIL changes detects a grade one cervical intraepithelial neoplastic lesion (CIN I), appropriate management is unclear, as the majority of CIN I lesions will spontaneously resolve over time. Although the chance of a significant underlying lesion is small in a woman with LGSIL cytologic abnormalities, further evaluation is indicated.

Patient compliance can play an important role in determining the appropriate type of follow-up for patients with LGSIL changes. If highly compliant, a patient can be followed with serial cytology alone, with colposcopy being reserved for those patients with persistent abnormalities. If patient compliance is uncertain, immediate colposcopy is indicated to minimize the chance of the patient being lost to follow-up. Finally, because the possibility of a significant premalignant lesion does exist with LGSIL changes, immediate colposcopy is an acceptable diagnostic option and currently represents the most common method of follow-up in the United States of women with low grade cytologic abnormalities.

The most difficult diagnostic category created by TBS is "atypical squamous cells of undetermined significance" (ASCUS). ASCUS Pap smears represent a category in which no clear diagnoses can be made. The term incorporates smears with cytologic changes that preclude their being placed in the "within normal limits" category but that do not fulfill the criteria required to be called "definitively preneoplastic." It is a category that has considerable interobserver vari-

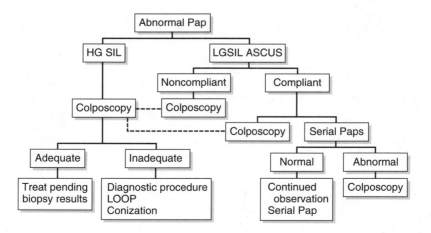

Figure 1.

ability. The creation of the ASCUS category in the TBS has resulted in a substantial expansion of the percentage of smears reported as abnormal nationwide. Investigators who have evaluated ASCUS patients with an immediate colposcopic examination have reported an underlying risk of CIN of 10% to 40%, with the large majority of these being CIN I. Although the majority of women with ASCUS Pap smears on examination will be normal, a risk of underlying CIN does exist. The best method for follow-up of women with ASCUS Pap smears remains controversial. Either frequent, serial Pap smears or immediate colposcopic examination is indicated. As discussed earlier, patient compliance is an important consideration when developing an individual patient plan.

In addition to assigning a diagnostic category to a Pap smear, TBS also comments on the quality of the smear. A Pap smear may be "unsatisfactory for evaluation." Inadequate sampling technique, the presence of obscuring blood, or inflammation with scant cellularity represents the most common causes. The response to an initial unsatisfactory Pap smear should be to repeat the smear after discerning and correcting the underlying cause. Importantly, a minimum of 6 weeks (and perhaps as long as 12 weeks) should separate the initial Pap smear and the repeat smear. If the repeat Pap smear again is unsatisfactory without a definite source, colposcopy should be considered. The presence of cellular debris or inflammation may decrease the sensitivity of the Pap smear to detect a significant neoplastic lesion. If abnormal cells are seen on either the initial or repeat Pap smear, colposcopy should be performed regardless of the adequacy of the smear.

Loop electroexcision is a technique commonly used to treat CIN. One advantage of this technique over ablative methods (cryosurgery, CO_2 laser) is the retrieval of a specimen that can be submitted for histologic evaluation. A worrisome finding sometimes encountered by a clinician is the involvement of the upper endocervical margin of the loop biopsy with CIN. It is likely that patients with such a finding are at increased risk for persistent CIN, as compared with similar patients with clear endocervical margins. It is not necessary to perform an immediate re-excision, however, as most women will not have persistent disease. In these patients, in addition to serial Pap smears, colposcopy may be helpful at the initial follow-up examination to help detect a persistent, significant preneoplastic lesion, if it is present.

Epithelial Architecture

Colposcopy is a technique based on pattern recognition of changes in the appearance of the cervical epithelium and its vascular plexus. To examine the cervix with a colposcope, it is important to understand the cytoarchitecture of normal and abnormal epithelium.

The majority of CIN originates in the cervical transformation zone (T-Z). The T-Z is a circumferential area at the cervical os that extends from the original squamocolumnar junction present in the prepubertal female, to the squamocolumnar junction present at the time of examination. In some women this junction is located in the endocervical canal. It is a dynamic area where columnar epithelium undergoes metaplasia to become mature squamous epithelium. It is probable that during this process, epithelial cells are particularly susceptible to various neoplastic stimulants (eg, HPV, infection), leading, in some cases, to conversion to preneoplastic epithelium.

Columnar epithelium in the normal T-Z grows in a villous, folded shape with a central vascular core creating a grapelike appearance when viewed through the colposcope. When exposed to the acidic environment present in the vagina at menarche, columnar epithelium undergoes metaplasia, eventually to become fully mature squamous epithelium. As both normal squamous and columnar epithelium are transparent, when the cervix is examined with a colposcope the underlying subepithelial vascular plexus is actually being viewed.

When atypical metaplasia occurs, the normal architecture is altered, and blood vessels begin to grow into the epithelium, forming characteristic patterns suggestive of a preneoplastic lesion. If these vessels remain as distinct capillary loops extending toward the epithelial surface, only the end of the vascular loop will be visible to the colposcopist who sees a "punctate" appearance. However, if the intraepithelial vessels form vascular connections, a tiled appearance will result, which is known as "mosaicism."

Atypical metaplasia also results in alteration of the appearance of the epithelium. During normal metaplasia, an increase in the nuclear-cytoplasmic ratio occurs, producing increased opacity of the epithelial cells. After the application of a dilute acetic acid solution (3–5%), this results in transitory opacification of the cells, producing a faint white appearance of the epithelium. Atypical metaplastic cells, for unknown reasons, are even more susceptible to opacification with acidic acid and turn bright white with sharp borders, becoming easily visualized by the colposcopist. Recognition of atypical epithelial vascular patterns allows a colposcopist to obtain directed biopsies of the suspicious areas to detect the presence of preneoplastic lesions.

Colposcopy Technique

A colposcope is a low power binocular microscope with magnification ranging from 2 to 40×, with the range 4 to 15× most commonly used. A long focal length of approximately 30 cm allows the entire depth of the vagina to be examined and also provides adequate room for the introduction of biopsy instruments for specimen collection. A coaxial light source produces illumination. A green filter is an important accessory. This allows better visualization of blood vessels. Standard photographic equipment can be attached easily to make a permanent record of significant findings. More recently, a video camera and monitor have become important accessories. The video camera is an excellent tool for educating the patient regarding detection and diagnosis of lower genital tract disease. Visualization by the patient of suspicious lesions usually helps allay fears that often arise after being informed of an abnormal Pap smear result. Additionally, by allowing visualization of a cervical lesion through the video camera, the reluctant patient is more apt to accept treatment and follow-up of this otherwise asymptomatic condition. Utilization of the video camera at colposcopy also a functions as an excellent educational tool for other health care providers learning the technique.

After visualizing the cervix for signs of a frankly invasive lesion, 3% to 5% acetic acid is applied with a cotton swab. Over a 30 to 60-second period, this solution causes opacification of atypical epithelium, which lasts for several minutes before it fades. When a suspicious lesion is seen, a directed biopsy can be obtained. Although many cervical biopsy devices are commercially available, double cutting edged instruments are preferred.

There are three components of an adequate colposcopic examination: First, the entire transformation zone must be seen; second, all suspicious lesions must be seen in their entirety; and third, the endocervical canal must be adequately evaluated.

Most CIN is located in the T-Z. If the colposcopist visualizes the squamocolumnar junction, the entire T-Z has been seen, and the examiner can be comfortable that the area of the cervix most at risk has been evaluated for CIN. It is essential to view the entirety of any suspicious lesion in the T-Z. Visualization of the complete lesion allows a colposcopist to obtain a biopsy from the lesion's most suspicious area and thus minimize the chance of missing an early invasive lesion. Usually it is easy for the entire T-Z and any suspicious lesions to be fully visualized. However, when examining a postmenopausal woman or a woman previously treated with ablative therapy for CIN, the existing squamocolumnar junction may not be seen fully. An endocervical speculum or dry cotton-tipped applicator may be used to evert the external cervical os, and both are very useful in improving visualization. This often allows an adequate examination to be completed successfully.

The final component of an adequate colposcopic examination is the evaluation of the endocervical canal. This is accomplished when one visualizes the normal grapelike columnar epithelium, and by sampling the canal with either an endocervical curette or an endocervical brush. The latter has the advantage of being less painful to the patient and more sensitive in detecting occult endocervical lesions. If any one of these three components is absent, the colposcopic examination is inadequate and further diagnostic procedures are indicated.

Conclusion

Colposcopy is a simple technique for evaluating women with abnormal Pap smears. Although straightforward, diagnostic and therapeutic errors can occur if it is improperly utilized. A good colposcopist must have extensive experience with the technique, a thorough knowledge of the pathophysiology of CIN, and an understanding of the indications for its use. When utilized appropriately, colposcopy is extremely sensitive in detecting cervical disease in the preneoplastic stage, thus allowing early treatment and cure and prevention of significant lower genital tract disease.

Disorders of Pelvic Support

David H. Nichols, MD*

Because there are more older women living among us, preservation or restoration of quality of life has become increasingly important. Disorders of pelvic support may detract considerably

*Deceased.

from quality of life. Sexual interest and activity are often retained among older women. From a combination of circumstances, including congenital defect, obstetric trauma, and the involution of aging, a sizeable number of these women develop various forms of genital prolapse. When these interfere enough with the quality of life, women seek their physicians' help to restore their genital comfort. It is now more widely understood that a dropped uterus is the result of a genital prolapse and not the cause. Although vaginal hysterectomy is often an important ingredient in the surgical treatment of genital prolapse, the most important surgical step is the repair of the various endopelvic defects that permitted the uterus to fall. All of these are surgically correctable provided that each has been accurately diagnosed.

There are at least six different anatomic systems concerned with providing pelvic support, and any one or combination of these can be damaged. From the top downward these systems include the following:

1. The bony pelvis—the ultimate attachment of all the soft tissues of the pelvis.
2. The broad ligament and round ligament complex, including the vast subperitoneal retinaculum, and the peritoneal fusion fascia of Denonvilliers (the rectovaginal septum).
3. The cardinal-uterosacral ligament complex, including the attachments of the vaginal portion or fornices to the white line (arcus tendineus) of the pelvic diaphragm.
4. The urogenital diaphragm and its pubourethral ligament portion.
5. The pelvic diaphragm.
6. The perineal body, which separates the lower vagina from the rectum and upon which normally rests the lower anterior vaginal wall, including the urethra.

Etiology

Damages can be the result of three general etiologic circumstances that may occur singly or in any combination and should be recognized for each individual patient, correlating both the damage and the patient's symptoms. These causes are the following:

1. Congenital defect of either the structure itself or its intrinsic nerve supply.
2. Trauma from damage during pregnancy, labor, and delivery or lifestyle, such as a lifetime of lifting heavy things; coexistent disease such as chronic respiratory problems, emphysema, asthma, or hay fever may traumatize the pelvic supports.
3. Aging—due to either loss of hormone support or failure of tissue replication among the elderly, as the mechanisms of cellular repair become exhausted.

A careful history should uncover the particular symptoms relevant to pelvic relaxation, including the general ones of a feeling of pelvic heaviness and of falling out, and consciousness of the protrusion of pelvic tissues beyond the vulva, all of which are made worse as the day goes on and are relieved by lying down. Specific symptoms related to the genitourinary system include periodic episodes of cystitis, inability to completely empty the bladder, and the various forms of urinary incontinence, including overflow incontinence from chronic high residual urine volume and urinary stress incontinence consequent to loss of urethral tone and therefore pressure. Relevant gastrointestinal symptoms are related to evacuation and to rectal continence. Symptoms of rectocele are primarily those of inability to completely empty the bowel (often requiring digital pressure for evacuation) and aching after a bowel movement. Constipation may be present but is not necessarily caused by rectocele, as there are many women with rectoceles who are not constipated and there are many women who are constipated who have no rectoceles. Anal continence of either gas or stool is controlled by both the muscular and the neuromuscular integrity of the voluntary external anal sphincter system, which in combination with the pelvic diaphragm is innervated by the pudendal nerve and by the involuntary internal anal sphincter, which is a continuation of the smooth muscle of the lower bowel wall. Disorders of pelvic support may produce dyspareunia or impaired coital satisfaction.

The examiner should note the presence of any scars or herniations of the anterior abdominal wall, and if a quick glance reveals a moderate or excessive number of striae, some interference of connective tissue elasticity involving the pelvic supporting tissues should be assumed.

Examination

Pelvic examination should be performed first while the patient is at rest in the lithotomy position on the examining table, then while she is straining, to see what portion of the prolapse appears first, as this may indicate the site of primary damage. (Appearance of a cystocele and rectocele followed by the cervix or vault of the vagina suggests primary damage to the lower supporting structures of the pelvis, whereas the appearance first of a prolapsed vault or cervix followed by cystocele and rectocele suggests primary damage to the upper suspensory system. It is a rule that the primary site of damage should be established if possible, so that it may receive the greatest emphasis during surgical reconstruction.) The patient should then be asked to cough, to see whether urine is involuntarily lost, either immediately or after a delay of several seconds, the latter suggesting a detrusor instability rather than stress incontinence.

When there is prolapse of the cervix, a tenaculum should be applied to the posterior lip of the cervix and traction gently exerted, which will stretch the uterosacral ligaments, clearly demonstrating their length and strength, the location of the cul-de-sac of Douglas at a midline point between their attachment to the cervix, and the degree of any cervical elongation that may be present, all of which should be noted. The operator should observe the surface of the vagina, seeking evidence of atrophy or hypertrophy of the vaginal membrane.

Since gravity accentuates both the symptoms and findings of the disorders of pelvic support, the patient should be examined next while she is standing, often with one foot supported on the shelf at the foot of the examining table. She should be examined in this standing position first at rest and then asked to strain, as by a Valsalva maneuver. This often reveals an unexpected enterocele, demonstrable as a palpable bowel-filled sac between the rectum and vagina, or partial vault eversion. The position of the vaginal vault is determined; the pull of gravity may often identify a partial prolapse of the vault. The patient should be asked to voluntarily tighten the muscles of her pelvic floor (pubococcygei and external anal sphincter) to determine their integrity.

It must be remembered that the normal axis of the upper vagina is in a more or less horizontal plane. This is brought about because the vagina normally sits on an empty rectum, which in turn rests on an intact levator plate; that is, the axis is formed by the midline fusion of the bellies of the pubococcygei behind the rectum.

The vaginal depth and axis should be identified both at rest and with the patient straining.

The axis of the urethra should be identified, as well as the presence of cystocele, and a notation made as to how far down the cystocele comes below the inferior margin of the pubis when the patient is standing and straining.

Treatment

When the findings on physical examination have been correlated with the patient's symptoms, treatment should be planned and offered. If the patient is postmenopausal and tissue atrophy is evident, estrogen replacement should be suggested to increase tissue elasticity and blood supply. Both local (intravaginal estrogen cream) and systemic doses of replacement estrogen can be offered. Constipation should be treated by the addition of daily bran to the patient's breakfast, adequate amounts of fluid intake during the day, prompt attention to a feeling of rectal fullness, and the use of bowel bulk producers, softeners, or stimulants as indicated.

Abnormalities in the patient's lifestyle should be corrected, including heavy lifting, weight reduction when appropriate, and cessation from smoking, along with treatment of chronic respiratory disease. If voluntary pubococcygeal contractions are of poor quality, a program of Kegel-type perineal resistive exercises of the pelvic muscles should be recommended and explained; this should include 15 isometric squeezes of 3 seconds' duration each, performed six times a day (first thing in the morning, mid-morning, lunchtime, mid-afternoon, suppertime, and bedtime). Alternatively, a course of biofeedback with or without electrical stimulation may be used. For the relief of symptoms in a patient in whom surgery is not appropriate, the use of an intravaginal pessary, generally of the Gellhorn type, or a plastic ring can be tried, although the patient must be made aware that this is only a temporary help and is by no means curative. A pessary must be removed, cleaned, and replaced at monthly and then trimonthly intervals as long as it is being used.

Appropriate pelvic reconstructive surgery should be offered to the majority of patients who are symptomatic. This should include correction of *all* demonstrable defects, even if certain individual components of structural weakness appear at the time to be asymptomatic. This relaxed tissue is regarded as hernial tissue, and all weaknesses should be corrected at the initial operation, lest they progress and require future reoperation.

The goals of reconstructive surgery include the relief of symptoms and the restoration of normal anatomic and functional relationships between the pelvic organ systems, the latter divided into urinary, genital, and rectal components.

When there is prolapse of the uterus, vaginal hysterectomy is most often the first part of the operation. It removes the endometrium as a source of future and possibly troublesome bleeding, particularly if the patient is to receive postoperative hormone supplementation. For this reason, the Manchester operation, which preserves the endometrium and the potential for future uterine bleeding, is but rarely performed. The feasibility of safe vaginal hysterectomy is determined mostly by the mobility of the uterus, confirmed by the findings of examination under anesthesia preceding the initial incision. The movable leiomyomatous uterus of up to 10 to 12 weeks' gestational size can still be removed vaginally, often incorporating a process of coring or of morcellation or bisection, quite useful once the cardinal ligaments and uterine arteries have been clamped, transected, and ligated. It is imperative that the operator identify preoperatively the length and strength of the uterosacral ligaments, because when these are long and strong they may be shortened by use of a McCall culdoplasty carefully incorporated into the operative support of the vaginal vault. On the other hand, when these ligaments are thin and weak and insufficient to support the vaginal vault postoperatively with confidence that it will remain in place, alternate methods of vault support should be planned as part of the primary surgery, such as coincident sacrospinous colpopexy or sacral colpopexy. Lack of surgically usable cardinal-uterosacral ligament complex support is evident in 5% to 20% of the patients with procidentia. This weakness can be determined or confirmed with reasonable certainty by examination of the pelvis while traction is applied to the posterior lip of the cervix, as described earlier.

Defect of the anterior vaginal wall for the most part arises in the midline connective tissue supports, and anterior colporrhaphy should include the full length of the anterior vaginal wall, including plication of the urogenital diaphragm beneath the urethra at the vesical neck and the elimination by plication of any urethral funneling that may be demonstrated. In an occasional patient (5% of those with cystocele), a lateral or paravaginal support defect can be predicted by disappearance of the anterior sulci, accentuated when the patient is asked to voluntarily contract her pubococcygei. This may be remedied by the transvaginal reattachment of the anterior fornix to the "white line" of the arcus tendineus of the pelvic diaphragm on each side, as described by George R. White in 1909, or to the fascia of the obturator internus muscle at the site of the arcus.

The occasional patient will have both midline and lateral defects, and each should be repaired.

The normal position of the urethra is maintained by both suspension from above (the pubourethral ligament portion of the urogenital diaphragm) and support from below (the anterior vaginal wall and its attachments to the arcus tendineus). Defects of the former are identifiable as weaknesses in the midline of the vagina and of the latter as weaknesses evident by disappearance of the anterior sulcus, accentuated when the patient voluntarily contracts her pubococcygei.

Operative blood loss requiring replacement transfusion is not popular with either surgeon or patient and can be reduced considerably by the paracervical injection of a "liquid tourniquet," using about 50 mL of either 0.5% lidocaine in 1:200,000 epinephrine, Neo-Synephrine, or saline, with descending degree of effectiveness. Intravascular injection can be avoided by periodic aspiration.

Successful posterior colporrhaphy requires that all of the rectocele be repaired, beginning at a point cranial to the upper limit of the rectocele.

Both cystocele and rectocele are generally caused by defects of the vagina and its support and basic integrity, rather than by primary damage of the wall of the bladder or rectum; the latter organs only follow the defects in the vagina. Primary corrective surgery of cystocele and rectocele should be directed to the vaginal wall and its supports, with secondary attention given to the plication of the connective tissue capsule and fascia and muscularis of the bladder and the rectum. Perineorrhaphy corrects demonstrable weakness of the perineum, which is quite separate and distinct from that of rectocele, the former requiring perineorrhaphy and the latter posterior colporrhaphy. A patient with both rectocele and perineal defect requires both posterior colporrhaphy and perineorrhaphy.

A widened levator hiatus is usually the consequence of either obstetric damage to the pelvic diaphragm or damage from the wedge-like effect of the prolapsing cervix during development of procidentia. It should be emphasized that the medial borders of the pubococcygei, which constitute this levator hiatus, for the most part come together *behind* the rectum rather than in front of it. Reconstructive perineorrhaphy can be accomplished by bringing together the connective tissues attached to the medial borders of the pubococcygei rather than the pubococcygei themselves, avoiding unanatomic and painful ridges that may be a source of future troublesome dyspareunia.

When the integrity of the levator ani has been

compromised through damage either to the muscle itself or to its pudendal nerve supply, or both, the support of the perineum may be severely compromised, giving rise to the perineal descent syndrome in which the anus is readily recognized as the lowest point in the perineum of the patient both at rest and while straining. Early in its development this is asymptomatic, but when moderately well advanced it may be productive of obstipation and significant reduction in the diameter of the stool, both a consequence of pathologic funneling of the pelvic diaphragm. Ultimately, pudendal neuropathy, probably caused by stretching of the pudendal nerve from either childbirth or chronic straining at stool, produces permanent damage to the neuromuscular integrity of the pelvic diaphragm, which may undergo consequent atrophy. The final result is loss of voluntary sphincter control of both the external anal sphincter and the pelvic diaphragm, and continence is maintained solely by action of the smooth muscle of the internal anal sphincter. When this too has been exhausted, total anal incontinence results. When perineal descent syndrome is recognized as a component of pelvic relaxation, surgical restoration directed to the retrorectal area by appropriate levatorplasty should be included in the operative reconstruction. Retrorectal levatorplasty is accomplished with entry into the retrorectal space through a Kraske type of incision between the tip of the coccyx and the anus. The posterior surface of the rectum is plicated, and these plication stitches are sewn to the periosteum of the hollow of the sacrum, carefully avoiding the vessels within the sacral foramina. When these have been tied, the rectum is effectively resuspended to the hollow of the sacrum; re-establishment of an intact and strong levator plate may be brought about by bringing together the pubococcygei posterior to the rectum.

Because the supports of the rectum are independent of the supports of the vagina, weakness of rectal supports may bring about rectal prolapse, which is an actual intussusception of the rectum. Remedy, therefore, requires surgical reconstruction distinctly different from that required for weaknesses of support of the birth canal. The most effective treatment of rectal prolapse is by the transabdominal route using a suspensory or Ripstein-type of operation, or if markedly elongated, a low bowel resection with anastomosis and proximal fixation.

Posthysterectomy vaginal vault prolapse or eversion may exist with or without coincident enterocele, just as enterocele may occur with or without eversion of the vaginal vault, although in most cases, enterocele and posthysterectomy eversion of the vaginal vault coexist, and each should be repaired. The enterocele component requires opening of the sac, high double ligation of its neck, and resection of the excess peritoneum. Vault prolapse exists because of a fundamental weakness in the cardinal-uterosacral ligament complex supporting the vault, which generally has undergone atrophy by the time the vault prolapse develops and therefore is not a reliable site for support of a prolapsed vault with confidence that it will remain where it has been placed. Posthysterectomy vaginal vault prolapse often requires the use of a strong nongynecologic structure for support, such as that offered by the sacrospinous ligament. The latter runs as the aponeurosis of the coccygeus muscle, one of which extends on each side of the pelvis from the ischial spine to the lower sacrum and coccyx. For the surgeon who is comfortable with the anatomy of the pelvic connective tissue planes and spaces, the sacrospinous ligament–coccygeus muscle complex will be found in the lateral wall of the pararectal space. It can be safely penetrated by the tip of a ligature carrying suture punch, a modified long-handed Deschamps ligature carrier, holding a strong synthetic suture. This penetration is accomplished on one or both sides, usually the patient's right if unilateral, at a point one and one-half to two fingerbreadths medial to the palpable ischial spine, safely away from the pudendal nerve and artery, which lie immediately beneath the spine. After appropriate excision of any enterocele that may be present, the vault of the vagina is narrowed, then is sewn directly to the surface of the coccygeus muscle and through the sacrospinous ligament contained within it. Although unilateral colpopexy pulls the vaginal vault somewhat to the patient's right, this has not been a source of dyspareunia. With bilateral colpopexy, the vagina remains in the midline. Appropriate coincident anterior and posterior colporrhaphy and perineorrhaphy should be added.

A transabdominal support may be employed when there is some indication for opening the abdomen (eg, an adnexal tumor, or if the operator is inexperienced with or uncomfortable using a transvaginal approach) and a transabdominal sacral colpopexy performed in which the vault of the vagina is attached to the periosteum immediately caudal to the sacral promontory, by a bridge of intermediate material such as fascia lata or Mersilene mesh through a retroperitoneal tunnel. Anterior and posterior colporrhaphy to relieve any coincident cystocele and rectocele must then be performed as a separate transvaginal operation.

Any surgical procedure that changes the normal axis of the vagina by moving it in an anterior direction (such as a suprapubic vesicourethral pinup procedure) exposes the now vulnerable and unprotected cul-de-sac of Douglas to increases in intra-abdominal pressure, which may result in prolapse of the vaginal vault (with the uterus if it is present), generally with coincident enterocele.

When defects in pelvic support are symptomatic, they should be accurately diagnosed preoperatively so that an appropriate surgical reconstruction can be planned for the particular patient. When any element of defective support is to be repaired, any and all coincident defective areas of weakness should be repaired at the same time, even though they are at the moment asymptomatic, to lessen the likelihood of future progression and development of symptoms. Possible elective oophorectomy should be given the same consideration with vaginal hysterectomy as with abdominal hysterectomy. When this cannot be safely accomplished transvaginally, it may be done by coincident operative laparoscopy either before, or preferably after, the hysterectomy when the peritoneal cavity has been closed. When estrogen is deficient, it should be offered both pre- and postoperatively. Correction of contributory medical defects and disorders of the patient's lifestyle should be advised and undertaken as part of the treatment program.

A surgical goal should be cost-effective treatment that provides adequate pelvic reconstruction, done correctly the first time, avoiding the need for future reoperation with its attendant discomfort, risks, and expense.

Dysfunctional Uterine Bleeding

Peter G. McGovern, MD
A. Brian Little, MD

Definition

Dysfunctional uterine bleeding refers to abnormal uterine bleeding from the endometrium in response to abnormal hormonal stimulation. The majority of these cases are due to anovulation, which is seen most commonly at the extremes of reproductive life (puberty and perimenopause). It is important to first consider complications of pregnancy (predominantly in younger women) and pathologic lesions (more often in older women), which may present with abnormal bleeding patterns (Table 1). Depending on their probability in the clinical circumstances, anatomic lesions should be ruled out at once or after hormonal treatment has proved unsuccessful.

Abnormal Ovulatory Bleeding

Midcycle bleeding is associated with ovulation and is likely caused by the fall in circulating estrogen just prior to ovulation. Treatment is necessary only in the patient who is troubled by the bleeding. Low-dose estrogens (conjugated equine estrogens [CEE] 0.625 mg PO or its equivalent) from cycle days 10 to 20 is the simplest treatment, although regular cycling with low-dose oral contraceptive pills (OCPs) may also be used.

Persistence of the corpus luteum (Halban's disease) is a rare cause of abnormal bleeding. Continued hormone production by the corpus luteum in the subsequent follicular phase of the next menstrual cycle leads to continued or prolonged irregular bleeding. The diagnosis is made by an endometrial biopsy on the fourth day of menses (cycle day 4), which usually shows persistence of both secretory and proliferative components. Treatment is to cycle the patient with OCPs for 2 to 3 months. This treatment may have to be repeated because the cause is unknown and the problem often recurs.

Menorrhagia, heavy or prolonged bleeding at the time of regular menses, often has different

TABLE 1. Nonhormonal Causes of Abnormal Vaginal Bleeding

Vaginitis/atrophy
Vaginal lesions, foreign bodies
Vaginal/vulvar neoplasms
Cervicitis, cervical polyps
Cervical dysplasia/neoplasia
Endometritis
Endometrial hyperplasia/neoplasia
Endometrial polyps
Submucous myomas
Adenomyosis
Fallopian tube carcinoma
Ovarian neoplasms

etiologies in the adolescent than in the adult. In the adolescent, menorrhagia may be associated with systemic diseases (up to 20% of cases) that interfere with normal coagulation and platelet function. Examples include immune thrombocytopenic purpura, von Willebrandt's disease, and leukemia. Often these conditions are already diagnosed and are part of the patient's history. A complete blood count (CBC) with a platelet count and a test of the patient's bleeding time will detect most of these problems and should be performed on all adolescents with menorrhagia.

In the adult, menorrhagia is more likely due to structural uterine abnormalities, such as an enlarged cavity secondary to intramural myomas, submucus myomas, endometrial polyps, or adenomyosis. Most of these conditions may now be detected by vaginal sonography (with or without the aid of saline infusion). Operative hysteroscopy is therapeutic in most cases but should rarely be necessary for diagnostic purposes alone. The diagnosis of adenomyosis is suggested by the physical finding of a tender, globular, enlarged uterus at the time of menses and is most often confirmed only by the pathologic diagnosis on a hysterectomy specimen. A T_2-weighted magnetic resonance imaging scan shows some promise in the diagnosis of this disorder but remains an expensive test.

Anovulatory Bleeding

Anovulation is likely the most common cause of dysfunctional uterine bleeding, although this may depend a little on the demographics of one's practice. It is seen most frequently at the extremes of reproductive life, due to either immaturity or aging of the hypothalamic-pituitary-ovarian axis. An exception to this would be the syndrome of chronic anovulation in polycystic ovarian syndrome, with or without associated hyperandrogenism. This syndrome is usually easily diagnosed by history, with a (silent) perimenarcheal onset and lifelong persistence. It may first manifest later in life, often in conjunction with significant weight gain. Anovulation leads to a state of chronic, unopposed stimulation of endometrial growth by estrogens, which can cause endometrial hyperplasia and unpredictable, often heavy, bleeding due to the uncoordinated endometrial sloughing. In the absence of progesterone, the cellular mechanisms leading to controlled, efficient loss of the upper two endometrial layers (compacta and spongiosa) do not take place, as in secretory endometrium. Thus, estrogen stimulation followed by progesterone-induced changes lead to both synchronous sloughing and the cessation of bleeding. The basis of therapy for these patients is the provision of progesterone, whether using cyclic progestins (medroxyprogesterone acetate [MPA] or micronized progesterone for 12 days per month) or using OCPs (which will provide progestin 21 days per month). This replacement of progesterone allows the secretory development of the endometrium to occur, and its withdrawal is followed by a more "normal" menstrual flow.

Perimenopausal women with abnormal bleeding often have oligovulation and endometrial exposure to low, irregular levels of estrogen secreted by aging ovaries. It is important to remember this, as patients with low estrogen secretion will not respond to progestins alone, but may require both estrogen and progestin replacement.

Diagnosis

The history should detail the pattern of bleeding. In this regard, many patients are poor historians, and the use of menstrual diaries may be helpful. (These diaries may also be quite useful when following the patient's response to treatment.) The general physical and nutritional state of the patient should be observed, and one should inquire about symptoms of abnormal coagulation (easy bruisability, gum bleeding), of hypothyroidism, and of hyperprolactinemia. A medication history with special attention to the use of aspirin, psychiatric medications, or hormones should be elicited, because aspirin is known to affect coagulation, psychiatric medications often impair gonadotropin function, and small doses of hormones, as appear in some "vitamins," may be enough to cause bleeding in older patients.

The physical examination should include a careful inspection of the lower genital tract and a Pap smear. In virginal adolescents, a digital rectal exam may be substituted for the pelvic examination. This may be augmented by abdominal ultrasonography, if necessary. Bimanual palpation should record uterine enlargement or adnexal masses. An endometrial biopsy should be performed in most patients age 35 or older and in young patients suspected of having prolonged chronic anovulation and unopposed estrogen exposure.

Laboratory testing for all patients should include a CBC with a platelet count and a sensitive serum test for beta-human chorionic gonadotropin. In adolescents, a normal bleeding time will rule out significant coagulopathy. This simple test can be performed easily in the office. Briefly, a blood pressure cuff is inflated to 40 mm Hg and three forearm punctures are made with a lancet. The three bleeding sites are *touched* with filter paper (not blotted) every 15 seconds to remove visible blood. The time when the last site no longer bleeds is the patient's bleeding time (normal is 2 to 8 minutes). Anovulatory patients should also have thyroid-stimulating hormone, prolactin, follicle stimulating hormone, and luteinizing hormone assayed. Follicle-stimulating hormone and luteinizing hormone levels may reveal unexpected premature menopause (if high) or hypothalamic amenorrhea (if low). Patients with ovulatory menorrhagia require the addition of a thyroid-stimulating hormone level, as this complaint may be the only manifestation of early thyroid disease.

Vaginal sonography is a sensitive method for the detection of anatomic abnormalities of the uterus and adnexa. Saline infusion sonography (hydrosonography, saline ultrasonography) is a recently described technique providing improved visualization of the uterine cavity. Briefly, a one-sided speculum is inserted and the cervix and vagina cleaned with a povidine solution. An intra-uterine insemination catheter (such as a Tomcat) or a balloon catheter (such as is provided in disposable hysterosalpingography kits) is connected via extension tubing to a 20 mL saline-filled syringe and is threaded into the uterine cavity. The catheter is held in place against the lateral vaginal wall with one finger while the speculum is removed. Then a vaginal ultrasonographic probe is inserted and the endometrial cavity is visualized longitudinally and transversely while saline is gradually infused. Anywhere from 2 to 60 mL of saline may be necessary, depending on the size of the uterus and how rapidly fluid is lost through the fallopian tubes and cervix. We find the late follicular phase (cycle days 6–10) to be an ideal time for the test, but the test can be performed at any time except during menses (when uterine contractions tend to prevent adequate distension of the cavity). Antibiotic prophylaxis or nonsteroidal anti-inflammatory drugs (NSAIDs) to prevent cramping have been suggested by some authors, but we have not found these to be essential. Saline infusion distends the cavity and allows clearer visualization of polyps and submucus myomas. Using this technique, sessile polyps as small as 5 mm can be readily seen. Although an isolated focus of endometrial cancer could be missed, in large part saline infusion sonography may obviate the need for hysteroscopy for diagnosis alone.

Treatment
Adolescent

Most cases in the adolescent are due to anovulation, but it is first important to rule out a more serious disorder. A history and physical examination (including pelvic and rectal examinations), along with some simple laboratory testing (CBC with platelet count, bleeding time and beta-human chorionic gonadotropin), should detect causes other than anovulation. If these steps reveal no abnormalities, treatment for anovulation with OCPs or cyclic MPA should be used. If these are unsuccessful, the etiology should be reconsidered; further testing at this time should include a Pap smear, office endometrial biopsy, vaginal sonogram or saline infusion sonography, and basal body temperature recording.

Adult (Fig. 1)
Ovulatory Dysfunctional Bleeding

Midcycle spotting, if treated at all, is best treated with midcycle estrogen supplementation, as described earlier. Ovulatory menorrhagia can be treated with OCPs; however, as menorrhagia is associated with prostaglandin release, NSAIDs such as naproxen sodium (500 mg PO bid–tid) or ibuprofen (400–800 mg PO tid–qid) may also be given. Both groups of agents have been shown to decrease menstrual blood loss by about 50% in patients complaining of heavy menses. The mechanisms are different: NSAIDs decrease the production of vasodilatory prostaglandins in the endometrium, while the progestin component of OCPs limits endometrial growth. Because these medications act differently, there may be a synergistic effect when both are utilized.

If these agents are contraindicated or are ineffective, a variety of second-line medications may be employed. The progestin-containing intra-uterine devices effectively decrease menstrual blood loss and can be useful in appropriate patients who also require contraception. Depo-Provera (150 mg IM q 3 months) acts in a similar manner, but its use can be complicated by irregular spotting or amenorrhea. It should not be used in patients contemplating pregnancy in the near future, as its contraceptive effects can persist for some time after discontinuation. Danazol, in a dosage as low as 200 mg daily, may be useful, but its cost and occasional side effects, such as acne and hair growth, limit its appeal to patients. Long-acting preparations of gonadotropin-releasing hormone agonists (Lupron Depot 3.75 mg

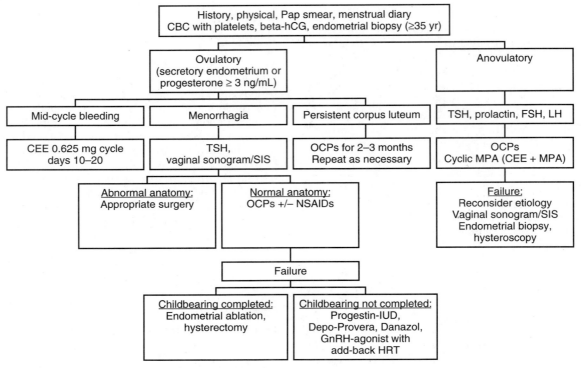

Figure 1. Treatment algorithm: abnormal bleeding in the adult. CBC, complete blood count; CEE, conjugated equine estrogen; FSH, follicle-stimulating hormone; GnRH, gonadotropin-releasing hormone; hCG, human chorionic gonadotropin; HRT, hormone replacement therapy (see text); IUD, intrauterine device; LH, luteinizing hormone; MPA, medroxyprogesterone acetate; NSAID, nonsteroidal anti-inflammatory drug; OCP, oral contraceptive pill; SIS, saline infusion sonography; TSH, thyroid-stimulating hormone.

IM monthly) along with low dose "add-back" estrogen/progestin hormone replacement therapy may be useful for the perimenopausal patient. The cost of gonadotropin-releasing hormone agonists and concerns about associated bone loss make it inappropriate for long-term use.

In patients for whom the results of medical therapy are unsatisfactory, endometrial ablation may be indicated. Results are variable, but decreased bleeding or amenorrhea are often achieved. Hysterectomy is the final definitive therapeutic solution, which may be required.

Anovulatory Bleeding

The treatment of anovulatory bleeding resulting from abnormal hormonal function is primarily medical. Dilatation and curettage should be reserved for the uncommon case of uncontrolled hemorrhage. Most patients with acute bleeding who are hemodynamically stable will respond to oral or intravenous estrogen in high doses (CEE 25 mg IV q4h or 10 mg PO q4h). Estrogen alone is often a better choice in these cases because the heavy bleeding may signify that most of the endometrium has sloughed, leaving the raw, denuded basalis layer only. In this circumstance, the addition of progestin acutely is relatively ineffective, and estrogen alone will better promote endometrial regeneration. Once the bleeding has abated, progestins will be necessary to promote secretory transformation. We recommend following the 28-day high-dose estrogen treatment with OCPs for one package, with four pills taken daily for seven days. On the fifth day following the last pill, the patient should begin the next package of pills (one per day) and continue for 2 to 3 months; her menses will become progressively lighter with each package. After this, she can be treated for the chronic control of anovulatory bleeding (see later).

Several agents are available for the chronic control of anovulatory bleeding. OCPs or the cyclic use of progestin (MPA 10 mg PO on calendar days 1–12 each month) are both excellent choices to control bleeding and prevent endometrial hyperplasia. The patient must be aware that

MPA is not a contraceptive, and failure to bleed following its withdrawal should lead to a pregnancy test. For the patient desiring pregnancy, ovulation induction may be appropriate.

In the special circumstance of the perimenopausal patient (or in other cases of low and irregular estrogen production), hormone replacement with estrogen and progestin (CEE 0.625–1.25 mg PO daily and MPA 5–10 mg PO on calendar days 1–12) is a useful regimen. It is important to continue CEEs every day, not to stop for several days each month as some have suggested.

Dysmenorrhea

M. Yusoff Dawood, MD

Dysmenorrhea refers to painful menstrual cramps. Although many women during the reproductive years can feel their uterus contracting during menstruation, the term *dysmenorrhea* should be applied only when painful contractions are present. Until the advent of the oral contraceptive pill and, more recently, nonsteroidal antiinflammatory drugs (NSAIDs), dysmenorrhea was one of the most common gynecologic complaints and a major cause of lost work hours. Among those with the severe form of the condition, approximately 600 million working hours were lost annually from 1 to 2 days' absenteeism a month.

Dysmenorrhea should be classified as *primary* or *secondary*. In primary dysmenorrhea, there is no underlying visible pelvic pathology to account for the pain; in secondary dysmenorrhea, a visible lesion is readily identifiable. However, in primary dysmenorrhea, it is now clear that a biochemical derangement accounts for the pathogenesis of pain in most of the patients.

Primary Dysmenorrhea

Primary dysmenorrhea affects as many as 50% of postpubescent females, 10% of them severely enough to result in absenteeism. In addition, both work and school performance are found to be poorer in women on their days with dysmenorrhea. Primary dysmenorrhea is more frequent in nulliparous females, 20 to 24 years of age, and in women with a higher stress score of their daily activities (presumably reflecting their reaction to the pathologic process rather than the cause of

dysmenorrhea). It is noteworthy that primary dysmenorrhea improves with advancing age rather than with vaginal delivery. Although exercise does not appear to reduce the incidence of dysmenorrhea, it is reported to be improved after athletic activity with a lower incidence found in adolescents with intense sports activity.

Clinical Features

Occurring almost invariably in ovulatory cycles and starting within 6 to 12 months after menarche, primary dysmenorrhea is characterized by suprapubic spasmodic pain. The pain is usually most severe on the first or second day of menstrual flow. Associated symptoms include nausea and vomiting, fatigue, diarrhea, low backache, and in severe cases syncope and collapse. The diagnosis of primary dysmenorrhea should be made on the basis of a characteristic history, with the absence of any disease responsible for the pain on pelvic examination. The characteristic hallmarks of primary dysmenorrhea are the following:

1. The initial onset of primary dysmenorrhea is at or shortly after menarche. Dysmenorrhea starting 2 or more years after menarche should arouse suspicion of secondary dysmenorrhea.
2. The duration of dysmenorrhea is usually 48 to 72 hours, with the pain starting no earlier than a few hours before the onset of menstrual flow and usually at its worst on the first or second day of the menstrual flow. Dysmenorrhea occurring several days before the onset of menstrual flow and lasting through the menstrual flow is unlikely to be primary.
3. The pain is usually suprapubic, crampy or spasmodic in nature, and sometimes described as labor-like. Backache may be a component.
4. Pelvic examination is almost invariably normal.

The differential diagnosis of primary dysmenorrhea includes all the causes of secondary dysmenorrhea: endometriosis; presence of an intrauterine device (IUD); pelvic inflammatory diseases and infection; adenomyosis, uterine myomas, polyps, and adhesions; congenital malformations of the müllerian system (bicornuate and septate uterus, transverse vaginal septum); cervical strictures and stenosis; ovarian cysts; pelvic congestion syndrome; and Allen-Master syndrome. One should always try to exclude endometriosis, even when the history is remarkably consistent with primary dysmenorrhea, because endometriosis can mimic this condition very closely and can also begin with the onset of menarche or shortly thereafter. In patients who have a strong index of suspicion for endometriosis, such as those with a history of endometriosis in their female siblings or mothers, laparoscopy should be considered early in the management after medical therapy has failed.

To understand the therapy of primary dysmenorrhea, it is important to comprehend its pathophysiology. Current evidence suggests that primary dysmenorrhea, which occurs only during ovulatory cycles, is largely due to excess endometrial prostaglandin production and release during menstruation, giving rise to increased and abnormal uterine activity. This activity in turn results in uterine hypoxia. Thus the afferent stimuli for the uterine cramps are due to (1) uterine hypercontractility, (2) uterine hypoxia or ischemia, and (3) hypersensitization of the pain fibers from the pelvis due to excess prostaglandin production and release, in particular prostaglandin E_2 and cyclic endoperoxides. The precise basis for increased uterine prostaglandin production and release is not currently known.

Limited studies have also suggested that in women with primary dysmenorrhea there is increased vasopressin release during menstruation, which is believed to cause abnormal uterine activity. (This could possibly be inhibited by the use of vasopressin antagonists acting through competitive inhibition with vasopressin at its receptor level in the myometrium. However, this approach is still under investigation and cannot currently be employed for routine practice.) Ongoing research also suggests that in some patients with primary dysmenorrhea, there is an increase in leukotrienes, which are products of the 5-lipooxygenase pathway and which also induce uterine contractions. This could explain the pathophysiologic basis of primary dysmenorrhea in the small percentage of patients who have a laparoscopically proven normal pelvis but poor or no response to NSAIDs. (It is noteworthy that prostaglandins are synthesized from arachidonic acid via the cyclo-oxygenase pathway; NSAID inhibits the cyclo-oxygenase pathway but not the 5-lipooxygenase pathway through which leukotrienes are synthesized from arachidonic acid.)

It is tempting to hypothesize that endothelin-derived relaxing factor, which is nitric oxide, or even endothelins may be involved in the blood flow of the uterus and therefore in dysmenorrhea. However, no direct data on changes in these substances have been reported in women with primary dysmenorrhea or in those with chronic pelvic pain.

Management

With a careful, thorough history and a negative pelvic examination, the diagnosis of primary dysmenorrhea can be readily made without resorting to laboratory investigations. There is no single diagnostic laboratory test currently available to confirm the diagnosis of primary dysmenorrhea. Laboratory tests and invasive investigative procedures are reserved for diagnosing the cause of secondary dysmenorrhea or ruling it out when medical therapy of primary dysmenorrhea has failed.

The overall approach to the treatment of primary and secondary dysmenorrhea should include psychological and behavioral factors as well as specific therapy, be it pharmacologic or surgical. Careful assessment of the proportions of the various components (organic versus psychological) of the patient's pain experience is also necessary. The efficacy of any treatment for either type of dysmenorrhea can be greatly enhanced by patient-physician dialogue, explanation, and reassurance, all of which contribute to reduction of the reactive component (which constitutes part of the overall psychological component) of the pain.

Treatments used for primary dysmenorrhea are listed in Table 1. Currently two groups of drugs, oral contraceptives and NSAIDs, are used. The choice of medication depends on whether the woman wants oral contraceptives for birth control and whether there is any contraindication to the use of oral contraceptives or NSAIDs. The choice of agents and subsequent steps in the management of primary dysmenorrhea are briefly outlined in the algorithm in Figure 1.

If the patient desires birth control with the oral contraceptive, this is the agent of first choice. The effectiveness of oral contraceptives is believed to be due to their inhibition of ovulation. Current evidence shows that menstrual fluid prostaglandin levels are reduced below normal levels in women who use oral contraceptives, probably because endometrial tissue growth is suppressed and therefore menstrual fluid flow is reduced. More than 90% of women with primary dysmenorrhea experience complete relief in response to oral contraceptives. A trial of this treatment for 3 to 4 months is worthwhile; if the dysmenorrhea is not adequately relieved, an effective NSAID can be added.

If the woman does not wish to use oral contra-

TABLE 1. Available Treatment Modalities for Primary Dysmenorrhea

Treatment Modality	Specific Agent or Mode	Comment
General measures	Reassurance, physician-patient dialogue	All patients
Surgery	Presacral neurectomy, uterosacral ligament division	Rarely. Avoid in nullipara
	Dilatation and curettage	Seldom by itself. Combine with laparoscopy
Tocolysis	Alcohol	Side effects; not practical
	Betamimetics	Terbutaline only, but side effects
Endocrine therapy	Oral contraceptives	Effective; best for contraceptive need or when patient has ulcers or NSAID hypersensitivity
Prostaglandin synthetase inhibitors	NSAIDs	Medication of first choice, highly effective, up to 80–90% success rates. Use only those proven to work
Nerve block or stimulation	Alcohol or anesthetic injection of nerves	Usually for secondary dysmenorrhea or pelvic pain
	Transcutaneous electrical nerve stimulation	For those preferring no medication, to reduce dose of NSAID required, and when NSAID contraindicated
Analgesics	Non-narcotics, narcotics	Nonspecific, can be effective. Use when NSAID and oral contraceptives ineffective and laparoscopy negative
Calcium blockade	Calcium channel blocker (nifedipine)	Use only when NSAID and oral contraceptives ineffective and laparoscopy negative; experimental therapy

NSAID, nonsteroidal anti-inflammatory drug.

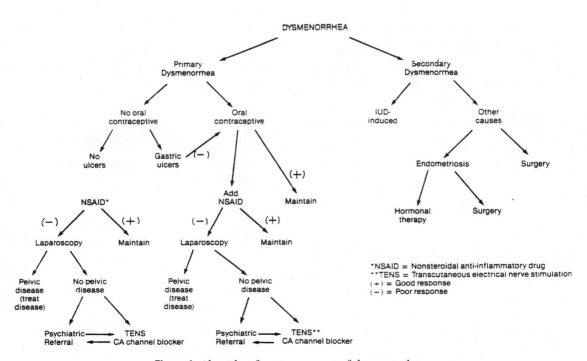

Figure 1. Algorithm for management of dysmenorrhea.

ceptives as a method of birth control, the drug of choice for the treatment of primary dysmenorrhea is an NSAID. Table 2 shows the types of NSAIDs, the doses employed, and their effectiveness in relieving primary dysmenorrhea in clinical trials. NSAIDs should be taken only during the first 2 to 3 days of menstrual flow when primary dysmenorrhea occurs. To obtain maximum therapeutic efficacy, the NSAID should be given on a continuing basis as soon as menstrual flow begins for at least 48 hours and in practice during the first 3 days of menstrual flow. There are numerous NSAIDs available; the choice should be based on clinical evidence of its efficacy and its ability to block cyclo-oxygenase effectively in the uterus; rapid absorption after oral intake to achieve therapeutic blood levels quickly; low tendency to induce ulcers; minimal, tolerable, and inconsequential side effects; and long-term safety. A trial of up to 6 months with NSAIDs, with changes in dosage and agent as needed, will be sufficient to demonstrate whether relief can be obtained through this form of therapy.

NSAIDs appear to relieve primary dysmenorrhea through suppression of menstrual fluid prostaglandins. These compounds also have direct analgesic properties; it is currently unclear how much, if any, of the relief of dysmenorrhea is mediated through that effect. NSAID treatment is necessary for each menstrual cycle, as this is a cyclic phenomenon. Because many NSAIDs are rapidly absorbed, treatment prior to the onset of dysmenorrhea is not necessary, obviating the risk of inadvertently giving the drug in an early pregnancy cycle. Contraindications to the use of NSAIDs include gastrointestinal ulcers and hypersensitivity to aspirin or similar agents. In such cases, oral contraceptives must be used for the treatment of primary dysmenorrhea. Side effects of NSAIDs include gastrointestinal (indigestion, heartburn, nausea, abdominal pain, constipation, vomiting, anorexia, diarrhea, melena), central nervous system (headache, dizziness, vertigo, visual disturbances, hearing disturbances, irritability, depression, drowsiness, sleepiness), and other symptoms (allergic reactions, skin rash, edema, bronchospasm, hematologic abnormalities, eye effects, fluid retention, effects on liver and kidney). Fortunately, very few of these side effects occur with only 3 days of NSAID therapy. The usual side effects encountered during the treatment of primary dysmenorrhea with NSAIDs are gastrointestinal, primarily nausea, indigestion, and heartburn.

If the patient does not respond to NSAIDs for up to 6 months of therapy, secondary dysmenorrhea must be ruled out even if the clinical features and history are strongly indicative of primary dysmenorrhea. A laparoscopy should rule out or confirm pelvic disease; if pelvic disease is discovered, therapy should be directed to its underlying lesion and the dysmenorrhea will usually be alleviated. In addition, during laparoscopy, dilatation of the cervix should be undertaken, since this will contribute to pain relief in primary dysmenorrhea, albeit temporarily for a small number of cycles after the treatment. However, dilatation of the cervix is not indicated as a primary form of therapy in primary dysmenorrhea.

If a pelvic pathology is not found after laparoscopy, patients may have to try more experimental forms of pharmacotherapy. These include the use

TABLE 2. Nonsteroidal Anti-inflammatory Drugs That Are Effective for Relief of Primary Dysmenorrhea

Group	Example	Dose (mg; times/day)	Relief Provided (%)
Indole-acetic acid derivatives	Indomethacin	25; 3–6	73–90
Fenamates	Flufenamic acid	100–200; 3	77–82
	Mefenamic acid	250–500; 4	93
	Tolfenamic acid	133; 3	88
Arylpropionic acid	Ibuprofen	400; 4	66–100
	Naproxen sodium	275; 4	78–90
	Ketoprofen	50; 3	90
		25; up to 4	88
		12.5; up to 4	87
Miscellaneous	Piroxicam	20; 2	60–80
	Nimesulide	50–100; 1–2	78–83

of calcium channel blockers (nifedipine), which have been shown in a small preliminary trial to be effective. In limited studies, magnesium has been found to be effective. Magnesium given as Mg 5-Longoral reduces menstrual blood prostaglandin $F_{2\alpha}$ to less than half the levels before treatment and may therefore correct the pathophysiology of primary dysmenorrhea. Another alternative is to employ terbutaline, which is the only betamimetic agent thus far tested that has been shown to be more effective than placebo in relieving primary dysmenorrhea. However, there is a high incidence of side effects, some of which are troublesome.

Another approach has been the use of transcutaneous electrical nerve stimulation (TENS), which we have found can relieve primary dysmenorrhea, eliminate the need for medication in about one-third of the patients studied, and reduce the total dose of NSAID required for relief of the primary dysmenorrhea. TENS appears to relieve pain through two mechanisms. First, by saturating the afferent nerve pathway and dorsal root ganglion with electrical impulses, conduction of the pain stimuli is blocked (gate control therapy). Second, electrical stimulation of the afferent nerve induces release of endogenous opiates such as endorphins.

Alcohol is certainly effective, as it has a direct relaxation effect on uterine muscle contraction and blocks the release of neurohypophyseal hormones, including vasopressin (which can induce uterine contractions), and thus decreases the perception of pain. However, the accompanying state of inebriation induced by alcohol does not restore function to the woman.

Finally, psychiatric help may be appropriate in those instances in which the psychological component of the pain plays a significant role.

Surgical treatment is rarely indicated for primary dysmenorrhea today. Such procedures include presacral neurectomy and uterosacral ligament division, which interrupts the postganglionic fibers supplying the lower portion of the uterus. Presacral neurectomy is best reserved for patients with chronic pelvic pain for whom other methods of pain relief have failed, those with pelvic malignancy, and those with pelvic pathology such as endometriosis that impinges on or involves the presacral plexus. Presacral neurectomy has been shown to be effective only in centrally located pelvic pain. Similarly, uterosacral ligament division with either translaparoscopic laser or cautery, widely advocated by some, should be reserved for very few patients.

The efficacy of uterosacral nerve ablation is yet to be convincingly demonstrated in a large,

well-controlled, randomized study of a homogeneous population of women with primary dysmenorrhea. At best, in uncontrolled, nonrandomized descriptive reports of the personal experience of enthusiasts, this surgical procedure provides no better relief than the less expensive and less invasive treatment with NSAIDs or analgesics. The procedure can result in bleeding as well as postoperative adhesion involving the tubes and ovaries, which are in close proximity to the uterosacral ligaments, and therefore has potentially adverse effects on the fertility of nulliparous young women. Additionally, uterine dislocation and descensus has been reported following uterosacral ligament denervation.

Secondary Dysmenorrhea

The appearance of dysmenorrhea years after menarche or in women with anovulatory cycles suggests the secondary form of the disorder. Frequent causes include endometriosis, the use of intrauterine devices (IUDs), chronic pelvic inflammatory disease, pelvic adhesions, and uterine myomas. Although the patient's age at the onset of dysmenorrhea often distinguishes primary from secondary dysmenorrhea, an endometriosis has also been known to occur soon after the onset of menarche. Physical examination, especially a pelvic examination that includes a rectovaginal examination, is likely to reveal the most common causes of secondary dysmenorrhea. In women over 35 years of age adenomyosis should be considered, but the final diagnosis can be made only on the basis of uterine specimen evaluation.

Other investigations to determine the cause of secondary dysmenorrhea include a complete blood count, erythrocyte sedimentation rate, pelvic ultrasonography (particularly vaginal ultrasonography, which is more informative than the abdominal approach), hysterosalpingography, and genital cultures for pathogens. However, the single most useful investigation for establishing or confirming the diagnosis is diagnostic laparoscopy combined with hysteroscopy and dilatation and curettage.

Management

The treatment of secondary dysmenorrhea should be directed to the underlying pathology and therefore varies depending on its cause. IUD-induced dysmenorrhea is due to increased uterine prostaglandin production and release.

Therefore, in women using the IUD, relief should be obtained specifically with NSAIDs, which should be taken throughout the duration of their menstrual flow or dysmenorrhea. (An additional benefit of relieving their dysmenorrhea with NSAIDs is correction of the IUD-induced menorrhalgia.) Dysmenorrhea due to endometriosis is best relieved with hormone therapy such as danazol, oral contraceptives, or one of the gonadotropin-releasing hormone (Gn-RH) agonists such as buserelin, leuprolide, goserelin, and nafarelin. Danazol and the Gn-RH agonists are the most effective in relieving dysmenorrhea as well as pelvic pain associated with endometriosis. Pain relief progresses gradually, with maximum relief seen about 3 months after initiating therapy. Danazol should be given 200 mg orally three times a day or 400 mg twice a day; the three Gn-RH agonists available in the United States for endometriosis treatment are nafarelin acetate (400 mg intranasally daily), leuprolide acetate (3.75 mg intramuscular depot every 28 days), and goserelin (3.6 mg subcutaneous pellet every 28 days). Medical therapy with analgesics, including the NSAIDs, will provide only partial and temporary relief in most other forms of secondary dysmenorrhea and should not be resorted to except as a temporizing measure while waiting for surgery or to provide additional relief in addition to specific medical therapy such as that for endometriosis. In most cases of secondary dysmenorrhea, surgery becomes a primary approach to treatment. Hysterectomy is indicated for adenomyosis, and myomectomy or hysterectomy for uterine myomas. Congenital malformations of the uterus require surgical correction if dysmenorrhea is sufficiently severe. Similarly, uterine polyps, transverse vaginal septum, ovarian cyst, and pelvic adhesions require surgical intervention.

Dyspareunia

John F. Steege, MD

Dyspareunia, or pain during or resulting from sexual intercourse, is one of the most common complaints heard in gynecologic practice. Although women are now perhaps less reticent about voicing such complaints than they were a generation ago, it is still useful to include screening questions about pain during sex in your routine history. As with other clinical problems, it helps to have in mind a hierarchy of problems:

those you will be able to solve at a routine visit, those that will require serial visits, and those that will need professional counseling help.

Problems with dyspareunia are not easily categorized as physical or psychological. Indeed, in many situations of any duration, both factors are present in varying degree. It is more fruitful to design treatment for all the components simultaneously than to direct all attention to the most obvious factor. For example, a gynecologist might provide to a patient preventive care to reduce the frequency of yeast infections and suggestions on how best to use vaginal dilators for vaginismus, while a marriage counselor could provide some help to the patient and her partner on maintaining and improving their sense of emotional intimacy while dealing with a difficult problem of dyspareunia. Ongoing cooperation between the health professionals involved is certainly desirable.

Designing a therapeutic approach often begins with a careful history and physical examination. Routine questions might include, "Are you having any sexual discomforts?" Although this is vague, it allows response from women whose sexual expression may range from self-stimulation, to intercourse, to activity with a same-sex partner. Often a patient may not feel at ease reporting such a complaint during the first visit. If the question is routinely included in your history, however, she will soon perceive that you ask this of every patient and that you consider it important. She may then become comfortable enough to voice her concerns.

Pain during intercourse can be assessed using a strategy similar to that applied to any other pain complaint. That is, one needs to know about site, intensity, duration, regularity of occurrence, associated physical signs, chronology of development, ameliorating or aggravating factors, and impact on emotional and physical function. The answers to a few of these questions will allow you to perform immediate triage to the single visit problem, the multi-visit problem, or the multi-visit and mental health referral problem. Screening questions include the following:

1. Is the discomfort at the opening of the vagina, along the sides, or deep inside?
2. Does it occur on all occasions of intercourse or just some?
3. How long has this been going on?
4. How big a problem is it?
5. What have you and your partner/husband tried to do about it?

Questions about physical changes such as vaginal discharge might be included, although most women will report this as a chief complaint when it is present, and will later add the complaint of dyspareunia on their own or when specifically asked. The remainder of this discussion presumes that you already are aware of many elements of routine gynecologic history that may be relevant, such as the patient's age, marital or relationship status, menstrual history, degree of dysmenorrhea, history of disorders such as pelvic infection or endometriosis, and surgical history.

The less dramatic the responses to questions 2, 3, and 4, the more likely the problem can be handled briefly, regardless of the location of the pain. With problems that are a bit more involved, the answer to question 5 will tell you much about the resources your patient and her partner bring to the problem. Of course, in addition to the mechanical or technique-oriented details, you need to understand the emotional atmosphere surrounding any attempts at self-help.

Before continuing your evaluation, it is useful to create realistic expectations by suggesting, as appropriate, "This may not be as difficult a problem as you might fear," or "We'll be able to get started on this today, but it may take some time and some more visits to get the best results." For example, the woman with a baseline of sexual comfort who experiences vaginal tightening over several weeks following a urinary tract infection may be vastly reassured by the first response, and better able to hear the rest of your questions and advice. In contrast, the patient with a year-long problem who has struggled to get the courage to seek help will understand that a single, simple answer may not be possible.

The following discussion of history, physical examination, and treatment will be outlined by the anatomic site of the pain complaint. For the sake of brevity, conditions likely to be diagnosed by each question or examination technique will simply be listed parenthetically, with more detailed discussion deferred to the treatment section.

History

Introital Pain

Does the whole area around the vagina hurt (vulvadynia, fungal vulvitis, vulvar dystrophies, atrophy) or just the area right around the vaginal opening itself (vaginitis, vestibulitis syndrome, poor lubrication, vaginismus)? Is the whole opening of the vagina sore (fungal disease, extreme cases of vestibulitis syndrome) or just certain spots (urethral: urethritis or diverticulum, ure-

thral syndrome; 3 to 9 o'clock area of vestibule and/or hymen: mild to moderate vestibulitis syndrome)? Is there soreness of the tissue only (inflammatory conditions mentioned above) or is there tightness as well (vaginismus, atrophy)? Which is worse? Is there any problem with lubrication during sex (hypoestrogenism, oral contraceptives, chronic vaginitis, insufficient sexual arousal)?

Vaginal Barrel Pain

Is there any sense of dryness or too much friction along the vagina (same as above)? Is there any tightness or pain along the vagina (levator spasm, atrophy, postoperative stricture, urethral diverticulum)?

Deep Pelvic Pain

Do you feel pain deep inside during sex (endometriosis, pelvic adhesions, uterine retroversion, adnexal prolapse into cul-de-sac)? Is it in the middle or to one side (central vs. adnexal pathology)? Do you feel as though something is being "bumped" (insufficient sexual arousal, uterine retroversion with/without adnexal prolapse)?

Physical Examination
Vulva and Introitus

Careful inspection of the epithelium will reveal pigment changes, ulcerations, general erythema, and the focal sensitivity of vulvar vestibulitis. Ask the patient to show you where it hurts, especially if her history indicates focal or unilateral discomfort. Retract the labia carefully and walk over the vaginal vestibule and hymen with a cotton-tip applicator. The woman with vestibulitis will report exquisite sensitivity over a sharply demarcated area of the vestibule, with normal sensation in closely adjacent normal areas. Then place the applicator in a small amount of saline to do a hanging drop examination after the physical examination is completed. Examination with a colposcope offers confirmatory information (punctation, aceto-white and papillary changes, well-demarcated erythema) in cases of vestibulitis, although the significant discomfort reported on application of the acetic acid solution is virtually diagnostic in itself.

Place the index finger in the introitus to the first knuckle, assess the degree of muscular tension, and ask for one or more cycles of contraction/relaxation of the introital muscles (principally the bulbocavernosus). Vaginismus (involuntary spasm) typically involves these muscles, with or without additional spasm in the levators. About 25% of women will experience involuntary spasm during sexual encounters, but not during pelvic examinations. In these instances, the diagnosis is made by history.

Then introduce the index finger a bit further to assess tone in the levator plate. Ask again for contraction/relaxation, and ask whether palpation of the tensed levators reproduces any part of her symptoms. In cases of levator spasm, this often reproduces part of the dyspareunia as well as the aching pain present during the day that radiates to the low back. Supinate the hand and trace the index finger tip gently along the bladder base and urethra. Women with trigonitis will often report pain to palpation in this manner, and focal tenderness from a urethral diverticulum (perhaps with chronic infection or stone formation) can be detected as well.

Speculum examination, complemented by hanging drop examination of vaginal secretions, will then detect estrogen deficiency, focal ulceration (herpes), or vaginal pathogens (yeast, trichomonas, bacterial vaginosis).

Deep Pelvis

The cervix varies greatly in its sensitivity. In some women, a normal-appearing cervix will be quite tender to palpation. Often this seems to be a conditioned pain that follows episodes of cervicitis. Insufficient sexual response (failure of the vagina to lengthen and widen during sexual response) will result in this tender cervix being painfully struck during coitus.

The uterus may become tender in some cases of adenomyosis. In this condition, comparing follicular phase with premenstrual examinations may reveal a significant increase in uterine tenderness and size premenstrually. The dyspareunia may be cyclic as well.

Tenderness in the cul-de-sac often betrays endometriosis, although this diagnosis should be confirmed by laparoscopy prior to embarking on any intrusive hormonal manipulations (medroxyprogesterone, danocrine, or gonadotropin-releasing hormone agonists). The patient will often be able to identify a tender palpated spot as the location of her deep discomfort during coitus.

Similar careful, stepwise palpation of the adnexa will often suggest localized pathology that can be the source of focal deep dyspareunia. For

many women, discomfort will start out being focal and may spread to the whole pelvis over time even if the pathology remains limited. This does not mean that the pathology is meaningless, but speaks rather to the complex nature of pain perception and the tendency of pain to be more difficult to treat when present chronically.

Causes and Treatments

Many of the entities described here appear in varying degrees of severity. The number of visits and type of help required will differ on the basis of individual patient characteristics rather than the pathophysiology involved.

Vulvar Dystrophies

Lichen sclerosus and other forms of vulvar dystrophy should be documented by punch biopsy prior to starting any form of treatment. Since many pathologic vulvar changes can be subtle, and truly precancerous lesions can have many appearances, the clinician should maintain a high index of suspicion and should perform a biopsy if there is any doubt. For proven lichen sclerosus, testosterone propionate in eucerin or petrolatum will cause gradual improvement when applied daily for months.

Atrophy

A more common problem is atrophy that occurs gradually after a number of years of menopause without estrogen replacement therapy (ERT). The atrophic changes may become a clinical problem when a new relationship begins and sexual intercourse is once again desired. The vaginal lining and introitus continue to show improvements in blood flow (and, presumably, lubricating capacity) during the first 6 months of ERT, although improved comfort may be achieved after as little as 4 to 6 weeks. In some instances, vaginal diameter may need to be increased with the use of dilators after estrogen replacement has improved mucosal vascularity and elasticity, but before coitus is attempted. ERT may be given either in the traditional form of estrogens for 25 days each month and a progestin for the last 10 days of estrogen, or in a continuous regimen of estrogen (eg, conjugated estrogens 0.625 mg qd) and progestin (eg, medroxyprogesterone 2.5 mg qd). The latter pattern has the advantage of avoiding uterine bleeding in the majority of cases.

Vulvovaginitides

Despite the increased variety of antimonilial agents and their easier accessibility as over-the-counter drugs, chronic recurrent vulvar and vaginal irritation remain the bane of women and their gynecologists. In addition to the usual well-publicized regimens, a few suggestions based only on clinical observation may be useful.

Many refractory cases can be traced to one or more of the following causes: (1) "vicious cycles" of oral or intravaginal antibiotics followed by antifungal agents followed by mechanical or chemical douching; (2) recurrent transmission of infectious agents (yeast, *Trichomonas*, bacteria) from your patient to her partner and back again; and (3) increased awareness of and sensitivity to any hint of increased vaginal secretion, even if clearly physiologic. Over the course of time, vaginal spasm (vaginismus) may be superimposed even in women with no prior history of sexual trauma or other sexual problems.

Treatment begins with both patient and physician acknowledging that this will be a long-term management problem, not one that has a single permanent cure. Begin with review of basic vaginal hygiene (bathe with nonperfumed soap; avoid medicated douches, bubble baths, scented or tinted toilet paper, vaginal deodorants; avoid constant wear of panty-liners and other occlusive forms of protection or dress; use pure cotton underwear only; and above all, avoid wearing underwear during sleep), and add other measures as needed: carefully patting dry after bathing and completing drying with a handheld hairdryer; applying unscented talc or cornstarch to the vulva prior to dressing; taking a single dose of antibiotic such as nitrofurantoin prior to coitus to diminish the need for full antibiotic courses; voiding before and after coitus; supplemental coital lubrication; prophylactic pre- and/or postmenstrual single doses of an antifungal agent; and regular (one or two times weekly) use of an acidifying vaginal gel. Vinegar douching may be used temporarily, but can be quite drying with long-term or frequent use.

Cases in which recurrent transmission between partners is suspected can be more difficult. Simultaneous treatment of both partners is, of course, indicated in the presence of an identifiable and treatable pathogen such as *Trichomonas*. Treatment of the male with topical antifungals is sometimes helpful, especially with uncircumcised men. In the case of bacterial vaginosis, the benefits of partner treatment are less certain, and the relapse rate is high regardless of treatments used. The best compromise can be reached with vigorous application of the vaginal hygiene measures described together with occasional vinegar douching or antibiotic courses.

Vulvar Vestibulitis Syndrome

Although human papillomavirus was the leading suspect as the cause for this disorder, many clinicians now view it as a neuroinflammatory disorder not caused by any particular infectious agent. Pathologic specimens obtained by biopsy or at surgery routinely reveal chronic inflammation.

With passage of time, usually about 6 months, partial or complete remission of symptoms sometimes occurs. Some cases of longer duration that resolve spontaneously may exist, but they would not come to the attention of a referral center, since most women wish treatment sooner. Symptomatic relief can be obtained with xylocaine 5% ointment, although the alcohol in the preparation causes some stinging for a minute or so after application. Combination ointments with topical anesthetics and steroids may also be helpful in about half of cases. Since the condition is not known to directly affect health adversely, if symptoms can be tolerated or diminished by symptomatic treatment, there is no medical necessity to do anything further. Although this may seem obvious, this information is often received with welcome relief.

Other topical agents that have been tried include estrogen creams, vegetable oil (with massage), and three or four applications of trichloroacetic acid. Although systemic comparisons have not been made, each of these methods seems to help 30% to 50% of affected women.

If further treatment is needed, removal of the tender tissue involved is the next step. Laser ablation and surgical excision each have their advocates, with each method resulting in about 70% or greater success, depending on the definition of "success." In our hands, using a surgical approach in 36 patients, all but 2 felt the operation to be worthwhile, with 74% enjoying at least 80% improvement. The surgical technique generally used involves excision of a crescent of vestibular tissue, using a mobilized flap of vaginal mucosa to cover the defect. Recovery time until comfortable coitus is about 2½ to 3 months for either the laser or the excisional approach. Concomitant vaginismus must be looked for and treated.

Vulvadynia

When discomfort is more generally present over the entire vulva and no infectious agents or epithelial changes can be identified, this term is often applied. The etiology is obscure, although psychological factors are often suspected and, in fact, treatment with amitriptyline, a tricyclic antidepressant, often relieves this condition. The drug may have central effects that alter pain perception in those with some evidence for concomitant affective disorder, despite the absence of proof that the affective change is a direct cause for the discomfort. Nevertheless, coupled with the vaginal hygiene measures described earlier, amitriptyline can help in many cases. It is not yet known whether the newer serotonergic antidepressants (fluoxetine, sertraline), which are better tolerated, will have similar beneficial effects.

Urethritis

Chronic intermittent urethral infection can occur with chlamydia as well as many urinary tract pathogens. Insufficient coital lubrication due to estrogen deficiency or poor sexual response may lead to increased coital trauma to the urethra, resulting in traumatic inflammation as well as increased vulnerability to ascending bacteria. Complete treatment addresses all apparent risk factors and may include supplemental lubrication (lubricating jelly, Astroglide, vegetable oil), pre- and postcoital voiding, and precoital antibiotic, usually nitrofurantoin. Vaginismus should be discussed and treated with vaginal relaxation exercises if present.

Urethral Syndrome

Frequency, urgency, and dysuria in the absence of bacteria define this troublesome problem. A close cousin is "interstitial cystitis," and indeed many authors speak of them synonymously. Although the location of the discomfort may be focused in a slightly different location, the two problems act similarly. Etiology remains essentially unknown, although histologically mild inflammation is believed to be often at the root, augmented by reactive muscular spasm, anxiety, and the debilitating effects of chronic bladder

discomfort. Detailed review of interstitial cystitis is beyond the scope of this discussion.

The same evaluation and treatment factors listed for urethritis apply to these problems in terms of vaginal lubrication and sexual function. In addition, tricyclic antidepressants are sometimes helpful, as are commonly employed urinary antispasmodics. When habitual frequent voiding has resulted in small bladder capacity, a "bladder drill" may help: suggest that the patient record voiding times for a day while maintaining relatively constant fluid intake; then have her void on a schedule of gradually increasing intervals. Over several weeks, considerable progress can often be made at no risk or expense.

Poor Lubrication

Secondary reduction in lubrication due to altered sexual response is the most common element in a vicious cycle: poor response—poor lubrication—more discomfort (with or without focused urethral, vaginal, or bladder symptoms)—worse response. The problem can develop over time on its own but is certainly aggravated by events such as intermittent vaginitis, cystitis, and so on. The larger risk is that a primary lubrication problem will be overlooked while the aggravating factors get the most attention.

In my experience, increasing the dose of estrogen in oral contraceptives may sometimes help, despite the lack of evidence for any general detrimental effect of these drugs on sexual response. Clearing up as many aggravating factors as possible also helps, as outlined earlier (see Vulvovaginitides), and supplemental lubrication is essential. Vegetable oils will degrade latex products (condoms, diaphragms), but have the advantage of not being spermicidal, which is a problem with most water-based commercial lubricants.

Levator Spasm

The levator plate does not develop intrinsic pathology, except in the case of severe pelvic relaxation, which is not usually directly painful. Spasm may frequently develop as a reaction to pelvic discomforts of many other kinds and can remain as a lingering problem after correction of the precipitating difficulty. Endometriosis, chronic pelvic inflammatory disease, chronic vaginitis, and chronic cystitis are perhaps the most common instigators. A high anxiety state may predispose to developing the problem, but this is by no means essential. The discomfort of levator spasm is often likened to "something falling out," even if support is good, and often radiates to the very low back.

Treatment starts with explaining the problem and offering reassurance about its benign nature. When the patient can identify the "falling out" sensation, it often helps to simply suggest that during normal activities she simply "let it fall out." Functionally, this lets the muscles relax, and relieves the pressure sensation. Frequent hot baths, reclining with the feet elevated, and pelvic floor contraction/relaxation exercises will also help. When present with generalized anxiety, anxiolytic medication or relaxation training supervised by a psychologist, or both, may help.

Vaginismus

Spasm of the introital (bulbocavernosus) muscles characterizes this disorder, although the levators may be involved as well. Unresolved conflict about sexuality in general may be present, but more often the spasm begins as an appropriate response to understandably painful stimuli (eg, vaginal penetration during a bout of vaginitis), and continues as a conditioned response when the inciting problem is resolved.

Behavioral treatments work well, but the patient and her partner may require psychological help from a marriage or sex counselor when emotional conflict hinders comfortable implementation of the behavioral suggestions. Having demonstrated vaginal contraction and relaxation during the pelvic examination, you may simply suggest that the patient do the same thing on her own, with the goal of learning comfortable control over the vaginal muscles. Once learned, the contraction/relaxation skills will need to be practiced with her partner present, then during cautious attempts at intercourse, gradually moving toward less guarded coitus over time.

Vaginal Stricture or Shortening

Most such cases develop after pelvic surgery, during menopause, or following radiation. Occasional cases have followed intravaginal application of 5-fluorouracil.

Treatment begins with estrogenization and continues with the use of graduated dilators. Various types of dilators are commercially available (Young's dilators, Milex), but creative clinicians and patients have fashioned reasonable facsimiles from syringe barrels, candles, and the like. A more elegant approach involves the use of Plexi-glas stents of graduated lengths and diameters, and a bicycle seat. A stent just slightly longer and wider than the starting anatomy is placed in the vagina, beneath underclothes. The patient then sits on a bicycle seat mounted on a pedestal (an exercise bike does nicely) for 1 to 2 hours nightly. Over weeks to months, the vagina will increase in depth and diameter. Once desired dimensions are reached, maintenance dilator use can be continued at empirically derived intervals.

Endometriosis

Although treatment of early stage (American Fertility Society stage 1 or 2) disease at the time of laparoscopic diagnosis may have little or no value in terms of increasing fertility, it may have significant value in reducing dyspareunia. Unfortunately, this has not received much attention in the literature. There is no clear evidence to favor one mode of laparoscopic treatment over another (laser vs electrocautery vs excision) for the relief of dyspareunia per se, although I have personally come to favor a surgical excision approach. Hormonal therapies can also be effective, but again, analyses of treatment results have not often focused on dyspareunia.

Pelvic Adhesions

The long-standing controversy about the relationship of adhesive disease to pain has been brought to the foreground again by the progress made in operative laparoscopy. It appears that laparoscopy will prove more effective than laparotomy in reducing adhesion burden. While the effect of laparoscopic adhesiolysis on pain requires more study, it does appear that up to 75% of patients may get long-term relief. Further, in one series, dyspareunia was relieved in every case in which adhesiolysis resulted in relief of general pelvic pain.

Uterine Retroversion

In a minority of women with uterine retroversion, the pelvic bony configuration (platypelloid especially) or generally diminutive stature may leave relatively little room in the posterior pelvis. The uterus may be uncomfortably struck during deep vaginal penetration. The presence of pelvic pathology such as endometriosis or adhesions will make the problem worse.

Adjustments in coital position to allow penile entry in a more anterior direction will take advantage of the fact that, when the uterus is retroverted, vaginal expansion during sexual response involves mostly the portion of the vagina anterior to the cervix; the retroverted fundus does not elevate out of the pelvis as does the anteverted uterus. In addition to correcting pelvic pathology, the laparoscopic approach can be used to perform uterine suspension as well.

Adnexal Pathology

Less commonly, unilateral adnexal pathology may be associated with dyspareunia that localizes to the affected side, especially when the uterus lies in a midposition or retroverted position. Pelvic inflammatory disease may sometimes result in asymmetric damage to the adnexa, and localized adhesions can be the sequel of a ruptured and/or hemorrhagic ovarian cyst as well as endometriosis.

For adhesive disease, laparoscopic diagnosis and treatment can usually be done simultaneously. Removal of the adnexa can usually be accomplished as well, if this is indicated by the patient's clinical situation. In the case of uterine retroversion with adnexal disease, adding uterine suspension to the procedure may be useful.

Diminished Sexual Arousal

Last, but by no means least, in this long list is the problem of decreased sexual response. For whatever reasons of personal history, naivete, or relationship difficulties, when sexual response is absent or significantly diminished, coitus can be at least uncomfortable if not painful at the level of the introitus, vaginal barrel, the deep pelvis, or all three. As described, other problems may develop with time, such as urethritis, cystitis, vaginitis, and vaginismus. The challenge in taking a history is to sufficiently attend to the chronology to understand the evolution of the problem.

Treatment of the associated conditions may be minimally or only temporarily successful in the absence of improvement in the underlying sexual response problem. Discussion of the treatment of sexual dysfunction is well beyond the scope of this review. In general, problems that began after a period of good sexual adjustment and have been going on a relatively short period of time (6 months to a year) may be amenable to an educational and office counseling approach, assuming that the individual and her partner have the emotional resources to comfortably and cooperatively employ the suggestions made. More complicated or long-standing problems commonly require the assistance of professionals skilled in marital and sex counseling. Ideally, if trained sex counseling help is not available, a collaborative relationship between the gynecologist and the therapist can be successful in helping the couple.

Conclusion

Dyspareunia is often a time-consuming problem. A careful history and pelvic examination is needed to elucidate as many of the contributing factors as possible. A generation ago, it was generalized that deep dyspareunia was often based on physical pathology and superficial problems were often psychologically based. Interestingly, exactly the opposite formulation has been voiced more recently. Such generalizations are not really clinically useful, however. It may serve the patient better to limit one's preconceptions and keep an open mind to the information offered.

Endometrial Hyperplasia

Alberto Manetta, MD

Endometrial cancer is the most common type of gynecologic malignancy, and certain types of endometrial hyperplasia may ultimately progress to cancer. Identification of hyperplasias with poor prognosis is critical for the prevention of endometrial cancer as well as the avoidance of overtreatment of patients with hyperplasias not associated with adverse prognoses.

Hyperplasias of the endometrium constitute a group of conditions characterized by noninvasive endometrial proliferations. Any endometrial proliferation associated with a stromal invasion ceases to be considered an endometrial hyperplasia and represents a carcinoma. This heterogeneous group of pathologic entities ranges from reversible to truly preneoplastic conditions. Kurman, Norris, and colleagues[*] have greatly clarified this difficult subject by offering a classification with significant clinical correlation. In general, hyperplasias may be classified as simple, complex, and atypical.

Simple hyperplasia is characterized by an in-

[*]Norris HJ, Connor MP, Kurman RJ: Preinvasive lesions of the endometrium. Clin Obstet Gynaecol 13:725–738, 1986; Kurman RJ, Kaminski PF, Norris HJ: The behavior of endometrial hyperplasia. A long-term study of "untreated" hyperplasia in 170 patients. Cancer 56:403–412, 1985.

crease in the number of endometrial glands. The glands may show a little crowding, which is referred to as cystic or mild hyperplasia, or, on occasion, substantial crowding, referred to as adenomatous hyperplasia.

Complex hyperplasia is distinguished by significant structural complexity with irregular outlines of the glands and back-to-back crowding.

Atypical hyperplasia indicates the presence of cytologic atypia in addition to structural changes. Thus, simple hyperplasia with cytologic atypia is simple atypical hyperplasia, and complex structural change in the presence of cytologic atypia is designated complex atypical hyperplasia.

Prognosis

Overall, a large percentage of these lesions will regress. It is the occasional patient with simple or complex hyperplasia in whom lesions will not regress spontaneously. Although patients with simple atypical hyperplasia may develop adeno-

carcinoma of the endometrium, a large percentage will not. Patients with complex atypical hyperplasia are at higher risk and their disease should be managed more aggressively.

Management (Fig. 1)

Most patients with endometrial hyperplasias will seek medical attention for menstrual disorders (in the premenopausal woman) or for abnormal vaginal bleeding (in the postmenopausal woman). The clinician should be particularly suspicious in cases of patients at high risk for the development of hyperplasias, such as patients with anovulatory cycles, those receiving unopposed exogenous estrogen, or those who are obese. Patients receiving long-term tamoxifen for treatment or prevention of breast cancer may also be at an increased risk for hyperplasia of the endometrium.

Diagnosis should be established by endometrial biopsy. This office procedure has almost completely replaced the need for in-patient dilatation and curettage.

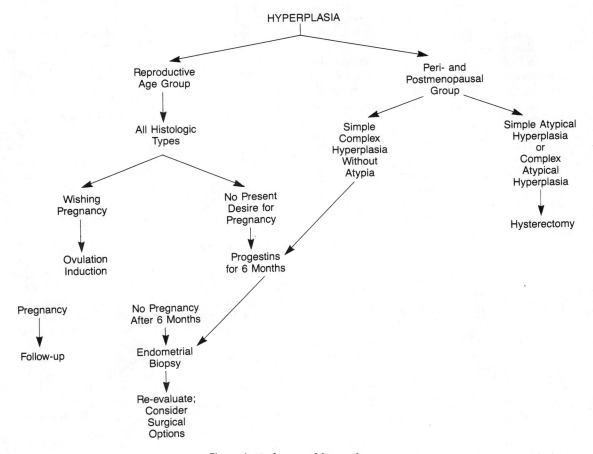

Figure 1. Endometrial hyperplasia.

Women within the reproductive age group who wish to preserve their fertility are candidates for conservative treatment, regardless of the type of hyperplasia, but particularly in the case of those without significant atypia. Anovulatory patients wishing to become pregnant should be managed by induction of ovulation. If the patient fails to become pregnant within 6 months, another endometrial biopsy should be performed. A woman interested in preserving her fertility, but not interested in pregnancy at the time of the diagnosis, should be treated with progestins such as megestrol acetate 40 mg twice daily for 6 months. The endometrium should be reassessed and further treatment will depend on the degree of cytologic atypia found.

Peri- and postmenopausal patients with atypical hyperplasia, especially complex atypical hyperplasia, should be managed with hysterectomy. Patients with simple or complex hyperplasia without atypia should be treated with progestational therapy, as indicated previously. The endometrial cavity should be sampled after 6 months of treatment. Peri- and postmenopausal women with hyperplasia receiving estrogen replacement therapy should be advised to discontinue this medication. They should be treated with progestins, and appropriate re-evaluation should be performed. Patients who fail under conservative management or in whom the hyperplasia recurs should be evaluated for a functional ovarian tumor such as granulosa cell and should be managed surgically.

In the future, advances in ultrasonograms, methods to quantitatively analyze the distribution pattern of nuclei and nucleoli, and flow cytometry may allow us to further refine the management of patients with hyperplasia. However, using our present knowledge, we should be able to significantly reduce the number of patients overtreated without failing to detect patients with true premalignant conditions.

Endometriosis and Adenomyosis

Eric S. Surrey, MD

Endometriosis is defined as the presence of endometrial tissue implanted in ectopic locations. The predominant extrauterine sites in which endometriosis has been isolated are, in order of frequency: ovaries, fallopian tubes, uterus, cul-de-sac, vesicouterine fold, uterine ligaments, rectovaginal septum, gastrointestinal tract, cervix, vagina, and vulva. More rarely, implants have been identified in incisional scars, skin, pelvic lymph nodes, pleura, lungs, and retina. On pathologic examination, endometriotic implants are composed of endometrial glands and stroma in addition to hemosiderin-laden macrophages and occasional fibrotic elements.

Several hypotheses have been proposed to explain the pathogenesis of this disorder: retrograde flow of endometrial tissue through the fallopian tubes during menses with subsequent deposition and implantation on pelvic organs, hematogenous or lymphatic metastasis of endometrial tissue, and metaplastic transformation of coelomic epithelium. None of these proposed mechanisms adequately describes all manifestations of endometriosis. For instance, retrograde menstruation has been described in normal women with patent fallopian tubes who have no evidence of endometriosis.

Recently, several investigators suggested that endometriosis may have a more complex etiology. After measuring increased levels of circulating antiendometrial antibodies in patients with endometriosis, one group of researchers proposed that endometriosis may represent an autoimmune process. Others have demonstrated that local immunologic mechanisms within the peritoneal cavity, perhaps mediated by activation of macrophages and associated cytokines, are an inherent part of the pathophysiology of this disorder.

Endometriosis most commonly afflicts women in their late 20s and early 30s with an incidence ranging from 5% to 15%. (It should be noted that this disorder may occur in adolescents as well.) Patients with endometriosis may present with pain, infertility, or a combination of the two. The classic symptom attributed to endometriosis is dysmenorrhea, which most typically begins just prior to the onset of menses and ceases before the end of menstrual flow. However, patients often have more localized pain or severe dyspareunia that may not be cyclic in nature. A host of other symptoms can also be associated with this disorder, particularly those related to gastrointestinal tract dysfunction including cyclic constipation, diarrhea, hematochezia, or melena. Additionally, cyclic urinary tract symptoms such as hematuria, dysuria, or urinary frequency or urgency may be secondary to endometriosis on the vesicouterine fold or invading the bladder wall.

Establishing a diagnosis must begin with taking a careful sexual, menstrual, gynecologic, and pain history as well as attempting to rule out other etiologies of chronic pelvic pain including gastrointestinal disorders, chronic salpingo-oophoritis, pelvic adhesions, musculoskeletal abnormalities, and other mass lesions in the reproductive tract. Physical examination is vital and must include a careful abdominal, pelvic, and rectovaginal exam. Induration and tender nodularity of the uterosacral ligaments classically is associated with the presence of endometriotic implants. Careful palpation of the ovaries and uterus to assess enlargement, tenderness, or cul-de-sac fixation is crucial. Pelvic ultrasonography has a role only as an auxiliary tool to assess adnexal masses. Its correlation with the specific diagnosis of endometriosis is poor; however, the typical "ground glass" appearance of an endometrioma on transvaginal sonography is extremely suggestive. The use of nuclear magnetic resonance imaging may have application in the future, but its value as a research tool has not yet been clearly demonstrated.

Levels of CA-125, a cell-surface antigen derived from coelomic epithelium, have been shown to be elevated in patients with endometriosis to an extent that appears to correlate loosely with disease severity. Unfortunately, CA-125 levels are also elevated in the presence of epithelial carcinomas of the ovary, as well as in a host of nonmalignant gynecologic and nongynecologic conditions including pelvic inflammatory disease, adenomyosis, menstruation, ovarian hyperstimulation syndrome, pregnancy, uterine leiomyomata, acute pancreatitis, chronic liver diseases, and peritonitis. However, serial measurement of this antigen may have some value as a means of assessing responsiveness of disease to therapeutic interventions and as an indication of recurrence.

Visualization of implants is crucial in making the diagnosis. Both typical and atypical appearances have been described. The more classic powder-burn implants and ovarian endometriomas or "chocolate" cysts do not represent the only appearance of this disease and, in fact, may represent more chronic states. Vesicular, petechial, hemorrhagic, polypoid, and white lesions have been correlated histologically with the presence of endometriosis, the first three of which may be more biologically active.

It is also important to note that symptoms often fail to correlate with disease extensiveness. Thus, laparoscopy remains the only definitive tool for assessment of the extent of endometriosis. The use of near-contact laparoscopic techniques with accessory probes has proven extremely helpful. A thorough and complete evaluation of the entire abdominal cavity, including an inspection of the regions lateral to the ovaries, must be performed before ruling out endometriosis. If the ovaries cannot be lifted medially, then one can assume that there is some pathologic process limiting their mobility.

The extent of endometriosis is currently quantified by the revised staging system of the American Society for Reproductive Medicine. According to this system, points are assigned on the basis of distribution and invasiveness of peritoneal implants, ovarian disease, tubal occlusion, pelvic adhesions, and cul-de-sac obliteration at laparoscopy. The disease is classified from stage I (minimal) to IV (severe), based on a summation of these scores.

The association of endometriosis with infertility is an issue of debate and controversy. The severe distortion of pelvic anatomy associated with stage IV disease, resulting in interference with ovum pick-up and tubal function by dense pelvic adhesions and loss of tubal motility, represents an obvious anatomic cause of infertility. However, in patients with lesser forms of disease it is less easy to explain the etiology of infertility or to even demonstrate a clear association. Several hypotheses have been put forward to explain infertility in patients with minimal amounts of endometriosis. These include abnormalities in follicular development or luteinizing hormone surges, luteal phase deficiencies, and hostile peritoneal environment including local elevations of prostaglandins and macrophage-derived secretory products that may impair fertilization processes. Reports of abnormal hamster and mouse egg fertilization and embryo development after exposure to peritoneal fluid obtained from patients with endometriosis support the latter point. Others have suggested that abnormalities in implantation may be related to an alteration in endometrial integrin subfractions. However, previously described increases in spontaneous abortion rates in patients with endometriosis have not been confirmed in properly controlled studies.

Options for treating symptomatic endometriosis include observation, medical therapy, surgical therapy, and combinations of surgical and medical therapy. The choice of appropriate intervention depends on patient age, as well as fertility desires. Certainly expectant management or observation is not appropriate in patients with severe pain or advanced disease, but it may be reasonable in young patients with lesser forms of asymptomatic disease and relatively short-term infertility.

Medical management of endometriosis is based on the assumption that exogenous sex steroids influence endometriotic tissue in the same way that they influence the endometrium. Since implants and symptoms tend to regress after menopause and after oophorectomy, and seem to abate during pregnancy, it is presumed that endometrium and endometriosis proliferate as a result of increased estrogen. Estrogen deficiency and androgens cause atrophy of both tissues, while progestins and progesterone arrest the growth and development of a decidual reaction in both endometrium and endometriosis.

Traditional medical therapies for endometriosis include pseudopregnancy, progestins, and danazol. Pseudopregnancy is obtained by the administration of high-dose oral contraceptives in a continuous rather than cyclic fashion. Although this therapy creates a progestin-dominant milieu, there is a high incidence of breakthrough bleeding responsive only to increasing estrogen doses.

The progestin most commonly used in this country for the treatment of endometriosis is medroxyprogesterone acetate. When administered orally in a minimal daily dose of 30 mg, a percentage of patients do note improvement. A patient who tolerates oral medroxyprogesterone acetate well may then be offered the option of switching to a longer-acting depot preparation in doses of 150 mg administered intramuscularly every 8 to 12 weeks. It should be noted that the depot preparation is not ideally suited for patients who wish to attempt conception immediately after therapy since post-therapy amenorrhea may be prolonged and onset of return of menses unpredictable. Weight gain, dysfunctional bleeding, and mood swings have been reported with both preparations.

Danazol is an isoxazol derivative of 17-alpha ethinyltestosterone that acts to suppress endometriosis on several levels. There appears to be a direct atrophic effect on endometriotic implants by its interaction with progesterone and androgen receptors. In addition, several steroidogenic enzymes are inhibited. Although basal gonadotropin levels are not affected by danazol, preovulatory luteinizing hormone and follicle stimulating hormone surges are inhibited. Free testosterone levels are inhibited by a decrease in hepatic production of sex hormone building globulin (SHBG) levels as well as by direct binding to SHBG with subsequent displacement of testosterone. The drug is administered orally in an initial divided dose of 400 to 600 mg daily and increased to a maximum of 800 mg daily until amenorrhea is achieved. The effectiveness of this agent in the suppression of symptoms associated with the disease is unsurpassed by other agents. Unfortunately, patient acceptance is reduced by hyperandrogenic side effects that include hirsutism, acne, and seborrhea, as well as depression, vasomotor symptoms, and abnormal lipoprotein changes. In addition, should the patient conceive, the masculinization of a female fetus is a theoretic possibility.

Gonadotropin-releasing hormone (Gn-RH) agonists have more recently been shown to represent an attractive alternative to other forms of medical therapy. These agents act by down-regulating pituitary gonadotropes, resulting in the induction of a reversible hypoestrogenic state or "medical oophorectomy." The currently approved agents are administered either in short-acting nasal or subcutaneous forms or in longer-acting intramuscular depot preparations. In most patients, menses return 30 to 90 days after completing a course of therapy. Several prospective randomized multicenter trials have demonstrated the similar effectiveness of intramuscular (leuprolide and goserelin) and intranasal (nafarelin) preparations. No untoward lipoprotein changes have been noted in patients receiving these agonists. The most common side effects are secondary to chronic hypoestrogenism and include hot flushes, vaginal dryness, libido changes, and reversible loss in bone mineral density. Investigators have recently published data to suggest that the combination of Gn-RH agonists with such progestins alone or in combination with low-dose estrogens may eliminate both vasomotor symptoms and bone mineral density loss without compromising the effectiveness of the Gn-RH agonist in treating endometriosis.

Surgical intervention can be conservative or radical. Radical surgery, designed for patients who no longer desire fertility, includes removal of the uterus with or without bilateral oophorectomy. All visible disease should be excised. The effect of posthysterectomy estrogen replacement on potential recurrence of disease with an ovary left in situ is extremely controversial, although the incidence is fairly small, particularly with complete excision of the disease.

Conservative surgical therapy is designed to restore normal pelvic anatomy and ablate or excise all visible manifestations of endometriosis. This has traditionally been performed at laparotomy, but the introduction of new endoscopic techniques, including the use of laser, has allowed reproductive surgeons to perform major pelvic reconstructive procedures with a significant decrease in morbidity, hospitalization, and patient cost. Superficial implants may be ablated or cauterized. Deeper implants should be excised in their entirety. Given the great potential for distortion of normal anatomy with severe disease, careful attention should be given to identification of the ureters, pelvic vessels, and bowel. Adhesions should not only be lysed, but excised in their entirety, since there is a high incidence of active endometriosis within these fibrotic structures. Endometriomas represent a primary surgical disorder, the regression of which is minimal with medical intervention. The capsule of the endometrioma should be completely excised or ablated since mere drainage of these cysts results in rapid recurrence. When residual disease is noted after extensive surgical ablation, patients may be treated postoperatively with suppressive medical therapy in the form of danazol or GnRH agonists to achieve an optimal result.

The value of transection of nerve bundles to the reproductive tract by either presacral neurectomy or bilateral uterosacral nerve ablation performed endoscopically or at laparotomy remains extremely controversial. The long-term effectiveness of these procedures has not been demonstrated clearly in well-designed controlled clinical trials. In performance of these procedures, careful attention must be paid to the location of the venous plexus at the sacral promontory and to the location of the ureters and associated vascular plexuses just lateral to the insertion of the uterosacral ligaments.

The management of infertility associated with endometriosis is not clearly defined. In the event of severe endometriosis, restoration of normal pelvic anatomy, with careful maintenance of hemostasis using magnification and meticulous microsurgical technique, is vital. Raw surfaces should be minimized with adhesion protection barriers. Ablation of minimal amounts of endometriosis has been shown to result in improved pregnancy rates in one controlled randomized study. Similarly, there are data to suggest that administration of danazol or GnRH agonists to infertile patients with stage I or II disease yields pregnancy rates that are no better than those followed expectantly. It is interesting to note that patients in both groups still show fertility rates that are below those of the normal fertile population. Unfortunately, very few well-designed controlled randomized prospective trials have been completed to truly assess the management of these difficult patients. In addition, our lack of complete understanding of the natural history of this disease often forces us to intervene in cases of minimal endometriosis to theoretically arrest progression. Patients with refractory infertility and concomitant endometriosis are successfully treated with such assisted reproductive technologies as in vitro fertilization/embryo transfer after all other etiologies for infertility have been ruled out. (This should include a thorough assessment of the male.)

Adenomyosis

Adenomyosis represents direct myometrial extension of endometrial tissue and therefore is a unique form of endometriosis. Pathologically, adenomyosis is defined as the presence of endometrial glands and stroma distal to the junction of the endometrium and myometrium. The diagnosis of adenomyosis can only be made histologically and thus only after hysterectomy has been performed. Recent studies have examined the role of magnetic resonance imaging, ultrasonography, hysterogalpingography, and transmyometrial biopsy as better diagnostic tools. It is interesting to note that adenomyosis is also noted in otherwise asymptomatic patients after hysterectomy is performed for other indications.

Adenomyosis occurs primarily in patients of reproductive age who are parous, a significant percentage of whom have dysmenorrhea and menorrhagia. It is also reported, however, in nulliparous women without prior history of uterine manipulation and thus may result from some form of metaplastic process of myometrial cells. Patients present with symptoms compatible with essential dysmenorrhea, and on physical examination the uterus is often tender, boggy, and slightly and symmetrically enlarged. These patients may often be treated effectively with nonsteroidal, anti-inflammatory drugs. Empiric therapy with agents used specifically for the treatment of endometriosis could theoretically result in improvement in symptoms. However, no controlled studies have been performed to date. Similarly, hysterectomy is performed only for intractable symptoms. The disorder subsides or regresses following menopause.

Endoscopic Surgery

Michael P. Diamond, MD

The role and scope of endoscopic surgery has been revolutionized over the past two decades. Whereas it used to be most commonly utilized by gynecologists for diagnostic assessments and sterilizations, it is now utilized by surgeons of nearly all specialities, with procedures ranging from arthroscopy to bowel resection, nephrectomy, and even cardiac surgery. For some obstetricians and gynecologists, procedures commonly performed endoscopically include hysterotomy, bladder suspensions, lymphadonectomies, neosalpingostomies, and treatment of severe endometriosis and pelvic adhesions. Perhaps even more impressive than a list of what a few of the most highly skilled surgeons can perform endoscopically is the realization that operative endoscopy of varying extent is commonly performed by so many gynecologic surgeons. The conversion from laparotomy to laparoscopy has been greatly facilitated by the rapid improvement in equipment and instrument availability. Clearly, there is no longer a question of what can be done endoscopically; rather the question is when, in which patients, and under what circumstances (and perhaps by whom) should operative endoscopy be utilized?

Several generalizable advantages of endoscopic surgery have been touted in comparison with "conventional approaches," including shorter hospital stays, reduced cost, and less postoperative morbidity (thereby allowing more rapid resumption of presurgical activities, including work). Under certain circumstances, each is likely to be true; however, important caveats exist for each. For most operative gynecologic procedures, patients come in, undergo their procedure, and are discharged all on the same day. For procedures requiring extensive dissections such as a laparoscopically assisted vaginal hysterectomy (LAVH), overnight stay is usual and may commonly extend to several days. However, this length of stay must be looked at in comparison to the altered perception held by clinicians of the required length of stay following a vaginal or abdominal hysterectomy. Although in the not-too-distant past it was common for these patients to be hospitalized postoperatively for 3 to 4 and 4 to 5 days, respectively, it is no longer unusual for patients undergoing these vaginal or abdominal procedures to go home in 2 days. It seems that, as clinicians recognize that many patients may be able to go home so quickly, patients are being so counseled, and it therefore can become a self-fulfilling prophecy. (This trend of course is not true for all patients, particularly those with confounding chronic health disorders or complicated surgical procedures.) In fact, in a recently published manuscript, a blinded comparison was made of postoperative morbidity in individuals undergoing cholecystectomy. Patients had a bandage placed so that they were unaware whether the gallbladder had been removed endoscopically or by an open procedure. No differences were noted in such factors as length of hospital stay, time to reinitiating eating, and other factors related to postoperative morbidity.

With regard to cost, there is the potential of surgical procedures. However, a review of reports documenting cost savings usually demonstrates that the savings comes from a reduction in the length of stay (and its associated expenses such as intravenous lines and medications) as opposed to a financial advantage in the operating room. In fact, due to the cost (and cost markup) associated with the disposable instruments and equipment, it is not uncommon for the operating room portion of care to actually cost more for endoscopic surgical procedures than corresponding operations performed by an abdominal or vaginal approach.

Reductions in postoperative morbidity procedures performed endoscopically is most likely to be attributable to a reduction in size of skin incisions or tissue retraction. However, to the extent that abdominal procedures can be performed through "mini-laparotomy" incisions, the potential advantage of multipunctured laparoscopic procedures may be lost. Furthermore, for hysterectomy that could be performed vaginally, inclusion of a laparoscopic component to the procedure may actually contribute to increased morbidity.

Thus, while the advantages to laparoscopic surgery may seem on the surface to be inherent, in fact this is not always true. Consequently, we must look closely at individual circumstances, including the procedure, the patient, the surgeon, and anticipated efficacy and complications, to determine the appropriate role of endoscopic surgery. In view of these observations, the remainder of this chapter deals primarily with the role of laparoscopy in the performance of individual surgical procedures. It first must be emphasized, however, that many of the comments that follow are thoughts that are unfortunately not based on well-designed and conducted studies, as such studies do not exist. Further, unlike the gold standard of randomized, double-blind, placebo-controlled protocols for drug studies, such protocols are extremely difficult, if not impossible, to utilize for surgical procedures, if for no other reason than that surgeons are differentially skilled in endoscopic versus nonendoscopic approaches, and thus are not even good controls for themselves.

Currently, probably the most discussed endoscopic surgical procedure is LAVH. LAVH has been described to encompass variable components of the procedure to be performed laparoscopically, from looking at the pelvic cavity to assess whether concomitant pelvic disease exists, to performing the entire extirpative procedure laparoscopically, and anywhere in between. This diversity has made comparison of different techniques for LAVH, as well as comparison of LAVH with conventional methods of access, difficult. In view of the reduced morbidity and complications of vaginal hysterectomy as opposed to abdominal hysterectomy (although the latter many be greatly biased because of adverse patient selection for abdominal hysterectomies), I believe an LAVH should be a method of converting what would have been an abdominal hysterectomy into a vaginal hysterectomy. Thus comparative studies seeking to determine the appropriate role of LAVH should make comparisons involving patients who may otherwise have undergone abdominal hysterectomies. However, such comparisons are further complicated because the relative contraindications for vaginal hysterectomy (ie, when an abdominal hysterectomy would be performed) are variable based on such factors as training and experience of the surgeon. The issue was recently highlighted to me at a postgraduate course at which I asked the participants which of the following was a contraindication to vaginal hysterectomy: nulliparity, history of pelvic inflammatory disease, pelvic adhesions, uterine fibroids, endometriosis, lack of uterine descensus, all of the above, or none of the above. Each of the individual factors were chosen by up to 8% of participants, while 29% said all of the above, and 35% said none of the above.

Other than complications associated with entry into the abdominal cavity, the complications that has probably been most commonly identified with LAVH is ureter damage at the level of the uterine vessels. Some surgeons have tried to minimize this complication by performing a supracervical hysterectomy. This has been criticized by others, however, because of the potential of problems from retaining the cervix, including the risk of cervical cancer and the difficulty of trachelectomy.

Although I am unaware of official numbers, it is my impression that probably well over half of stable ectopic pregnancies are now treated endoscopically, either by salpingectomy or salpingostomy (or medically). The feasibility of this endoscopic approach has been repeatedly demonstrated in descriptive series, as well as comparative studies with treatment on laparotomy. Choice of treatment at laparoscopy versus laparotomy should be based on such issues as surgeon experience and expertise, as well as availability of endoscopic instrumentation and equipment, and assistants trained in their use.

Endometriosis treatment by laparoscopy is performed for patients with infertility or pelvic pain, or both. Adequacy of therapy requires the ability to recognize endometriosis, which will not always have a characteristic purplish-black appearance, but can appear also as clear blebs or lesions that are yellow, red, or black. Additionally,

at times the presence of endometriosis will be identified by whitish scarring or abnormal vascular patterns. Endometriosis, and the scarring it causes, can result in extensive tissue distortions. Additionally, endometriosis can invade normal anatomical structure such as the bowel, bladder, rectovaginal septum, and ovary. Therapy, which can be conducted by laparotomy or laparoscopy, may involve removal or destruction of endometriotic implants; choice of vaporization or excision can be determined by the surgeon. However, particularly if the former is chosen, care should be taken to ensure complete obliteration of diseased tissue. The potential for incomplete treatment is suggested by the observation that the most common site for "recurrence" of endometrosis is the site of the lesion at the time of the initial surgery, which suggests that treatment was not deep enough or not wide enough. For patients with bowel symptoms, preoperative bowel preps are often recommended.

Over the past several years, a laparoscopic approach has been increasingly utilized for women with stress urinary incontinence. Multiple descriptive series now exist, although well-designed comparative studies are needed. Also important will be good documentation of patients' follow-up and the success for this procedure, based on their initial presentation and preoperative evaluation findings. The surgical approaches that have been employed include both a transabdominal laparoscopic approach and a retroperitoneal approach into the space of Retzius without traversing the abdominal cavity. In the future, the outcomes from these approaches will need to be compared not only with similar procedures performed at laparotomy but also with less invasive needle suspension approaches.

Pelvic adhesions are treated endoscopically in patients with pelvic pain and infertility, in the hope of alleviating these disorders. While this is often successful, particularly in patients who initially had distortion of normal organ relationships (eg, an ovary adherent to the anterior abdominal wall, and a tube and ovary adhered separately from each other), efficacy of these procedures is greatly hindered by postoperative adhesion development. In one study evaluating the entire pelvis, adhesions were identified in 97% of 68 women who had undergone laparoscopic adhesiolysis within the previous 3 months. Thus, in contrast to suggestions from animal studies, operative laparoscopy per se is not a cure-all for prevention of postoperative adhesions. Further, de novo adhesions formed in 12% of these patients, and at 23% of available sites in these women. While there are many inherent difficulties in comparing these numbers to ones following laparotomy, such comparisons do suggest that de novo adhesion formation (but *not* adhesion reformation) is less after laparoscopic surgery. Clearly, adjuvants to help reduce adhesion development are needed for endoscopic surgery.

In addition to adhesiolysis, which has already been addressed, fertility-promoting laparoscopic procedures that have been performed include neosalpingostomy, fibrinoplasty, and tubal anastomosis. Most reports of these procedures have described outcomes or used historical controls rather than comparative trials. While results may appear to be equivalent in the hands of some surgeons, in the absence of adequate control for other infertility factors I believe the gold standard for these procedures remains performance of an open procedure. In those patients who desire an endoscopic approach, laparoscopic attempts may be initiated. For patients who require neosalpingostomies, knowledge of the tubal lumen status may help determine whether to perform the procedure or to refer the patient for assisted reproductive technology procedures. Currently, this requires creating a neostomy and placing the viewing scope at the distal end of the tube; under such circumstances its value is extremely limited at best. However, if in the future it is possible to place a tuboscope transcervically in the office, it would potentially be of much greater value. It is important that the role for tubal surgery for infertility therapy (whether by laparotomy, laparoscopy, or transcervically) be continually reappraised as advances are made in both surgery and assisted reproductive technology.

Laparoscopic myomectomy has been performed by a variety of techniques, including electrosurgery, laser, and harmonic scalpel. The biggest difficulties with performance has not generally been excising the myomas or controlling bleeding (although many hospitals have reports of excessive bleeding requiring transfusions), but rather adequate closure of the uterus and removal of the myoma from the abdominal cavity. In one series by experienced surgeons, a fistula rate of 25% between the abdominal and uterine cavity was identified following laparoscopic myomectomy. As a result, some now advocate laparoscopic myomectomy followed by mini-laparotomy for fibroid removal; others question why the entire procedure is not performed by mini-laparotomy. The difficulty with uterine closure is also a concern regarding subsequent integrity of the uterus throughout pregnancy in

those wishing to conceive. This concern underscores the difficulty many physicians have had with laparoscopic suturing, although new devices are now becoming available to facilitate this process. Also, automated "morcellators" are becoming available that are likely to facilitate tissue removal. Recently, several surgeons have advocated "myolysis," or the repeated placement of a narrow energy source into the fibroid with the hope that it will disrupt the blood supply sufficiency to cause resorption. While this has primarily been performed under endoscopic guidance, there is the potential that in the future it could be performed under imaging guidance, thereby eliminating the need for an endoscopic procedure.

In summary, laparoscopic surgery has come a long way in a short time, and rightfully so. It offers the potential for reducing morbidity and cost, and has provided opportunities for improved efficacy and reduced complications. It has also changed the way in which "conventional" approaches have been performed, with the goals being the same: to improve efficacy, reduce complications, and provide for treatment of disease with less morbidity and cost. It appears that human imagination is the only limit to what can be done laparoscopically; it is now time to determine when the laparoscopic approach will be best, a decision which undoubtedly will often vary based on unique aspects of each patient, each surgeon, and the operative setting in which the procedure is performed.

Female Genital Tuberculosis

George Schaefer, MD

Since 1985, the incidence of tuberculosis has increased in the United States, owing in part to immigration from Asian, African, eastern European, and Latin American countries. In addition, in the past decade, homelessness, drug abuse, and acquired immunodeficiency syndrome (AIDS) have left a large population defenseless against the germ that causes this disease. More than one third of the world's population now carry tubercle bacilli; over 8 million new cases of tuberculosis occur worldwide annually and nearly 3 million people die annually from the disease. The increase in pulmonary tuberculosis has been accompanied by an increase in extrapulmonary tuberculosis. One may anticipate that female genital tuberculosis (FGT) will also become more prevalent.

In South Africa and India, large series of patients with FGT have recently been reported as a result of specific screening for this condition in infertility clinics. FGT is uncommon in the United States and is usually discovered in the course of an infertility examination, although many asymptomatic cases remain undiscovered.

Female genital tuberculosis should be differentiated from pelvic or peritoneal tuberculosis, which presents as tuberculosis of mesenteric or pelvic lymph nodes usually with miliary spread to the omentum and serosal surface of intestines and pelvic viscera. It does not involve the mucosa of the pelvic organs and may not impair reproduction. FGT involves the mucosa of the fallopian tubes, with or without spread to the uterus and ovaries. The peritoneum may or may not be involved. It is always secondary to tuberculosis elsewhere in the body, usually the lungs. The usual routes of infection are the blood stream, the lymphatics, and direct extension from a neighboring viscus. The frequency of involvement of the genital organs by tuberculosis are fallopian tubes, 100%; endometrium, 50% to 80%; ovaries, 15% to 25%; cervix, 5% to 15%; and vulva and vagina, 1%. About 85% of FGT cases are first diagnosed in patients aged 20 to 40 years, usually during an investigation for infertility, although the disease probably existed for many years before it was detected.

Diagnosis

Female genital tuberculosis is rarely considered in the differential diagnosis of pelvic inflammatory disease. It is usually discovered postoperatively from the histologic examination of endometrial curettages or from serial sections of the fallopian tube removed at operation. A diagnosis of FGT will more frequently be made if a high index of suspicion is used with the following patients:

1. A patient who gives a past history or family history of tuberculosis. About 20% of patients with FGT give a history of tuberculosis in their family. About 50% of our patients have had tuberculous pleurisy; peritonitis; erythema nodosum; renal, osseous, or pulmonary tuberculosis. A few of our patients were operated on for appendicitis in childhood, and a review of the pathologic findings revealed a tuberculous appendix.
2. A patient with primary sterility in whom

examination reveals no apparent cause and who gives a past or family history of tuberculosis, particularly if she has recently immigrated from a Third World country.
3. A patient with "chronic pelvic inflammatory disease" who does not respond to the usual antibiotic therapy.

The five most frequent symptoms in FGT are sterility, pelvic pain, poor general condition, menstrual disturbances, and vaginal discharge. None of these conditions is specific for FGT, and, indeed, the patient may have no complaints and seek advice only because of infertility. If she does present three or more of these complaints, a thorough examination for FGT is warranted.

Pelvic Examination

On bimanual examination, there may be no palpable disease or only slight induration in both adnexal regions. Large bilateral tuberculous tubo-ovarian masses are not commonly found in the developed countries. Early diagnosis and treatment of pulmonary tuberculosis may prevent progression of tuberculous salpingitis to large adnexal masses. Other pelvic lesions may coexist with genital tuberculosis. The presence of bilateral tubo-ovarian masses in a virgin who gives a history of pulmonary or extrapulmonary tuberculosis is highly suspicious of genital tuberculosis.

Laboratory Aids

Female genital tuberculosis can be ruled out if the tuberculin test is negative. However, a positive tuberculin test does not confirm a diagnosis, since the tuberculin test does not differentiate genital tuberculosis from pulmonary or extrapulmonary disease. It may also sometimes be falsely positive in fever, pregnancy, influenza, brucellosis, or measles.

The most common method of diagnosing genital tuberculosis is by endometrial curettage performed shortly before the menstrual period. Half of the specimen should be sent for histologic examination and the other half for bacteriologic examination for tubercle bacilli.

Some investigators have reported that menstrual fluid collection and culture (repeated) proved to be a reliable diagnostic procedure.

A hysterosalpingogram done in the course of an infertility work-up may reveal changes suggestive of tuberculosis of the uterus and tubes; however, a definitive diagnosis cannot be made from radiographic studies alone and must be confirmed by histologic or bacteriologic examination.

Although laparoscopy has been used in the diagnosis of FGT, this procedure is not without danger; perforation of the bowel or bladder with the laparoscope has been reported. Open laparoscopy is a safer procedure. In addition, laparoscopy cannot always differentiate between pelvic tuberculosis and FGT, since involvement of the serosa of the tubes does not necessarily mean involvement of the mucosa.

One investigator used diagnostic laparoscopy in 687 cases. Of these, 101 were suspected of having pelvic tuberculosis from appearance alone. When this was correlated with other criteria, definite evidence was found in 70 cases.

Treatment

General Aspects

As a rule, active extragenital foci of tuberculosis are rarely present when the genital lesion is discovered, since the original pulmonary or extrapulmonary disease has usually been arrested. However, a chest roentgenogram, repeated sputum analyses, and examination of the urine for tubercle bacilli are performed routinely.

Any treatment instituted must include general therapeutic measures such as mental and physical rest, proper nutrition, dietary supplements when indicated, and careful personal hygiene.

A pulmonary physician or infectious disease specialist should be consulted in the management of gynecologic tuberculosis. Liver function test, examination by an ophthalmologist, and, when possible, drug susceptibility tests should be carried out before starting antituberculosis drugs.

Antituberculosis Drugs

A 9-month regimen of isoniazid and rifampin, usually supplemented by ethambutol, streptomycin, or pyrazinamide for the initial 2 months, has been recommended by the American Thoracic Society as standard therapy for tuberculosis in the United States and Canada, regardless of the age of the patient or the site of involvement. Others recommend only isoniazid and rifampin for short-course (9-month) therapy for pulmonary tuberculosis. Whether to use two or three drugs initially depends on the resistance of the tubercle bacilli to the antimicrobial agents used.

It has recently been shown that short-course chemotherapy for extrapulmonary tuberculosis has an overall success rate of over 95%.

A 1-year treatment of FGT with isoniazid, rifampin, and ethambutol (discontinued after 90 days) has been reported with a success rate of 97.5% after 2½ years' follow-up.

In general, the key to successful short-course therapy is patient compliance. Therapy that extends 18 to 24 months is not completed in 30% of developed countries and up to 50% of Third World countries.

On the basis of the excellent results described, I suggest a modification in the treatment of FGT to isoniazid and rifampin for 9 to 12 months with ethambutol for the initial 2 months. (If drug sensitivity studies indicate no resistance to isoniazid and rifampin, ethambutol may be omitted.) If isoniazid or rifampin is contraindicated because of previous liver disease, alcoholism, or toxicity, ethambutol may be substituted for either drug, in which case treatment should be continued for 18 months.

Extent of the Disease

Minimal disease is usually asymptomatic, except for sterility, and is diagnosed by finding tuberculous endometritis on curettage or biopsy, or tubercle bacilli on culture of the curettages of menstrual blood. Advanced genital tuberculosis is diagnosed by the presence of palpable tuboovarian masses plus histologic or bacteriologic evidence of tuberculosis. Different regimens are suggested for each.

Minimal Genital Tuberculosis

The patient is given isoniazid 300 mg daily plus rifampin 600 mg daily orally in the morning for 9 months and ethambutol 15 mg/kg for 2 months. She is examined at monthly intervals, and after 6 months, a dilatation and curettage is done and the endometrial curettages are examined histologically and bacteriologically. If these are negative for tuberculosis, chemotherapy is continued for a additional 3 months. Six months after cessation of antituberculosis drugs, the endometrium is again examined for tuberculosis.

The patient should be followed annually for an indefinite period of time. Before the combined use of rifampin and isoniazid, exacerbations had been reported up to 10 years after apparent cure. This is highly unlikely with current therapy, although long-term follow-up is not available. At present, any patient whose tuberculosis recurs should be tested for AIDS.

Advanced Genital Tuberculosis

For advanced genital tuberculosis, isoniazid 300 mg and rifampin 600 mg are given orally daily for 6 months and ethambutol 15 mg/kg is given orally for 2 months. The patient is examined at monthly intervals. If the adnexal masses resolve, chemotherapy is continued for 1 year, provided endometrial curettages are negative for tuberculosis at 6 months and at 1 year. If palpable adnexal masses persist after 9 months, a total abdominal hysterectomy and bilateral salpingo-oophorectomy are performed. Isoniazid and rifampin are continued for an additional 6 months postoperatively.

I now recommend isoniazid and rifampin for 9 months before performing surgery in patients with palpable adnexal masses. The effectiveness of concomitant isoniazid and rifampin in healing pulmonary and extrapulmonary lesions in 6 to 9 months leads me to believe that a similar result can be expected in FGT. Nontuberculous pelvic infection may be responsible for adnexal enlargement, in which case conventional antimicrobial therapy should be used.

Surgery

Surgery should not be performed in a woman known to have genital tuberculosis until she has had a course of antituberculosis drugs. These make the surgical procedure technically easier and reduce the risk of operative and postoperative complications.

Surgery has not often been necessary in the past 10 to 15 years because of the effectiveness of the combined use of isoniazid and rifampin and because large adnexal masses are infrequently found at the initiation of therapy.

Indications for surgery are:

1. Persistence or increase in pelvic masses after a 9-month course of antituberculosis drugs.
2. Recurrence of positive endometrial culture or histology after 9 months of isoniazid and rifampin. (This is most unusual and would indicate resistance to isoniazid and/or rifampin.)
3. Persistence or recurrence of pain or bleeding after 9 months of antituberculosis therapy.

At Operation

When genital tuberculosis is first discovered at operation, overzealous attempts to remove all tuberculous tissue may lead to intestinal or bladder injury. Tissue should be removed for biopsy and antituberculosis drugs started immediately using isoniazid, rifampin, and ethambutol. If the masses do not resolve in 9 months, they should be surgically removed. Isoniazid and rifampin should be continued for 6 months after surgical removal of tuberculous tissue.

Tuberculous salpingitis discovered at tuboplasty should be treated with antituberculosis drugs for 9 months, and the patient should be investigated for tuberculosis elsewhere in the body. I do not recommend tuboplastic procedures on tuberculous tubes. Meningeal and miliary tuberculosis have been reported after such procedures in patients not suspected of having tuberculous salpingitis.

Postmenopausal Tuberculosis

When endometrial tuberculosis is first discovered at curettage for postmenopausal bleeding and no adnexal disease is palpable, the patient is given isoniazid 300 mg, rifampin 600 mg orally daily, and 15 mg/kg of ethambutol, and investigated for evidence of extragenital tuberculosis in the lungs, intestinal tract, kidneys, and osseous systems. If no active tuberculosis is found, treatment is continued for 9 months (ethambutol is discontinued after 2 months). Curettage is repeated at 9 months before discontinuing treatment. If pelvic symptoms persist after 9 months of antituberculosis drugs, a total abdominal hysterectomy and bilateral salpingo-oophorectomy should be performed. Antituberculosis drugs are given for 6 months postoperatively.

I have previously avoided the concomitant use of isoniazid and rifampin in the elderly patient for long periods of time because of the danger of hepatitis, particularly in patients with a history of hepatitis or in alcoholics. However, clinically and laboratory confirmed hepatitis has been reported in only 1.4% of elderly patients with extrapulmonary tuberculosis treated with short-course therapy using isoniazid and rifampin. I advise this short-course regimen for the postmenopausal patient. The patient should be checked at monthly intervals for clinical symptoms, and, if these appear, liver function tests should be done.

If concomitant isoniazid and rifampin are contraindicated, ethambutol may be given in place of rifampin. Ethambutol 20 mg/kg daily orally with isoniazid 300 mg/daily should be administered for 18 months. If pelvic symptoms persist after 9 months of therapy, the uterus, tubes, and ovaries should be surgically removed. Isoniazid and ethambutol should be given for 9 months postoperatively if all tuberculous tissue has been removed.

Toxicity

Toxic side effects have been reported in patients receiving antituberculosis drugs. In 350 patients receiving short-course therapy for extrapulmonary tuberculosis, 5.4% had minor side effects and 1.4% developed a major reaction such as hepatitis.

Patients taking isoniazid should be advised about the symptoms of hepatitis and should be advised to consult their physician immediately if these occur. Although hepatic toxicity from isoniazid is rare, it may occur in elderly patients and alcoholics, in combination with rifampin, or in patients with a history of previous hepatitis. Hepatic toxicity can usually be diagnosed on history alone in approximately 85% of cases. If clinical symptoms do appear, liver function tests should be done; if positive, treatment with rifampin or isoniazid should be discontinued.

Rifampin may cause hepatitis in patients with prior liver disease and in those taking isoniazid. Minimal abnormalities of liver function tests are common, and they usually disappear while the patient continues to take the drug. Patients must be observed carefully for more substantial degrees of elevation of enzymes and for jaundice, which occurs in 0.6% of patients who take rifampin. If these side effects occur, use of the drug should be discontinued.

Ethambutol is a relatively safe drug. Ocular toxicity is dose related and occurs in less than 2% of patients who receive 25 mg/kg daily. This toxic effect is usually reversible when the drug is promptly discontinued. Patients should be tested for visual acuity and green color perception before and periodically during therapy.

There are conflicting views as to whether a successful pregnancy may be expected after treatment for FGT. My experience is that a full-term pregnancy rarely occurs in a woman who has had genital tuberculosis. However, a few full-term pregnancies following treatment in early minimal cases with current therapy have been reported recently.

Tuboplasty operations should not be performed in patients with female genital tuberculosis. The probability of a full-term pregnancy is extremely unlikely and the risk of miliary spread is present.

I have had no experience with in vitro fertilization after treatment of FGT. If there are no signs or symptoms of pelvic disease 1 year after successful completion of treatment, in vitro fertilization may be considered. In 1994, a few cases of full-term pregnancy were reported after in vitro fertilization and embryo transfer.

Female Sterilization

Gerald I. Zatuchni, MD, MSc

Tubal sterilization is one of the most frequently performed gynecologic operations. It is estimated that by 1992, over 28% of women of reproductive age in the United States had been sterilized. A tubal sterilization procedure is relatively simple to perform and teach, very safe, and extremely effective. A variety of operative procedures are now available that will achieve permanent female sterilization. The procedure may be performed on an out-patient or in-patient basis, by the abdominal or vaginal route, using local or general anesthesia, in the postpartum or postabortal period, or as an interval operation. There is no one best procedure; each has its own advantages, disadvantages, and appropriateness. The choice of a specific procedure, the surgical approach, and the type of anesthesia must depend on the experience of the gynecologist and the facilities available. Most importantly, because female sterilization is an elective procedure, the patient's wishes must have a paramount place in the decision concerning which procedure, if any, would be best.

Patient Counseling

Proper patient counseling and informed consent are mandatory in preparing the patient for a sterilization procedure. The woman's decision for sterilization must be made on an entirely voluntary basis following appropriate discussion with the physician regarding the risks, benefits, and alternatives for fertility regulation.

The large number of women sterilized in the United States attests to the perception that female sterilization offers significant benefits. The methods are extremely effective, involve a one-time-only surgical procedure that is immediately effective, can be performed on an ambulatory basis, are cost-effective, and rarely have serious complications. Female sterilization has a mortality rate of 1 to 2 per 100,000 procedures.

Although the risks associated with voluntary sterilization are minimal, in the individual case they can be profound. As most procedures are carried out under general anesthesia, there is an obvious but fortunately rare risk of life-threatening consequences. Similarly, the use of the laparoscope carries with it certain risks. Accordingly, in the informed consent discussion, the patient must be told of the potential risks of anesthesia and of the operative procedure itself. Specific risks such as perforation of organs, occasional need for emergency hospitalization, bleeding, and infection should be mentioned. Risks vary with the type of procedure.

Regardless of the exact procedure employed, the patient must fully understand that the tubal obstruction is permanent. Should she have any doubts about her wish for permanence, then this patient should not be offered tubal sterilization. Sterilization reversals can be done, some quite successfully, depending on the original type of sterilization procedure performed, but the question of reversibility should be in the surgeon's mind and not in the patient's.

The patient should be informed that there is no guarantee that the procedure will prevent pregnancy. There is a failure rate with each surgical procedure, varying from 1 to 3 per 1000 for tubal electrocoagulation/cauterization techniques, to 4 to 6 per 1000 for Silastic rings, clips, and suture ligations. The patient should be informed also that there is a possibility of later ectopic pregnancy.

The physician must document in office records the informed consent procedure and patient counseling, including the use of written materials or videotape. In these days of medicolegal concerns, some physicians have the patient write one or two paragraphs about her understanding of the sterilization procedure and its risks. Additionally, just prior to the performance of the procedure, the consent form for sterilization must be read, understood, and signed by the patient and a witness. This surgical consent form must include all elements of the informed consent discussion that took place in the office.

Surgical Approach

Tubal sterilization may be performed by the abdominal or vaginal route. The abdominal entry may be through a mini-laparotomy incision in the suprapubic or the infraumbilical area, or with a laparoscopic approach. Most interval sterilization procedures are done via laparoscopy, although a significant number are accomplished by means of a suprapubic mini-laparotomy approach. In the postpartum period, the usual surgical approach is through a small infraumbilical incision. A posterior colpotomy approach to the tubes as an interval procedure only is usually simple and quite safe. It avoids the risks of laparoscopy but has its own risks, including a somewhat higher incidence of postoperative infection.

For a mini-laparotomy approach in the interval situation, the most satisfactory incision is a suprapubic transverse one made approximately 3 cm above the pubis and 5 to 6 cm in length. The underlying fascia is divided, the rectus muscles are retracted, and the underlying fascia and peritoneum are then incised. Usually, a uterine-elevating device is inserted preoperatively to bring the uterus forward to the anterior abdominal wall. Once the tubes are identified, a variety of sterilization procedures can be easily accomplished.

In the postpartum period, the usual mini-laparotomy incision is infraumbilical, either vertical or transverse, and 4 to 6 cm in length. Once entry into the peritoneal cavity is obtained, the tubes can be brought into the incision most easily by the surgeon's exploring finger. Occasionally, a sponge stick may be useful in bringing the tube into the incision. Because of the size of the fallopian tubes in the postpartum period, rings and clips are not recommended. One or another type of suture ligation and excision technique can be employed.

In the colpotomy approach, the peritoneal cavity is entered via an incision in the posterior vaginal fornix between the uterosacral ligaments. Most often, a transverse incision is easily done. The tubes are then brought into the incision and the selected sterilization procedure is performed. This may be the application of a ring or clip or suture material. Since infection is a concern following colpotomy, prophylactic antibiotics should be administered during the immediate postoperative period.

Surgical Sterilization Procedures

Tubal Ligation and Resection

There are a multitude of successful tubal ligation and excision procedures, each having its proponents. Probably the most common type is the modified Pomeroy technique. This technique is popular because of its simplicity and efficacy. The basic procedure consists of tying an absorbable suture around a knuckle of tube and excision of the tube distal to the suture. In approximately 4 to 6 weeks, the cut ends of the tube become fibrotic and the suture is absorbed, leaving a gap in tubal continuity. This procedure can be utilized in the puerperal and nonpuerperal patient. It also can be performed through a colpotomy incision.

Historically, there have been other types of tubal ligation and resection techniques, including the Madlener technique, in which the midsection of the tube is crushed with a clamp and ligated with nonabsorbable suture material. Some surgeons have modified this technique and excised that portion of the tube distal to the suture. The failure rate for the Madlener technique is higher than for the Pomeroy technique. The Irving technique is more complicated, in that the tube is divided between two absorbable ligatures and the proximal stump is buried in the uterine myometrium. This procedure has a high effectiveness rate, but owing to its complexity it is not widely employed. Other techniques include the Uchida and the Kroener fimbriectomies. The fimbriectomy is associated with high failure rates and lack of opportunity for reversal.

Tubal Occlusion

Tubal sterilization may be accomplished by simple ligation in several places on each tube using nonabsorbable suture or by the application of various occlusive devices such as Silastic rings or tubal clips. The most popular tubal occlusive procedure in the United States is the application of Silastic rings. The rings are placed on the tubes by means of a specially designed applicator, used with laparoscopy. Tubal clips are applied in a similar manner. The Silastic ring should be applied at least 1.5 to 2 cm from the cornual end of the tube to obtain a good knuckle of tube that will not soon retract out of the ring. Similarly, the tubal clip should be applied in the middle third of the tube. Occasionally, a second ring or clip may be applied to the same tube if the surgeon believes the first application was inadequate. The anticipated failure rate for rings or clips is approximately 4 to 6 per 1000 procedures. The major advantage, besides simplicity and safety, is the minimal amount of tubal destruction required for effective sterilization. Indeed, should the need arise, a successful surgical reversal can be anticipated in as many as 80% of patients.

Tubal Cauterization

Electrocauterization or thermocoagulation of the tubes is popular because of the simplicity of the procedure and its great effectiveness. The failure rate is estimated to be 1 to 3 per 1000. Laparoscopy is the preferred approach for tubal cauterization. In the past several years, there has been a shift in use from unipolar fulguration to bipolar fulguration. The latter procedure is far safer, because there is no errant electricity to injure the bowel or other organs. On the other hand, bipolar electrocoagulation requires more intensive electricity to ensure that the inner tubal epithelium is completely coagulated. If the bipolar apparatus does not put out sufficient wattage, the failure rate may be significantly increased. Accordingly, it is wise to follow the manufacturer's recommendations regarding the generating equipment and the specific instruments to be employed. As with any mechanical system, the surgeon should confirm that all parts of the system are functioning in an appropriate manner prior to their being employed on the patient.

Failures

Every patient must be informed that the sterilization procedure has a failure rate of at least 1 to 6 per 1000, depending on the exact procedure performed. Surgical failures can result from inappropriate technique, misidentification of the fallopian tube, incorrect or faulty application of the ring or clip, or faulty equipment. The gynecologist always must bear in mind these potential causes for failure and institute immediate corrective measures when they occur. A later hysterosalpingogram can be done, should the gynecologist be concerned with the efficacy of the procedure. In this situation, the patient should be advised to refrain from intercourse until the determination is made.

If a failure (intrauterine pregnancy) occurs within the first year after sterilization, most probably it is due to a technical problem that occurred at the time of the sterilization. On the other hand, failures that occur more than 1 year after sterilization are most likely due to spontaneous recanalization of the tube or tuboperitoneal fistula formation.

Complications

Complications of female sterilization include general anesthetic problems and intraoperative problems. The latter includes inappropriate laparoscopic trocar insertion causing injury to the bladder, bowel, or blood vessels; intraoperative bleeding associated with mesosalpingeal tears; postoperative bleeding; and infection. Fortunately, these complications are not common and can be reduced even further by strict adherence to appropriate surgical techniques.

A considerable number of papers have been published regarding the long-term effects of tubal sterilization on the female reproductive system, especially with regard to abnormal uterine bleeding—the so-called post–tubal ligation syndrome. Several retrospective studies have indicated that women undergoing tubal sterilization seem to have a higher incidence of hysterectomy for abnormal uterine bleeding. On the other hand, several prospective studies involving thousands of women undergoing tubal sterilization have indicated no significant differences in menstrual patterns, abnormal bleeding, or dysmenorrhea before and after tubal sterilization.

Hysterectomy

Hysterectomy should not be performed merely as a sterilizing procedure, owing to its risks of morbidity and even mortality. However, many women desiring voluntary termination of their fertility have gynecologic problems that may be best treated by vaginal or abdominal hysterectomy. These associated conditions may include uterine disease, such as leiomyomata, pelvic relaxation syndrome, and pelvic inflammatory disease. Should hysterectomy be advised, the physician is obligated to inform the patient of the increased risks of the procedure. It is wise for the physician to obtain a second opinion regarding the need for hysterectomy.

Reversibility

The tubal sterilization procedures described here should be offered to the patient as a permanent and irreversible method of fertility regulation. The gynecologist should refuse to do the procedure if the patient expresses any doubts as to her contemplated fertility termination. Nevertheless, a small percentage of sterilized women (estimated at 1%) will request a surgical reversal owing to unexpected changes in life situations. The results of surgical reversal with the aid of the operating microscope depend primarily on the type of sterilization procedure performed—the greater the amount of tubal de-

struction, the less the opportunity for successful reversal. Accordingly, sterilization procedures that destroy only a minimal amount of tube, for example, rings, clips, and suture ligation/excision, have high potential for reversibility, whereas the opposite is true for electrocoagulation techniques. These facts must be understood by the gynecologist, so that the patient is appropriately counseled.

Galactorrhea and Hyperprolactinemia

Howard A. Zacur, MD, PhD
Endrika L. Hinton, MD

Discharge of milk from the breasts unrelated to pregnancy and breast feeding is called galactorrhea. A circulating plasma or serum concentration of prolactin exceeding the upper limit of normal is called hyperprolactinemia. This chapter discusses the diagnosis and management of these conditions, which may occur together or separately.

Galactorrhea

The existence of a nipple discharge may be brought to the attention of the examiner by the patient or detected by the examiner at the time of physical examination. Nipple discharge may exhibit one of several colors, including white, clear, green, brown, black, and red. Galactorrhea may be distinguished from other types of nipple discharge by the presence of lipid-laden spheroids on microscopic examination of the discharge. Sudan red dye staining is not required for this test. When the diagnosis of galactorrhea is made, the patient should be reassured that an underlying breast malignancy is unlikely. The patient should be advised that an underlying endocrine disturbance such as hyperprolactinemia may exist.

Secretion of breast milk is galactorrhea. Postpartum lactation requires that the breast be primed during pregnancy by the hormones estradiol and progesterone, which stimulate growth of the ducts and alveoli within the breast. Stimulation by prolactin of epithelial cells lining the alveoli results in the synthesis and secretion of the milk proteins casein and α-lactalbumin. Although priming of the breast by estrogen and progesterone is usually required before breast milk is secreted, high levels of these hormones during pregnancy block prolactin from acting on the breast. After delivery, the levels of estradiol and progesterone fall, allowing prolactin to function unopposed. During full lactation, it is possible for a woman to produce 1000 mL of breast milk per day even with a normal prolactin level.

When galactorrhea is detected, it is appropriate to request that a plasma/serum prolactin level be drawn to determine if hyperprolactinemia is present. The chance of making a diagnosis of hyperprolactinemia for the patient with galactorrhea will depend on the menstrual cycle status. For individuals with galactorrhea who are menstruating, only 30% will be found to be hyperprolactinemic. For individuals with galactorrhea who are amenorrheic, the chance of detecting hyperprolactinemia will be approximately 70%.

Diagnosis of Hyperprolactinemia

Prolactin is a protein hormone secreted by lactotrophs in the anterior pituitary gland. Its existence in humans has been known only since 1971, when a radioimmunoassay to detect the presence of this hormone was developed. Prolactin is involved in many biologic activities, but its role in initiating and maintaining lactation is well known.

Prolactin levels vary in response to many pharmacologic and physiologic stimuli. Discrimination between an expected state of prolactin elevation and one that is unexpected is required before a diagnosis of pathologic hyperprolactinemia can be made. Sleep or ingestion of food at lunch or dinner but not breakfast will cause a rise in the prolactin level. Nipple or breast stimulation or chest wall irritation, such as in herpes zoster, will provoke a rise in prolactin. Controversy exists over whether a normal breast examination may induce transient hyperprolactinemia, with some authors reporting an effect and others reporting no effect. A rise in prolactin during the periovulatory interval at the time of the luteinizing hormone surge has also been reported, presumably resulting from gonadotropin-releasing hormone stimulation of pituitary lactotrophs. Physical and emotional stresses evoke rises in prolactin levels. Measurement of an elevated serum prolactin level on at least two different occasions under standardized conditions, as in a nonstressed individual during the follicular phase of menstrual cycle (if menses occur) who is fasting

and has been awake for over 2 hours, has been advised as a necessary requirement before making the diagnosis of hyperprolactinemia.

Evaluation of the Hyperprolactinemic Patient

Once hyperprolactinemia has been diagnosed, it is necessary to exclude drug ingestion, hypothyroidism, pregnancy, and hypothalamic-pituitary anomalies. A careful history is usually all that is required to exclude drug-induced hyperprolactinemia. Medications that diminish the hypothalamic release of dopamine, such as the antihypertensive agent methyldopa, or those that block dopamine receptors, such as the antiemetic metoclopramide, are capable of causing hyperprolactinemia. Thyrotropin-releasing hormone may stimulate pituitary prolactin release, so hypothyroidism should be excluded by measuring the serum thyrotropin-stimulating hormone (TSH) level. Measurement of a thyroxine level will be necessary if the TSH level is low, to exclude central hypothyroidism. Because pregnancy is a well known cause of hyperprolactinemia, a pregnancy test should always be obtained.

When drug ingestion, hypothyroidism, or pregnancy cannot explain hyperprolactinemia, the hypothalamus and pituitary gland should be imaged to exclude hypothalamic or pituitary lesions. A plain radiograph of the skull provides limited information, since only very large or calcified lesions will be seen. Use of computed tomography provides more information, but the patient is exposed to radiation in this test and normal variations of the bony sella have been mistaken for pituitary lesions using this method. Use of magnetic resonance imaging (MRI) without and particularly with contrast displays an exquisite anatomic view of the pituitary gland and hypothalamus. Small, noncalcified lesions may be diagnosed using this method and an accurate estimate of lesion size determined. Suprasellar expansion and encroachment on the optic chiasm can easily be determined.

The possibility of detecting a pituitary anomaly is significant, since approximately 10% of normal menstruating women will be found to have a small intrapituitary lesion on MRI. This is to be contrasted with a 40% chance of detecting a pituitary lesion if the prolactin concentration is elevated above normal. Reliance on a particular prolactin concentration, for example, 100 ng/mL, before ordering an imaging study is not advantageous. Verification of a prolactin concentration of any value above normal is the only requirement before requesting an imaging study. Should any abnormality be identified, its proximity to the optic chiasm should be determined. Patients with lesions not encroaching on the sella do not require visual field testing.

When a pituitary lesion is detected in a patient with hyperprolactinemia, an effort should be made to determine whether the lesion is directly or indirectly responsible for hyperprolactinemia. Lesions secreting hormones other than prolactin, such as growth hormone, gonadotropic hormones (luteinizing hormone or follicle-stimulating hormone), adrenocorticotropic hormone, or thyrotropin stimulating hormone will often disrupt the regulation of adjacent lactotrophs, causing simultaneous hyperprolactinemia.

To determine the true identity of a pituitary lesion in a hyperprolactinemic patient, screening tests for elevations of other pituitary hormones should be performed, as indicated in Table 1.

A discussion with the patient about the pituitary lesion identified by imaging should include reassurances that the patient does not have a "brain tumor." Prolactin-secreting lesions within the pituitary gland are almost always benign, as they do not exhibit nuclear or cytoplasmic atypia. These lesions do not metastasize, and, since they are not encapsulated, they should not even be called adenomas. Prolactin-secreting pituitary lesions are best described as exhibiting nodular hyperplasia. Use of the term "prolactinoma" to describe these lesions may be advantageous. If the pituitary lesion is less than 1 cm in diameter it is called a microadenoma, but if it is greater than 1 cm in diameter it is called a macroadenoma.

Management of the Hyperprolactinemic Patient

Once the hyperprolactinemic patient has been evaluated and obvious causes of hyperprolactin-

emia identified and treated, such as correction of hypothyroidism, management of this endocrine disturbance can commence. In general, management will be influenced by the following four variables: (1) presence or absence of a pituitary lesion, (2) desire to conceive, (3) concern about bone density and heart disease, and (4) ability to take prescribed medication. Hyperprolactinemic patients can be classified into four categories: (1) no evidence of pituitary lesion, pregnancy not desired, (2) no evidence of a pituitary lesion, pregnancy desired, (3) evidence of a pituitary lesion, pregnancy not desired, and (4) evidence of a pituitary lesion, pregnancy desired. Specific management recommendations will depend on the particular classification.

No Evidence of Pituitary Lesion, Pregnancy Not Desired

The hyperprolactinemic patient without a pituitary lesion who does not desire to conceive may be managed either by observation or by medical treatment. If the patient is observed without medical therapy, there is a 34% chance that the prolactin concentration may return to a normal value within 5 years. For hyperprolactinemic amenorrheic women, the consequences of hypoestrogenism in terms of reduced bone density and increased risk of heart disease should be included in the decision-making process.

Medical therapy to lower the prolactin concentration to normal values may be prescribed. Two drugs approved by the Food and Drug Administration (FDA) are available for this purpose. Bromocriptine (Parlodel, Sandoz Pharmaceuticals) is an ergot-derived dopamine agonist. It is a short-acting drug given daily either as a single tablet of 2.5 mg or as a 2.5 mg tablet given on a twice daily or three times daily schedule. Dosage of the medication should be titrated to the prolactin concentration. The majority of patients taking this drug will experience minor side effects such as nausea, dizziness, and nasal stuffiness. Some patients may experience orthostatic hypertension. After the initiation of drug therapy, ovulation may resume within 8 weeks after normalization of the prolactin level. Recently, another ergot alkaloid-derived drug, cabergoline (Dostinex, Pharmacia-Upjohn Co.) has become available. It is a long-acting dopamine agonist reported to cause fewer side effects. The starting dose of this drug is 0.25 mg given twice weekly with increasing doses up to 1 mg twice weekly as required to normalize the prolactin concentration. If the patient has difficulty tolerating either

---

TABLE 1. Screening Tests

Hormone Type	Test
Growth hormone	Elevated plasma insulin-like growth factor-1
Adrenocorticotropic hormone	Elevated 24-hour urinary free cortisol
Follicle-stimulating hormone, luteinizing hormone	Elevated levels as well as an elevated α subunit level
Thyrotropin-secreting hormone	Elevated level with elevated thyroxine level

medication taken orally, intravaginal administration of either drug may be attempted.

Estrogen replacement or oral contraceptive pill therapy has been recommended by some practitioners for hyperprolactinemic women who cannot tolerate or do not wish to take dopamine agonists. Estrogen may stimulate prolactin-producing cells within the pituitary, and the development of microadenomas and macroadenomas when none had existed before has been reported following estrogen therapy. Patients should be cautioned about this possible risk and monitored appropriately if estrogens are to be prescribed.

No Evidence of a Pituitary Lesion, Pregnancy Desired

For hyperprolactinemic patients desiring pregnancy, normalization of the prolactin level using a dopamine agonist is quite effective. Bromocriptine has been approved by the FDA as specific dopamine agonist treatment for infertility. Dostinex does not currently have this FDA approved indication, but it has been safely used for this purpose in Europe. Patients unable to tolerate dopamine agonists may be treated with other ovulation-inducing drugs, such as clomiphene citrate or menotropins. If pregnancy occurs, there is no need to monitor the patient by using pituitary imaging or visual field testing.

Prolactin measurements during pregnancy are not helpful since the prolactin level is normally quite elevated as a consequence of pregnancy.

Evidence of a Pituitary Lesion, Pregnancy Not Desired

When pituitary imaging discloses an anomaly, the existence of other hormone-producing adenomas or tumors within the gland should be excluded. Patients with prolactinomas that are microadenomas should be reassured that rapid growth of the lesion is unlikely. Periodic monitoring by MRI is recommended for patients with macroadenomas. Visual field testing is required only if the adenoma impinges on the optic chiasm.

These patients may be offered no therapy or treatment with dopamine agonists in a manner similar to that discussed for hyperprolactinemic patients without a pituitary lesion.

Evidence of a Pituitary Lesion, Pregnancy Desired

Excluding other hormone-producing lesions of the pituitary is essential. After this has been accomplished, the patient may be treated with dopamine agonists to lower the prolactin concentration or with ovulation-inducing drugs.

When pregnancy is diagnosed, dopamine agonist drug therapy should be discontinued, but not abruptly. Tapering the drug dosage is recommended to avoid adenoma infarction. Risk of pregnancy loss is not increased by discontinuing dopamine agonist therapy.

Visual field testing during each trimester of pregnancy, particularly if the patient has a macroadenoma, is helpful. If optic nerve compression is encountered, dopamine agonist therapy may be restarted. Prophylactic dopamine agonist therapy during pregnancy is not routinely recommended to avoid adenoma expansion. Delivery should be determined by obstetric indication.

Management of Galactorrhea

The patient with galactorrhea who has hyperprolactinemia should be managed similarly to the patient who has only hyperprolactinemia. Normalization of the prolactin concentration will usually be quite effective in causing cessation of galactorrhea.

For the patient with galactorrhea who has a normal prolactin concentration, reassurance is usually all that is required. These patients should be advised not to check themselves for nipple discharge, as nipple stimulation could perpetuate the galactorrhea. Dopamine agonist therapy may be attempted, but frequency and intensity of side effects are increased when dopamine agonist therapy is given to individuals with normal prolactin levels. The expense of medical therapy for euprolactinemic galactorrhea must also be considered.

Imaging of the pituitary gland for an individual with galactorrhea who has a normal prolactin level is not informative, as the chance of finding a pituitary anomaly in this situation is not increased. Periodic measurement of the serum/plasma prolactin level may be performed if galactorrhea persists. Measurement of serum/plasma insulin-like growth factor-1 to screen for acromegaly may be considered for patients with galactorrhea and a normal prolactin level, since growth hormone can also stimulate prolactin receptors.

Summary

Diagnosis of galactorrhea is possible by performance of a physical examination and microscopic inspection of any nipple discharge. Hyperprolactinemia is diagnosed by measurement of an elevated serum prolactin level. Galactorrhea and hyperprolactinemia may exist separately or together. When hyperprolactinemia is diagnosed, a careful medical history must be taken to exclude expected physiologic causes of hyperprolactinemia. Drug ingestion and hypothyroidism must also be excluded. If a cause for hyperprolactinemia cannot be readily found, imaging of the pituitary and hypothalamus by an MRI scan using contrast is advised. If a pituitary anomaly is detected, other hormone-producing tumors of the pituitary gland should be excluded. Treatment of the hyperprolactinemic patient will depend on the presence of a pituitary anomaly and the patient's desire to conceive. Dopamine agonist therapy with either Parlodel or Dostinex is available. Patients with galactorrhea and hyperprolactinemia should be treated using recommendations for the patient who only has hyperprolactinemia. Patients with galactorrhea who have a normal prolactin level rarely require further therapy.

Genital Prolapse

John O.L. DeLancey, MD

Prolapse of the pelvic organs is a distressing and debilitating condition that prevents many women from being as active as they would like. It involves protrusion of the vaginal walls through the urogenital hiatus, accompanied by descent of the urethra, bladder, uterus, cul de sac, and rectum. These displacements are often accompanied by functional problems such as urinary incontinence or difficulty with defecation. Each patient presents with a specific combination of defects in pelvic support and symptoms related to these defects. Therapy must, therefore, be targeted toward addressing the particular problems found in each individual woman.

Incidence

One in every nine American women will require surgery for pelvic organ prolapse. In addition, many women suffer from incontinence and prolapse but do not seek care for this problem. This is, therefore, a major health problem for women and one that deserves careful attention.

Pathophysiology

Pelvic organ prolapse is caused by a combination of pelvic floor muscle damage and injury to the endopelvic fascia. The constant action of the levator ani muscles lifts the pelvic organs and closes the urogenital hiatus. This activity protects the endopelvic fascia from the constant load placed on the pelvic connective tissue by the tremendous weight of the abdominal contents. Pelvic floor muscle damage caused by vaginal birth weakens the muscles and puts the ligaments at greater risk. A combination of age-related connective tissue loss and accumulated injury then leads to ligament failure and prolapse.

Stretching of the endopelvic fascia had long been thought to cause pelvic organ prolapse. It is now evident that connective tissue rupture rather than connective tissue stretching is responsible for causing prolapse. The specific location of this damage determines the type of prolapse that is present. At the uterine cervix and upper third of the vagina (Level I), there are relatively long vertically oriented fibers that suspend the genital tract from the pelvic side-walls. These fibers are clinically referred to as the cardinal and the uterosacral ligaments. Failure of these tissues results in uterine or vaginal apex prolapse. In the middle of the vagina, Level II, the vaginal walls are attached laterally. The pubocervical fascia of the anterior vaginal wall is attached laterally to the arcus tendineus fasciae pelvis, and the posterior rectal vaginal fascia is attached to the rectal pillars. Damage here results in cystocele or rectocele. In the distal third of the vagina, Level III, the vagina is fused with the surrounding structures, being attached to the medial margins of the levator ani muscle laterally, the perineal body posteriorly, and the urogenital diaphragm anteriorly. Damage in this region relates to poor support of the urethra and perineal body.

Classification

There are five areas where vaginal support defects occur. These defects result in the vagina and adjacent organs prolapsing downward under the force of abdominal pressure. Even though it is the support of the vagina and not the support of the adjacent organ (eg, bladder in cystocele) that is primarily at fault, it has become customary in America to discuss support loss by calling attention to the pelvic organ that has prolapsed. Support classification involves the regions of the vagina adjacent to the (1) urethra, (2) bladder, (3) vaginal apex or uterus, (4) posterior cul de sac, and (5) lower rectum. Success in treating pelvic organ prolapse comes from carefully determining which areas are damaged and by ensuring that this damage is repaired at the time of surgery.

The degree to which each element has prolapsed must also be graded. A variety of systems are currently in use and can be confusing because different degrees of prolapse may be designated as "moderate" or "II/III," for example. A simple description of the distance in centimeters that each element of the prolapse lies above or below the hymen is simple and unambiguous (eg, a cystocele that protruded 4 cm below the hymenal ring with the cervix 2 cm below and a normally supported rectum and cul de sac).

Diagnosis

Diagnosis of pelvic organ prolapse is made on physical examination. All abnormally supported areas can be detected only with the patient straining forcefully enough that the prolapse protrudes to its maximum extent. Although this can usually be done in the supine position, a standing examination may be necessary if the patient is unable to perform a strong enough Valsalva maneuver to cause the prolapse to protrude. Asking the patient how large her prolapse is when it is maximally extended allows the examiner to assess whether or not the full extent of the prolapse has been detected.

Once the prolapse is visible, each of the five areas of support must be individually assessed. The urethral carina occupies the lower 3 cm of the anterior vaginal wall. Because the urethra and vagina are fused, descent of the distal 3 cm of vagina reflects loss of urethral support. Examination of bladder base support that lies between the urethrovesical junction and the uterine cervix or vaginal apex is next determined. Next, the position of the cervix or vaginal apex is similarly assessed.

To evaluate the posterior vaginal wall, with the prolapse maximally developed, a rectal examination can be performed to trace the outline of the anterior rectal wall to see whether it protrudes below its normal position. Simultaneous vaginal and rectal palpation will detect the presence of the small intestine between the vagina and rectum, indicating an enterocele. It should be emphasized that this examination must be performed with the patient straining forcefully enough that the prolapse is maximally expanded.

With the woman supine and not straining, the small intestine may not occupy the posterior cul de sac, and therefore an enterocele could be missed.

In women who have previously undergone a hysterectomy, the location of the vaginal cuff should be carefully noted because the obvious landmark of the uterine cervix is no longer present to call attention to the loss of Level I support.

Symptoms

Discomfort from the distended vagina is the most characteristic symptom of pelvic organ prolapse. This causes a sense of pressure and pain that is often difficult for patients to describe. In addition, lower back pain resulting from traction of the supportive ligaments on their attachments to the sacrum is quite common. In certain individual women, urinary stress incontinence is present, and in the absence of stress incontinence, the patients may have urinary urgency and frequency because of the pressure that the cystocele exerts on the urinary trigone. Paradoxically, with large cystocele, urinary retention may occur, with elevated post-void residual urine volume or inability to urinate. Although difficulty with defecation is considered the hallmark of a rectocele, there is often little correlation between the size of a rectocele and the presence or absence of symptoms. There are no symptoms of enterocele other than the typical symptoms of prolapse.

When the prolapse is large, complications may arise. Ulceration of a large prolapse is not uncommon and may give rise to bleeding. Ureteral dilation with hydronephrosis is common in women with advanced uterine prolapse and can be diagnosed by having an intravenous pyelographic study performed with the patient in the standing position. Incarceration of the prolapse is a rare but serious event. This is occasionally associated with a bladder stone, or pelvic abscess, and these possibilities should be kept in mind when evaluating a woman with a prolapse that cannot be easily replaced into the pelvis. Infection of the exposed vagina does not occur in the absence of ulceration.

Treatment

Treatment of pelvic organ prolapse is indicated when patients are sufficiently symptomatic that they request relief from specific problems. It is not uncommon for women to seek medical advice because they have noted something protruding from the vaginal opening. Unless the prolapse is large (several centimeters below the hymen) treatment is not necessarily required. The prolapse can be monitored and treated if it becomes progressive. There is no particular advantage to repairing prolapse "before it gets any worse," since the success of repair does not seem to depend on the size of the prolapse when it is corrected.

Pessaries

For symptomatic women whose medical condition precludes surgery, or who prefer nonsurgical management, vaginal pessaries provide an effective treatment for pelvic organ prolapse. Pessaries come in a wide variety of shapes and sizes and practitioners typically become familiar with the use of small subset of these. Pretreatment of severe vaginal atrophy, with topical estrogen prior to pessary fitting, often increases the resistance of the vagina to erosion and helps the vagina tolerate the pessary. Gellhorn and doughnut pessaries are the most commonly used types. After the patient is fitted properly with a supportive pessary, she should be re-examined within the first week to make sure that the vagina is tolerating the pessary and then re-examined after a month. Once the absence of ulceration is confirmed, then re-examination is required less often.

Surgical Therapy

Surgical management must address each of the several defects that are present in any individual woman. A variety of techniques are available for each site, and the patient's pathologic anatomy as well as the surgeon's training and experience will guide the choice of operation.

When urethral support is defective, but stress urinary incontinence is not a problem, the endopelvic fascia is plicated under the urethra. Because urethral support loss is usually caused by detachment of the suburethral endopelvic fascia from the pelvic wall, care must be taken to achieve a wide enough dissection so that the tissues that remain attached at the inner surface of the pubic bone may be used for the fascial plication. If stress incontinence coexists with pelvic organ prolapse, the most successful treatment for this symptom is achieved with retropubic operations (eg, Marshall-Marchetti-Krantz, Burch, paravaginal repair). Of these, the paravag-

inal repair best corrects the coexistent cystocele in addition to correcting urethral support and stress incontinence. Needle suspension operations (Pereyra, Stamey, Raz) can be used with less morbidity than a retropubic operation, but the long-term results in curing stress incontinence are not as good. Plication of the endopelvic fascia can also be carried out and does cure stress incontinence in some women, but the results are inferior to retropubic and needle suspension procedures.

When a cystocele is present, the bulging of the anterior wall can be reduced by plicating the pubocervical fascia together under the midline of the bladder. When combined with a plication of the suburethral fascia and elevation of the vaginal cuff (which contains the upper margin of the pubocervical fascia), this decreases the sagging of the anterior vaginal wall. Alternatively, an abdominal or vaginal paravaginal repair can be used to reattach the pubocervical fascia to the arcus tendineus fasciae pelvis from which it has become detached.

Uterine prolapse is treated with a vaginal hysterectomy and elevation of the vaginal cuff. Because the vaginal cuff is pulled down with the uterine cervix, steps must be taken to elevate the vaginal cuff to a normal level. Simple removal of the uterus does nothing to accomplish this. Shortening the cardinal and uterosacral ligaments at the time of the hysterectomy, reattaching these shortened ligaments to the vaginal cuff, and placing a high McCall culdoplasty are the elements of the operation that successfully elevate the vaginal apex.

In women with vaginal vault prolapse following hysterectomy, suspending the vaginal apex is necessary when the vaginal apex lies below the level of the introitus. This can be accomplished by attaching the vaginal apex to the sacrospinous ligament or by sacral colpopexy. In this latter operation the vagina is attached to the sacrum by a synthetic mesh. High McCall culdoplasty and suspension to the iliococcygeus fascia are also effective treatments for vaginal prolapse.

Enteroceles form when the upper vagina is not in a position where abdominal pressure can push it against the rectum and levator plate. In this case, the peritoneum of the cul de sac becomes distended with bowel. Repair of an enterocele involves elevating the vaginal apex through one of the techniques previously described for treating uterovaginal prolapse and closing the peritoneal sac. This can be accomplished abdominally with purse string sutures that include the closure of the perineal sac and shortening of the uterosacral ligaments (Marion-

Moschcowitz culdoplasty) or with reefing sutures placed along the sagittal plane (Halban culdoplasty). The repair must not focus exclusively on the peritoneum. As is true in inguinal hernia, the peritoneal sac is the sign of the enterocele, not its cause. Restoring the normal mechanics of the cul de sac is the most important aspect of the operation.

Repair of a rectocele involves dissecting laterally within the rectal vaginal septum to grasp the separated edges of the endopelvic fascia and reconstructing the perineal body. This brings the diastasis of the levator ani muscles into closer proximity. Reconstruction of the perineal body to bring the separated edges of the urogenital diaphragm back together is also needed.

GIFT Procedure

Pasquale Patrizio, MD
Omid Khorram, MD, PhD

In recent years there has been extraordinary progress in the treatment of human infertility. GIFT, an acronym for *gamete intrafallopian transfer*, is one of the recently developed technologies for overcoming cases of long-term infertility in which the female partner has at least one normal, patent, and accessible fallopian tube. This procedure involves the direct placement of both gametes, sperm and oocytes, into the ampullary portion of the fallopian tubes, allowing fertilization to occur in vivo, at the site where it naturally occurs in humans.

The religious acceptance of GIFT has been a topic of debate. GIFT can be viewed as compatible with the teachings of Roman Catholicism and Halakhic Judaism. A widely held view in the Roman Catholic church is that GIFT would be acceptable provided the sperm was that of the husband and was not collected by masturbation but rather through a marital act with a condom perforated to retain some of the ejaculate while allowing a reasonable deposition of the remainder in the vaginal vault. Like Roman Catholicism, Halakhic Judaism condemns masturbation, and the preferred method of semen collection is from the vagina following intercourse. If this is impractical, then semen may be collected by the use of a condom.

Preliminary work-up required to determine if a couple is suitable for GIFT involves (1) proof of tubal patency either by hysterosalpingography or by laparoscopy, and (2) at least two semen analyses with preparation of the sample showing a recovery of greater than 1.5 million total motile sperm, with normal forms being greater than 30%.

Indications

The main indications for GIFT include (1) unexplained or idiopathic infertility, (2) pelvic endometriosis, (3) mild male factor infertility, (4) periadnexal adhesions, (5) failure of previous cycles of artificial insemination either by husband or donor, (6) cervical factors, (7) immunologic causes, and (8) premature ovarian failure in which oocyte donation is desired. Unexplained infertility and mild endometriosis encompass the vast majority of candidates for GIFT.

Preparation for GIFT

The following procedures are necessary in preparation for GIFT.

Controlled Ovarian Hyperstimulation

By inducing multiple follicular development, a greater number of oocytes than in a spontaneous cycle are obtained. Different therapeutic regimens are available to induce controlled ovarian hyperstimulation. The most frequently used regimen involves a combination of leuprolide acetate, an analogue of luteinizing hormone-releasing hormone, to suppress the pituitary, and the use of pure or recombinant follicle-stimulating hormone, and human menopausal gonadotropins to stimulate the ovaries.

Monitoring of Follicular Growth

Serial assays of plasma estradiol and serial transvaginal ultrasonography are used to assess and monitor the follicular development.

Human Chorionic Gonadotropin Administration

Human chorionic gonadotropin replaces the mid-cycle luteinizing hormone surge and is given when at least two follicles have attained a diameter of 18 mm and the serum estradiol levels are in the range of 250 to 350 pg/mL for each follicle.

Oocyte Retrieval

Thirty-six hours after the injection of 10,000 IU of human chorionic gonadotropin, the oocyte recovery is carried out. The follicular aspirations can be performed with a suction needle under transvaginal ultrasonographic guidance or by laparoscopy. If a laparoscope is used, it is placed through a subumbilical entry; a second entry site allows the passage of a grasping forceps to hold the utero-ovarian ligament, while a third entry is used for the suction needle. Once all the follicles have been aspirated, the oocytes retrieved are numbered and classified and the most mature are selected to be transferred.

Sperm Preparation

Two hours before a scheduled case of GIFT, the male partner produces a semen sample in a sterile container. After allowing time for liquefaction, the sample is examined for count, motility, and morphology, washed with culture medium to remove the seminal plasma, and finally, by a technique called "swim-up," the most motile fraction of sperm is obtained and used for the transfer.

Transfer of Gametes

The sperm and up to four of the most mature oocytes (two per fallopian tube) are loaded into a special catheter in the following order: aliquot of sperm—air space—two oocytes—air space—aliquot of sperm—air space. The presence of air spaces serves to avoid the mixing of the gametes in vitro. Once loaded, the tip of the catheter is inserted approximately 3 cm into the fimbriated end of the fallopian tube and the contents are gently injected. The same procedure is then repeated for the other tube.

In special cases, such as patients with only one fallopian tube or those in whom the accessibility of the tube is difficult, up to four oocytes can be transferred in one tube. When dealing with infertility due to male factor, a larger number of sperm (more than 500,000 per tube) are transferred to increase the chances of fertilization, whereas for other indications the number of sperm utilized is between 300,000 and 500,000 per tube.

After the gametes have been deposited into the ampullary portion of the fallopian tube, the catheter is returned to the laboratory, where it is examined to ensure that all the oocytes have been injected. More recently, hysteroscopy has been used to transfer the gametes into the fallopian tube. With this technique, CO_2 is used to distend the endometrial cavity. The gametes are loaded into the transfer catheter and fed into the fallopian tube through the operating channel to a depth of 2 to 4 cm. The CO_2 distension is then stopped, and the gametes are gently injected into the tube. Advantages of hysteroscopic GIFT are that it does not require general anesthesia or the operating room, thus reducing costs. Furthermore, it is viewed as a less invasive technique than laparoscopic transfer.

Luteal Phase Support

Although the need for supporting the luteal phase is still uncertain, 25 to 50 mg of progesterone in oil is given daily starting on the second day after surgery until the day of the pregnancy test 2 weeks later. If the patient is pregnant, the administration of progesterone is then continued for another 6 weeks.

Results

The GIFT procedure has an overall pregnancy rate of 33%. Pregnancy rates with hysteroscopic GIFT are comparable to those with laparoscopic GIFT according to some studies, and lower according to others. Currently there are no randomized prospective studies comparing the two methods of transfer. Success rates are also dependent on the etiology of infertility. In patients with unexplained infertility, mild endometriosis, or periadnexal adhesions, the pregnancy rate is 37%, whereas in the group with male infertility, the pregnancy rate is 17%. The apparently higher success rate of GIFT in the former cases could be related to the fact that the procedure overcomes possible mechanical deficiencies in the transport of the gametes to the site of fertilization, where there is a more natural environment. The most recent application of GIFT in patients with premature ovarian failure utilizing oocyte donation has yielded a pregnancy rate of 75%.

In cases of severe oligospermia or immunologic causes, the pregnancy rate is lower, possibly because of a reduced rate of fertilization in vivo of gametes that are somehow defective. In these cases and also in cases of previously failed GIFT attempts, a different approach, called tubal embryo transfer, is proposed. It represents a hybrid of the GIFT and in vitro fertilization procedures in which the fertilization of the gametes occurs in vitro and the resulting cleaving embryos are transferred to the fallopian tubes 44 to 48 hours later.

The importance of well-controlled ovarian hyperstimulation in the success of a GIFT procedure is well documented. The pregnancy rate when four mature preovulatory oocytes are transferred is 41%, versus 20% when immature oocytes are utilized.

The overall rate of spontaneous abortion after GIFT is 20% and the risk of ectopic pregnancy is 4%. When up to four oocytes are transferred, the incidence of multiple pregnancies is 28%. If more than four oocytes are replaced, the pregnancy rate is not increased; however, the chance of multiple pregnancy is higher.

Congenital malformations and genetic disorders may occur in less than 5% of live births. This rate is not significantly higher than that occurring in spontaneous pregnancy.

Conclusions and Future

The GIFT procedure has found definitive and worldwide recognition in the treatment of infertile couples. Today in the United States alone, approximately 130 centers of reproductive medicine offer the GIFT procedure as one of the main treatments for long-standing infertility.

The simplicity of this technique would suggest its widespread application. However, the following points should be evaluated carefully. First, centers offering GIFT should be prepared to offer in vitro fertilization and embryo transfer if unexpected problems such as impaired tubal accessibility should arise. Second, to increase the chances for future pregnancies, it will be of considerable benefit for the couple to have extra embryos frozen for use at a later date. Third, a program of oocyte donation will be helpful for patients with premature ovarian failure or patients who have undergone chemotherapy or who are carriers of chromosomal abnormalities.

The future is directed to a further simplification of the technique by transfer of gametes via cannulization of the fallopian tubes by a flexible hysteroscope or with a special catheter passed through the cervix and inserted in the isthmic portion of the tubes under ultrasonographic guidance.

Gonadal Dysgenesis

Paul McDonough, MD

Gonadal dysgenesis is represented by a relatively broad spectrum of clinical phenotypes. They all have in common the absence of the entire or a portion of the X-chromosome. These deleted or structurally abnormal X-chromosomes may be present as single cell lines (eg, 45,X, or 46,XXqi), or as mosaics (eg, 45,X/46,XX). Most individuals with X-chromosome aneuploidy are functionally agonadal from birth. When therapy is being considered, it is important to remember that 12% to 14% of these patients may have spontaneous puberty with brief or protracted menstrual lives and, rarely, pregnancy. Pregnancies have been reported in approximately 150 subjects with X-aneuploidy. Individuals with sex chromosome aneuploidy and gonadal failure are referred to in this text as having chromosomally incompetent ovarian failure (CIOF). The designation indicates that the condition is present at birth and is causally related to the privation or deletion of the X-chromosome. This serves to distinguish this group of patients from individuals with functional ovarian failure and normal peripheral blood karyotypes. The latter condition is referred to as chromosomally competent ovarian failure (CCOF) and has a heterogeneous etiology ranging from X-chromosome molecular mutations through autoimmune ovarian failure to multiple acquired causes (Table 1). Since the cytogenetic findings in the CCOF group are by definition normal 46,XX or rarely 46,XY (Swyer's syndrome), the clinical phenotype is consistently a normal or tall female.

Chromosomally Incompetent Ovarian Failure (X- and Y-Chromosome Aneuploidy)

Therapeutic considerations in the young prepubertal girl with X-chromosome aneuploidy revolve around two principal issues. A careful search should be made to identify cardiovascular-renal malformations that might benefit from surgical correction. The principal anomaly in this category is coarctation of the aorta and tricuspid aortic valve. Echocardiography should be part of the initial work-up and repeated at 3-year intervals. In recent years, otolaryngologic and plastic surgeons have been more aggressive in correcting the micrognathism and neck webbing that occurs in some patients with gonadal dysgenesis.

TABLE 1. Etiologies of 46,XX Ovarian Failure (Chromosomally Competent Ovarian Failure)

Molecular deletions of X-chromosome material
Single gene—autosomal recessive (familial)
Environmental factors
    Virus
    Radiation therapy
    Cytotoxic drugs
Autosomal abnormalities
Autoimmune disease (Schmidt's syndrome)
Infectious process
Myotonia dystrophica
Ataxia telangiectasia/DiGeorge syndrome
17-alpha-hydroxylase deficiency
Resistant ovary syndrome/Albright's
    osteochondrodystrophy
Kennedy's disease
Galactosemia
47,XXX usually with a cryptic 45,X cell line
    Non-mosaic 47,XXX probably do not develop
        ovarian failure

The second principal consideration is the risk for dysgenetic ridge tumor. The clear presence of a cytologically normal Y-chromosome in the karyotype (eg, 45,X/46,XY) dictates immediate prophylactic extirpation of the gonadal structures, usually streak gonads. Retention of the uterus is suggested so that the patient can still be a gestational mother through embryo transfer at some future date. If a sex chromosome fragment is present that cannot be clearly determined to be X or Y, then DNA studies are indicated. The most practical Y DNA probe for this purpose is one that is specific for Y centromeric sequences. The precise molecular or biochemical culprit in gonadal oncogenesis is currently unknown. The only common denominator in tumor subjects is the presence of Y DNA. No specific DNA sequences on Y, including the testicular determining region, have been incriminated to date. There is a locus on the long arm of the Y-chromosome, called gonadoblastoma on Y that seems to be consistently present in subjects with tumor formation. Since these fragments are mitotically stable, one can anticipate the retention of centromeric sequences regardless of the cytologic deformity of the Y fragment. One should also be aware of a growing trend to perform DNA screening on all 45,X gonadal dysgenesis subjects to exclude the presence of low-level mosaicism for Y-cell lines. This trend has received additional momentum with the automation of techniques to amplify the DNA sequences of a single cell by a factor of 10^6 in a matter of several hours. This technique, recently refined with a heat-stable copying enzyme, is called polymerase chain reaction (PCR). Gynecologists may identify or be referred more gonadal dysgenesis subjects for surgery in the future on the basis of these newer detection techniques for covert Y DNA. More recently, fluorescent in situ hybridization (FISH) with fluorochrome-labeled DNA probes for Y has been used to identify a chromosomal fragmental Y or to detect covert Y-chromosomes in resting interphase cells. Although this approach is frequently valuable in detecting cryptic Y-chromosomes, it is less sensitive than PCR amplification of a Y DNA sequence. Annual serum measurements of alpha-fetoprotein and human chorionic gonadotropin combined with pelvic imaging should be performed on all gonadal dysgenesis subjects who are at risk for dysgenetic tumor.

A growing area of debate in the unusually short prepubertal child with gonadal dysgenesis is the use of recombinant growth hormone or very low dose estrogen therapy. Children with gonadal dysgenesis who are even below the customary 5th to 10th percentile on linear growth charts require careful evaluation before these two therapeutic options are discussed. Systematic evaluation for rare associated deficits in growth hormone secretion, diabetes mellitus, Crohn's disease, renal failure, and primary hypothyroidism should be performed. Children with isochromosome for the long arm of X (Xqi) in single or multiple cell lines are almost universally prone to autoimmune thyroiditis with resultant primary hypothyroidism.

The empiric use of recombinant growth hormone therapy in gonadal dysgenesis subjects has met with only moderate success. This is not surprising, since growth hormone deficits have been identified infrequently in these children. The lack of dramatic results, prohibitive cost, and still uncertain long-term sequelae limit this drug to children with bona fide growth hormone deficiencies. The current cost of treating a 30 kg child with 9 mg per week is about $20,000 a year.

At the same time, two or three small studies suggest that small doses of ethinyl estradiol, 4 to 5 µg/day in a 40 kg girl or 100 ng/kg/day, may provide for gradual growth prior to puberty. In our experience, the former dose of ethinyl estradiol or Premarin 0.3 mg every third day does augment growth and, except for slight breast budding, is devoid of other estrogenic side effects. Care must be taken to titrate growth with growth velocity charts to be certain that the rate of growth is not excessive in the early stages leading to premature closure of epiphyses and further compromise of final height. Until long-term follow-up is achieved, it will be difficult to know whether the final resultant height in gonadal dysgenesis subjects is improved by either of these therapeutic modalities. Currently, these two therapeutic options should be considered only in prepubertal patients with gonadal dysgenesis who are unusually short for their age.

Once the child approaches chronologic age 8 to 9 years, serum follicle-stimulating hormone (FSH) and luteinizing hormone (LH) levels should be obtained. At this point, 90% of patients who are truly agonadal demonstrate elevations in serum gonadotropins consistent with ovarian failure. These measurements provide a screen to identify the 10% to 14% of patients who have sufficient residual ovarian function to experience spontaneous puberty and perhaps continued endocrine function. If the serum FSH and LH values at this time are not in the agonadal range, then continued follow-up and observation without therapy are indicated.

Elevated gonadotropins, on the other hand, clearly indicate ovarian failure. Substitution therapy should be initiated after obtaining baseline bone age, blood sugar, and lipid levels. Starting at chronologic age 9, one can initiate therapy with ethinyl estradiol, 4 to 5 µg or 100 ng/kg on a daily basis. These dose levels must be prepared by the pharmacist. An alternative to ethinyl estradiol is Premarin 0.3 mg every third day to continue for 2 years. The parameters of linear growth need to be followed on a growth velocity chart. At chronologic age 11 years, Tanner I breast budding becomes evident, and therapy can be increased to ethinyl estradiol 20 µg/day or Premarin 0.625 mg/day. If the pattern of growth spurt seen on the growth velocity chart is too accelerated compared with normal, then the dose of estrogen should be titrated downward. An attempt should be made to extend the steroid growth phase over a period of time that will ensure maximum final height. A rapid acceleration and deceleration of growth may compromise final adult height. Approximately 2 years after increasing the estrogen dosage to a standard Premarin 0.625 mg/day or its equivalent, one can begin to add 5 days of progestational agent each month. This regimen, with or without a further increase in estrogen dosage, usually brings about satisfactory sexual and somatic development. Maximum increases in sitting height are usually marked by the complete ossification, lateral to medial, of the iliac apophysis, which is seen on standard anteroposterior films of the pelvis. Once an adult female phenotype has been reached, bone centers are closed, and growth velocity is at zero, the patient is switched to a combined low-dose oral contraceptive, usually a 1/35 micro-

gram preparation. At that time the principal concerns center around endometrial neutralization and maintenance of bone density. These goals are achieved most effectively with this type of combined steroid preparation. Endometrial biopsies on these patients over time reveal little if any endometrial tissue when combined hormonal preparations of this type are used. An additional benefit for certain patients is consistent gonadotropin suppression and avoidance of ovarian cysts. Some subjects with gonadal dysgenesis who have residual secretory elements in the ovarian streak may experience painful ovarian cysts and breakthrough bleeding if erratic gonadotropin surges occur. These are more likely to occur with lower-dose triphasic and transdermal estrogen formulations. Gonadal dysgenesis subjects on long-term combined regimens should be monitored for hypertension and serum lipid alterations.

Occasionally, patients with gonadal dysgenesis may experience disproportionate development of the breast areola compared to the breast mound, or less than optimal breast size, on estrogen therapy. Augmentation mammoplasty has been very helpful in these patients as soon as it is apparent that this nonresponsive situation is present. Perhaps in the future studies of the estrogen receptor in genomic DNA may clarify the role of molecular mutation in this unique phenomenon of estrogen insensitivity.

In our experience, anabolic steroids have limited comparative value in the treatment of gonadal dysgenesis. Although their use is associated with similar increases in linear growth, they tend to augment weight gain. When they are given with estrogen, breast development and achievement of a feminine phenotype are delayed. Since they afford no advantage over estrogen for linear growth, their masculinizing and more pronounced anabolic effects may interfere with appropriate psychosexual development in some patients.

Probably one of the most important therapeutic points is early diagnosis and early therapy. A firm feminine psychosexual identity depends in part on reaching developmental landmarks at the same time as one's peers. Given current technology, this is possible for every young girl with gonadal dysgenesis. To date the only limitation of their genotype is the lack of exocrine function and consequently the inability to achieve genetic motherhood. Current techniques of assisted reproduction with donor oocytes provide the opportunity for gestational motherhood for women with sex chromosome aneuploidy.

The therapeutic aspects of aging in individuals with sex chromosome aberrations, specifically X and Y aneuploidy, are just becoming apparent. Apart from individuals with cardiovascular anomalies, there is increased evidence of labile hypertension starting in the fourth decade of life. The use of estrogen delivery systems that provide for liver bypass to avert increases in renin substrate have not been remedial. Consequently, oral steroid preparations are continued indefinitely in these individuals. The long-term follow-up of a sufficient number of gonadal dysgenesis subjects will take several more decades to see whether there are any unique aspects to aging in this patient population.

Chromosomally Competent Ovarian Failure

By definition, individuals with CCOF have high gonadotropins due to gonadal failure and normal intact 46,XX or, rarely, 46,XY karyotypes. Their phenotype is consistently female in appearance, except that 20% to 50% of these individuals may never experience spontaneous puberty. Unlike individuals with CIOF, these individuals are normal or tall in stature. Given this phenotype and the range of ovarian function, one may anticipate that the etiologies of 46,XX ovarian failure are diverse. With rare exceptions, therapy is substitutional in nature and similar regardless of whether the cause is genetic or acquired. Except for the 46,XY variety (Swyer's syndrome), the use of the term *gonadal dysgenesis* is something of a misnomer for this group of patients with diverse causes of ovarian failure. Except for a recently reported molecular mutation located on Xq segregating with 46,XX ovarian failure, genetic etiologies in this group may be much less frequent than was originally thought two decades ago.

Rare individuals with normal female phenotypes, normal müllerian systems, high serum gonadotropins, and sexual infantilism at puberty may turn out to have an intact peripheral blood karyotype that is 46,XY rather than 46,XX. Further studies are not necessary, but immediate prophylactic extirpation of both rudimentary streak gonads is indicated in the 46,XY Swyer's subject. The uterus and fallopian tubes may be left in place for assisted reproduction at a later date. Since the diagnosis cannot be suspected prior to puberty, endocrine substitution does not need to be graduated. After 1 to 2 years of a standard sequential regimen of estrogen and progestin, these patients are switched to a standard 1/35 oral contraceptive. Long-term follow-up is similar to that for CIOF; however, these individuals are not prone to complications of cardiovascular-renal anomalies or enigmatic labile hypertension. Unusually tall stature may be viewed by some as a complication of 46,XY Swyer's syndrome.

The vast majority of the chromosomally competent group have normal 46,XX karyotypes and are identified only at the time of pubertal arrest or later with secondary amenorrhea. The former group can be placed initially on a sequential regimen of 1.25 mg of Premarin daily, with superimposition of Provera 10 mg daily for the first 5 or 10 days of each calendar month. After sexual development is stabilized, they can be switched to a standard 1/35 steroid formulation to provide substitution therapy and maintain endometrial neutralization. Rare individuals in this group with residual secretory elements may develop a coordinated LH surge, ovulate, and become pregnant. This seems to occur more frequently when a "permissive" regimen of low-dose estrogen (Premarin 0.3 mg) is given. For those hoping for pregnancy, vigorous ovulation-induction regimens with human menopausal gonadotropin and clomiphene citrate have been less successful than low-dose estrogen and serendipity.

Dysgenetic tumors almost never occur in this group, but one must still provide careful periodic pelvic examination. A Sertoli-Leydig cell tumor producing alpha-fetoprotein occurred in 46,XX patients with ovarian failure several years ago. Until the molecular basis for oncogenesis in these subjects is understood, prudent periodic surveillance is the best management.

The precise etiology of 46,XX ovarian failure is most frequently obscure, and specific therapy is not available. In some subjects there may be associated autoimmune disorders, especially thyroiditis requiring therapy. All 46,XX ovarian failure subjects should have thyroid studies, prolactin level assessment, blood sugar assessment, and a serum cortisol drawn initially. They should be monitored periodically to identify the development of a potential multiple endocrinopathy, such as polyendocrinopathy II (Schmidt's syndrome). Resumption of menses and pregnancy has been reported with prednisone therapy in some subjects with presumed autoimmune oophoritis. Subjects with 46,XX ovarian failure and an enzymatic block in 17-hydroxylation have somewhat elevated serum gonadotropins and secretory type of ovarian failure. Such subjects theoretically may have restoration of normal ovarian endocrine and exocrine function with adrenal substitution therapy. Other diverse and rare causes of CCOF such as galactosemia, myotonic dystrophy, viral infections, chemotherapy, and radiation therapy should receive the same type of replacement therapy long term and "permissive" expectant low-dose estrogen therapy if pregnancy is a desired goal.

The therapeutic approach to gonadal dysgenesis over the past decade has been augmented by the development of probes for Y DNA, gene amplification techniques (PCR), FISH and the varied techniques of assisted reproduction. It is possible that before the year 2000, new proteins manufactured by recombinant DNA technology may provide an approach to the stature problem in gonadal dysgenesis that is uniquely beneficial.

Herpes Genitalis

David A. Baker, MD

Genital herpes is one of the most common sexually transmitted viral diseases in the United States. It is estimated that 500,000 new cases of genital herpes occur in the United States each year, and serologic data suggest that 45 million persons are infected with herpes simplex virus (HSV-2) in the genital tract. Newer information is becoming available concerning viral transmission, shedding of virus either with symptoms or without symptoms (asymptomatic shedding), and the clinical course of this disease. Eighty-five percent of genital herpes is caused by HSV Type 2 and 15% is caused by HSV Type 1. It is impossible to differentiate on clinical grounds which type of virus is infecting the genital tract, and in most clinical situations this is not an important fact to determine. HSV-1 can infect the genital tract (15% of cases), but individuals who have HSV-1 in the oral cavity do not acquire genital infection with Type 1 virus. In addition, HSV-2 is rarely found in the oral cavity in immunocompetent patients.

Epidemiology and Diagnosis

Asymptomatic acquisition of genital herpesvirus occurs in approximately 25% of patients infected with this disease in the United States. In addition, once an individual acquires this infection, the virus becomes dormant and there is a pattern of recurrent disease. Recurrent disease can be symptomatic, whereby there is a clinical lesion with viral shedding, or, as has been demonstrated in several papers, can be asymptomatic or subclinical, whereby the individual sheds virus from the genital tract without any clinical lesions.

Much of the diagnosis of genital herpes relies on clinical examination and the clinical recognition of a herpetic lesion in the genital tract. It is clear that genital herpes is the most common ulcerative sexually transmitted disease (STD) in the United States. It is clear, however, that relying solely on clinical examination, looking for classic vesicular and ulcerative lesions, would underdiagnose genital herpes. In those patients who give a history of genital herpes from a large group of randomly selected women attending a sexually transmitted disease clinic, characteristic ulcerations of the genital tract were present in only two thirds of women with positive HSV cultures. One third of women had atypical genital lesions or were shedding virus symptomatically and did not present with any clinically recognizable disease.

Transmission

Patients acquire genital herpes when they become sexually active, and 80% of patients with their first episode of genital herpes are between 18 and 36 years of age. In women, the highest annual incidence of genital herpes is in the age group of 20 through 24. In a population of women of reproductive age, approximately 5% will give a history of having genital herpesvirus infection. However, upwards of 30% of the population is seropositive for HSV-2 using type-specific antibody testing. The symptomatic patient with genital herpes is just the "tip of the iceberg" compared with the total number of individuals who are seropositive. From 65% to 90% of seropositive persons may be unaware of their infection. Newer epidemiology clearly shows a significant association with genital herpes and the age of the patient, years of sexual activity, race, one or more episodes of other genital infections, lower annual family income, and multiple sexual partners. Therefore, any patient who has or is diagnosed as having genital HSV needs to have testing for other STDs, including human immunodeficiency virus (HIV), and needs to be counseled in safe sex practices.

Once a patient acquires genital herpes, this disease will become latent and the patient will have symptomatic or asymptomatic recurrent disease. There is a direct correlation between an initial symptomatic HSV primary genital infection and the patient's having symptomatic recurrences. About 35% of such patients who have a primary symptomatic HSV infection will have frequent recurrences (more than six per year) of genital herpes.

New data have been reported about asymptomatic herpesvirus shedding. This is defined as the isolation of infectious herpesvirus from the genital tract in the absence of clinical lesions. This has been reported to be a significant factor in the natural history and transmission of herpes. In addition, it has been found to be more frequent in the first 3 months after primary infection. Several studies have clearly documented asymptomatic shedding in patients who give a history of genital herpes. Asymptomatic shedding is clearly directly related to the frequency of sampling (days in which cultures are obtained) and adversely related to the time since the onset of the first episode of genital herpes. In a large study in which cultures were taken every 4 to 6 weeks from patients who were infected with either HSV-1 or HSV-2 in the genital tract, asymptomatic cervical shedding was three times more frequent during the first 3 months after the resolution of the primary HSV-2 infection. Among patients with Type 2 infection in the genital tract, previous HSV-1 antibody was associated with a lower rate of asymptomatic vulvar shedding. After primary HSV-1 infection, asymptomatic reactivation occurred in approximately 12% of women. However, after primary HSV-2 infection, it occurred in over 18% of women sampled. In patients who had nonprimary, first-episode genital HSV-2, recurrent disease occurred symptomatically in almost 23% of patients.

It must be emphasized that current commercially available tests cannot differentiate between HSV Type 1 and Type 2 antibodies. Therefore, testing patients with insensitive antibody assays is not clinically useful at this time. The seroepidemiologic data reported here are from studies in which type-specific antibody testing was used.

Primary infection of genital herpes has a short incubation period of approximately 6 days. In the 75% of patients with symptomatic primary infection, there can be numerous genital lesions covering much of the perineum. Patients will present to a health care provider, usually within 4 to 6 days after the onset of symptoms, and complain of significant local pain, burning and irritation, dysuria, and systemic symptoms of low-grade fever, myalgia, and fatigue. Numerous published reports clearly show the benefit of antiviral therapy in the treatment of primary genital herpes. As with other viral infections, therapy initiated at the earliest possible time gives the greatest therapeutic benefit. Current therapy for primary genital herpes is acyclovir 200 mg five times a day for 10 days. Numerous studies clearly show that different dosage schedules can be used; one that may be more acceptable to patients is 400 mg three times a day for 10 days. This therapy shortens the duration of primary infection, reduces pain, markedly reduces viral shedding, and significantly shortens time to healing of lesions. It must be clearly emphasized that antiviral therapy for primary genital herpes does not alter the natural history of this disease, nor does it alter the chances of recurrent disease. Numerous antiviral agents have been shown to be as effective as acyclovir in treating primary infection with a less frequent dosing schedule, including valacyclovir and famciclovir.

Patients who present with genital herpes need extensive counseling and education concerning this disease entity. In the majority of patients who will experience recurrent disease, this can be not only a medical but also a psychological problem, and these two aspects need to be addressed by the clinician. The patient needs to be fully informed of the associated problems of transmitting genital herpes as well as the risks of contracting other STDs. There is a clear indication to test the patient with HSV for chlamydia, gonorrhea, human papillomavirus, and syphilis. In addition, numerous studies show that there is an association between having the antibody to HSV-2 and acquiring HIV. Therefore, all patients with the diagnosis of genital herpes should be encouraged to have HIV testing.

Therapy

The clinician has several options in managing patients with genital herpes. Newer information shows that symptomatic and asymptomatic shedding after primary infection can be significant within the first 3 months after acquisition of genital HSV. In addition, asymptomatic shedding will decrease after the first 2 years from the acquisition of primary infection.

Antiviral therapy has been shown to be effective and safe in treating recurrences of genital herpes and suppressing outbreaks of recurrent genital herpes. Acyclovir is the first drug shown to be safe and effective in treating genital HSV, and, because the drug requires activation by a viral thymidine vinase, it has little or no effect on noninfected cells. Over more than a decade, numerous preclinical and clinical studies have proved the safety of acyclovir in the therapy of genital herpes. The medication is safe and well tolerated, with minimal side effects, and has been shown to change the course of this disease for many patients. Currently, oral therapy is recommended for the treatment of genital herpes in most patients. Topical therapy is cumbersome, and significantly less effective and should not be used to treat genital disease. The clinician needs to assess the patient with primary infection who has severe disease or has some underlying immunocompromising condition (uncontrolled diabetes, on steroid therapy) who may require intravenous acyclovir therapy and hospitalization. Perineal hygiene needs to be considered in that there is a risk of superimposed bacterial infections of the genital area with *Streptococcus* and *Staphylococcus* bacteria. Therapy for each recurrence can be used in treating genital herpes. This therapy has been shown to be safe and effective but does not stop or prevent the outbreaks or recurrences.

It is usually recommended that therapy be patient-initiated (the patient should have medication available when the first signs of recurrent disease appear) and that the medication be taken in a dose of 200 mg five times a day for 5 days. However, a dosing regimen of 400 mg three times a day for 5 days seems to have better patient compliance. Numerous studies of this therapeutic regimen have shown that there is a shortening of the recurrence with decreased viral shedding. It must be emphasized, however, that this form of therapy does not prevent recurrent disease.

Long-term daily suppressive therapy has been shown to be safe and highly effective in suppressing genital herpes. Numerous reports from the United States, Canada, and Europe show that daily oral doses of acyclovir at 400 mg twice a day can significantly reduce recurrent disease in a patient with frequent outbreaks of genital herpes. The clinician needs to select patients who would benefit from suppressive therapy. The medical condition and severity of recurrent disease are important in the assessment of patients. The clinician needs to take into consideration the psychological and social impact of this viral STD in the therapy of patients. Recent reports on long-term suppressive therapy show that long-term therapy is safe. The major side effects of acyclovir therapy are headache, nausea, and some dizziness. These are usually mild and transient, and patients usually do not discontinue medication because of them. In a long-term study in more than 1100 men and women with frequent recurrences of genital herpes, suppressive therapy with acyclovir 400 mg twice a day significantly reduced outbreaks from more than 12 recurrences per year to less than one recurrence, with patients maintained on medication over 3 to 5 years. Newer data reported in abstract clearly show that suppressive therapy can be extended for upwards of 10 years and be effective and well tolerated. Patients can be informed that while on suppressive therapy they have a 50% to 70% chance of not having any recurrent disease. If they have a recurrence, it is usually mild and transient. Approximately 3% of patients will require a higher dose of acyclovir than the initial dose of 400 mg twice a day to suppress their recurrent disease.

Other antiviral agents have been approved for the treatment of episodic recurrent genital herpes. Valacyclovir is an ester of acyclovir that has significantly greater bioavailability and, when absorbed through the gut, is identical to acyclovir in the serum. The dosage for treating episodic therapy is 500 mg twice a day. Therefore, the same safety and efficacy can be obtained in a drug with a less frequent dosing schedule. Famciclovir has also been approved for episodic therapy. There is less information about this drug.

Herpes in Pregnancy

The majority of babies who contract neonatal herpes are borne by mothers who did not give the clinician a history of herpes prior to delivery. In addition, the emphasis in observing only those patients who give a history of genital herpes misses the major population of patients with genital HSV disease. Current recommendations fall short in the prevention of neonatal disease. It is clear that the patient who has a visible clinical lesion when in labor requires a cesarean section. This is the case regardless of the time of ruptured membranes, but consideration needs to be given to the time at which delivery will be accomplished. Certainly, if the patient presents in active labor well into the course of her labor with an imminent delivery, vaginal delivery is appropriate, with subsequent prophylactic therapy of the newborn. However, if the patient is early in labor with a visible herpetic lesion, cesarean delivery is indicated.

There is a developing body of information concerning herpes in pregnancy. It suggests that managing the patient only by observation without the use of culturing and perhaps serologic testing is not adequate to decrease the incidence of this severe neonatal disease. In patients who give histories of genital herpes, it is clear that asymptomatic shedding will occur in about 1% of women while they are in labor. However, in a population of randomly selected women, asymptomatic shedding occurs in approximately 3 per 1000 women who are in labor. Therefore, these babies are at risk of developing neonatal herpes even though mother has no clinical history and there are no clinical signs or symptoms that she is shedding infectious virus. Viral culture in labor may be a useful tool when applied to a select population, such as those individuals who give a history of recurrent disease.

Obtaining culture samples from all women in labor still requires further study. Taking a culture from the newborn directly after delivery has not been shown to be predictive of which babies will develop neonatal herpes. Further studies need to be performed to determine whether culture sampling of the baby on the first or second day of life may be predictive of the development of neonatal disease, as well as whether using other, more sophisticated tests such as polymerase chain reaction may be helpful. Type-specific HSV-2 serology may have a role in determining which patients are at risk for shedding virus while in labor. The use of antiviral medications is indicated in pregnancy in women with genital HSV disease. Acyclovir, valacyclovir, and famciclovir are not approved for use in pregnancy. A study with acyclovir used in the first trimester did not show any increased incidence of congenital anomalies or neonatal problems. Therefore, treatment of all patients with primary genital herpes in pregnancy with acyclovir or valacyclovir is suggested. In addition, because of the incidence of asymptomatic and symptomatic shedding, suppressive therapy for patients with primary infection until their delivery is indicated.

Results of initial studies of the use of suppressive acyclovir therapy in the last 4 weeks of pregnancy are being reported. Certainly, more detailed studies need to be performed to determine whether suppressive therapy can reduce the incidence of cesarean delivery, decrease the incidence of symptomatic and asymptomatic shedding and decrease neonatal herpes. The current recommended dose of acyclovir is 400 mg three times a day. Care needs to be taken in the selection of patients for this therapy and in obtaining consent from these patients. In addition, it must be realized that with suppressive therapy there can still be viral shedding, and therefore the pregnant women is still at risk for having a baby with neonatal herpes.

Hypopituitarism

Janice Andreyko, MD

Hypopituitarism is defined as a deficiency of one or more of the pituitary hormones, either from the anterior or posterior pituitary gland. Panhypopituitarism refers to generalized anterior pituitary insufficiency. Presenting symptoms reflect the specific hormone deficiency as well as the severity and duration of the deficiency. Causes of hypopituitarism are listed in Table 1. In adults, the most common causes are a mass lesion in the pituitary (eg, tumor or infiltrating or inflammatory disease), head trauma with a pituitary stalk-section effect, or pituitary radiation. In the postpartum woman who presents with lack of lactation, one must consider pituitary necrosis (Sheehan's syndrome) or lymphocytic adenohypophysitis. Most causes of pituitary insufficiency affect the hormones of the anterior pituitary. The posterior pituitary, which is responsible for antidiuretic hormone (ADH) and oxytocin production, is less vulnerable, since the cell bodies of the neurons lie in the hypothalamus. The anterior pituitary depends on trophic hormones reaching it via the portal circulation and is thus more vulnerable if this blood supply is interrupted.

Patients with destructive lesions of the anterior pituitary may lose the anterior pituitary hormones in a serial manner, often beginning with

---

TABLE 1. Causes of Hypopituitarism in Adults

Pituitary adenomas
Brain tumors, eg, craniopharyngioma, meningioma, glioblastoma, cholesteatoma
Metastatic carcinoma
Autoimmune adenohypophysitis (especially postpartum)
Sheehan's syndrome (postpartum pituitary necrosis)
Granulomatous disease, eg, sarcoidosis, tuberculosis, Wegener's granulomatosis
Aneurysm or arteriovenous malformation
Head trauma
Surgical or radiation injury to pituitary/hypothalamus
Hemochromatosis
Kallmann's syndrome (congenital follicle-stimulating hormone and luteinizing hormone deficiency with anosmia)
Noonan's syndrome (congenital)
Laurence-Moon-Bardet-Biedl syndrome (congenital)
Myotonic dystrophy
Idiopathic (sometimes associated with empty-sella syndrome)

growth hormone (GH), then luteinizing hormone (LH) and follicle-stimulating hormone (FSH). Thyroid-stimulating hormone (TSH) and adreno-corticotropic hormone (ACTH) are affected later. The exception to this is postpartum lymphocytic hypophysitis, in which there is a preference for destruction of ACTH and TSH secreting cells initially. It is extremely important to recognize symptoms of deficiencies of these hormones, particularly since the thyroid and adrenal glands are so important for homeostasis and loss of these hormones can be fatal.

Other presenting symptoms of hypopituitarism may have to do with the presence of a mass lesion, and thus a patient may complain of headaches or of visual loss. Loss of peripheral vision may be detected only on specific testing (Goldmann's fields), indicating compression of the optic chiasm.

In adults, GH deficiency may be associated with decreased muscle strength and exercise capacity, increased abdominal adiposity, impaired psychological well-being, reduced bone density, and elevated total and low-density lipoprotein cholesterol. Prolactin deficiency causes inability to initiate or maintain lactation in the postpartum period. There are no known symptoms of prolactin deficiency in men.

Deficiency of LH and FSH in women is associated with loss of ovarian function, which results in amenorrhea, hot flushes, loss of bone density, and of course infertility. In Kallmann's syndrome (isolated congenital gonadotropin deficiency) patients may also report anosmia due to olfactory nerve hypoplasia. Men experience decreased libido and impaired spermatogenesis. The differential diagnosis of isolated FSH and LH deficiency in women also includes systemic disease, severe weight loss (as seen in anorexia nervosa), and hyperprolactinemia. Severe stress or very vigorous exercise, both of which are associated with increased endorphin levels, may also be associated with FSH and LH suppression and amenorrhea.

Hypothyroidism is associated with cold intolerance, decreased energy, constipation, dry skin, bradycardia, weight gain, and eventually mental torpor. Adrenal insufficiency results in fatigue, hypotension, nausea, vomiting, and loss of axillary and pubic hair.

Posterior pituitary insufficiency with decreased ADH production causes diabetes insipidus, with polydipsia, polyuria, and nocturia. Urine osmolality cannot be concentrated above plasma osmolality. If polyuria is severe, urine output may be more than 6 L per 24 hours.

Diagnosis

Laboratory evaluation should include baseline serum levels of pituitary hormones (FSH, LH, TSH, prolactin, GH, ACTH), morning and evening cortisol, and estradiol. Since low levels of these hormones can be within normal limits, provocative testing should be performed to assess pituitary reserve and confirm the diagnosis of hypopituitarism. The hypothalamic releasing hormones are used for this purpose. This testing should be done under the supervision of an endocrinologist. The patient fasts overnight and an intravenous line is placed to administer the trophic hormones. Venous blood samples of the anterior pituitary hormones are drawn twice prior to and usually 20, 40, 60, 90, and 120 minutes after injection of the trophic hormones. These tests are summarized in Table 2. In a normal patient, there will be a significant rise in the pituitary hormone levels in serum in response to the boluses of trophic hormones; in a patient with pituitary failure this rise will not occur, thus helping to establish the diagnosis of hypopituitarism.

It is extremely important, particularly in a postpartum female with hypopituitarism, to perform radiologic imaging of the pituitary by magnetic resonance imaging (MRI). This valuable tool allows differentiation of a pituitary tumor from lymphocytic adenohypophysitis. With hypophysitis, there is diffuse homogeneous contrast enhancement, as opposed to the mass lesion one sees with a tumor.

Treatment

Management of hypopituitarism is determined by its cause and by the extent of pituitary compromise. If postpartum lymphocytic adenohypophysitis is diagnosed, there have been some reports of the beneficial action of corticosteroids in this condition, and there has also been evidence of spontaneous resolution. These patients, though treated with hormone replacement, should be periodically re-evaluated for return of pituitary function and resolution of abnormalities on MRI scanning.

Pituitary hormones are not practically available for replacement therapy, so treatment of hypopituitarism consists of supplying replacement doses of end-organ hormones (Table 3). The two most critical for sustaining life are cortisol and thyroxine. A patient in addisonian crisis (hypotension, nausea, vomiting) should be given intravenous or intramuscular cortisone acetate

TABLE 2. Diagnostic Testing for Suspected Hypopituitarism in Women

Provocative Test	Dose	Rationale
Gonadotropin-releasing hormone (GnRH)*	100 µg IV bolus	Stimulates LH, FSH secretion
Corticotropin-releasing hormone (CRH)*	1 µg/kg IV bolus	Stimulates ACTH, cortisol secretion
Growth hormone–releasing hormone (GHRH)*	1 µg/kg IV bolus	Stimulates GH secretion
Thyrotropin-releasing hormone (TRH)*	200 µg IV bolus	Stimulates TSH, prolactin secretion
Insulin tolerance test	0.1 U/kg regular insulin IV	Stimulates ACTH, cortisol secretion by inducing hypoglycemia, used when CRH unavailable
Metyrapone test	750 mg PO q4h for 6 doses	Blocks 11-β-hydroxylase in the cortisol synthesis pathway, causing an elevation in ACTH and increased secretion of 11-deoxycortisol and urinary 17-hydroxycorticosteroids
Dehydration test	Water deprivation followed by vasopressin 5 U SC	A deficiency of antidiuretic hormone will result in failure to concentrate urine osmolality greater than plasma osmolality

ACTH, adrenocorticotropic hormone; FSH, follicle-stimulating hormone; GH, growth hormone; LH, luteinizing hormone; TSH, thyroid-stimulating hormone.
*These hypothalamic releasing hormones can be given simultaneously.
Modified from Liu JH: Hypopituitarism. In Zuspan FP, Quilligan EJ: Current Therapy in Obstetrics and Gynecology, 4th ed. Philadelphia: WB Saunders, 1994.

TABLE 3. Hormone Replacement Regimens

Deficient Hormones	Replacement Hormones	Doses
FSH, LH	Estrogen, progestin	Micronized 17-β-estradiol 1–2 mg daily PO or conjugated equine estrogens 0.625–1.25 mg daily with medroxyprogesterone acetate either 10 mg/day × 12 days each month or 2.5 mg daily
ACTH	Cortisol	Cortisone acetate 20 mg q AM, 10 mg q PM or prednisone 5 mg q AM, 2.5 mg q PM
TSH	Thyroxine	L-thyroxine 0.05 mg/day. Increase by 0.05 mg q 2 weeks until euthyroid. Maintenance dose usually 0.15 to 0.20 mg/day
Prolactin, GH		Routine replacement not required
Vasopressin	Arginine vasopressin	DDAVP, 2–4 μg/day SC or IV in two divided doses, or 0.1–0.4 mL/day intranasally as a single dose or in two to three divided doses

ACTH, adrenocorticotropic hormone; FSH, follicle-stimulating hormone; GH, growth hormone; LH, luteinizing hormone; TSH, thyroid-stimulating hormone.
Modified from Liu JH: Hypopituitarism. In Zuspan FP, Quilligan EJ: Current Therapy in Obstetrics and Gynecology, 4th ed. Philadelphia: WB Saunders, 1994.

100 mg, then 50 mg q 6 hours until stabilized. The dose is then tapered until a maintenance dose is reached, usually 20 mg of cortisone acetate each morning and 10 mg each evening. The patient should carry a Medicalert bracelet, and, for illnesses not requiring hospitalization, the patient should triple the usual replacement dose. The patient should see a physician within 3 days, especially if nausea or vomiting occurs.

Thyroxine is replaced as levothyroxine, starting at 0.05 mg/day. The dose is increased by 0.05 mg every 2 weeks until the patient is clinically euthyroid and serum thyroxine is in the normal range. Most patients require doses of 0.15 to 0.20 mg per day. Prolactin and growth hormone do not routinely require replacement in adults. Some recent studies have used biosynthetic human GH replacement in adults. GH replaced as a once-daily subcutaneous injection has been reported to improve psychological well-being and exercise capacity in GH deficient adults. Some investigators believe that all adults with GH deficiency should be considered for biosynthetic GH replacement therapy. This has not yet been applied in routine practice.

In women with gonadotropin deficiency, hormone replacement therapy is the equivalent to that used in menopause, and for the same reasons—to treat hot flushes, to prevent osteoporosis, to reduce the risk of cardiovascular disease, and to prevent genital atrophy. Estrogen must be administered with a progestin in women with an intact uterus, to prevent endometrial hyperplasia and carcinoma. The progestin may be given on an intermittent basis (eg, 12 days of the calendar month) or on a continuous basis.

If a woman with gonadotropin deficiency wishes to conceive, follicle development may be induced with human menopausal gonadotropins (Pergonal, Humegon), which are the hormones FSH and LH. Once mature follicles are seen on ultrasonogram and serum estradiol levels are appropriate for the number of mature follicles seen, ovulation is induced by human chorionic gonadotropin (hCG; 5000 or 10,000 IU), which binds to LH receptors on the ovary and triggers ovulation. In these patients, there is no pituitary LH support to the corpus luteum after ovulation, so luteal support should be given. This may be in the form of three times per week hCG injections (1500 IU), progesterone injections 25 mg daily, progesterone vaginal suppositories 50 mg twice daily, or progesterone vaginal gel (Crinone, 8%) once daily. If the patient conceives, placental hCG will support the corpus luteum, but it is helpful to continue the luteal support until 9 weeks' gestation, at which time the placenta is self-sufficient in progesterone production.

Finally, in the patient with posterior pituitary insufficiency who is hypernatremic and not drinking, treatment consists initially of intravenous fluids, usually 0.45 N NaCl. Electrolytes, blood pressure and weight should be carefully monitored. Parenteral arginine vasopressin (DDAVP) may be tried empirically at doses of 1 to 2 μg (4 μg/mL) every 8 to 24 hours. For chronic treatment, DDAVP may be administered as a nasal spray 0.05 mL to 0.2 mL twice daily.

Hysteroscopic Evaluation and Therapy of Müllerian Anomalies

Eli Reshef, MD

Joseph S. Sanfilippo, MD

Congenital anomalies of the müllerian tract affect 0.5% to 3% of women. While most of these anomalies are not clearly associated with failure to conceive, some are related to an increased incidence of pregnancy loss. It is important to discern which anomalies are relevant to poor obstetric outcome, so that appropriate surgical correction, if indicated, can be performed. One should keep in mind that the mere presence of an anomaly, even one that is categorically associated with poor obstetric outcome, does not necessarily indicate future reproductive failure. However, those patients with müllerian anomalies who experience repetitive pregnancy losses are very likely to experience further losses and are candidates for surgical intervention. The incidence of müllerian anomalies in women who habitually abort is approximately 15%, the majority of which are due to the presence of a uterine septum. These patients will derive the most benefit from surgical correction.

Diagnosis and Evaluation

Clinical clues to the presence of müllerian anomalies can be obtained from the history and the physical examination. A history of two or more first- or second-trimester pregnancy losses is suggestive of the presence of a septate or bicornuate uterus. Menstrual irregularities often accompany other müllerian anomalies such as uterus didelphys with obstructed hemivagina or diethylstilbestrol (DES)-associated abnormalities. Amenorrhea, especially if primary, is often associated with congenital absence of the vagina and uterus (Meyer-Rokitansky-Kuster-Hauser syndrome). Maternal DES exposure is related to vaginal adenosis, narrow, deformed, and polypoid uterine cavity (often T-shaped), and various fallopian tube abnormalities. Pelvic pain and dysmenorrhea are common symptoms of endometriosis, which is quite often noted in women with müllerian anomalies, especially of the obstructive type.

On physical examination, absence of the vagina can be readily detected. The presence of vaginal skin tags or a septum is highly suggestive of associated uterine anomalies such as septate, bicornuate, or didelphic configuration. A pelvic mass is often palpated in postpubertal patients with obstructive vaginal or uterine anomalies, representing hematocolpos or mucocolpos, hematometra, hematosalpinx, or an endometrioma.

A hysterosalpingogram (HSG) is useful in outlining the endometrial cavity and evaluating tubal patency in patients with nonobstructed müllerian anomalies. The most common anomalies likely to be detected by HSG are septate, bicornuate, didelphys, and unicornuate configurations. Despite attempts to define radiographic criteria, the HSG procedure alone will not establish the distinction between the bicornuate and the septate uterus with a high degree of confidence. Laparoscopy enables the clinician to distinguish between these two entities. Ultrasonography, including the fluid-enhanced scan (sonohysterogram), magnetic resonance imaging, and computed tomography have not yet proven to be adequate substitutes for the HSG in determining the exact nature of the müllerian anomaly. They are useful, however, in obstructive müllerian anomalies such as absent vagina or uterus, obstructed hemivagina, transverse vaginal septum, or congenital cervical atresia.

Hysteroscopy alone will not establish whether the divided cavity is associated with a septate or a bicornuate configuration. The combination of laparoscopy and hysteroscopy is still considered the procedure of choice for diagnosing and correcting a septum in a single anesthesia session. In the case of septum resection, laparoscopy allows monitoring of the progression of hysteroscopic metroplasty as well as avoidance or detection of uterine perforation (see discussion following).

Obstetric Consequences of Müllerian Anomalies

Symmetric fusion failures of the uterus (septate, bicornuate, didelphic) are the most common müllerian anomalies. DES-associated defects of the reproductive tract (hypoplastic uterine cavity, uterine polyps, vaginal adenosis) are still commonly recognized today. Septate, bicornuate, didelphic, and DES-exposed uteri have a higher incidence of cervical incompetence, which often results in poor obstetric outcome. Although approximately 80% of patients with symmetric uterine anomalies will carry their pregnancies to term without difficulty, the incidence of pregnancy wastage among patients with a prior history of adverse obstetric outcome in the presence of bicornuate or septate uteri is 80% to 90%, and in the presence of didelphic uterus it is 40%. Obstetric complications range from first- and second-trimester spontaneous abortions to preterm labor, malpresentations, pre- and postpartum hemorrhage, and dystocia due to vaginal obstruction (Table 1).

Hysteroscopic Management
Hysteroscopic Metroplasty

The mere presence of a uterine septum does not automatically indicate surgical correction. However, if the patient has already experienced at least one first- or second-trimester loss, metro-

TABLE 1. Reproductive Outcome with Müllerian Anomalies

Type of Reproductive Tract Anomaly	Pregnancy Outcome
Vertical fusion septum defects	50% term pregnancy
Congenital absence of cervix	One pregnancy in 20 reported cases
Lateral fusion defects Obstructive Rudimentary horn (75% do not communicate with normal hemiuterus) Uterine duplication with unilateral vaginal obstruction	64–85% term pregnancy in normal horn
Nonobstructive Asymmetric: Uterus unicollis	Intrauterine growth retardation
Symmetric: Septate Bicornuate Didelphic	Overall fetal wastage 31% Increase in spontaneous abortion Malpresentation Premature labor Postpartum hemorrhage Term pregnancy before surgery: Septate 15% Bicornuate 10% Didelphic 57% After surgery: Septate >80% Bicornuate (rarely surgically corrected) Didelphic 75%

Adapted from Rock JA, Schlaff WD: The obstetric consequences of uterovaginal anomalies. Fertil Steril 1985;43:681–692. Reproduced with permission of the publisher, The American Fertility Society.

plasty should be considered. The patient with three or more losses would certainly benefit from hysteroscopic metroplasty.

Preoperative Preparation

Minimal thickness of the endometrial lining facilitates an unobstructed view during the procedure. A uterus with late luteal phase shaggy endometrium or late follicular phase thick endometrium may pose technical difficulties because of loose endometrial tissue and increased bleeding. Under these circumstances, the hysteroscope may create "burrows" upon insertion and iatrogenic "pseudopolyps." Ideally, the procedure should be performed during the early follicular phase after cessation of the menstrual flow. Preparation of the endometrium with gonadotropin-releasing hormone (GnRH) analogues is currently the preferred method of (medical) endometrial preparation. One dose of intramuscular depot gonadotropin-releasing hormone analogue, or a single subcutaneous implant, 3 to 4 weeks prior to surgery is usually adequate. Mechanical preparation with a small-gauge suction curette may also be performed, alone or in combination with medical agents. An intravenous pyelogram should be obtained in all patients, since associated renal anomalies are present in 5% to 55%.

Anesthesia

The procedure may be performed under regional or general anesthesia, but general anesthesia may be preferred with laparoscopy. The anesthesiologist should be advised about the nature of the procedure and the distension medium. Careful hemodynamic monitoring with strict attention to fluid intake and output is mandatory to avoid fluid overload and electrolyte imbalance. If the procedure lasts over 1 hour or if distension medium intake is greater than output by more than 500 to 1000 mL, hematocrit/hemoglobin values, as well as serum electrolytes, should be assessed intraoperatively and postoperatively.

Uterine Distension

To avoid embolization, carbon dioxide insufflation should be avoided with operative hysteroscopy unless the septum is small or very thin. If the metroplasty is carried out with hysteroscopic scissors, a liquid medium is preferred. If resection by electrocautery is planned, a nonconducting medium such as 1.5% glycine or 3% sorbitol is preferred. If the procedure is expected to last more than 30 minutes, liquid solutions, such as glycine or sorbitol, that are least likely to cause fluid and electrolyte imbalance should be used. (Nevertheless, in excess, even these solutions can cause fluid overload and hyponatremia.)

Surgical Technique

A laparoscopy may be performed first to visualize the pelvis, in particular outlining the uterine fundus. The posterior surface of the uterus must be adequately visualized, since perforations most commonly will occur in this location. One begins the hysteroscopy by sounding the uterus to assess the depth and direction of the cavity as well as the length of the septum. The cervix is then dilated to accommodate the appropriate-sized hysteroscope (24 French). Either a diagnostic hysteroscope with a port allowing introduction of hysteroscopic scissors or a resecting hysteroscope with continuous flow may be used. A 0-degree scope may be appropriate for visualizing the septum, which is a midline structure. Then either a 0-degree, 12-degree, or 30-degree telescope can be used for the resection.

Visualization of the cavity should start from the endocervical canal cephalad. The hysteroscope must not be inserted too deeply, since entry into one of the two uterine compartments may confuse the anatomy, and undue trauma to the endometrium may produce bleeding and create misleading tracks.

The septum is then divided in its midline, with care taken not to stray too far posteriorly during resection to avoid uterine perforation. (Uterine perforation does not often cause significant bleeding, but it may dictate termination of the case due to escape of distension medium through the perforation and suboptimal visualization.) The metroplasty is terminated at the fundus when viable fundal myometrium is reached. This region, which is more vascular than the septum, can be identified by increased bleeding during the final portion of the resection and by uniform transillumination of the uterus with concomitant visualization by the nonilluminated laparoscope.

It is unclear whether complete excision of the septum provides any advantage over simple division, and it may prolong the operative time and increase bleeding. Often, the endometrial cavity will expand immediately following septum division, thus obviating the need for complete excision. If the resectoscope is used, a resecting loop or knife blade is helpful. Resection in a forward direction must be avoided, since the risk of perforation is significant. The knife or loop should be advanced forward into the cavity and only then applied to the septum. Resection is performed while moving the blade outward toward the operator. The current parameters are 30 to 100 watts for a pure cutting current, or a combination of 60 watts cutting and 30 watts coagulation for a blended current.

The neodymium-yttrium-aluminum-garnet (Nd:YAG) laser, the potassium-titanyl-phosphate laser (KTP), or the argon laser may be used for metroplasty. With the Nd:YAG laser, the bare fiber—not the sapphire tip—should be used. The air-cooled sapphire tip has been associated with increased operative morbidity and with at least one fatality attributed to intravascular air injection. An intraoperative hysterosalpingogram may be performed under fluoroscopy to assess the extent of septum resection.

Postoperative Management

Strict hemodynamic monitoring should be exercised during and after the procedure. Hemoglobin/hematocrit and serum electrolytes should be obtained postoperatively. Significant hemodilution or hyponatremia may necessitate overnight observation. Uterine bleeding is usually infrequent, since the septum has decreased vascularity. Immediate and delayed postoperative bleeding, however, has been described and may be treated with oral or intravenous estrogen administration or with intrauterine insertion of a 12 or 14 Foley catheter left in place for up to 7 days. Routine postoperative administration of estrogen and progestin has been advocated (eg, conjugated equine estrogen 1.25 to 2.5 mg for 30 to 60 days, followed by medroxyprogesterone acetate, 5 to 10 mg, in the last 5 to 10 days of the estrogen course). However, a number of surgeons choose to forgo postoperative hormonal treatment.

Hysteroscopy in the Diethylstilbestrol Uterus

The DES uterus may pose a special challenge to the surgeon because of the small and very rigid cavity and often sharp angulation of the cornual areas (T-shaped configuration). Endometrial polyps are quite common in the DES uterus. While it is likely that those polyps that are strategically situated (eg, at the tubal ostia or in the lower uterine segment) contribute to infertility, the role of endometrial or endocervical polyps in pregnancy loss is unclear. Hysteroscopic surgery in the DES-exposed patient is limited to removal of polyps, when indicated. This can be performed through a small-diameter hysteroscope (5 mm or 15F) with rigid, semirigid, or flexible polyp forceps or scissors. Alternatively, a flexible hysteroscope with biopsy forceps or ureteral stone wire basket may be used to remove polyps in difficult locations.

Outcome Following Hysteroscopic Management

The live birth rate following hysteroscopic metroplasty has been reported to be 68% to 87%, with term delivery being 80% to 90%. These statistics are similar to those for abdominal metroplasty, which is done via a laparotomy and has greater morbidity. In fact, with the advent of sophisticated hysteroscopic instruments, hysteroscopic metroplasty, with a low complication (20.7/1000) and morbidity rate, has replaced traditional wedge metroplasty. It is unclear whether and to what extent endometrial polyp removal in DES uteri improves fertility or pregnancy outcome.

In summary, hysteroscopy has an important role in the evaluation and therapy of certain müllerian anomalies. Its therapeutic benefits in the treatment of uterine septum have been substantiated, although its utility in the treatment of other congenital müllerian anomalies is yet to be established. The key to the successful management of müllerian anomalies lies in the complete evaluation of the patient and careful selection of the appropriate diagnostic and therapeutic hysteroscopic procedure.

Induction of Ovulation

Douglas C. Daly, MD

The identification of anovulation or dysovulation and the pharmacology to induce ovulation are at the core of our ability to treat infertility and to enhance fertility. Historically in the era of descriptive endocrinology, identification was limited by a lack of precision in measuring ovulation quality. Therefore, only major dysfunctions such as amenorrhea or Stein-Leventhal syndrome were readily identified. Once identified, the lack of pharmacologic options made therapy other

than ovarian wedge resection a moot point. The description by Noyes and colleagues in 1950 (Noyes RW, Hertig AT, Rock J: Dating the endometrial biopsy. Fertil Steril 1:3:1950) of normal luteal endometrial maturation improved the precision of diagnosis by providing objective evidence for both luteal phase defect (LPD) and anovulation associated with menstruation. It was not until the introduction of cortisol as a therapeutic agent in the mid 1950s that medical therapy of anovulation first became a reality. The response rate of 30% for LPD and 15% for anovulation by today's standards would leave much to be desired. Yet with the alternative being 0% or surgery, cortisol therapy seemed miraculous.

The introduction of cortisol was one of the first salvos of the revolution in endocrinology from description to biochemistry. In the 1950s, 1960s, and 1970s, the major hormones were identified, purified, and synthesized and their mode of action described. This allowed for the development of clinical assays that improved diagnosis and allowed for therapy to be monitored. These assays for estradiol, progesterone, prolactin, follicle-stimulating hormone (FSH), lutenizing hormone (LH) and so on remain the mainstay of diagnosis and treatment. This revolution brought the discovery and synthesis of compounds that replaced or competed with the natural hormones. By 1967, the trickle that had started with cortisol had become a pharmacologic torrent—a torrent that included clomiphene citrate and FSH, the drugs that for 30 years have been the first-line therapy for anovulation. But before we treat, it is important to define how patients are evaluated and selected for treatment.

Patient Evaluation and Selection

Before therapy is initiated for any specific cause of infertility, a general evaluation of the couple is performed. This includes a complete history and pertinent physical on both female and male. A semen analysis should be performed in a specialized andrology lab. Pelvic anatomy is evaluated by ultrasonography to identify stage III or IV endometriosis or congenital anomalies. A *Chlamydia trachomatis* immunoglobulin G antibody is obtained. If positive or if there is a history of pelvic infection, then a hysterosalpingogram is indicated. A significant finding of sperm abnormality or pelvic-tubal disease warrants assessment of the best approach to therapy. Frequently the patient is better off with in vitro fertilization (IVF).

The etiology for anovulation should be sought in all patients. Usually this will fall into one of five categories:

1. *Premature or perimenopause, resistant ovary syndrome, and autoimmune resistance.* These conditions are characterized by an elevated FSH level and are not amenable to standard ovulation induction. Clomiphene is contraindicated and FSH therapy ineffectual. Estradiol (1 mg) is the most effective treatment when oocytes persist. Patients less than 30 years of age should be karyotyped. Evidence of generalized or endocrine autoimmune disease should be sought.

2. *Hormonal disorders in other systems,* including tumors, thyroid disorders, hyperprolactinemia, and adrenal dysfunction are sought with thyroid-stimulating hormone, prolactin, and dehydroepiandrosterone sulfate assays. Any abnormality is evaluated and treated. Frequently the anovulation will then resolve. For example, a recent patient with ovarian mass was found to have an FSH level of less than 1 and a high inhibin B level. Removal of the granulosa tumor resulted in normal ovulation and pregnancy.

3. *Weight loss or low weight anovulation.* Ovulation is often lost when weight drops below 90% of ideal body weight (IBW). General medical and psychological health is evaluated. Since failure to gain weight during pregnancy is detrimental to the fetus, anorexia/bulimia or other health problems should be adequately treated. Weight gain to above 90% of IBW should be required before ovulation induction medications are used.

4. *Excess weight.* As patients gain weight above 130% of IBW, an increasing number become anovulatory. In part this may be due to individual predisposition (see point 5) but the majority is due to the impact obesity has on peripheral steroid metabolism and to insulin resistance. Skin and the stromal cells of adipose tissue are active in the metabolism of weak sex steroids to the strong sex steroids normally produced by the gonads. Since insulin-generated growth factors are involved in folliculogenesis, the insulin resistance associated with obesity has a detrimental effect on ovulation quality. This is particularly true in those patients with a genetic predisposition for insulin resistance. Family history is, therefore, very important. Since our primary goal is the delivery of a healthy child and since pregnancy in markedly obesewomen is at higher risk for diabetes, hypertension, premature delivery, and preeclampsia (all of which would be worsened by multiple pregnancy—risk for clomiphene 5–10%, for FSH 10–20%), weight loss should be a mainstay of treatment. In my practice, clomiphene is not used until a patient weighs less than 175% of IBW and FSH is not used until the patient weighs less than 150% of IBW. In those patients with proven insulin resistance (abnormal glucose tolerance test result), treatment of the insulin resistance with oral agents may be of benefit.

5. *Idiopathic anovulation.* This group of patients has no hormonal abnormalities except anovulation at or near normal weight and has normal to low normal FSH levels. Most common in the teen years and decreasing with age, it has frequently been attributed to "hypothalamic immaturity." My own belief is that there is a more mundane explanation that also explains the propensity of these patients to hyperstimulate. They simply have too many follicles/oocytes available for maturation. This may result in an elevated inhibin B level, keeping the FSH level too low to mature any of the follicles. I refer to this as polyfollicular ovaries.

Clomiphene Citrate

Clomiphene citrate is a very weak estrogen that primarily functions as an anti-estrogen. It occupies the estradiol receptor for extended periods and has a half-life of up to 5 days. Clomiphene binds to estradiol receptors in all tissues and this nonspecificity accounts for both its actions in promoting ovulation and in the side effects that limit its efficiency. The beneficial activity presumably occurs in the hypothalamus and in the anterior pituitary either by decreasing luteinizing hormone (LH) or by increasing FSH, or both. The detrimental activity can occur in the ovary (perhaps by down-regulating the FSH receptor), in the endometrium by blocking endometrial proliferation, and in the cervix by preventing adequate hydration of the mucus. Any of these side effects can prevent pregnancy, and any of them can be abnormal in a treatment cycle. Hot flashes can occur if the hypothalamus is completely estradiol blocked; further increase in the dose of clomiphene in this circumstance is ineffectual. Visual disturbances are an indication to discontinue clomiphene.

Clomiphene is initially administered 1 tablet on days 4 to 8, and a temperature chart (basal body temperature) is used to assess response. When the dehydroepiandrosterone sulfate level is greater than 2500 ng/mL then 0.25 to 0.5 mg dexamethasone at bedtime will improve clomiphene response in most patients. If an ovulatory response is obtained, then in the second cycle a pre- and postovulation ultrasonogram and a postcoital test (PCT) are performed to rule out side effects (if only the PCT result is abnormal, then intrauterine insemination is indicated). Once normal ovulation is documented, the dose is repeated for a total of four to six cycles without monitoring.

If ovulation does not occur at the initial dose, the clomiphene is increased to 2 tablets on days 4 to 8. An ultrasonogram and PCT are performed on cycle day 15 or 16. If one or two dominant follicles are present, they are followed and ovulation (hopefully) confirmed. If three or four follicles are present, 10,000 units of human chorionic gonadotropin (hCG) are given and confirmation of ovulation sought 2 days later. If no dominant follicle is seen, a progesterone withdrawal is given, the dose increased to 3 tablets, and the process repeated (unless the patient has had hot flashes). If an adequate response does not occur with 3 tablets, an increase to 4 can be attempted but in my experience it is seldom successful. Likewise, adding hCG without assessing for dominant follicles or for whether only a single dominant follicle is present will not be productive.

When clomiphene is used to treat LPD, it should be started on day 2 or 3 and used for 5 days. It is seldom beneficial to exceed 1 tablet a day. The same monitoring pattern is used.

Follicle-Stimulating Hormone/Human Menopausal Gonadotropins

Gonadotropins have been extracted from the urine of menopausal women for several decades. However, the increase in the use of estrogen replacement in menopausal women has lowered the LH level in this urine, making the Food and Drug Administration (FDA) approved ratio for the combined FSH/LH product difficult to obtain. For this reason and because genetically engineered FSH was in the product pipeline, the traditional supplier began to market FSH-only products. In our experience, all of the urinary human menopausal gonadotropins (FSH and LH) are equally potent, although they are all subject to some degree of lot-to-lot variability. The same was true of the initial urinary FSH (Metrodin) that is no longer available. Urinary FSH-HP (Fertinex) in our experience is consistently less potent. Genetic engineering has now come to reproductive endocrinology. Two competing products are now available and are at least as potent as urinary FSH/hMG in our early data and more potent than urinary follicle-stimulating hormone-highly purified (UFSH-HP). There does not appear to be a potency difference between these two genetically engineered FSH products. Both products are expensive.

For monitoring purposes, I believe some LH is desirable. When hypothalamic pituitary activity is present, the LH produced is adequate. When this activity has been suppressed, the addition of LH may be desirable for monitoring. Excessive LH (more than 150 IU) is detrimental.

When treating anovulation, the FSH is started after a progesterone withdrawal on cycle day 2 or 3. A baseline ultrasonogram is obtained to assess residual follicle activity and the number of early follicles. While the traditional starting dose is 2 amps (150 IU) a day, patients with a polyfollicular ovary pattern (see earlier discussion) are started at 1 to 1.5 amps. Monitoring by ultrasonography and estradiol is started after 4 days of treatment and FSH doses modified and revisits scheduled based on the results. The estradiol needs to be available on a same-day, 7-days-aweek basis.

Ideally, the physician performs the ultrasonogram himself or herself. As ovulation approaches, the patient is seen at 24- or 48-hour intervals. When the lead follicle is 17 mm in average diameter, I recommend that 17-OH progesterone levels (an LH-dependent hormone produced by a mature dominant follicle) be measured on that day's sample and the sample from after 4 days of medication. An increase of 1 ng/mL or more confirms follicular maturity, and 10,000 IU of hCG should result in ovulation. (If no rise occurs, FSH can be continued for 1 or 2 more days, but if still no rise occurs, the induction is suboptimal.) Although not proven, the use of additional progesterone in the second week of the luteal phase may be beneficial.

If the estradiol exceeds 2000 pg/mL, the number of follicles larger than 14 mm is five or more, or there are a large number of immature follicles, hCG is contraindicated. Two undesirable outcomes are possible: hyperstimulation syndrome and high-order multiple pregnancy. The former is due to excessive immature follicles and is characterized by large ovaries, ascites, and fluid imbalance. It can be life-threatening. Over 80% of quadruplet and higher pregnancies are the result of the use of FSH **without** IVF or gamete intrafallopian transfer. These pregnancies cost 0.5 million dollars or more and can result in children with long-term disabilities. As it is a potentially dangerous drug, FSH use is both art and science. FSH should be used only by those with experience in its use or under direct supervision. **If you are reading this chapter to learn how to use FSH, then you should not be using FSH without supervision.**

I have found no advantage to combining FSH with gonadotropin-releasing hormone (GnRH) agonists when treating anovulation, although some physicians recommend this for patients who hyperstimulate. In some patients, an induction that is both safe and effective cannot be achieved. IVF can be used to reduce the risk of both hyperstimulation and multiple gestation. Alternatively, ovarian wedge resection is making a comeback, though I view this as a last resort.

Gonadotropin-Releasing Hormone

In a small number of patients with hypothalamic insufficiency, the use of gonadotropin-releasing hormone by automated pump at 75- to 90-minute intervals will achieve a single ovulation that mimics the natural cycle. Best given intravenously in 5 μg doses, it can be given subcutaneously at 10 to 20 μg. However, few patients have anovulation due to hypothalamic insufficiency. Of those that do, weight loss amenorrhea is the primary cause and this should be treated by weight gain.

Ovulation Induction in Normally Ovulating Patients

In those patients with unexplained infertility or moderate male infertility, multiple ovulation has been used to accelerate conception. Clomiphene is given, 1 to 2 tablets on cycle days 3 to 7, and ultrasonography performed on cycle day 11 or 12. If three or more dominant follicles are present with an 8 mm endometrial echo and a normal PCT documented or an intrauterine insemination planned, hCG is given. If fewer than three follicles are present, the clomiphene is not repeated. In this circumstance, FSH can be used as described for anovulatory patients, although the number of follicles allowed to ovulate may

be increased based on the duration of the unexplained infertility.

Infertility

Samuel J. Chantilis, MD
Bruce R. Carr, MD

Initial Evaluation

Infertility is a disorder that affects approximately 15% of married couples. The standard and time-honored definition of infertility is failure to achieve pregnancy after 1 year of unprotected intercourse. In general, the evaluation of infertility proceeds after the diagnosis is made, which would normally require a duration of 1 year to achieve pregnancy. However, the standard definition may be inadequate for all patients. For example, women who are at least 35 years of age or older may be considered for an evaluation earlier than 1 year, as would patients with obvious barriers to achieving pregnancies such as known tubal obstruction, severe oligospermia or azoospermia, or amenorrhea.

The basic evaluation of an infertile couple is generally agreed upon (Fig. 1). The evaluation consists of a detailed history, physical examination, an assessment of ovulation, semen evaluation, and uterotubal assessment. The methods used to assess ovulation include basal body temperature charts, midluteal progesterone levels, a luteal phase endometrial biopsy, home testing of luteinizing hormone (LH) levels and serial ultrasonograms to evaluate follicular growth; each of these methods has advantages and disadvantages. The basal body temperature charts are inexpensive, requiring only the patient's constant vigilance to remember to obtain and record the basal temperature; however, they are ineffective for prospectively determining the day of ovulation. Midluteal progesterone levels are simple for patients to obtain and give the physician a general assessment of ovulation and adequacy of the luteal phase. The major disadvantage of the midluteal progesterone level is that progesterone levels vary and provide no assessment of the endometrium. Endometrial biopsies are generally performed in the late luteal phase and are considered the gold standard for assessing the luteal phase. Unfortunately, endometrial biopsies are expensive and painful, and the histologic interpretation is often inconsistent. Many studies have reported a marked variation in histologic

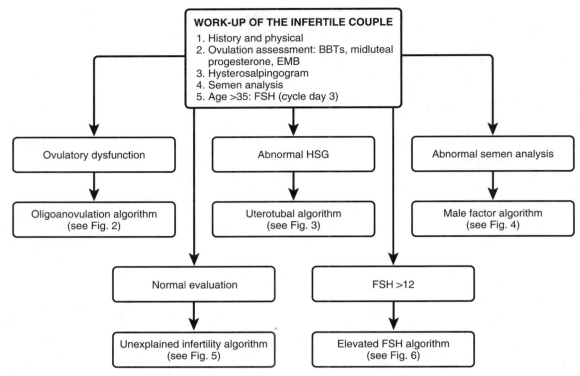

Figure 1. Diagnostic algorithm for the basic evaluation of an infertile couple. BBT, basal body temperature; EMB, endometrial biopsy; FSH, follicle-stimulating hormone; HSG, hysterosalpingogram. (Reproduced with permission from Bradshaw KD, Chantalis SJ, Carr BR: Diagnostic evaluation and treatment algorithms for the infertile couple. *In* Carr BR, Blackwell RE (eds): Texbook of Reproductive Medicine, 2/E. Stanford, CT: Appleton and Lange, 1998, pp 533–564.)

dating of similar endometrial biopsies among different pathologists. Additionally, regardless of which method is used for assessing adequacy of the luteal phase, a second abnormal value (midluteal progesterone or endometrial biopsy that lags) is necessary to establish the diagnosis. This practice is expensive and impractical and, more importantly, may not alter treatment plans. LH testing predicts the onset of ovulation but does not provide information regarding the quality of follicular development or luteal phase adequacy. Serial ultrasonograms are very predictive of adequate follicular growth and documentation of ovulation but are expensive.

In summary, ovulation assessment includes determination of the regularity of ovulation (defined as spontaneous, regular, predictable menses), establishing the adequacy of a luteal phase, which is generally defined as a length of greater than or equal to 12 days, midluteal progesterone greater than 10 ng/mL, or an endometrial biopsy that is dated within 2 days of the predicted cycle day.

Assessment of the uterus and fallopian tubes initially consists of the hysterosalpingogram (HSG). This provides a screening test for the endometrial cavity as well as tubal patency. Although the HSG may be associated with tubal spasm, artifactual filling defects in the uterus, and the inability to assess peritubal adhesions, the HSG remains critical in the basic fertility evaluation and provides the clinician a wealth of information. In the future, sonohysterography with the use of sonolucent injection material may be a viable option to assess the uterine cavity and tubal patency.

The semen analysis is the primary screening test for male factor fertility. The correlation between sperm density and motility with pregnancy is reasonably established, although men with oligoasthenospermia can produce pregnancies, whereas men with normal semen analyses may have a male factor that is not assessed by the semen analysis.

Additional consideration can be given for an evaluation of the cervix, which may include an evaluation of any previous cervical surgery and physical examination of cervical mucus at ovulation. Although still performed by many clinicians, the postcoital test has been a source of ongoing controversy owing to the poor predictive value of a negative test and the poor repeatability of the test. Unfortunately, there is no universally agreed upon method for conducting a postcoital test and, therefore, there is a lack of consensus for a definition of cervical factor infertility. A follicle stimulating hormone (FSH) level (and estradiol) obtained on cycle day 3 is correlated with ovarian reserve and pregnancy rates, as demonstrated with data from in vitro fertilization treatment cycles. An FSH level may be helpful in determining prognostic value in a woman who is 35 years old or older. The initial evaluation of the infertile couple is presented in Figure 1.

Treatment Algorithm for Ovulatory Dysfunction

Women with amenorrhea, oligoanovulation, or ovulatory dysfunction and infertility are initially assessed for thyroid disease and hyperprolactinemia with measurement of thyroid-stimulating hormone and prolactin levels (Fig. 2). An FSH level is obtained if amenorrhea or ovarian failure or hypothalamic disease is suspected. Abnormal values warrant further investigation and treatment as indicated. If normal, treatment is initiated with clomiphene citrate at an ovulatory dose for three cycles monitored by urinary LH testing and intercourse. A progesterone level to assess luteal phase adequacy in the first treatment cycle may be helpful. Additionally, some clinicians will consider postcoital testing which, if results are abnormal, is suggestive that intrauterine insemination using husband sperm (IUH) may be beneficial. If pregnancy has not been achieved after three cycles of minimal intervention, three more treatment cycles with clomiphene citrate are indicated, with more intensive monitoring. Sonography, to confirm follicular development in response to clomiphene citrate, and human chorionic gonadotropin (5000–10,000 units, intramuscularly) to accurately time inseminations, are combined with IUH.

There is some debate over whether one versus two inseminations is best; one guideline may be to use two inseminations with a normal semen analysis, and one insemination with a male factor considering the consistent poor sperm density and motility with the second specimen in male factor patients. If pregnancy is still not achieved at this time, then one must consider laparoscopy. However, one may argue that a woman without symptoms of endometriosis, a normal HSG, and a completely normal physical examination may be better served by proceeding with treatment rather than diagnosis. Menotropin therapy, moni-

tored with sonography and estradiol levels, and IUH are employed if clomiphene citrate is unsuccessful. If pregnancy is still not achieved after three cycles of menotropin therapy, then in vitro fertilization is indicated.

Treatment Algorithm for Uterotubal Abnormalities

If an abnormal HSG is found during the basic infertility evaluation, further testing to diagnose the uterotubal etiology is indicated (Fig. 3). Office hysteroscopy is performed to further delineate the presence of a polyp or submucous leiomyoma in the event that a uterine defect is detected. Further hysteroscopic surgical removal of the detected pathology is generally warranted, although the extent of infertility impairment with a minimal lesion, that is, a 1 to 2 mm filling defect, is unknown. Tubal occlusion on a hysterosalpingogram may be unilateral or bilateral, and proximal or distal. Although tubal spasm is a cause of tubal occlusion, one should consider further diagnosis and treatment with laparoscopy. A woman with unilateral proximal tubal occlusion on an HSG believed to be secondary to tubal spasm and without risk factors for occlusion may be a candidate for treatment before proceeding with laparoscopy. Bilateral proximal tubal occlusion is usually best treated with laparoscopy for diagnosis and possible hysteroscopic tubal cannulation. Bilateral distal tubal occlusion that is considered mild (i.e., minimal dilation of the fallopian tubes, or with possible partial spilling of dye) may be treated with laparoscopy and tuboplasty. Severe bilateral distal tubal occlusion, that is, bilateral hydrosalpinx with enlarged (>3 cm dilation) distal fallopian tubes, is probably best treated with in vitro fertilization.

Treatment Algorithm for Male Factor Infertility

The semen analysis is the gold standard for evaluation of the male. The semen analysis is an easy test to obtain and is relatively inexpensive. The semen is evaluated for volume, pH, and sperm density, motility, and morphology. Although a normal semen analysis does not ensure the absence of a male factor, and an abnormal semen analysis does not preclude pregnancy, potential for pregnancy is decreased with sperm density less than 20 million/mL and less than 50% forwardly progressive, motile sperm. If abnormal results are found, the semen analysis should be repeated at least 4 weeks after the initial speci-

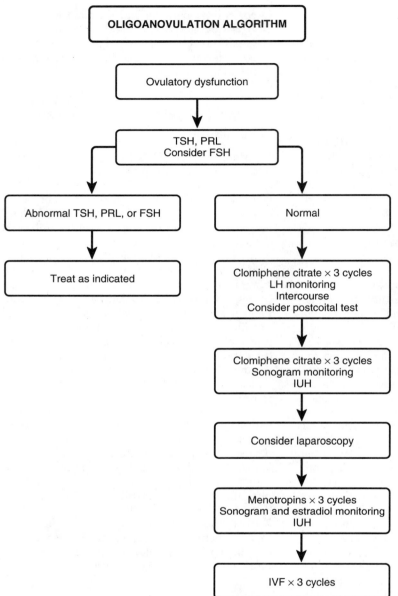

Figure 2. Treatment algorithm for infertile couples with oligoanovulation. FSH, follicle-stimulating hormone; IUH, insemination using husband sperm; IVF, in vitro fertilization; LH, luteinizing hormone; PRL, prolactin; TSH, thyroid-stimulating hormone. (Reproduced with permission from Bradshaw KD, Chantalis SJ, Carr BR: Diagnostic evaluation and treatment algorithms for the infertile couple. *In* Carr BR, Blackwell RE (eds): Texbook of Reproductive Medicine, 2/E. Stanford, CT: Appleton and Lange, 1998, pp 533–564.)

men (Fig. 4). If the second specimen is normal, the couple may have a borderline male factor, and continued observation of semen during treatment should be conducted. Upon confirmation of an abnormal semen analysis, consideration for referral to a urologist should be made. Clear indications for referral include persistent low volume (<1 mL) which may indicate an obstructive disease, azoospermia, or signs or symptoms of decreased masculinization. While some controversy exists regarding the efficacy of the correction of asymptomatic or subclinical varicocele with respect to infertility, symptomatic varico-

celes should be treated. Although no standard definition to differentiate mild, moderate, and severe male factor exists, we define these categories as follows:

mild: 15–20 million sperm/mL, 35–50% motility
moderate: 5–15 million sperm/mL, 20–35% motility
severe: <5 million sperm/mL, or <20% motility

Many other parameters have been used to categorize degrees of severity of male factor and

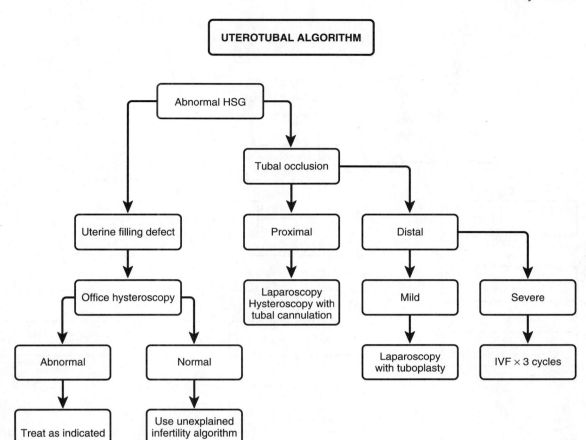

Figure 3. Treatment algorithm for uterotubal infertility diagnosed by an abnormal hysterosalpingogram (HSG). IVF, in vitro fertilization. (Reproduced with permission from Bradshaw KD, Chantalis SJ, Carr BR: Diagnostic evaluation and treatment algorithms for the infertile couple. *In* Carr BR, Blackwell RE (eds): Texbook of Reproductive Medicine, 2/E. Stanford, CT: Appleton and Lange, 1998, pp 533–564.)

are certainly appropriate. Some clinics use an enhanced sperm penetration assay to further evaluate the ability of sperm to penetrate a hamster egg and undergo nuclear decondensation. The value of this test relies on its positive and negative predictive values for fertilization of human oocytes. Mild and moderate male factors are best treated with artificial insemination using husband sperm for up to six cycles. Failed IUH and severe male factor infertility are probably best treated by in vitro fertilization with the intracytoplasmic sperm injection procedure. Of course, donor insemination is an option for couples not wishing to pursue advanced reproductive techniques.

Treatment Algorithm for Unexplained Infertility

Perhaps one of the more difficult areas for couples and physicians alike is that of unexplained

infertility (Fig. 5). The most challenging question for infertility treatment today, given constraints and infertility coverage, is the decision to undergo laparoscopy. Depending on which diagnostic category in which a patient is placed, as well as the signs and symptoms such as pelvic pain or pelvic masses, laparoscopy may be indicated to evaluate the presence or absence of endometriosis, pelvic adhesions, or other peritoneal factors. With often limited resources, there has been a trend toward spending less on diagnostic evaluation to determine the etiology of infertility, and an allocation of more resources toward treatment. This issue is most important with respect to the role of laparoscopy and a working diagnosis of unexplained infertility after the initial evaluation. Given the cost, the decision to perform a diagnostic laparoscopy may be questioned in a woman with a normal history and physical examination, for whom resources could be applied

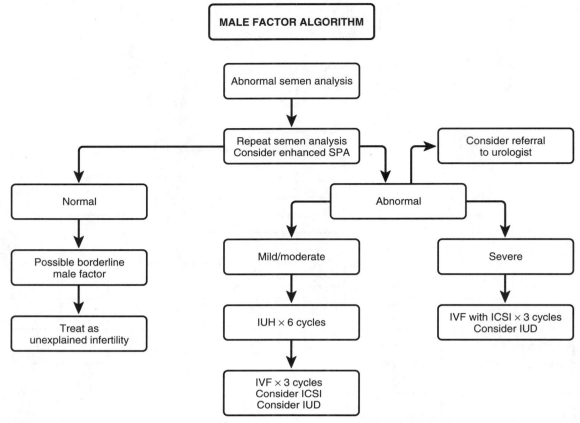

Figure 4. Treatment algorithm for male factor infertility. ICSI, intracytoplasmic sperm injection; IUD, intrauterine device; IUH, insemination using husband sperm; IVF, in vitro fertilization; SPA, sperm penetration assay. (Reproduced with permission from Bradshaw KD, Chantalis SJ, Carr BR: Diagnostic evaluation and treatment algorithms for the infertile couple. *In* Carr BR, Blackwell RE (eds): Texbook of Reproductive Medicine, 2/E. Stanford, CT: Appleton and Lange, 1998, pp 533–564.)

toward treatment instead of diagnosis. Although up to 30% of women with infertility have endometriosis, and approximately 85% of women undergoing fertility evaluation have some atypical finding, only 10% to 15% of patients undergoing diagnostic laparoscopy for fertility (with normal HSGs) will have significant pelvic pathology. With further attention to cost and benefit ratios, one could argue that a traditional diagnostic laparoscopy for the purposes of infertility could be economically replaced with an in vitro fertilization or gamete intrafollicular transfer (GIFT) treatment cycle, resulting in pregnancy in approximately 33% to 50% of these patients. On the other hand, microlaparoscopy, with the use of intravenous sedation and local anesthesia, is a more affordable diagnostic procedure that may play an important role in treatment before a relatively expensive menotropin-stimulated treatment cycle is attempted. We believe that this

cost-benefit issue will encourage diagnostic laparoscopy in a nonoperative setting, which is less expensive than the traditional laparoscopy in an operating room or will discourage the use of diagnostic laparoscopy in favor of therapeutic measures.

Often couples with unexplained infertility are treated with supraovulation induction, with artificial insemination using husband sperm. We feel that treating couples with unexplained infertility with clomiphene citrate stimulation monitored with sonography, ovulatory "triggering" with human chorionic gonadotropin, and IUH has some benefit, given the difficulty in diagnosing subtle ovulation defects and cervical factors. Clomiphene citrate monitored with LH-surge testing and intercourse in an ovulatory woman is a simple initial treatment, although it remains unproven. If pregnancy is not achieved at this time, or if history and physical examination are sugges-

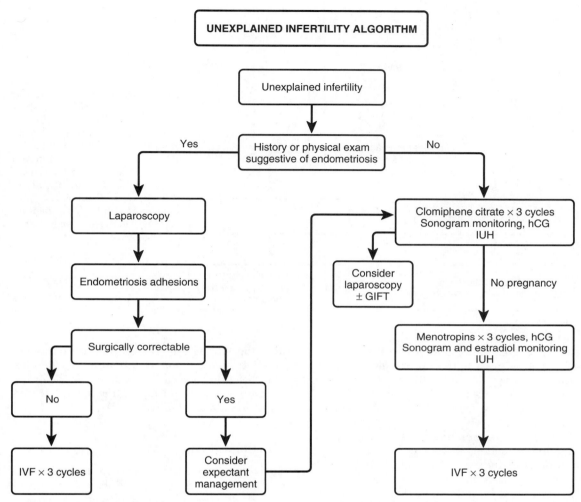

Figure 5. Treatment algorithm for unexplained infertility. GIFT, gamete intrafallopian transfer; hCG, human chorionic gonadotropin; IUH, insemination using husband sperm; IVF, in vitro fertilization. (Reproduced with permission from Bradshaw KD, Chantalis SJ, Carr BR: Diagnostic evaluation and treatment algorithms for the infertile couple. *In* Carr BR, Blackwell RE (eds): Texbook of Reproductive Medicine, 2/E. Stanford, CT: Appleton and Lange, 1998, pp 533–564.)

tive of endometriosis at initial consultation, consideration should be given for laparoscopy. If endometriosis, pelvic adhesions, or tubal disease is diagnosed, surgical correction should be instituted if possible. Depending on the severity of the disease and the age of the couple, a period of expectant management may be recommended for up to 6 months before the patient undergoes clomiphene citrate ovulation induction with IUH. If pelvic factor is diagnosed that is not surgically correctable, in vitro fertilization is recommended. Couples with unexplained infertility who fail initial clomiphene citrate treatment are treated with menotropins, monitored with sonography and estradiol level, and IUH for three

cycles. Should pregnancy not ensue, then in vitro fertilization is considered.

Treatment Algorithm for Elevated Follicle-Stimulating Hormone

In couples in which the woman is more than 35 years of age, we obtain a cycle day 3 FSH level and, perhaps, estradiol level in an effort to evaluate ovarian reserve (Fig. 6). Using most immunoassays, a value of greater than 12 mIU/mL, or an estradiol level greater than 75 pg/mL, may indicate a poor prognosis with respect with reproductive potential. Persistently elevated early follicu-

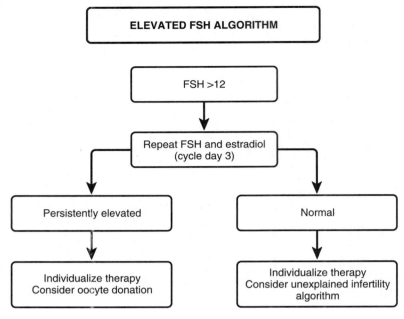

ELEVATED FSH ALGORITHM

FSH >12

Repeat FSH and estradiol
(cycle day 3)

Persistently elevated

Normal

Individualize therapy
Consider oocyte donation

Individualize therapy
Consider unexplained infertility
algorithm

Figure 6. Treatment algorithm for elevated cycle day 3 follicle-stimulating hormone (FSH). (Reproduced with permission from Bradshaw KD, Chantalis SJ, Carr BR: Diagnostic evaluation and treatment algorithms for the infertile couple. *In* Carr BR, Blackwell RE (eds): Texbook of Reproductive Medicine, 2/E. Stanford, CT: Appleton and Lange, 1998, pp 533–564.)

lar phase FSH and estradiol levels may warrant a more progressive approach and, ultimately, may warrant oocyte donation. Repeat values in the normal range offer some hope, but continued surveillance is certainly prudent and a more aggressive approach is generally considered.

While we have outlined a basic algorithm for fertility evaluation, this by no means is an attempt to include every permutation possible. Certainly, there are many instances in which therapy must be individualized. Nevertheless, this serves as a basic guideline for diagnostic and treatment issues for the infertility physician.

Intrauterine Adhesions

Robert Israel, MD

Prior to the advent of hysteroscopy, intrauterine adhesions (IUA, Asherman's syndrome) were a significant diagnostic and therapeutic problem. Although IUA can be strongly suspected in a woman with postcurettage amenorrhea who has evidence of luteal phase activity, eccentric echogenic areas on transvaginal ultrasonogram, filling defects on hysterography, or persistent amenorrhea despite sequential estrogen-progesterone administration, these classic features are not always seen and not definitive in confirming the diagnosis. The hysteroscope can not only confirm

that the intrauterine defects seen on ultrasonogram or hysterogram are intrauterine adhesions, but the endoscope can accurately map the extent of the pathology and be the therapeutic instrument to eliminate the IUA.

Diagnosis

If the patient presents with postcurettage amenorrhea and evidence of luteal phase activity (sustained elevation of basal body temperatures or serum progesterone elevations in one or more weekly samples, or both), IUA is the presumptive diagnosis and one proceeds to hysteroscopic assessment and therapy. Although uterine sounding can be a diagnostic aid when the endometrial cavity is obliterated totally, it may not be helpful in lesser degrees of IUA. The routine use of transvaginal ultrasonography may permit the diagnosis of IUA, especially if the endometrial echo pattern is observed carefully in women who have had prior endometrial curettages. Even patients with normal, cyclic menses can have IUA, which is detected usually by hysterosalpingography in the course of an infertility work-up.

With anything less than the obvious IUA presentation, hysterography remains the primary presumptive method of diagnosis. Slow instillation of the contrast medium by the gynecologist, or an understanding radiologist, and visualization with image intensification fluoroscopy will increase the delineation of IUA immeasurably. Typically, IUAs present as single or multiple, soft, lake-like filling defects of variable size and configuration within the endometrial cavity. They may be located centrally or peripherally but should be present on each film to differentiate them from polyps. In some cases, the uterine cavity may appear to be obliterated completely with endocervical canal fill only. Eventually, when hysteroscopy is carried out, the obstruction turns out to be lower uterine segment/upper endocervical canal adhesions only and, once cleared away, the main part of the endometrial cavity is free of adhesions. Why these patients present with amenorrhea and not hematometra remains a mystery, but it has been postulated that even minimal adhesions may decrease myometrial activity, thus reducing sex steroid perfusion to the endometrium, which contributes to endometrial atrophy. In those cases in which the well-performed screening hysterogram reveals a normal uterine cavity on a complete anterior-posterior view, hysteroscopy need not be performed.

Treatment

With the diagnosis strongly suspected, the hysteroscope confirms, delineates, and treats the IUA. As most patients present with secondary amenorrhea or hypomenorrhea, cycle timing of hysteroscopy may not be an issue. However, in normally cycling women, visualization is best when the endometrium is thin, within 2 to 3 days after the end of menstruation. Various media can be utilized to distend the endometrial cavity. With minimal pathology, carbon dioxide or 5% glucose in water are fine, but with any significant pathology a 32% dextran solution in 10% glucose in water (Hyskon, molecular weight 70,000 daltons) is preferable. It provides excellent clarity, and, as the dissection proceeds, its immiscibility with blood becomes a major advantage. In most instances, however, the total volume of Hyskon absorbed should not exceed 250 mL. Noncardiogenic pulmonary edema and disseminated intravascular coagulation may occur after large amounts of Hyskon are absorbed, causing platelet dysfunction and inhibition of factors V, VIII, and IX. Since a continuous-flow resectoscope is unnecessary, and possibly contraindicated with IUA, glycine, or sorbitol (low viscosity media requiring high flow rate), high volume systems are not needed.

With minimal IUA, hysteroscopy may be performed safely in an office setting under sedation and a paracervical block (10 mL of 1% lidocaine injected at 3, 5, 7 and 9 o'clock). For brief procedures, 600 mg of ibuprofen should suffice, but meperidine (50 mg), midazolam (2–5 mg), or diazepam (5–10 mg) may be given intravenously, if necessary. With moderate or severe IUA, involving more than one half of the uterine cavity or obliterating the upper endometrial cavity where laparoscopic guidance may be useful, general or conduction anesthesia in an out-patient surgical unit is necessary.

Following a pelvic examination, uterine sounding, and cervical dilatation to between 4 and 7 mm, the hysteroscope is introduced through a 7 or 8 mm sheath. Depending on the extent of the IUA, the endometrial cavity is distended as much as possible, and the cavity and adhesions are assessed. Utilizing hysteroscopic scissors, the IUA are lysed under direct vision, a process that is safer and more complete than the old method of IUA therapy, blind curettage. Scissor dissection cuts scar only and does not traumatize normal endometrium. Each adhesive band is identified and divided. Complete lysis of adhesions can be achieved even in women with extensive scarring. Attempting to excise the adhesions is unnecessary. As mentioned earlier, when the adhesions obliterate the upper endometrial cavity, simultaneous laparoscopy is used to reduce the risk of uterine perforation. To aid laparoscopic visualization of the hysteroscopic dissection, the laparoscope light should be turned off so the transmitted light of the hysteroscope can be seen and incipient perforation anticipated. As hysteroscopic scissor dissection works so well, use of the laser or the resectoscope is unnecessary, and, in the case of the resectoscope, may incite further adhesion formation.

After lysis, two ancillary techniques have been important in producing fine results. To keep the uterine cavity walls apart, an intrauterine splint, inserted immediately post-lysis and left in situ for 2 months, is important. An intrauterine contraceptive device (IUD) that has a good surface area, such as, the old Lippes loop, is ideal. If you do enough of these procedures, you can acquire these devices from physicians' offices that have them but are not using them. Copper-bearing IUDs and the Progestasert IUD have too small a surface area to prevent adhesion reformation, and those that contain copper may induce an excessive inflammatory reaction. Therefore, their use is not advised. Although an 8 French Foley catheter with a 3 mL balloon can be used and a broad-spectrum antibiotic prescribed, it can remain in situ for only 2 weeks because of the potential for infection. As 2 weeks is too short a time to prevent adhesion reformation, a Foley catheter is utilized only with a uterine perforation occurring at the end of the lysis in an attempt to get some benefit from the surgical procedure.

The other ancillary postoperative therapy involves 60 days of high-dose estrogen use (conjugated estrogens, 2.5 mg bid) with 10 mg of medroxyprogesterone acetate added during the last 5 days of estrogen therapy to induce a withdrawal menses. The intrauterine splint is removed during this menstrual flow. High-dose, sequential estrogen-progestin treatment maximally stimulates the endometrium so that the scarred surfaces are re-epithelialized. The adequacy of therapy should be assessed by hysterography following the hormonally induced withdrawal bleeding. If hysterography is normal, complete resolution may be presumed. However, if the original dissection was less than complete or the follow-up hysterography is abnormal, repeat hysteroscopy for diagnosis or repeat therapy, or both, should be carried out.

Results

With secondary amenorrhea as the presenting complaint, post-therapy cyclic menses should resume in 99% of patients. With hypomenorrhea as the presenting complaint, normal flow can be expected in 100% of patients. After one hysteroscopic treatment, 90% of the patients should have a normal follow-up hysterography or hysteroscopy. Most of the others will require only a second hysteroscopic procedure to restore normal uterine architecture, but a few women will require three to five operations. The importance of a postoperative study to verify uterine cavity normalcy prior to permitting conception cannot be overemphasized. Severe obstetric complications, such as a 5% to 31% incidence of placenta accreta, have been reported in patients who conceived prior to having postoperative studies performed to document complete resolution of the adhesions. With a visualized normal, post-treatment uterine cavity, there have been no reports of abnormal placentation.

The pregnancy results are excellent and surpass other types of outdated treatment regimens such as blind disruption of adhesions by a sound or curette. Patients with a desire to conceive do so 60% to 75% of the time, and over 85% of these pregnancies go to term. With a normal postoperative hysterogram or hysteroscopic examination, gestational outcome should be very good, irrespective of the pretreatment extent of pathology, that is, minimal, moderate, or severe IUA. In this one small area of gynecologic pathology, hysteroscopic therapy reigns supreme.

Intrauterine Devices

Phillip G. Stubblefield, MD

Development of the Intrauterine Device

Intrauterine contraceptive devices (IUDs) are thought to have evolved from stem pessaries, intracervical devices used in Europe and the United States in the late 1800s (Fig. 1). The efficacy of these devices is unknown. They were linked to infection and disappeared from use early in the 20th century. From these devices evolved versions that were completely intrauterine. Coils of silkworm gut and metal wire and rings of metal were developed in the 1930s. Modern flexible plastic versions were devised in the 1960s; these could be pulled into a narrow tube for insertion without dilatation, and pushed into the uterine cavity where they resumed their preconfigured shape. A string was added to allow confirmation that the IUD was still present and for easy removal.

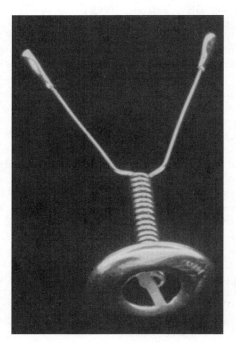

Figure 1. Stem pessary made from gold wire.

Intrauterine devices were soon widely distributed and thoroughly studied. Small plastic IUDs were better tolerated because they produced less pain and bleeding but had higher pregnancy rates than larger versions of the same device. Thus, the next advance in intrauterine contraception was the addition of an active substance to improve the efficacy of small IUDs. Intrauterine copper was found to have an important antifertility effect. The addition of copper wire to the plastic T device reduced the pregnancy rate for that device from 10 or more per 100 women-years to 2 per 100. In another approach, a polymer reservoir containing progesterone was added to the stem of a T device (Alza Corporation, Palo Alto, CA). Intrauterine progesterone also increased efficacy.

A third generation of devices has been developed. The initial copper T and a similar device, the copper 7, had a surface area of 200 to 220 mm. A newer device, the Copper T380A, has sleeves of copper on the cross arms of the T in addition to the wire on the stem and provides a total surface area of 380 mm of copper, theoretically enough to last over 20 years (Fig. 2). This device is sold in the United States as the "ParaGard" (GynoPharma, Inc., Somerville, NJ). It is the most effective commercially available IUD and is approved by the US Food and Drug Administration for 10 years of use. Several other third-generation IUDs are available in Europe and Canada. None is more effective than the T380A.

A further development in hormone-releasing third-generation IUDs was the substitution of levonorgestrel for progesterone in the stem of an IUD. Levonorgestrel is much more potent than natural progesterone, and the intrauterine source provides sufficient hormone for systemic absorption and blockade of ovulation. The levonorgestrel IUD is sold in Europe and is approved for 7 years of continuous use. Women wearing hormone-releasing IUDs have reduced menstrual bleeding, and with the levonorgestrel device, may develop amenorrhea. The levonorgestrel IUD has been used successfully to treat menorrhagia. Women wearing other IUDs have increased menstrual bleeding.

Mechanism of Action

The mechanism of IUD action is not entirely clear. It is currently thought that the presence of the IUD in the uterus produces a low-grade chronic inflammatory response, with an outpouring of white cells and fibrin. The resultant

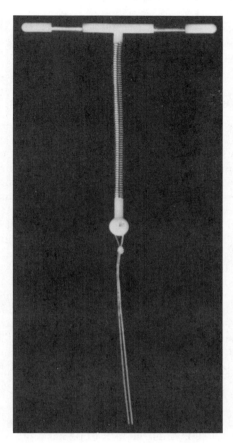

Figure 2. Copper T380A (ParaGard).

"biologic foam" is a mesh of fibrin, phagocytic cells, proteolytic enzymes, and cytokines, which are toxic to sperm. Physicians managing women on immune suppression, as after renal transplant, have reported much higher than expected pregnancy rates with IUDs, suggesting that the inflammatory response in the uterus is the key to IUD efficacy.

It is not true, as formerly thought, that the IUD acts primarily as an abortifacient. IUD-wearing women do not test positive for pregnancy hormone, with the exception of an occasional positive beta-human chorionic gonadotropin at the midcycle that represents detection of the luteinizing hormone surge preceding ovulation. In women not using contraception, studies of peritoneal fluid obtained at midcycle by laparoscopy revealed living sperm; no sperm were found in the peritoneal fluid of IUD-wearing women. The levonorgestrel IUD has the additional mechanism of action of blocking ovulation in as many as one third of wearers. Additionally, the changes in cervical mucus induced by levonorgestrel could be expected to prevent sperm penetration of cervical mucus, as has been demonstrated in women wearing the levonorgestrel-releasing subdermal implant, Norplant.

Outcomes

The T380A (ParaGard) has a very low pregnancy rate, approximately 0.5 per 100 women-years in the first year of use, and totalling only 2 per 100 women-years after 8 years of use. A limiting factor is the development of pelvic pain and increased bleeding, which lead to discontinuation by a few percent of patients each year. At the end of 8 years, approximately one third will have requested removal for this reason, an additional 11% to 12% will have expelled the device, and another 9% will have had it removed for other medical or personal reasons. A woman who has tolerated an IUD for some time is very unlikely to develop problems with pregnancy or pain and bleeding in subsequent years. After 8 years, only about 30% of those who started use of the T380A will continue with it. This rate is actually as good or better than long-term continuation rates for oral contraceptives and progestin implants, and the IUD costs much less. The Progestasert has a 1-year pregnancy rate of 1 to 2 per 100 women and must be replaced at that time. The levonorgestrel IUD available in Europe has a pregnancy rate of 0.2 per 100 women-years.

Associated Infection

Several events in the early 1970s had a major impact on the use of IUDs and on the women wearing them. First, the Dalkon shield was introduced. This device has a tail made of multiple fibers encased in a sheath, in contrast to the monofilament nylon used on all other IUDs. Soon, cases of severe sepsis were described in women who became pregnant while wearing Dalkon shields and developed fulminant gram-negative bacterial septicemia. Several deaths occurred before this problem was appreciated. Subsequently the Dalkon shield was implicated in severe pelvic inflammatory disease (PID) in nonpregnant women as well. The Dalkon shield was withdrawn from the market.

During the same years, sexual customs had changed in the developed countries. Rates of sexually transmitted diseases were rising year after year, and soon rates of ectopic pregnancy also increased. When these events occurred in IUD-wearing women, the IUD was blamed and lawsuits ensued. Other manufacturers withdrew

their devices from the market, and for a time only the Progestasert remained available in the United States. Subsequently the ParaGard was introduced. Both devices are now available for our patients.

Formal study has considerably clarified the connection between IUDs and sepsis. Under laboratory conditions, the multifilament string of the Dalkon shield acts as a wick, pulling water and bacteria up to where the string is knotted on the IUD. Devices with monofilament strings do not do this. Epidemiologic studies of women hospitalized for PID revealed the Dalkon shield to be very highly associated with PID, while all other devices are only weakly associated. When the Dalkon shield was excluded, IUDs were associated with infection only during the first 30 days after insertion. They were not related to infection in women who were married or cohabitating and who said they had had only one sexual partner in the previous 6 months. A very large review of IUD experience from the World Health Organization confirmed these findings. The incidence of PID was minimal beyond the first 21 days after insertion. PID rates were highest in young, nulligravid women. Whether this is a truly biologic phenomenon or simply that youth and nulliparity are associated with having more partners and hence more risk of sexually transmitted disease has not been clarified. Only one type of infection is clearly related to IUDs. Women who wear plastic IUDs for several years may become colonized with actinomyces. Actinomyces pelvic infection appears to have been reported only in plastic IUD-wearing women. Copper probably inhibits actinomyces, as this problem appears not to have been associated with the copper devices. Copper in the concentrations released by the IUD inhibit the growth of chlamydia organisms in cultured endometrial cells.

Associated Ectopic Pregnancy

Intrauterine devices prevent pregnancy better in the uterus than in other locations. When pregnancy occurs in an IUD-wearing woman, the probability that it will be ectopic is approximately 5 per 100 pregnancies, as compared with a general risk of approximately 1 in 100. However, with the T380A device and the levonorgestrel IUD, risk of pregnancy occurring anywhere is much reduced, so that the overall rate of ectopic pregnancy in women wearing these devices is actually considerably less than that of women using no contraception. The Progestasert increases the occurrence of ectopic pregnancy beyond that seen in the general population, as does the progestin-only oral contraceptive.

Intrauterine devices are frequently blamed for our present epidemic of ectopic pregnancies, but since so few women in our country have ever worn IUDs, they can be implicated in a very small proportion. Previous salpingitis is a far more important risk factor. An IUD-wearing woman who presents with pelvic pain or abnormal bleeding must be evaluated for ectopic pregnancy, but so must any women of reproductive age, even those who have had tubal sterilization.

Fertility

Normal fecundability is restored with removal of the device. Large studies show no difference in return to fertility between women discontinuing IUDs and those discontinuing barrier contraception. There is a weak association between past use of IUDs and infertility, although this is controversial and is strongly related to the number of sexual partners and to the acquisition of sexually transmitted infections.

Clinical Use

Patient Selection

The key to safe use of IUDs is the exclusion of women already at increased risk for salpingitis.

Other conditions we feel should exclude IUD use are listed in Table 1. We advise an initial visit to allow for thorough discussion of risks, benefits, and alternative methods and for testing for cervical gonorrhea and chlamydiosis. Vaginitis, if present, should be treated before insertion. The patient is given detailed written information about IUDs, such as that supplied by the manufacturer of the ParaGard, and is then scheduled for a second visit for insertion, usually during cycle days 5 to 12. Some would instruct the patient to take oral doxycycline just prior to the insertion visit. Since risk of pelvic infection appears related to insertion, use of prophylactic antibiotics makes sense. However, no study to date has been able to demonstrate a benefit, probably because the risk of infection in properly screened women is so low that a sample size larger than any studied to date would be needed. The patient may be advised to take 400 mg of ibuprofen or similar agent prior to insertion to reduce discomfort.

Insertion

A sensitive uterine pregnancy test is performed just prior to insertion. Pelvic examination is performed, noting uterine size and position. The upper vagina is washed with a germicidal solution. The cervix is grasped with a tenaculum and the depth and direction of the cavity determined with a uterine sound. A uterine sounding of less

---

TABLE 1. Contraindications to Intrauterine Device Use

Contraindications listed by manufacturer:°
  Pregnancy or suspicion of pregnancy
  Abnormalities of the uterus resulting in distortion of the uterine cavity
  Acute pelvic inflammatory disease or history of pelvic inflammatory disease
  Postpartum endometritis or infected abortion in past 3 months
  Known or suspected uterine or cervical malignancy including unresolved, abnormal Pap smear
  Genital bleeding of unknown etiology
  Untreated acute cervicitis or vaginitis, including bacterial vaginosis, until infection is controlled
  Wilson's disease or known copper allergy (for copper devices)
  History of ectopic pregnancy
  Patient or partner has multiple sexual partners
  Conditions associated with increased susceptibility to infections, including AIDS, IV drug use, and those
      requiring chronic corticosteroid therapy
  Genital actinomycosis
  A previously inserted IUD that has not been removed
We suggest the following additional contraindications:
  Chronic pelvic pain
  History of infertility
  Colonization with gonorrhea or chlamydia
  Chronic immune suppressive therapy, whether or not steroids are used

---

°Modified from prescribing information, ParaGard T380A Intrauterine Copper contraceptive. GynoPharma, Inc., Somerville, NJ, October 1991.

than 6.5 cm from external cervical os to fundus indicates a uterine cavity that is probably too small to comfortably accommodate currently available IUDs. A uterus that sounds to longer than 10 cm may not be well protected from pregnancy by the IUD.

Insertion technique varies somewhat with the type of IUD and its inserter. With the ParaGard device, the IUD is loaded into its inserter by compressing the side arms with sterile gloves. This should be performed just before insertion, as leaving the side arms compressed for more than a few minutes will result in slow return of the side arms to the extended position, and possible expulsion. The device inside its inserter is gently pushed into the uterine cavity and up against the fundus while maintaining downward traction on the tenaculum to straighten the angle between the cervical canal and the uterine cavity. While holding pressure with the push rod, the inserter's tubular outer sheath is partly withdrawn, just enough to release the side arms of the T. The sheath is then advanced into the uterus again to lift up the side arms and position the device at the top of the fundus before withdrawing the inserter. The patient is kept lying on the examination table for a few minutes to avoid syncope.

Insertion by an experienced practitioner is usually perceived as producing brief pain of moderate intensity. If the patient is fearful, paracervical anesthesia is offered, with 1% lidocaine injected into the cervix at 12, 4, and 8 o'clock positions to a total of 10 mL.

A similar but somewhat different technique is required for insertion of the Progestasert. It has a more complex inserter with an outer sheath that automatically folds the arms of the T. The manufacturer's instructions should be carefully studied prior to insertion.

Post-insertion instructions include a reminder to self-examine to confirm that the IUD strings are still present prior to intercourse, to come in promptly if pregnancy is suspected, and to report persistent pelvic pain or unexplained fever.

Follow-up

The patient is examined after her first menses to check for unnoticed expulsion, and then annually. She is asked about pelvic pain and bleeding and vaginal discharge. Purulent cervical secretions or pelvic tenderness on examination suggest the need for gonorrhea and chlamydia tests. The cytology laboratory should be instructed to search for actinomyces on the annual cervical cytologic examination. If found, we advise removal of the IUD and treatment with oral penicillin.

Pregnancy

Should pregnancy occur, the IUD should be removed immediately, while the IUD strings are still visible. Pregnancy with an IUD in situ does not produce fetal malformation, but it does place the patient at significant risk for septic abortion, premature rupture of the membranes with sepsis, and preterm labor. Delay and continued growth of the uterus may pull the strings up inside the uterus, complicating later removal. The patient should have the option of safe legal pregnancy termination. If she chooses to continue the pregnancy and the strings are not visible, an ultrasonographic examination is performed to locate the IUD. It may have been expelled, or an unnoticed perforation may have occurred at insertion. If the device is still in the uterus and is either lateral to the gestation sac or caudal to it, intrauterine removal under ultrasonographic guidance by an experienced person should be offered. A small alligator-type forceps is introduced through the cervix and guided to the IUD, which is then gently retrieved. Prophylactic antibiotics are administered. This maneuver will usually be successful, unless the IUD is rostral to (above) the gestational sac. If the patient declines removal of the device, she should be cautioned to report any early signs of developing sepsis at once: pelvic pain, fever, or bleeding. Emergency evacuation of the uterus and high-dose antibiotic therapy may be needed.

Pain and Bleeding

These symptoms usually indicate the development of an endometritis. The patient should be evaluated for gonorrhea, chlamydia, and bacterial vaginosis. Pregnancy must be ruled out. If symptoms are severe, or if uterine tenderness or fever is present, we would remove the device and treat with antibiotics. If these are not present and there is no uterine tenderness on examination, the patient can continue intrauterine contraception while attempts are made to treat the symptoms. Ibuprofen at the time of menses may provide sufficient pain relief and reduction of menstrual flow to allow continuation. If symptoms persist, removal of the device should be considered.

Perforation

Perforation is suspected when the strings cannot be seen and are not present in the cervical canal, or when pregnancy has occurred. Ultrasonography will confirm whether the device is in the uterus but can easily miss a device that is free in the abdominal cavity. A radiograph of the abdomen will be needed to exclude a perforated device. If the patient is pregnant and will continue the pregnancy, the radiograph can be deferred until after delivery. Because the IUD can provoke an intense intra-abdominal inflammatory response with adhesions, we advise laparoscopic removal of any perforated devices.

Use in Special Patients

Women with Heavy Menses or Dysmenorrhea

In contrast to the ParaGard device, which may increase menstrual bleeding and pain, the Progestasert often reduces these symptoms and could be considered for women with heavy menses or dysmenorrhea.

Cardiac Patients

In our opinion, IUDs provide an excellent alternative for long-term contraception for women with heart disease, provided the patient is otherwise suited for IUD use. The ParaGard device is an excellent choice, except in patients who take anticoagulants, in whom increased menstrual bleeding could be a problem. Although bacteremia has not been reported from IUD insertion, we would use prophylactic antibiotics for IUD insertion in cardiac patients and would pretreat them with atropine 0.5 mg IM to block "cervical shock," a form of vasovagal syncope that may provoke arrythmia. Continuous monitoring of the electrocardiograph during insertion is prudent.

Women with Diabetes

In our opinion, diabetes does not contraindicate IUD use, provided the patient is otherwise a good candidate at low risk for salpingitis and desires long-term contraception. Diabetic women are no more likely than other women to suffer complications with IUDs.

Other Uses

Postcoital Contraception

The copper IUD is a highly effective postcoital contraceptive. If it is inserted within 7 days of intercourse, it will prevent implantation in most cases.

Menopausal Hormone Replacement

The levonorgestrel IUD has been used as a way to conveniently provide progestin therapy to prevent endometrial hyperplasia in women receiving estrogen replacement.

Leiomyomata Uteri

Andrew J. Friedman, MD

Uterine fibroids, also known as leiomyomas or myomas, are the most common pelvic tumors in women. Fibroids develop only during a woman's reproductive years with a peak incidence between ages 30 and 50; they are not seen prepubertal girls, and new tumors do not develop after menopause. It is estimated that 25% of women have fibroids that are clinically detectable. Small (ie, clinically undetectable) or microscopic fibroids are present in approximately 75% of all uteruses. Approximately 20% to 50% of all women with clinically detectable fibroids have symptoms due to an enlarged pelvic mass or excessive menstrual flow, or both. Because of their high prevalence and potential to cause symptoms that can lead to a decreased quality of life, leiomyomas are of tremendous public health importance.

Composition, Nomenclature, and Etiology

Fibroids are benign neoplasms composed of smooth muscle cells and extracellular matrix (ECM). ECM consists primarily of collagen, proteoglycans, and fibronectin. The relative amounts of smooth muscle cells and ECM vary among fibroids, but ECM generally occupies a greater proportion of tumor volume.

Fibroids are categorized by their location within the uterine wall. Those located just under the serosa are called subserosal fibroids; those located primarily within the myometrium are called intramural fibroids; tumors that project into the uterine cavity are termed submucous fibroids. Since most fibroids span more than one anatomic space, accurate characterization of these tumors is often difficult.

Although the etiology of fibroids has not been elucidated, it is generally believed that these tumors result from somatic mutations. Once a somatic mutation has occurred, clonal expansion results in tumor growth and, often, symptom formation. It is unclear whether environmental or endocrine factors have a role in tumor initiation. Once a fibroid has developed, estrogen and progesterone modulate tumor growth either directly or indirectly via growth factors. It is the dependence of fibroids on these hormones that provides the rationale behind most medical treatments available today.

Symptoms

The majority of women with uterine fibroids are asymptomatic. The development of symptoms is related to tumor size and location within the uterus. Large tumors may cause extrinsic pressure on adjacent pelvic and abdominal organs, leading to pelvic discomfort, urinary frequency, and the sensation of bloating and pelvic fullness. Less commonly, women may present with constipation or early satiety. In rare instances, a large subserosal fibroid may cause partial ureteral compression, which in turn may lead to hydroureter and hydronephrosis and an increased likelihood of pyelonephritis and compromised renal function. Tumors located near, or in, the endometrial cavity may cause prolonged or excessive menstrual flow. In some cases, excessive menstrual bleeding may lead to the development of iron-deficiency anemia.

Infrequently, fibroids may contribute to reproductive dysfunction. It is estimated that 10% to 15% of infertile women have fibroids; however, in only 2% to 3% of all cases of infertility are fibroids thought to be the cause. Women with fibroids who conceive have an increased risk of spontaneous pregnancy loss, premature labor and delivery, malpresentation of the fetus (eg, breech presentation), abruptio placenta, and postpartum hemorrhage. The risk of these adverse outcomes is highest in women with tumors located in or near the uterine cavity.

When a patient presents with fibroid-related symptoms, it is important for the clinician to assess how these symptoms affect her quality of life. If symptoms are absent or only mild in intensity, the clinician may follow the patient with "watchful waiting," avoiding immediate medical or surgical intervention. Once symptoms progress to moderate-to-severe intensity (ie, when they affect a woman's quality of life on a daily basis), strong consideration should be given to medical or surgical intervention.

Leiomyomas During Pregnancy

After a woman conceives, estrogen and progesterone concentrations rise steadily throughout the gestation. The uterus grows under the influence of hormonal stimulation. Although it is commonly believed that all fibroids grow during pregnancy, this is not the case. Some tumors increase in size, some remain unchanged, and some actually regress. The majority of these changes occur during the first trimester. In addition to the above-stated problems caused by fibroids, these tumors may undergo degeneration during pregnancy, leading to the development of severe abdominal or pelvic pain. In rare cases, women with leiomyoma degeneration may require hospitalization and treatment with narcotics. Degeneration of fibroids may also contribute to the development of premature labor.

The presence of uterine fibroids increases the likelihood of cesarean section delivery. Should this occur, it is recommended that a myomectomy not be performed at the time of cesarean section because it may significantly increase the amount of intraoperative blood loss. Fibroids that are pedunculated (ie, attached to the uterus by a thin stalk) may be safely removed at cesarean section, however.

Diagnosis

The majority of women with fibroids are diagnosed at the time of pelvic examination. The clinician will appreciate an enlarged and, often, irregularly shaped uterus. A pelvic sonogram will confirm that the enlarged pelvic mass is of uterine origin. Magnetic resonance imaging may also help to elucidate the nature of the pelvic mass, but is often unnecessary and more costly. For women with heavy or prolonged menstrual bleeding, hysterosalpingography or sonohysterography may be performed to evaluate the uterine cavity for the presence of a filling defect suggestive of a uterine fibroid. Hysteroscopy may also aid in the diagnosis and, often, treatment (eg, resection) of a uterine fibroid discovered on a hysterosalpingogram.

Women who present with excessive menstrual flow should have an endometrial biopsy to rule out endometrial hyperplasia, carcinoma, or sarcoma. If an endometrial biopsy cannot be performed, a dilatation and curettage should be done.

Leiomyosarcomas

Leiomyosarcomas are malignant neoplasms that may be difficult to distinguish from leiomyomas in the early stages. Leiomyosarcomas often lead to uterine growth and irregular menstrual bleeding. It is estimated that 0.1% to 0.5% of uterine masses are leiomyosarcomas. It is unclear whether leiomyosarcomas arise from mutations in leiomyomas or in myometrium. The mean age of women with leiomyosarcomas is 55. The diagnosis is usually made on a hysterectomy specimen demonstrating a high mitotic index (usually greater than 10 mitoses/10 high-powered fields) and cellular pleomorphism.

Treatment Options

Watchful Waiting

In cases in which uterine fibroids cause no symptoms or symptoms of minor intensity, patients may be best served by close observation. Previous recommendations included the need for surgical intervention once the uterus is enlarged to the size of a 12-gestational-week uterus (approximately 280 g), but these guidelines have recently been challenged. Therefore, women with an enlarged uterus may be observed if there is no rapid growth in uterine size and minimal or no symptoms are present.

Although there is no uniformly accepted protocol for watchful waiting, a prudent approach may be to re-examine a woman 3 to 6 months after her initial visit to make certain that rapid uterine growth has not occurred and that new symptoms have not emerged or intensified. If a woman has remained stable during that time interval, she may be evaluated twice yearly. In cases in which uterine enlargement makes it difficult or impossible to palpate the ovaries on bimanual examination, a yearly pelvic ultrasonogram may be advised. The ultrasonogram will provide objective measurements of uterine/fibroid size as well as an assessment of ovarian size and architecture.

A baseline complete blood count with appropriate follow-up testing is also recommended. A number of studies have shown poor correlation between a woman's estimated blood loss during her menses and her hematocrit. When anemia is discovered, iron supplementation should be prescribed.

Medical Treatment

Gonadotropin-Releasing Hormone Agonists

The rationale behind medical therapy of uterine leiomyomas relies on the tenet that these tumors are sensitive to estrogen and progesterone. Modulation of these ovarian hormones will usually lead to changes in uterine and leiomyoma size. Induction of a hypoestrogenemic, hypoprogestinemic milieu with a gonadotropin-releasing hormone (GnRH) agonist will lead to regression of these tumors as well as shrinkage of the uterus.

The average reduction in uterine and leiomyoma volume is 40% to 50%, with maximum reduction usually achieved by 2 to 3 months. This "medical oophorectomy" will also induce endometrial atrophy, leading to amenorrhea. Anemic women will often have restoration of normal blood counts within 1 to 3 months. Thus, treatment with a GnRH agonist often leads to a reduction in symptoms due to an enlarged pelvic mass and excessive menstrual flow.

In the majority of patients, GnRH agonists cause side effects. Over 90% of women will experience hot flashes. Other women may experience vaginal dryness, headaches, muscle or joint stiffness or pain, transient hair loss, and mood changes. A major concern about long-term treatment with GnRH agonists is the effect of chronic hypoestrogenemia on bone loss. The average trabecular bone loss in patients treated for 6 months is approximately 3% to 6%. Although controversial, many investigators have reported that the loss of bone is not fully recovered after cessation of treatment. A treatment course of GnRH agonists is therefore limited to 3 to 6 months for preoperative therapy in most cases. The combination of GnRH agonists and hormone replacement therapy (ie, low doses of estrogen and progestin) is being investigated as a way to safely prolong the duration of treatment while avoiding many of the hypoestrogenic sequelae of GnRH agonist–only therapy.

Other

Progestins, androgens, and combination oral contraceptives may all be used to control excessive menstrual flow. Synthetic progestins and androgens will induce atrophy of the endometrium, causing endometrial thinning and resulting in a decrease in menstrual flow. These medications will not reliably decrease uterine or myoma size.

Surgery

Myomectomy

Myomectomy is a conservative surgical procedure in which uterine fibroids are removed from the uterus with subsequent uterine reconstruction. Myomectomy may be done endoscopically via hysteroscopy or laparoscopy in appropriately selected cases. Relatively small submucous fibroids can be resected with a resectoscope (operative hysteroscope); pedunculated and subserosal tumors can be resected via laparoscopy. It is occasionally beneficial to pretreat patients with a GnRH agonist or other medical therapy to induce myoma shrinkage, endometrial atrophy, and menstrual suppression leading to an increase in preoperative hemoglobin concentration and hematocrit.

More commonly, myomectomy is performed via a laparotomy. This is the safest approach for patients with large or multiple tumors. Myomectomy is highly successful in reducing or eliminating symptoms of an enlarged pelvic mass and excessive menstrual flow. Approximately four of five women undergoing myomectomy with preoperative complaints of menorrhagia will have resolution of this problem.

The effect of myomectomy on improving reproductive potential is less well studied, with inconsistent results reported in the literature. Some studies have reported enhancement of fertility after myomectomy in women with large submucous fibroids when no other etiology for infertility is discovered. Other case series have suggested that myomectomy may be helpful in treating some cases of recurrent miscarriage. The effectiveness of myomectomy in treating reproductive dysfunction is a difficult matter to study because of the large number of variables that affect fertility, the near impossibility of getting two relatively equal study groups, and the difficulty in conducting a randomized clinical trial.

Myoma Recurrence

The reported recurrence rates of myomas following myomectomy is quite variable. This reflects different study populations and different ways of assessing fibroid recurrence. For example, those studies that rely on bimanual examinations generally report a much lower recurrence rate than those that use ultrasonography to make the diagnosis.

In general, patients with a greater number of myomas at the time of myomectomy have a higher chance of recurrence. Patients with more than three or four myomas noted at myomectomy often have recurrence rates of 25% to 50% within 5 years. Only a minority of patients with recurrence will need a second major surgical procedure, but this possibility needs to be discussed with the patient before her first myomectomy. It is fibroid number, not size, that determines the chance of recurrence. Another factor that influences recurrence rates is the duration of follow-up after myomectomy. Thus, a 25-year-old woman undergoing myomectomy would be expected to have a higher lifetime recurrence rate than a 48-year-old woman undergoing the same surgical procedure.

Hysterectomy

Hysterectomy, the second most commonly performed major surgical procedure in the United States, is often performed for uterine fibroids. Approximately one third of all hysterectomies in the United States are performed with fibroids as the primary indication; among African-Americans, fibroids account for two thirds of all cases of hysterectomy.

Approximately 90% of all fibroid hysterectomies are performed abdominally. Abdominal hysterectomy gives the surgeon some flexibility with regard to the type and length of the incision. Very large tumors can be removed through an abdominal incision more easily and safely than through vaginal or laparoscopic approaches. An abdominal incision also gives the surgeon the ability to evaluate other organs in the pelvis and abdomen. Ovarian and or cervical conservation may be elected with this operation.

Although hysterectomy is the only cure for fibroids, the patient must be absolutely clear that this operation will render her unable to bear children. Even in cases in which a woman has completed her childbearing, the importance of preserving the uterus should not be underestimated and must be discussed when counseling a patient about treatment options.

A vaginal hysterectomy may be performed by a skilled surgeon when the uterine size is below his or her "uterine size threshold" to perform vaginal surgery. Other factors that must be taken into account are the location of the fibroids, anatomy of the patient's bony pelvis, her pelvic outlet including soft tissues, uterine mobility, the presence or absence of pelvic adhesions, and the patient's preference. Vaginal surgery, when performed by a skilled surgeon, will result in decreased morbidity compared with abdominal surgery. The mean recovery time for vaginal hysterectomy is 2 to 4 weeks compared to 4 to 6 weeks for abdominal hysterectomy.

Laparoscopically assisted vaginal hysterectomy (LAVH) is a relatively new technique that combines vaginal surgery with the assistance of laparoscopy to free the uterus from its uppermost attachments to the pelvis. The laparoscopic portion of the procedure is done first to maintain a pneumoperitoneum. The adnexa can be more easily resected when laparoscopy is used, especially when the uterus is large. Typically, the surgeon performs the laparoscopic portion of the procedure down to the level of the uterine vessels before starting the vaginal portion of the procedure. The recovery time for LAVH is approximately the same as for vaginal hysterectomy. Use of the laparoscope will help to increase the surgeon's "uterine size threshold" for performing vaginal surgery.

As preoperative medications, GnRH agonists may be appropriate in women seeking vaginal hysterectomy or LAVH. Decreasing the size of the uterus by 30% to 50% after 2 to 3 months may enable the surgeon to perform a vaginal hysterectomy or LAVH in selected cases. It must be remembered, however, that individual patients may have a wide variation in their response to a GnRH agonist, making it difficult to predict precisely the degree of uterine shrinkage.

Laparoscopic supracervical hysterectomy is a procedure done solely through the laparoscope with no vaginal incisions. This procedure is not performed widely but may become more popular as laparoscopic instrumentation and training improve.

Myolysis, the thermal coagulation of tumors performed with electrocautery or laser at laparoscopy, is an experimental procedure that has had some promising preliminary results. Other investigators are evaluating myoma freezing as another means to induce myoma necrosis. The efficacy and safety of these techniques have not yet been evaluated adequately or compared with other more traditional therapies.

Conclusion

Treatment options for uterine fibroids have grown steadily over the past 5 to 10 years with the advent of new medications and better surgical techniques. Although fibroids remain primarily a surgically treated disease, the possibility of using medications alone or in combination with minimally invasive or vaginal surgery is appropriate in selected cases. Proper counseling of patients involves a discussion of treatment options and the natural history of the disease.

Luteal Phase Defect

Georgeanna S. Jones, MD

A luteal phase defect (LPD) is an abnormality of progesterone production by the corpus luteum. Since ovulation occurs, it cannot be considered an ovulatory defect. Occasionally, a luteinized unruptured follicle is associated with a corpus luteum defect, but it may also have completely normal progesterone production. An endometrial defect of progesterone receptors, which is not a corpus luteum deficiency, also cannot be considered a luteal phase defect.

Symptomatology

A luteal phase defect is associated with both primary and secondary infertility. Its incidence in primary infertility or failure of implantation is between 5% and 15% of patients, depending on the population mix. Secondary infertility, or repeated first-trimester abortion, is due to shallow implantation or to failure of endometrial leukocytes to mount a reaction to the maternal rejection response. These miscarriages are usually widely spaced and with no, or poor, fetal development. The incidence of the luteal phase defect in these early miscarriages is approximately 35%, again depending on the population mix.

Anatomy

The corpus luteum differs from almost all other body structures in that it is renewed with every ovulatory menstrual cycle. It is a continuation of the graafian follicle, but when granulosa and theca cells luteinize to become a corpus luteum, they are morphologically and physiologically different from the same cells in the graafian follicle.

At the luteinizing hormone (LH) surge, the

granulosa cells, which have been the most rapidly replicating cells in the body, become fully differentiated and no longer replicate. Their major function, which during the follicular phase was protein synthesis for development and maturation of the oocyte, becomes steroid synthesis of progesterone, although protein synthesis of inhibin, oxytocin, and aromatase continues. (Production of aromatase is especially important for increased estrogen secretion in synergism with theca androgen.) The granulosa cell LH receptors, which were induced late in the follicular phase by follicle-stimulating hormone (FSH) and estradiol (E_2), differ from the endogenous receptors of the theca cells. Granulosa cell receptors are fully occupied by the LH surge and continue to translate the progesterone message for 10 days only, probably through their stable messenger RNA (mRNA). They do not respond to either the LH pulse or human chorionic gonadotropin (hCG) administration.

During luteinization, the theca retains its angiogenesis function and continues to regenerate as it incorporates into the interstices of the corpus luteum. Since the LH receptors of the theca are endogenous and do internalize and regenerate, the theca is responsible for the pulsatile pattern of progesterone, which appears approximately 3 days after ovulation. The theca responds not only to the LH pulses but also to the hCG stimulus from the trophoblast. Therefore, the theca "rescues" the corpus luteum if pregnancy occurs; the corpus luteum of pregnancy is composed of these luteinized theca cells.

Function

Both the theca and granulosa are important in preparing the endometrium for implantation. Although the luteinized granulosa cell is responsible for the major progesterone production during the first 7 days of the luteal phase, the pulsatile response of the theca, related to LH pulses, adds considerably to the progesterone pool after luteal day 4.

The major early response of the surface endometrial epithelium to progesterone—the formation of glycoproteins necessary for attachment of the zona pellucida of the fertilized eggs—is probably due to granulosa cell function. The theca component may be more important for inducing those elements that allow penetration and adherence of the trophoblast with dissolution of vessels. The theca furnishes the last 4 days of progesterone and stimulates the major progesterone-specific endometrial leukocytes. These are

"killer cells" that prevent the mounting of a maternal rejection reaction during the stage of trophoblastic penetration prior to complete villus formation. After this, the fetus is protected by the absence of human leukocyte antigen surface antigension villi. In effect, the conceptus is "hidden" from the maternal rejection reaction.

Depending on the time of the progesterone deficiency in relation to development of these elements necessary for proper embryo attachment and penetration and villus formation, the LPD causes primary infertility or early miscarriages. In addition, the empty sac syndrome would perhaps be related to failure of significant theca stimulation of the progesterone-specific endometrial leukocytes.

Diagnosis

Evaluation of the total corpus luteum progesterone production is necessary to make the diagnosis of LPD. An endometrial biopsy taken on day 26 of a hypothetical 28-day cycle is the only practical clinical technique for such an evaluation. Histologic dating by the Noyes and Hertig criteria should agree within 2 days on the theoretical date of ovulation, day 14, and onset of menses, day 28. A basal body temperature chart should be kept for an estimate of the length of the luteal span and a urine or serum LH assay should give an estimate of the date of ovulation. (If the LH surge is seriously abnormal, the urine LH may not be detected.)

Since the gland is renewed monthly, a repetitive defect should be documented. Two out-of-phase biopsies should assure one of the diagnosis. However, if the basal body temperature charts are indicative of a shortened luteal phase (12 days or less), a satisfactory clinical diagnosis can be assumed by a single out-of-phase biopsy. Because of the dual source and the changing pulsatile pattern of progesterone synthesis, a single or even multiple serum progesterone assays alone are unsatisfactory and may cause under- or over-diagnosis of LPD.

Etiology

The etiology of LPD is multifactorial, a fact that may contribute to the difficulty that many gynecologists have in accepting it as an important cause of reproductive problems. One can theoretically divide the etiology into three major categories, as follows.

Central Nervous System, Hypothalamic Pituitary Axis, and Neurogenic Control Mechanisms (β-Endorphins, Norepinephrine, Dopamine, Opioids)

These factors are the most common causes of LPD. If the LH surge is absent, no ovulation occurs and no corpus luteum is formed. (The only exception to this would be the luteinized unruptured follicle, the etiology of which is still unclear.) However, there are a number of factors that decrease the LH surge, which allows ovulation but is insufficient to fully luteinize the granulosa cell receptors. Among these are psychogenic stress, physical stress related to weight (either obesity or excessive weight loss), excessive compulsive exercise, and hyperprolactinemia (which probably exerts its action through increase in dopamine rather than excessive prolactin per se).

Any factor that decreases the LH surge will, in my experience, also decrease the LH pulse amplitude. Thus, both granulosa and theca cell production of progesterone would be reduced in proportion to the decrease in the LH surge. In the less severely affected surge, one would expect a normal 14-day span and reduced steroidogenesis; in the most abnormal surge, a short span and very poor steroidogenesis. This latter type of LPD is frequently associated with primary infertility.

Nutritional Factors, Drug Ingestion, Metabolic Disease, Immunologic Disease

A careful history and laboratory tests, if indicated, should screen for any one of the above intermediate factors, which may be causally related to LPD. Immunologic disease, specifically characterized by lupus, may act through immunologic damage to the luteinized granulosa or theca cells.

Ovarian: Smoking, Tetralogy of Fallot, Abetalipoproteinemia, and Possible Congenital Defects of Granulosa and Theca Cells

Smoking has a deleterious effect on the luteal phase, as on the total ovarian function, by constriction of the vessels in the ovarian pedicle. Tetralogy of Fallot (by reducing blood oxygenation) causes damage by decreasing steroidogenesis. Abetalipoproteinemia is an extremely unusual genetic disease in which cells are unable to internalize cholesterol because of the failure of lipid receptors. Because cholesterol is the primary substrate for progesterone by granulosa and perhaps theca cells, it causes defective progesterone production.

Finally, a congenital defect of granulosa or theca cells is a hypothetical category; it is difficult to document and probably makes up an extremely small proportion of cases. Granulosa cell defects would be clinically characterized by a normal 14-day luteal span, but very poor steroidogenesis, especially during the first 10 luteal days. In addition to complete failure of implantation, such defects might also be associated with unrecognized recurrent occult miscarriages that are interpreted as irregular, slightly prolonged menstrual cycles. The etiology of such a genetic defect might be a defective induction of LH receptors by FSH and E_2 stimulation during the follicular phase.

A defective production of progesterone by theca cells would be clinically characterized by a short luteal span of 10 or, at most, 12 days with reduced steroidogenesis, no or low progesterone pulse, and no corpus luteum rescue. The diagnosis is made by the absence of a progesterone response to administered hCG. This type of LPD would be associated with secondary infertility and recurrent first-trimester abortions. It is important to consider congenital defects, because such cases would be treated by progesterone substitution only, continued until the placental takeover has occurred.

Therapy

Therapy for LPD should be initiated only after a complete investigation for other factors related to infertility or repeated miscarriages and after therapy addressing the specific etiologic factors listed earlier.

Progesterone substitution therapy will bypass any factor causing a luteal phase defect and is, therefore, the treatment of choice. It has been used for 35 years successfully, with no complications, both at Johns Hopkins and at Norfolk. It has also been used in the Norfolk in vitro fertilization program in which over 2000 babies have been born with no increased incidence of or unusual associated congenital anomalies after postovulatory progesterone therapy. An in depth study of the first 100 in vitro fertilization babies showed that the only difference between the treated babies and a control cohort was a slightly increased intelligence quotient, related not to progesterone, but to their parents' DNA.

Progesterone should begin 2 days after estimated ovulation by basal body temperature or urine or serum LH test, or both; 12.5 mg in oil or 50 mg progesterone suppositories should be given nightly for 14 days, at which time, if no menses have occurred, a pregnancy test should be done. If the test is positive, 250 mg of 17-hydroxyprogesterone (17-OHP) is given intramuscularly and the progesterone continued during 5 days when the long-acting progesterone has developed a sufficient blood level to sustain a pregnancy. This should be continued through 15 weeks or until it can be shown by the serum progesterone levels that a placental takeover has occurred. (Since 17-OHP is not measurable in the serum as progesterone, one can estimate the patient's ovarian or placental progesterone function while it is being administered.)

In a rare disease like abetalipoproteinemia, in which the cells cannot internalize cholesterol to synthesize progesterone, or in the case of the tetralogy of Fallot, in which the blood oxygen radical is too low to support steroidogenesis, it is necessary to continue the long-acting progesterone throughout pregnancy. A dose of 250 mg of 17-OHP weekly is adequate; higher doses are not acceptable, as long-acting progesterone accumulates (unlike progesterone per se, which is rapidly excreted). High exposure to 17-OHP, which is an antiandrogen, has been associated with hypospadias in a male fetus.

Micronized progesterone vaginal suppositories, 100 mg taken three or four times during the day, or micronized oral tablets of 1000 mg a day may also cause a proper endometrial response. I have had no personal experience using this therapy, however.

If four satisfactory treatment cycles have been given without a pregnancy, re-evaluation of the treatment and diagnosis is necessary. Either a repeat biopsy on therapy and a renewed search for other infertility factors or a laparoscopic examination is indicated at this time, if not previously done. The mode of progesterone administration can be changed or the amount increased.

If there is no genetic abnormality of the theca cells, hCG can be used successfully. Ten thousand units of hCG will substitute for an LH surge, causing normal granulosa cell progesterone production and lasting through luteal days 8 to 10. It also substitutes for an inadequate LH pulse, ensuring a normal early stimulation of theca cells. A second injection of 5000 units 1 week after the first on approximately luteal day 9 will ensure a proper theca cell carryover to correct an LH pulse defect and allow adequate theca stimulation until trophoblastic hCG occurs.

Two major problems occur with hCG therapy. First, it is necessary to know that ovulation has occurred before initiating hCG therapy. If the injection is given prior to ovulation, it may cause a luteinized unruptured follicle or a lutein cyst. If the LPD is extremely severe, with a very short luteal phase and poor steroidogenesis, an LH surge may be difficult to identify. Second, hCG interferes with a pregnancy test. It is necessary to substitute with progesterone suppositories 25 mg on luteal days 14, 15, and 16. A day-16 pregnancy test should not pick up 5000 units of β-hCG from 7 days prior, but if a low positive value is obtained, a second test must be done to ensure that the beta level is rising rather than falling. I find that progesterone substitution is much simpler than hCG therapy; however, for the patient who has difficulty with daily medication, the hCG is sometimes more acceptable.

Clomiphene citrate is unacceptable therapy for LPD. In a patient who is ovulating, clomiphene citrate may cause a worse problem because it is an antiestrogen and blocks E_2 action at the cervical, endometrial, and ovarian levels. Even if the LH surge is improved and progesterone is thereby increased with perhaps a normal endometrial biopsy, it is of little value if the sperm cannot move, the endometrial receptors are not present, or the maturation of the oocyte is impaired. Likewise, progestational drugs are not useful, as they do not produce the same histologic changes in the endometrium. They also have a longer half-life than progesterone and therefore may be luteolytic to the corpus luteum.

The majority of pregnancies will have occurred by the fourth month of adequate progesterone substitution therapy. After six cycles, a 68% successful pregnancy rate should be expected in primary infertility and 90% in correction of repeated abortion.

Male Infertility: Intrauterine Insemination

Pasquale Patrizio, MD

Intrauterine insemination (IUI) is often the first procedure attempted in the algorithm of male infertility treatment. Despite its extensive use, however, the clinical efficacy of IUI in male factor infertility remains unclear, mainly because even after exhaustive work-up, the etiology of many forms of low sperm count, low motility, and low normal morphology remains unknown. Male factor infertility is assumed when on at least three different occasions a semen analysis showed that sperm count, motility, progression, and morphology were below a certain arbitrary minimum. This minimum has been revised many times during the last two decades. Today, it is assumed that a man is oligozoospermic if his sperm count is less than 20 million per milliliter; asthenozoospermic if the sperm motility is less than 50% with a progression less than 2 (on a scale of 0 to 4), and teratozoospermic if the normal sperm morphology is less than 30%. It is rare to find a patient with an isolated sperm problem. In general, two or three sperm defects are combined together with different degrees of severity. For this reason it is convenient to adopt the concept of sperm total motile count in the entire, unprocessed ejaculate and percent of normal forms for planning the best therapeutic approach. Total motile count is the product of total sperm count by percent motility. In general, the presence of a total number of motile sperm less than 3 million with a normal sperm morphology less than 14% gives a low chance of pregnancy (2% per cycle); therefore, in these instances it is recommended to proceed to a cycle of in vitro fertilization using intracytoplasmic sperm injection. When the total motile count is greater than 3 million and normal sperm morphology is greater than 14%, IUI with superovulation should offer a pregnancy rate per cycle of about 8% to 10%.

Likewise, performing IUI in women older than 42 years is associated with very poor pregnancy rates (3% per cycle); this outcome is worsened if compounded by the presence of male factor infertility.

The rationale for the use of IUI in infertility clinics is that sperm, once washed, concentrated, and capacitated, are deposited in the fundus of the uterine cavity, bypassing the cervical mucus, near to the tubal ostia and thus much closer to the site of fertilization. There are many indications for IUI (Table 1) and the results are mainly dependent on the etiology.

The highest pregnancy rates per cycle are obtained with anatomic factors, unexplained infertility, and the use of donor sperm (about 20% per cycle). However, to interpret the results correctly, it is necessary to look at lifetable analysis and to assess the cumulative conception rates after a minimum of four cycles. It is common to observe most of the pregnancies occurring in the first two cycles. After four cycles of IUI with donor sperm, the pregnancy rate is 70%, while in male factor infertility, it is about 30%. If no

TABLE 1. Common Indications for Intrauterine Insemination

Male factors
   Total motile sperm count >1 million and morphology greater than 14%
   Small (<1 mL) or large (>6 mL) volume of semen
   Seminal fluid of high viscosity (incomplete liquefaction)
Immunologic factors
   Poor postcoital test, with sperm immobilized in the endocervical mucus
   Antisperm antibodies produced in the male genital tract
Sexual dysfunction
   Anejaculation
   Status post spinal cord injury
   Electroejaculation
   Impotence
Retrograde ejaculation
   Diabetes
   Paraplegia
   Status post retroperitoneal lymph node dissection
Cryopreserved semen
   Autologous (before chemotherapy or radiotherapy; before vasectomy)
   Donor sperm (azoospermia due to complete testicular failure)
Anatomic defects
   Female: cervical stenosis, hypoplastic cervical canal thus poor mucus production
   Male: hypospadia, absence of ejaculatory ducts with sperm retrieved from the vas deferens
Unexplained infertility

pregnancy has been established after four cycles of IUI, it is time to proceed to a cycle of in vitro fertilization.

The variables that need to be controlled during a cycle of IUI are as follows:

1. Timing of the insemination with the ovulatory surge
2. Ovarian stimulation
3. Sperm preparation
4. Insemination procedure
5. Luteal phase support

Timing the Insemination

The timing of insemination in relation to the ovulatory surge, whether in natural or stimulated cycles, is very important. In general, this is accomplished by ultrasonography to measure the follicular size, the endometrial thickness and pattern and by correct use of ovulation predictor kits. In natural, unstimulated cycles, the IUI is scheduled between 36 and 40 hours from the beginning of the spontaneous luteinizing hormone (LH) surge. The patient is instructed to test her urine twice daily when the dominant follicle reaches a size of 16 mm in diameter. Poor results have been reported when IUIs are performed with natural cycles in male subfertility and unexplained infertility, thus it is recommended to time the insemination after the exogenous administration of human chorionic gonadotropin (hCG). As a rule, when the leading follicle in a natural cycle is 17 to 18 mm in diameter and the endometrial thickness is greater than 8 mm with a triple layer pattern, 5000 units of hCG are administered and the IUI is scheduled 36 hours later. In cycles in which clomiphene citrate is utilized, it is safe to wait until the leading follicle reaches a diameter of 20 mm before administering hCG. Even in this condition, it is recommended to instruct the patient to test the urine twice a day with the ovulation predictor kits to detect possible premature ovulatory surges.

Ovarian Stimulation

Using a variety of superovulation protocols, it is possible to enhance the number of eggs produced each month. Clomiphene citrate at doses varying between 50 mg and 100 mg is administered for 5 days starting on day 3 or day 5 of the menstrual cycle. Human menopausal gonadotropin (hMG) (75 or 150 IU) can be used as a single agent or in adjunct to clomiphene, usually added during the last 2 days of clomiphene therapy. Between clomiphene citrate and hMG, the latter has a much higher monthly fecundity rate (17% vs 10%). However, it is important to remember that use of gonadotropins carries an increased risk of multiple pregnancies (more frequent in cases of unexplained infertility than in oligoasthenozoospermia), a risk of ovarian hyperstimulation syndrome, and a significant increase in costs.

Sperm Preparation

Semen is collected by masturbation in a sterile container, after an abstinence period of 3 days and no longer than 5 days, especially for samples with low motility. In the event of sperm autoimmunity or extreme viscosity, it is recommended to collect the sample in medium (5 mL of modified human tubal fluid) and to process the sample within 20 minutes.

There are numerous methods of sperm processing, eg, swim-up, filtration through density gradients such as Percoll or mini-Percoll (polyvinyl pyrrolidone-coated silica particles), Sephadex columns. The goal is to choose the best method for each single case. In general, in male factor infertility the samples are usually contaminated by many cells (immature germ cells) and debris, thus it is preferable to prepare the specimen with a discontinuous density gradient. If the total motile sperm count is very low (<5 million), then to maximize the recovery rate the use of the mini-Percoll gradient is indicated. To accomplish this, three layers (0.3 mL each) of different concentrations of Percoll (50%, 70%, and 95% from the top to the bottom, respectively) are created in conical tubes. The washed sperm sample is carefully layered on the top of the 50% layer and the tube is placed in the centrifuge. After centrifugation, sperm are recovered from the 95% layer, cleaned of cells and debris. An additional washing of sperm is then required to remove the Percoll before sperm are utilized for IUI. If sperm concentration is more than 15 million per milliliter and the motility is greater than 30%, then a standard swim-up approach can be utilized. In this case, only the most motile sperm are able to swim out in medium layered on the top of the sperm pellet and thus are recovered for insemination.

The isolated fraction of motile sperm is then concentrated in 0.4 mL aliquot for insemination. In cases of retrograde ejaculation, it is important to (1) render the urine alkaline (pH between 7.4 and 7.8), (2) have the patient ejaculate in a container containing medium (10 mL), and (3) quickly separate sperm from the urine. The alkalization of the urine can be accomplished with sodium bicarbonate. The patient is instructed to drink water and to take sodium bicarbonate grains 2 hours before collection. After 2 hours, he is instructed to void, drink another glass of water, and then to masturbate. Once ejaculation has occurred, the patient is asked to void into the container prefilled with 10 mL of medium human tubal fluid. The specimen is quickly processed and centrifuged. If the pH is within the range of alkalization (7.4 to 7.8), it is common to find motile sperm in the pellet. The pellet is then filtered through a density gradient and the final sperm suspension can be used for IUI. Specimens obtained from electroejaculates in paraplegic men can also be utilized for IUI. Specimens obtained from electroejaculates, however, have very poor sperm motility and progression that ultimately limit the success of the IUI.

Occasionally, some groups have reported on exposing sperm suspensions with low motility to chemical stimulants such as pentoxifylline, caffeine, kallikrein, or follicular fluid. Pentoxifylline and caffeine are phosphodiesterase inhibitors, allowing accumulation of sperm intracellular adenosine triphosphate and this increases sperm motility. However, the clinical benefit remains to be proved.

Insemination Procedure

Some centers offer a single IUI 36 hours after hCG or LH surge, others select to perform two consecutive IUIs, 24 and 48 hours after hCG or LH surge. Data in literature are discrepant and it is unclear whether one or two IUIs should be carried out. In a recent prospective study, however, it was demonstrated that the pregnancy rate per cycle was better with two IUIs when clomiphene/hMG/hCG protocols were utilized (30% vs 13%), while there was no difference between one or two IUIs in cycles induced by clomiphene/hCG (12% vs 13% per cycle). Increasing the frequency of insemination can theoretically provide a higher chance of conception, since the ovulation of multiple oocytes may occur at different times from the hCG administration.

Many nontoxic, flexible catheters are available to perform the IUI. In brief, under sterile conditions, the sperm suspension (not to exceed 0.4 mL) is withdrawn in the catheter attached to a tuberculin syringe. The catheter is gently inserted through the cervix and the internal os up to 1 cm from the uterine fundus, where the content is slowly released. The catheter is then carefully removed, with plunging on the syringe to avoid any spill or "return" of fluid in the catheter. Whenever possible, it is the author's preference to involve the husband in the IUI procedure by directing him in the release of the sperm suspension and withdrawal of the catheter. After the IUI, the patient is instructed to remain recumbent for 15 minutes.

Luteal Phase Support

It is not clear whether luteal phase should be supported after IUI. However, after superovulation with hMG or with clomiphene citrate or both in women 37 years of age or older, it is preferable to add progesterone for luteal support. Progesterone can be used as vaginal suppositories at a dose of 50 mg twice a day, or as a vaginal gel at 8% concentration, or as an intramuscular injection (50 mg/day) from the day after IUI. Other practitioners prefer to use hCG at a dose of 1000 IU every 3 days until the day of the pregnancy test.

Male Sterilization

Mark J. Fallen, MD
William M. Kaylor, Jr, MD

Bilateral partial vasectomy is most frequently performed by a urologist but can be done by a properly trained non-urologist as well. An estimated 500,000 to 1 million vasectomies are performed annually and the procedure has been a simple, safe, reliable technique for male sterilization for decades. At present, no causal link between vasectomy and cancer has been found, including prostate and testicular malignancies. In addition, no increase in the subsequent risk of atherosclerosis or significant alteration of endocrine status has been revealed.

A thorough patient history is initially obtained to identify possible health risks of minor surgery. A genital examination is performed to determine the palpable presence of both vasa deferentia and to rule out scrotal or inguinal abnormalities. A prostate examination is recommended in men over the age of 40 years. The surgical technique is then fully described and all potential complications of the procedure reviewed. The most common early complications are generally bleeding or hematoma, superficial infection, and wound separation. Later complications include chronic scrotal pain, epididymitis, spermatocele, hydrocele, and vasectomy failure. The risk of vasectomy failure is stressed to ensure compliance with postoperative birth control and follow-up confirmatory semen analysis. Despite this risk of failure (less than 1%), the patient should be advised of the permanent nature of bilateral partial vasectomy since reversal is not only expensive but also fails to ensure subsequent pregnancy.

Bilateral partial vasectomy is typically performed as an out-patient procedure under local anesthesia with or without intravenous or oral sedation. Sodium bicarbonate can be added (3 mL in 30 mL 2% lidocaine) to the local anesthetic to prevent stinging discomfort associated with injection. The patient is shaved and the skin prepped with the patient in the supine position. The first vas deferens is palpated and manipulated to just beneath the skin surface and the skin, dartos, and perivasal tissues are infiltrated using a small-gauge needle. A 1 cm incision is made and carried through the skin, dartos, and the three fascial layers surrounding the spermatic cord. Bilateral or single midline incisions can be used. An alternative method known as the "no scalpel vasectomy" can also be used. This technique was first popularized in China and utilizes a specially designed hemostat that is sharpened at its tip to puncture the skin, dartos, and fascia and hook the vas. A second instrument (a vas ring forceps) is then used to secure the vas just prior to excision of a 1 cm segment. The vasal lumina are then electrofulgurated proximally and distally with a needle electrode cautery. A figure-eight 3–0 chromic suture closes the fascial layers over the testicular end of the vas and is held until hemostasis is assured. The suture is cut and the skin edge inspected. If good hemostasis is evident, then light pressure is applied and sterile gauze with an athletic supporter is applied. Skin sutures are used only if bleeding from the skin edge is problematic.

An ice pack is held to the scrotal area for 20 minutes in the recovery room to limit swelling. This can be repeated at home for discomfort and swelling over the next 24 to 48 hours. (A bag of frozen vegetables in a pillowcase works nicely.) Patients are encouraged to take Tylenol XS for minor pain, and Vicodin or similar narcotic is dispensed in a small quantity for higher level discomfort. The patient is advised to avoid sexual relations for 7 to 10 days and encouraged to limit strenuous physical activity for the same length of time. Postoperatively, the patients are seen at 4 to 6 weeks and specimen cups are given for semen analysis at 12 and 16 weeks. Patients are instructed to ejaculate 20 times or more prior to testing.

Menopause

Mary Evans, MD
Daniel A. Dumesic, MD

Our society is aging. Prolonged life expectancy and aging of women born immediately after World War II are contributing to the increased numbers of menopausal women in America. Women spend one third of their lives in the menopausal years, during which time they are susceptible to many of the consequences of estrogen deficiency, including urogenital atrophy, vasomotor instability, osteoporosis, and cardiovascular disease (CVD). Some women understand that the sequelae of estrogen deficiency can be prevented and that life style can be modified to promote health and prevent disease. Many do not. Therefore all women approaching the menopausal years need a health care system that prepares them for the transition to menopause, then constructs individualized preventive health care strategies, and finally initiates interventions when disease occurs.

Physiology of Ovarian Senescence

As ovarian function wanes during transition from reproductive life to menopause, the numbers of oocytes and their surrounding granulosa cells diminish. The resulting decrease in estradiol (E_2) production results in symptoms of estrogen deficiency, onset of menstrual irregularity, and changes in estrogen-dependent target tissues. As serum gonadotropins rise from the loss of estrogen's negative feedback on the hypothalamo-pituitary unit, a decrease in granulosa cell inhibin production causes preferential follicle-stimulating hormone secretion that temporarily shortens follicular development and menstrual cyclicity. Eventual loss of granulosa cell function with cessation of E_2 production induces permanent amenorrhea. Consequently, estrone derived from the peripheral conversion of adrenal androstenedione (A_4) becomes the major source of circulating estrogen.

Despite loss of granulosa cell function, the menopausal ovary continues to produce testosterone and A_4. Circulating levels of testosterone do not fall appreciably after menopause, and those of A_4 decrease by only 50%. Ovarian androgens may be involved with psychological and sexual functioning. Loss of ovarian function before the age of 40 years (normal age of menopause, 48–55 years) is referred to as premature menopause. Up to 50% of women with premature menopause have autoimmune disorders. Others may have a history of surgical castration, pelvic irradiation, chemotherapy (eg, alkylating antineoplastic drugs), viral infections, or galactosemia. Commonly, reproductive-aged women experience "medically induced menopause" while receiving gonadotropin-releasing hormone analogues ($GnRH_a$) for the treatment of estrogen-dependent diseases (eg, endometriosis, fibroids).

Symptoms of Estrogen Deficiency

The urogenital tract changes in response to the circulating estrogenic milieu. After menopause the uterus decreases in size and the endometrium undergoes atrophy. Atrophic vaginitis from thinning of the vaginal walls causes bleeding, pruritis, monilial infection, and dyspareunia. Stenosis of the upper vagina also occurs and may exaggerate the dyspareunia. Atrophy of the urinary tract and external genitalia are commonly associated with dysuria, urinary urgency, urinary frequency, and vulvar pruritis. All of these symptoms respond dramatically to exogenous estrogen.

Vasomotor instability, or the "hot flash," refers to the sensation of heat over the face, neck, and thorax, accompanied by reddening in these regions and profuse sweating. It is the most common complaint of the menopause, occurring in 50% to 76% of women. The hot flash lasts about 4 minutes and occurs at irregular intervals, often being preceded by palpitations and headache. Nocturnal hot flashes are particularly troublesome because they cause sleep deprivation with symptoms of insomnia, irritability, and mood change. Symptoms related to hot flashes are usually successfully treated with exogenous estrogen as described subsequently. Alternative therapies include medroxyprogesterone acetate (MPA), clonidine, bromocriptine, naloxone, and veralipride.

Osteoporosis

Osteoporosis affects 25 million Americans, most of whom are menopausal women and elderly people. It is the underlying cause of 1.5 million skeletal fractures annually, with vertebral fractures occurring in one third of women over age 65 years. Hip fractures account for 250,000 fractures annually in America and cause more deaths, greater disability, and higher costs than all other fractures combined. By the age of 90 years, 33% of women experience hip fractures that decrease expected survival by up to 20%. The annual costs of osteoporosis are 7 to 10 billion dollars.

Osteoporosis is a disease of decreased bone mass and increased bone fragility, particularly in the hip, vertebrae, and wrist regions. A greater degree of bone resorption than formation causes loss of bone mass. Primary osteoporosis is related to the circulating estrogenic milieu, peak bone mass, life style (eg, exercise, smoking, alcohol abuse, high caffeine intake), aging, heredity, and ethnicity (in decreasing order of risk: Northern European, Asian, black). Secondary osteoporosis refers to bone loss from an identifiable cause such as malnutrition, immobility, disease (eg, hypercortisolism, hyperthyroidism, hyperparathyroidism, diabetes mellitus, Paget's disease, rheumatoid arthritis, bone marrow disorders, intestinal malabsorption, connective tissue diseases) or drug use (anticonvulsants, glucocorticoids, heparin, lithium, aluminum antacids, $GnRH_a$).

Menopause-related osteoporosis results from excessive osteoclast-mediated bone resorption and accelerated loss of trabecular bone (2–5% annual loss for up to 10 years after menopause). Although prevention of this disease includes minimizing caffeine and alcohol intake, avoiding anticonvulsants when possible, and participating in weight-bearing exercise, menopause-related osteoporosis is best treated with antiresorptive agents that decrease excessive osteoclast activity and stabilize the structural integrity of trabecular bone. Antiresorptive agents are estrogen, calcium, bisphosphonates, and calcitonin.

Minimum effective daily doses of estrogen replacement therapy (ERT) for prevention of bone loss are conjugated equine estrogens (CEE), 0.625 mg; transdermal E_2, 50 to 100 μg; piperazine estrone sulfate, 1.25 mg; micronized E_2, 1 to 2 mg; and oral ethinyl E_2, 20 μg or less. If started within 5 years of menopause and used for 10 or more years, ERT prevents bone loss and reduces the incidence of bone fractures by 50%. If started when bone loss has already occurred, it may not confer as great a benefit on skeletal integrity but still can be used to reduce further bone loss, treat symptoms of estrogen deficiency, and prevent CVD as described subsequently. ERT must be continued indefinitely since the rate of bone loss after discontinuation of therapy is similar to that following oophorectomy. The addition of progestins or androgens to estrogen therapy does not appear to provide any additional antiosteoporotic effect.

Estrogen replacement therapy should be supplemented with daily intake of vitamin D (400 IU during winter months; 800 IU for elderly women) and calcium (1000–1500 mg elemental calcium [Ca^{2+}]). Generally, dairy products, such as milk, cheese, and yogurt, contain about 300 mg Ca^{2+} per serving. Over-the-counter oral calcium salts include calcium carbonate (500–1500 mg tablets, 40% Ca^{2+}), calcium citrate (950 mg tablets, 21% Ca^{2+}), tribasic calcium phosphate (800–1600 mg tablets, 38% Ca^{2+}), calcium lactate (325 mg tablets, 13% Ca^{2+}) and calcium gluconate (500–1000 mg tablets, 9% Ca^{2+}). Calcium carbonate is popular because it is usually well absorbed with meals and less expensive than other forms.

Bisphosphonates are synthetic analogues of inorganic pyrophosphate that bind to hydroxyapatite found in bone. They act as specific inhibitors of osteoclast-mediated bone resorption. Alendronate is one such bisphosphonate that is approved in the United States for treatment of osteoporosis. Oral administration of 10 mg Alendronate daily to menopausal women increases bone mineral density of the lumbar spine, femoral neck, and trochanter by 5% to 10% over 3 years. Because food interferes with its absorption, Alendronate should be ingested at least ½ hour before breakfast with plain water only. Its ingestion in the upright position reduces the risk of esophageal irritation. Alendronate is best suited for the treatment of osteoporosis in menopausal women who are unwilling or unable to use estrogen.

Subcutaneous salmon calcitonin, intranasal salmon calcitonin, and subcutaneous human calcitonin also are used to treat osteoporosis. Calcitonin induces an analgesic effect, possibly mediated by endorphins. Because it is expensive and may induce flushing, nausea, and drug resistance, calcitonin is often used to treat osteoporosis when ERT is not possible.

Bone mineral density (BMD) studies of the spine and hip may aid with decisions about therapy, particularly for women with suspected osteoporosis who are ambivalent about estrogen use. They also are useful for women who have vertebral abnormalities on plain radiographs, require prolonged glucocorticoid therapy, or have primary hyperparathyroidism. Several diagnostic techniques (eg, single-photon and x-ray absorptiometry, dual-photon and dual-energy x-ray absorptiometry (DEXA), radiographic absorptiometry, and quantitative computerized tomography) are available. DEXA currently is the method of choice for assessment of bone mass. It can be used to detect low BMD, defined as BMD between 1 and 2.5 standard deviations below the young adult mean value, and to monitor response to medical therapy. Repeat DEXA studies should be performed no sooner than 2 years after the initial measurement.

Cardiovascular Disease

Cardiovascular disease is the leading cause of death in American women over the age of 67 years. Approximately 250,000 deaths occur annually in women with coronary heart disease, and one in seven women between the ages of 45 and 64 years have some form of heart disease. Risk factors for CVD are menopausal status, smoking, family history, age, obesity, hypertension, diabetes mellitus, elevated serum low-density lipoprotein (LDL) cholesterol and total cholesterol levels, and suppressed serum high-density lipoprotein (HDL) cholesterol levels.

Estrogen replacement therapy reduces the risk of ischemic heart disease in menopausal women by up to 50%. Daily oral administration of 0.625 mg CEE to menopausal women lowers serum LDL cholesterol and total cholesterol levels by 15% to 16% and 4%, respectively; it also increases serum HDL levels by 13% to 16% owing to a 50% rise in the HDL_2 subfraction. These changes in serum lipoprotein levels account for only 25% to 50% of the reduced risk of CVD in estrogen users. The remaining cardioprotective effects of ERT include its ability to lower systolic and mean blood pressure, reduce fibrinogen levels, inhibit local platelet aggregation, induce vasodilation, increase cardiac stroke volume, and slow coronary artery atherogenesis.

Progestins antagonize some of the beneficial effects of estrogen on hepatic lipoprotein metabolism. 19-Nortestosterones (eg, norethindrone and norgestrel) have androgenic properties that lower serum HDL levels and raise serum LDL levels, although newer, less androgenic compounds (eg, gestodene, norgestimate, and desogestrel) may have less adverse effects on hepatic lipoprotein metabolism. The 17-hydroxyprogesterone derivative, MPA, and micronized progesterone affect circulating lipoprotein levels less than 19-nortestosterone derivatives or may have no adverse lipid effects. Oral administration of MPA in 5 to 10 mg daily doses for 12 to 14 days monthly (cyclic regimen) or in 2.5 to 5.0 mg daily doses continuously (continuous regimen) attenuates the estrogen-induced rise in serum HDL levels. It does not influence estrogen-dependent changes in serum LDL levels or significantly alter blood pressure, glucose-insulin homeostasis, or blood coagulation. Whether progestin action on hepatic lipoprotein metabolism is clinically relevant remains unclear, since ERT with or without progestin therapy appears to decrease the rate of myocardial infarction.

Hormonal Regimens

Oral estrogen therapy alleviates symptoms of estrogen deficiency and protects against both osteoporosis and CVD. The lowest effective dose of estrogen minimizes estrogen-related side effects, including mastalgia, nausea, and headache. Oral estrogens exert cardioprotective effects on hepatic lipoprotein metabolism because they are delivered to the liver in high concentrations via the enterohepatic circulation. Unfortunately, hepatic first-pass metabolism can cause erratic serum estrogen levels and rare cases of hypertension from increased renin-substrate production.

Transdermal E_2 therapy also treats symptoms of estrogen deficiency while protecting against osteoporosis. It is available in a variety of self-adhesive patches that are applied to the abdomen or buttocks once a week (Climara, Berlex Pharmaceuticals) or twice weekly (Estraderm and Vivelle, Ciba-Geigy Pharmaceuticals). Daily doses of transdermal E_2 range from 37.5 μg to 100 μg. Because nonhepatic markers of estrogen action respond similarly to the 50 μg transdermal E_2 patch and 0.625 mg CEE, and to the 100 μg transdermal E_2 patch and 1.25 mg CEE, the 50 μg transdermal E_2 patch is the minimum effective dose used to prevent bone loss. By avoiding enterohepatic circulation, transdermal E_2 is less likely to aggravate blood pressure in hypertensive individuals. It is also less likely to have cardioprotective actions on hepatic lipoprotein metabolism. Other disadvantages of transdermal E_2 are expense, local skin irritation, and inconsistent patch adhesion.

A dose of 0.5 g (0.3 mg) of CEE cream inserted vaginally at bedtime can be used to treat symptoms of vaginal atrophy. Vaginal use of estrogen cream does not protect against osteoporosis or CVD because serum estrogen levels are only 25% to 50% of that produced by comparable doses of oral estrogen. Moreover, estrogen used vaginally bypasses hepatic first-pass lipoprotein metabolism and, therefore, does not significantly alter serum lipoprotein levels. Vaginal estrogen cream is best reserved as an adjuvant to oral therapy in women with symptomatic atrophic vaginitis.

Estrogen replacement therapy alone increases the risk of endometrial hyperplasia, as evidenced by a 42% incidence of endometrial hyperplasia after administration of transdermal E_2 100 μg daily for 96 weeks. Consequently, women with a uterus require a combination of estrogen and progestin (combined therapy) to negate the risk of endometrial hyperplasia and carcinoma. The use of progestins in women without a uterus is unnecessary except perhaps in individuals with a history of stage I endometrial carcinoma, endometrioid ovarian cancer, or endometriosis. With combined estrogen/progestin therapy, cyclic progestin regimens with daily doses of MPA (10 mg), norethindrone (1 mg), norgestrel (150 μg) or micronized progesterone (200 mg) protect against endometrial hyperplasia when the duration of progestin therapy is at least 12 days monthly. Lower doses and shorter durations of cyclic progestins also reduce the rate of endometrial hyperplasia but do not eliminate it. Cyclic progestin regimens induce monthly menses in about 80% of estrogen users. They can be started on the first day of each month to avoid menses during most holidays. Alternatively, oral administration of MPA 10 mg daily for 14 days every third month can be used to induce infrequent, yet heavy, menses. The lowest dose of progestin that protects against endometrial proliferation reduces side effects (eg, headache, fatigue, mood change, bloating, mastalgia, menstrual bleeding, dysmenorrhea) and diminishes adverse effects on hepatic lipoprotein metabolism.

Continuous progestin regimens using daily doses of MPA (2.5 mg), norethindrone (0.35 mg), norgestrel (0.075 mg), or micronized progesterone (100 mg) also reduce the risk of endometrial hyperplasia in estrogen users. Continuous progestin regimens induce amenorrhea in up to 90% of estrogen users who continue therapy for 1 year. They also cause irregular vaginal bleeding for the first 6 months of therapy in about 50% of women receiving estrogen, although amenorrhea may occur sooner in women who start continuous combined estrogen/progestin therapy more than 2 years after menopause. Continuous progestin regimens are ideal for estrogen users who are willing to accept short-term irregular vaginal bleeding for the goal of permanent amenorrhea.

Some studies suggest that androgen/estrogen therapy is effective in the treatment of hot flashes, mastalgia related to estrogen use, loss of libido, and ill-defined psychological problems. Unfortunately, androgen/estrogen therapy has unwanted side effects, including hirsutism, acne, and negative effects on hepatic lipoprotein metabolism. Perhaps more importantly, the risks and benefits of long-term androgen/estrogen therapy for menopausal women are unknown. Since oophorectomized women have a greater loss of circulating androgens than women who undergo natural menopause, short-term androgen/estrogen therapy may be considered for women without ovaries, provided that they understand the risks of therapy and undergo periodic serum lipoprotein monitoring. Oral androgen/estrogen combinations, when used in women with a uterus, require progestin therapy to protect against endometrial hyperplasia.

Endometrial Surveillance

Outpatient endometrial biopsy is the preferred method of endometrial sampling. It is inexpensive and well tolerated, but it may miss up to 15% of endometrial disease, particularly focal lesions. Outpatient endometrial biopsy is recommended when women with a uterus receive ERT alone (before therapy and annually thereafter), when irregular uterine bleeding occurs beyond 6 to 12 months of continuous combined estrogen/progestin therapy, or when any unexpected uterine bleeding occurs. It also is recommended when women are at risk of endometrial hyperplasia from obesity, hepatic disease, or chronic anovulation (eg, diabetes mellitus, thyroid disease, and polycystic ovary syndrome).

Transvaginal ultrasonography can be used with outpatient endometrial biopsy to detect endometrial polyps and submucosal fibroids. Transvaginal ultrasonography also detects endometrial atrophy, defined as a total endometrial thickness less than 5 mm in the anterior-posterior plane. In menopausal women with abnormal uterine bleeding, the use of transvaginal ultrasonography alone, without outpatient endometrial biopsy, is not advised since a few endometrial cancers have occurred with endometrial thickness of 5 mm or less. Alternatively, out-patient hysteroscopy with directed biopsy is an acceptable, although expensive, technique that can be used to evaluate women with abnormal uterine bleeding and normal endometrial histology. The roles of Doppler color flow imaging and sonohysterography in detecting endometrial abnormalities remain to be elucidated.

Risk of Neoplasia

Estrogen users have an increased risk of developing endometrial cancer. Most endometrial cancers found in estrogen users are well-differentiated, superficially invasive tumors that do not affect survival if adequately treated. Furthermore, the risk of disease recurrence in women successfully treated for stage I endometrial cancer is not increased with ERT. Therefore, ERT can be given to selected women with a history of endometrial cancer for the same indications as for other women, except that patient selection should be based on prognostic indicators and the amount of risk the patient is willing to assume.

One in nine American women develops breast carcinoma during her lifetime. In other words, 175,000 new cases are diagnosed annually and about 44,000 women die of their disease each year. The relationship between estrogen use and breast cancer remains unclear, although some studies suggest that the relative risk of developing breast cancer may increase slightly after approximately 10 years of estrogen use. This finding has not been observed by other investigators. Breast cancer diagnosed in estrogen users appears to have a better prognosis than that of nonusers, perhaps reflecting a more well-differentiated tumor type or closer surveillance of the estrogen users. Withholding ERT from women with successfully treated breast cancer currently is under scrutiny because of the well-documented benefits of ERT in preventing osteoporosis and CVD. Meanwhile, tamoxifen, a nonsteroidal anti-estrogen used for breast cancer treatment, offers some estrogen-like effects on bone and hepatic lipoprotein metabolism but also increases the risk of endometrial proliferation.

Contraindications

Contraindications for ERT are known or suspected breast cancer or other estrogen-dependent neoplasia, undiagnosed abnormal uterine bleeding, active venous thrombosis, pregnancy, active liver disease or chronically impaired liver function, prior complications with ERT, and noncompliance.

Conclusion

Less than 15% of menopausal women use ERT. Of those who do so, most discontinue therapy within 6 months because of concerns about cancer and side effects, particularly uterine bleeding. Women should be counseled regarding the benefits of ERT in alleviating symptoms of estrogen deficiency and preventing osteoporosis. Furthermore, they should understand that oral estrogens alone, and perhaps in combination with progestins, protect against CVD. All estrogen users should consider the potential risk of breast cancer, while those with a uterus should receive progestins to avoid endometrial hyperplasia, even though progestin therapy may induce menses and negate some of the cardioprotective effects of estrogen. Educating women regarding the benefits and risks of ERT is the first step toward improving menopausal health care.

Microsurgical and Percutaneous Epididymal Sperm Aspiration (MESA/PESA)

Pasquale Patrizio, MD

Microsurgical epididymal sperm aspiration (MESA), combined with assisted in vitro fertilization (IVF) via intracytoplasmic sperm injection (ICSI), is now the state of the art technology for helping infertile men with irreparable obstructive azoospermia to father their own progeny. Briefly, this technique allows the microsurgical recovery of sperm "trapped" in any segment of the obstructed epididymis and their subsequent use for IVF-ICSI.

Lately it has been demonstrated that sperm can be retrieved without resorting to the microsurgical approach. This modification of the technique is called percutaneous epididymal sperm aspiration (PESA) and offers the advantages of local anesthesia, no need of scrotal incision, short operating time, quick recovery, and greater cost-effectiveness.

In 1988, the author reported the first two births from MESA and IVF in two couples in which the men had a diagnosis of congenital absence of the vas deferens. Since then, the technique of MESA, and since 1995, of PESA, has been applied to 300 men (for a total of 365 cycles) with a diagnosis of obstructive azoospermia. In general, it is reasonable to expect a 50% fertilization rate and a 30% pregnancy rate per transfer regardless of the etiology of the obstructive disorder.

Indications for MESA/PESA are (1) congenital absence of the vasa deferentia (CAVD), (2) postinflammatory epididymal obstructions with extensive scarring (eg, tuberculosis, gonorrhea),

(3) failure of vasectomy reversal attempts, (4) high ductal blockages (seminal vesicle neoplasm, sequelae of pediatric hernia repair with vas deferens ligation, ejaculatory ducts block), and (5) paraplegia not responding to electroejaculation. Congenital absence of the vasa deferentia has so far represented the most frequent indication for MESA/PESA and IVF-ICSI. Table 1 lists the major criteria to establish a correct diagnosis of congenital absence of the vas deferens. It is estimated that congenital absence of the vas deferens has an incidence of 1% to 2% of all the cases of male infertility and 25% of the cases of obstructive azoospermia. It is calculated that in the United States alone there are approximately 20,000 infertile men with infertility due to absence of the vas deferens. By adding the number of cases due to failed vasectomy reversal attempts, men potentially suitable for MESA/PESA and IVF-ICSI are in the range of 300,000.

Technical Aspects

The technical aspects involved in MESA and PESA with IVF and ICSI are directed toward a coordinated preparation of both partners and include ovarian hyperstimulation, transvaginal oocyte retrieval, microsurgical epididymal sperm aspiration, laboratory processing of the epididymal sperm for IVF and ICSI, and embryo transfer.

Ovarian Hyperstimulation

The aim of ovarian hyperstimulation is to induce a synchronous development of multiple follicles and to retrieve about 10 to 15 mature, metaphase II oocytes. Two protocols are mainly used, both consisting of a combination of leuprolide acetate, a gonadotropin-releasing hormone agonist used to suppress the pituitary, with human menopausal gonadotropin and follicle-stimulating hormone. The difference between these two proto-

TABLE 1. Diagnostic Criteria for Azoospermia due to Congenital Absence of Vas Deferens

Ejaculate of reduced volume (≤ 1 mL)
    No fructose
    pH acid
    Normal follicle-stimulating hormone
    Normal testicular biopsy
    Absence of vas on physical examination
    Positive screening for cystic fibrosis mutations

cols is the starting time of the gonadotropin-releasing hormone agonist: either late luteal phase (day 22) of the previous menstrual cycle or the beginning of the cycle (day 1).

When at least four to five follicles have reached a mean diameter of 20 mm on vaginal sonogram, human chorionic gonadotropin is administered to replace the mid-cycle luteinizing hormone surge, and the oocyte retrieval is scheduled 34 to 36 hours later.

Transvaginal Oocyte Retrieval

Oocyte retrievals are performed transvaginally with a suction needle under ultrasonographic guidance, with the patient in conscious sedation. The oocytes are then classified for degree of maturity and placed in an incubator until the time for ICSI. Before the advent of ICSI, a minimum of five mature oocytes were required to proceed with the epididymal sperm aspiration. Today, the epididymal sperm aspiration is postponed only if there are no oocytes available for ICSI.

Microsurgical and Percutaneous Epididymal Sperm Aspiration

Microsurgical epididymal sperm aspiration is performed with the patient under general anesthesia. Once the scrotum is opened and the tunica vaginalis incised, the testis and the epididymis are exposed. With the aid of an operating microscope at magnification between 6 and 20 times, an epididymal tubule is chosen for the epididymal sperm aspiration. It is recommended to proceed directly to the most proximal portion of the epididymis, since, in the condition of chronic obstruction, the most motile sperm are always found in areas closer to the testis.

Epididymal fluid is aspirated with a Medicut needle attached to a tuberculin syringe, and each aspirate is promptly handed to the biologist for the assessment of sperm presence, quality, and quantity. Careful attention must be paid to avoid blood contamination of the specimens since blood has a detrimental effect on the fertilization process. If no sperm are found or the sample is extremely poor, then another cut in a more proximal segment of the epididymis or, if necessary, in the vasa efferentia is carried out. If not enough sperm are retrieved from one side, then the contralateral testis and epididymis are exposed.

At the end of the aspiration the epididymal tubules and the tunica vaginalis are carefully re-closed to minimize scarring that could complicate further attempts at sperm aspiration.

Percutaneous epididymal sperm aspiration is technically easier. The patient requires conscious sedation and local anesthesia obtained with bupivacaine (Marcaine) injection of the spermatic cord. The aspirations are carried out by means of a 25G or 23G butterfly needle attached to a 20 mL syringe, used to create a vacuum effect, and inserted in the proximal portions of the epididymis.

If sperm are found, their number always exceeds those required for ICSI; thus, with both MESA and PESA, it is routine to cryopreserve sperm to avoid future surgeries in the male.

It is my recommendation that any epididymal sperm aspiration be begun as a PESA and proceed to MESA only if no sperm are found. At times, even with MESA, no sperm are retrievable from the epididymis or the vasa efferentia. In these instances, it is recommended to proceed to a testicular biopsy and then to extract sperm for ICSI. This very recent technique is called testicular sperm extraction (TESE).

Laboratory Processing of Epididymal Sperm for In Vitro Fertilization and Intracytoplasmic Injection

The laboratory processing of the epididymal sperm requires particular skill and expertise; this step ultimately limits the success rate of the entire procedure. Epididymal sperm are immediately diluted with human tubal fluid (HTF) medium supplemented with 0.5% of human serum albumin. Epididymal sperm are usually contaminated with blood, debris, and many amorphous and dead sperm; therefore, to clean and filter out the most motile sperm, the mini-Percoll technique is used.

The majority of laboratories are now equipped for the technique of ICSI since it has been shown to offer a higher fertilization rate than conventional IVF. After sperm have been processed, a drop is placed in polyvinylpyrrolidone solution to decrease sperm velocity. Then sperm are mechanically immobilized by stroking their tails with the tip of a micropipette. If sperm are not immobilized prior to their insertion into the egg cytoplasm, eggs can be damaged and the fertilization rates are low. The oocyte has to be prepared for ICSI as well. Only metaphase II oocytes with a visible polar body are selected for ICSI. The oocytes are first exposed to a solution of hyaluronidase to remove the cumulus-corona cells. Then, at the time of ICSI, each oocyte is positioned with a holding micropipette in such a way that the polar body is at either the 12 o'clock or the 6 o'clock position. The microneedle containing the single immobilized sperm is then inserted through the zona pellucida and the oolemma. When the oolemma has been pierced, the sperm is released into the egg cytoplasm and the oocyte is returned to the incubator.

To obtain sperm from the testicular biopsy, the testicular tissue is placed in HEPES (N-2-hydroxyethylpiperazine-N-2 ethone sulfonic acid)-buffered medium and has to be first finely minced with either microscissors or a blade. Second, the fluid is centrifuged at high speed for 5 minutes, and third, the pellet is examined for the presence of free testicular sperm. It is important to know that testicular sperm initially show minimal motility (twitching), which improves after 12 hours or more of culture or after exposure to pentoxifylline.

Embryo Transfer

If fertilization took place, 48 to 72 hours from the insemination, the embryos, up to a maximum of three, are transferred into the uterus. If the patient has patent fallopian tubes, some practitioners still prefer to perform a tubal embryo transfer via laparoscopy, since this technique has been shown to have a slightly higher implantation rate than the uterine transfer.

Excess embryos are cryopreserved and used for future transfer cycles.

Results

The first baby born after a MESA and IVF procedure was a healthy girl in May 1988. Since then, MESA and, lately, PESA and TESE have become the state of the art for treating obstructed azoospermic patients. The availability of different techniques has almost eliminated the risk of not finding sperm at the time of the aspiration, since, in the worst scenario, sperm can even be rescued from a testicular biopsy. The advent of the ICSI technology has remarkably improved the fertilization results. In the past, when only conventional IVF was available, 50% of the patients with congenital absence of the vas deferens and 65% of the patients with other forms of obstructive azoospermia experienced fertilization at a rate of 15% for men with CAVD and 30% for men with other kinds of obstruction. With ICSI, 95% of patients can expect fertiliza-

tion at a rate of about 45% to 50%. The pregnancy rate remained, for both IVF and ICSI, at about 30% per transfer. The use of ICSI has, however, allowed us to cryopreserve more extra embryos for future cycles.

Conclusion

The retrieval of sperm directly from the epididymis and their successful use for IVF represent one of the major therapeutic breakthroughs in assisted reproduction for male factor infertility. Infertile men with an established diagnosis of obstructive azoospermia can now benefit from PESA and IVF-ICSI to father their own progeny.

In developing this treatment, we were able to study some of the basic physiopathologic mechanisms that occur in the human epididymis when an obstruction exists. We learned that sperm located in the most proximal area of the obstructed epididymis are of better quality, and, although they have not travelled through any segment of the epididymis, they still have fertilizing potential. We demonstrated that sperm are disposed through a phagocytosis mechanism operated by giant macrophages. Further, by conducting immunologic studies, we have shown that antisperm antibodies are present in the serum of men with CAVD at a lower percentage than that of vasectomized men, and that the presence of antibodies of epididymal sperm do not affect their fertilization capacity.

Recently we identified the etiology of congenital absence of the vas deferens. By testing for known cystic fibrosis gene mutations in patients, their relatives, and their offspring, we found a solid link between these two apparently unrelated conditions. Men with isolated CAVD represent a variant, predominantly genital, form of cystic fibrosis and have been found to be carrying compound and rarer mutations for cystic fibrosis. Such information prompted us to perform genetic screening and counseling of the partners before PESA and IVF-ICSI procedures.

Future efforts are directed toward an improvement of the fertilization rate, and toward a better understanding of the biochemical composition of the epididymal milieu and its role in sperm-maturing or -nurturing capacity.

Non-neoplastic Epithelial Disorders of the Vulva

Raymond H. Kaufman, MD

In past decades, a whole range of different terms have been used to designate the various entities included under the title non-neoplastic epithelial disorders of the vulva. Because of the confusion existing over these various terms, the International Society for the Study of Vulvovaginal Diseases appointed a committee composed of gynecologists, pathologists, and dermatologists to review this terminology. Initially, in 1975, these various disease entities were included under the general term of vulvar dystrophies. Because of some disagreements between the disciplines making up the membership of this society, this classification was modified in 1987. In essence, it removed those lesions demonstrating cellular atypia from this group of diseases and placed them under the classification of intraepithelial neoplasia of the vulva. In addition, it included various other vulvar dermatoses under the overall umbrella of the non-neoplastic epithelial disorders. This classification is as follows:

1. Squamous cell hyperplasia (formerly hyperplastic dystrophy)
2. Lichen sclerosus
3. Other dermatoses (such as lichen planus, psoriasis, eczema)

Whereas the former classification relied on biopsy to establish a diagnosis, the newer more current classification evolved following 20 years of review, debate, discussion, and compromise between gynecologists, dermatologists, and pathologists. It has been accepted by the leaders of all three disciplines and has resulted in the uniformity of reporting of these disease entities. This is of considerable importance when one reviews the epidemiology, biology, diagnosis, and treatment of these disorders.

Of utmost importance, prior to attempting treatment of the non-neoplastic epithelial disorders, is that a precise diagnosis be established. Clinical history may be of some help to the clinician, but the primary complaint most often seen in women suffering from these conditions is that of pruritus. Pruritus is associated with a wide variety of diseases involving the vulva and does nothing more than draw the attention of the gynecologist to the source of this pruritus. Careful inspection of the vulvar tissues as well as of the vagina is imperative in establishing the diagnosis. Often, underlying fungal infections of the vulvar tissues or within the vagina are the source of the vulvar pruritus, leading to scratching and secondary changes on the vulvar tissues. Thus, specimens should be taken from lesions suspicious for fungal infections for examination in potassium hydroxide scrapings. This is easily accomplished by scraping the lesion with the sharp edge of a scalpel blade and depositing the debris accumulated on a glass slide, to which is added 10% to 15% potassium hydroxide solution. This is then cover-slipped and gently heated over a flame, resulting in the dissolution of keratinized material. This slide should then be carefully examined under the microscope using both low- and high-power magnification. In addition, a wet mount preparation should be taken from the vagina and examined in both saline and potassium hydroxide solutions, looking for various pathogens that could be the underlying cause of the vulvar pruritus.

Of paramount importance in establishing the correct diagnosis is vulvar biopsy. This is an easily performed office procedure that can be done under local anesthesia. The site to be biopsied should be infiltrated with 1% to 2% Xylocaine using a 30-gauge needle. A dermal punch is then used to provide a tissue sample for examination. In most instances, a 4-mm punch is adequate to obtain a specimen. Once the epithelium and dermis have been cut through, the specimen is lifted and the base cut utilizing fine scissors. Monsel's solution applied to the base is usually adequate to control bleeding. It is rarely necessary to place a suture for homeostasis. Once the specimen is obtained, it should be properly oriented before being placed in the fixative. This is easily done by placing the specimen bottom-side down on a small square of filter paper. This allows the pathologist to properly orient the tissue and cut sections in an accurate manner.

General Principles of Diagnosis and Management

As part of the history taken from the patient, it is important to inquire as to what local medications the patient has been using on the vulva. In addition, the types of soaps, toilet tissue, perfumes, and other substances coming in contact with the vulvar tissues should be listed. Not infrequently, the changes seen on the vulva are secondary to a contact irritant reaction. If this is the case, this needs to be identified and the patient instructed not to allow the substances or substance to come in contact with the vulvar tissue.

Careful inspection of the vulvar tissue should be done using a good light. A handheld magnifying glass ($2\times$–$3\times$) provides adequate magnification if this is necessary. Rarely is colposcopic examination of the vulva required.

As part of any treatment routine, it is important that the vulvar tissues be kept clean and dry. Often, it is useful to advise patients to discontinue the use of synthetic undergarments, not so much because they are a cause of irritation, but rather because they inhibit adequate circulation and evaporation of moisture. Either no undergarments or cotton undergarments are preferable. Often, if pruritus is intense, the use of compresses of 20% aluminum acetate (Burow's solution) will alleviate this symptom temporarily. Sitting in tap water is also useful in accomplishing this. Once the patient removes the compresses or leaves the sitz bath, the vulvar tissue should be carefully dried. The use of a hair dryer is often helpful.

Squamous Cell Hyperplasia

Most examples of squamous cell hyperplasia probably represent lichen simplex chronicus. In many instances, the changes seen on the vulvar skin are the result of chronic scratching and rubbing of the tissue secondary to pruritus. A vicious cycle develops in which the patient scratches, pruritus increases, and the patient continues to scratch. Thus, any hope for correction of this problem depends first on eliminating the source of pruritus if it can be identified and, second, on controlling the pruritus. On gross inspection, the findings associated with squamous cell hyperplasia include thickening of the tissue, lichenification (accentuation of the skin markings), often hyperemia, and more often, a white appearance to the vulvar tissue. Lesions may be localized or diffuse. A biopsy will confirm the diagnosis. The microscopic findings consist of an increase in thickness of the horny layer (hyperkeratosis) and irregular thickening of the malpighian layer (acanthosis) with associated elongation of the epithelial folds. A varying degree of inflammatory infiltration is present within the dermis, consisting of lymphocytes and plasma cells. There should be no evidence of cellular atypia. If there is, the lesion should then come under the category of a vulvar intraepithelial neoplasia.

Treatment

If an eczematous type of vulvitis is present as the result of chronic scratching or the use of poorly chosen medications, wet dressings with aluminum acetate (Burow's solution) should be applied frequently. The hallmark of treatment is the application of a corticosteroid. One of the high or medium potency corticosteroids, such as 0.025% or 0.01% fluocinolone acetonide, 0.01% triamcinolone acetonide, or similar preparation, is effective in alleviating the pruritus. It should be applied to the vulva two or three times a day. Occasionally, the use of one of the very high potency steroids such as clobetasol 0.05% is necessary to control the pruritus. The long-term use of such mid-range or high potency steroids should be avoided. Treatment should be continued for no longer than 2 to 3 consecutive weeks, following which application of the medication should slowly be tapered off. Occasionally, long-term use of this type of steroid will result in a rebound reaction, in which symptoms and physical findings become exacerbated when treatment is discontinued. Also, tissue atrophy and striae may develop following very long-term use of these medications.

Once pruritus is brought under immediate control, the potent steroids should be discontinued and replaced with a milder steroid such as 1% or 2.5% hydrocortisone cream. If an associated fungal infection is found, an appropriate antifungal agent such as clotrimazole 1% or ketoconazole 2% cream should be applied to the vulva twice daily for a period of 2 weeks. When the patient stops scratching, the gross changes seen on the vulva will often completely regress.

Occasionally, this therapeutic approach is unsuccessful and the patient continues to complain of persistent severe pruritus. Under these circumstances, a subcutaneous injection of triamcinolone suspension into the vulvar tissues will often produce dramatic relief of pruritus. Triamcinolone suspension, 5 mg, is diluted to 2 mL in normal saline. A 3-inch, 22-gauge spinal needle is used for the injection. The needle is inserted into the lower mons pubis and slowly passed subcutaneously beneath the skin of the labium majus until it reaches the perineum. Then, as the needle is slowly withdrawn, the suspension is injected. The same procedure is then followed on the opposite side of the vulva. Following injection, the tissue should be gently massaged to disperse the suspension through the subcutaneous tissues. This will often produce dramatic results that are permanent, but occasionally pruritus may return, under which circumstance a second series of injections can be carried out.

If use of subcutaneous steroids proves to be unsuccessful, as a last resort, subcutaneous alcohol injection can be attempted. It is rarely necessary to perform this procedure, but when it is carried out, it almost invariably results in complete relief of pruritus. The patient should be hospitalized and anesthetized for this procedure. Aliquots of 0.1 to 0.2 mL of absolute alcohol are injected subcutaneously at 1-cm intervals after the vulva has been carefully mapped out in a grid-like fashion. Following completion of all the injections, the tissue should be gently massaged to disperse the alcohol through the tissue. One of the complications of subcutaneous alcohol injection, especially if the alcohol is injected intradermally, is sloughing of the tissue. When this occurs, it usually does so focally, but will result in ulceration with severe vulvar pain.

It is important to keep in mind that although subcutaneous alcohol injection will relieve vulvar pruritus, it is of absolutely no value in the treatment of vulvodynia.

Lichen Sclerosus

Lichen sclerosus is seen much more commonly than is frequently appreciated. It occurs most often in the postmenopausal woman, but it is also seen in children, as well as during the reproductive years. Whereas most instances of lichen sclerosus in women are localized to the vulva, the changes of lichen sclerosus can also be seen elsewhere on the body. The etiology of this condition is not clearly understood, although it is suspected to be an autoimmune phenomenon.

Diagnosis

The gross lesions of lichen sclerosus are often classic in appearance. The lesions may be focal, but more often they are diffuse and involve large areas of the vulva, extending down over the perineum and around the anus in a figure-of-eight fashion. The tissue often has a crinkled "cigarette paper" appearance. Frequently, edema of the clitoral foreskin results in complete covering of the clitoris. Phimosis of the clitoris may be seen late in the course of the disease. The labia minora often disappear early in the course of the disease, seeming to fuse with the labia majora. Areas of telangiectasia and ecchymosis are very commonly noted in the vulvar skin. Occasionally, splitting of the skin may occur in the midline,

especially between the clitoris and urethra. In advanced stages of lichen sclerosus, the introitus may become so stenotic that the opening barely admits a finger. When present in children, the gross lesions are very similar to those seen in the adult. As with the other non-neoplastic epithelial disorders, the diagnosis should be confirmed by biopsy.

The microscopic features of lichen sclerosus are characteristic. Hyperkeratosis is usually present. The epithelium is frequently thin with flattening of the rete pegs. Cytoplasmic vacuolization of the basal layer of cells may be seen. Beneath the epidermis a zone of homogenized, pink-staining, collagenous-appearing tissue that is acellular can be seen. Occasionally, edema may be noted in this subepithelial zone. Immediately below this zone, in the mid-dermal area, a band of chronic inflammatory cells consisting of lymphocytes and plasma cells is often present. Occasionally, islands of squamous cell hyperplasia are seen intermixed with areas of epithelial thinning. Under the old classification, this was referred to as mixed dystrophy. It is generally believed, however, that the areas of squamous cell hyperplasia associated with lichen sclerosus are secondary to scratching and represent a reactive epithelial hyperplasia.

Treatment

Until recently, 2% testosterone ointment was considered the treatment of choice for lichen sclerosus. However, the use of clobetasol 0.05% has almost completely replaced testosterone in the management of this disorder. For unknown reasons, the relatively long-term use of these very potent steroids does not usually result in the same type of rebound phenomenon or vulvar atrophy that is seen when these steroids are used for long periods of time in treating other disorders of the skin. When clobetasol cream is utilized, it should be applied to the vulva twice daily for a period of 1 month. Following this, it should be applied at bedtime for 2 months followed by twice weekly for an additional 3 months. Not only will the patients often report complete disappearance of the pruritus, but in many instances, the gross changes of lichen sclerosus will regress. Following the completion of this routine, the clobetasol can be used on an as-needed basis, but no more than once or twice a week. Often, the use of a soothing ointment or even vegetable shortening applied to the vulva in a thin layer will keep the patient comfortable.

In the past, an association between lichen

sclerosus and vulvar carcinoma was suggested. However, more current prospective studies have suggested that although there is a frequent association of lichen sclerosus in patients with vulvar carcinoma, a very small percentage of individuals with lichen sclerosus, appropriately treated, ever develop carcinoma of the vulva. Somewhere between 2% and 5% of patients will develop vulvar carcinoma over a prolonged period of time. Often this occurs in patients who have not been adequately treated and who have continued to traumatize the vulva by scratching over a long period of time. In our own experience, we have seen vulvar carcinoma develop in 6 of somewhat over 200 women with lichen sclerosus who have been prospectively followed for up to 30 years.

Other Dermatoses

The other dermatoses are described elsewhere and will not be dealt with here.

Oral Contraceptives

Jayne A. Ackerman, MD
Mary Jane Gray, MD

Oral contraceptive pills (OCPs), first approved for contraceptive use in 1960, have been used by millions of women throughout the world, have been more extensively studied than any other medication, and remain one of the most effective, reversible methods of preventing pregnancy. Nonetheless, their use has been controversial from the beginning and new questions relative to safety emerge as old ones are put to rest.

Types of Pills

Oral contraceptive pills, with the exception of the so-called mini-pills, contain both synthetic estrogen and progestin. Most are composed of a fixed amount of these components in each of the active pills. The first pills contained 100 μg of mestranol as their estrogenic component. Currently lower estrogen–containing pills have largely replaced these. With the encouragement of the Food and Drug Administration (FDA), almost all of the 100 μg pills have been phased out by their manufacturers. The switch from 50 μg formulations to 30 to 35 μg has continued the reduction in estrogen; however, with the replacement of the weaker estrogen mestranol by the stronger ethinyl estranol, the change has been more apparent than real. Only two currently marketed pills (Ortho-Novum 1/50 and Norinyl 1 + 50) contain mestranol, and only a few contain less than 30 μg of ethinyl estradiol.

A decrease in progestin content has accompanied the reduction in estrogen. There are currently six synthetic progestins in general use in the United States (Table 1). Two new progestins—degestrel and norgestimate—are equally effective and less androgenic than previous ones. These progestins have less effect on carbohydrate and lipid metabolism and may, therefore, in individual users, side effects depend not only on the particular progestin a pill contains but also on variation in an individual's genetic make-up.

In an effort to reduce total drug ingestion without sacrificing control of menses, OCPs were introduced in which two (biphasic) or three (triphasic) different ratios of estrogen to progestin were combined within the same cycle. Although these are effective and produce a low incidence of side effects, there is little evidence that these OCPs are significantly safer than those combination pills containing a fixed dose of 30 to 35 μg of estrogen. Patients should usually be started on these low estrogen pills–whether fixed dose or triphasic.

Currently three progestin-only pills are available in the United States for use in women who have medical reasons for not taking estrogen or who do not tolerate it. Such pills are both less effective in preventing pregnancy (2 to 3 pregnancies per 100 women-years) and less effective in controlling bleeding. The progestin-only pills do not affect lactation and are, therefore, advised for postpartum use.

Often women who experience estrogen-produced side effects, such as headaches and breast tenderness, tolerate the 20 μg ethinyl estradiol pill. This preparation is associated with lower pregnancy rates and better cycle control than the progestin-only pills. If women do not do well on the 20 μg OCP, they may be given a choice of the mini-pill or another method of contraception.

Table 1 gives the oral contraceptive pills commonly used currently in the United States. All formulations containing more than 50 μg of estrogen are omitted. Current generic preparations are not included.

Choosing Pills

No physician can be clinically abreast of all the subtle variations in the effects of all the pills on

TABLE 1. Common Oral Contraceptive Pills

Manufacturer	Pill	Progestin (mg)	Estrogen (µg)
Wyeth-Ayerst	Ovral	Norgestrel 0.5	Ethinyl estradiol 50
	Lo Ovral	Norgestrel 0.3	Ethinyl estradiol 30
	Nordette	1-norgestrel 0.15	Ethinyl estradiol 30
	Triphasil	1-norgestrel 0.5/0.075/0.125	Ethinyl estradiol 30/40/30
	Ovrette	Norgestrel 0.075	
Berlex	Levlen	1-norgestrel 0.15	Ethinyl estradiol 30
	Tri-Levlen	1-norgestrel 0.05/0.075/0.125	Ethinyl estradiol 30/40/30
Parke-Davis	Loestrin 1.5/30	Norethindrone acetate 1.5	Ethinyl estradiol 30
	Loestrin 1/20	Norethindrone acetate 1	Ethinyl estradiol 20
Ortho	Ortho-Novum 1/50	Norethindrone 1.0	Mestranol 50
	Ortho-Novum 1/35	Norethindrone 1.0	Ethinyl estradiol 35
	Modicon	Norethindrone 0.5	Ethinyl estradiol 35
	Ortho-Novum 10/11	Norethindrone 0.5/1.0	Ethinyl estradiol 35
	Ortho-Novum 7/7/7	Norethindrone 0.5/0.75/1.0	Ethinyl estradiol 35
	Ortho Cept	Desogestrel 0.15	Ethinyl estradiol 30
	Ortho Cyclen	Norgestimate 0.250	Ethinyl estradiol 35
	Ortho Tri-Cyclen	Norgestimate 0.180/0.215/0.250	Ethinyl estradiol 35
	Micronor	Norethindrone 0.35	
Syntex	Norinyl 1 + 50	Norethindrone 1.0	Mestranol 50
	Norinyl 1 + 35	Norethindrone 1.0	Ethinyl estradiol 35
	Tri-Norinyl	Norethindrone 0.5/0.75/0.5	Ethinyl estradiol 35
	Nor-QD	Norethindrone 0.35	
Mead Johnson	Ovcon 50	Norethindrone 1.0	Ethinyl estradiol 50
	Ovcon 1/35	Norethindrone 0.4	Ethinyl estradiol 35
Searle	Demulen 1/50	Ethynodiol 1.0	Ethinyl estradiol 50
	Demulen 1/35	Ethynodiol 1.0	Ethinyl estradiol 35

the market. It is prudent to select one triphasic pill, one estrogen-dominant one, one progestin-dominant one, and one mini-pill or ultra-low estrogen pill and become familiar with these. By selecting among these, most clinical side effects can be countered.

Indications

The obvious and until recently only explicitly approved indication for OCP is contraception. Ever since the advent of the OCP, however, physicians have used these medications to treat dysmenorrhea and dysfunctional uterine bleeding. The decrease in dysmenorrhea has been recognized by almost all women taking OCPs. In part, this benefit reflects decreased bleeding; the passage of clots is almost always painful. Rarely, a woman experiences increased dysmenorrhea; changing the type of pill may reverse this undesirable effect. The incidence of symptomatic corpus luteum cysts is lower in women taking the OCP. An occasional woman with recurrent symptomatic cysts may, therefore, be helped by this medication. The triphasic pill may be less effec-

tive in preventing cysts than are the monophasic OCPs.

Dysfunctional or anovualtory bleeding in the adolescent, in whom there is scant risk of malignancy, can usually be controlled by the administration of two to four 50 µg progestin-containing pills daily for 2 to 3 days, to be followed by 3 weeks of one pill per day. Ovral is often used in this manner. If the patient is anemic, she should be kept on the pill for at least 2 to 3 months and given the opportunity to replace iron stores. Some young women revert to severe menorrhagia whenever taken off the OCP and may need to continue a low dose OCP for some years to prevent continuing disability. In all women, lighter periods decrease the loss of iron and reduce the likelihood of anemia.

The use of Ovral as a morning-after pill or emergency contraceptive has been reported in numerous series. Only recently has the oral contraceptive pill been approved by the Federal Drug Administration for this indication. The standard dose is two tablets taken together followed by two tablets 12 hours later if the woman is seen within 72 hours of unprotected intercourse. Four tablets of Lo-Ovral or other low-dose OCP may replace the two tablets of Ovral. Nausea is frequent, and promethazine may be required before the second dose. The total amount of hormone is less than that contained in one cycle of the pill as a contraceptive, and only the rigid contraindications for the OCP need apply. The mid-cycle risk of pregnancy in this circumstance is reduced to about 5 per 100 women, less than if there is no intervention. In addition to decreasing the risk of pregnancy, the search for morning-after contraception brings self-designated "at risk" women to the professional for care. In this setting, follow-up with counseling about effective contraception is extremely important.

Premenstrual syndrome (PMS) has been reported by some women to worsen and by others to improve with OCP use. Overall, the incidence is less in women taking oral contraceptives. If reduction in caffeine, salt, and sugar together with vitamin B6 supplements and increased exercise do not bring sufficient relief, the woman may be willing to try an estrogen-dominant pill such as Demulen. Many find significant improvements with this therapy.

Dermatologists early noted that estrogen-dominant OCPs such as Demulen improve acne, and that strongly progestational/androgenic pills make acne worse. Thus it is important to note the character of the skin before starting a woman on the OCP.

Contraindications

Absolute contraindications to the OCP are detailed by the FDA and include thrombophebitis or thromboembolic disease or a history of these, cerebrovascular or coronary vascular disease, known or suspected carcinoma of the breast or other estrogen-dependent neoplasms, undiagnosed abnormal genital bleeding, known or suspected pregnancy, and benign or malignant liver tumors that developed during pregnancy or while using the OCP or other estrogen-containing products.

There are a number of relative contraindications to the use of the contraceptive pill. The physician and patients must discuss risks and alternatives and come to an informed decision as to whether this method of contraception is justified. Note that cardiovascular risks and risks of malignancies are greater in smokers; therefore, smoking should tip the balance away from OCP use in women over the age of 35 years. The pill can activate the renin-angiotensin system and trigger hypertension in women with predisposing factors as well as increase blood pressure in those with preexisting hypertension. Glucose tolerance is decreased by the pill, and diabetic or prediabetic patients require special monitoring.

Experience with current low-dose pills has indicated relative safety for their use in nonsmoking women over 40 years of age. These women can be continued on the OCP until the menopause and then switched to estrogen replacement therapy as indicated.

Underlying medical condition such as congenital heart disease and sickle cell anemia must be evaluated on a case by case basis. Active liver or gallbladder disease is a risk factor because the steroids in the pill are metabolized in the liver. Since an increase in vascular headaches may precede the occurrence of stroke, a history of migraine headaches is to be considered a relative contraindication to use of the OCP. These patients should be taken off the pill promptly if headaches worsen. The occurrence of menstrual migraines in women not taking OCPs underlines the intrinsic link between hormones and vascular reactivity.

Depression can be increased by the OCP, especially by the formulations with strong progestins, and women with a history of depression should be monitored closely. Mental retardation, major mental illness, or alcoholism or drug abuse may make it impossible for a woman to take prescribed medication correctly. These women may be better served by Norplant or Depo-Provera. The increased risk of thrombophlebitis in women on the OCP suggests that the pill be stopped 4 weeks before elective surgery or if a cast or traction will impede adequate circulation in the lower extremities. Similarly, the pill should not be started sooner than 2 weeks postpartum. Lactation is a relative contraindication to the combination OCP because it may be associated with decreased milk supply; however, progestin-only pills may be used.

Side Effects

There are numerous minor and mostly transient effects of the OCP, which are often responsible for women discontinuing pills with resultant pregnancy. The most common side effect, breakthrough spotting or bleeding, should be discussed in advance so that the woman is not alarmed. If such symptoms continue more than 3 months, a pill containing a stronger progestin will usually stop the breakthrough bleeding.

Nausea and tender breasts are minor estrogen-related symptoms that are usually transient.

Fluid retention can relate to either estrogen or progestin intake but is rarely severe. Weight gain usually reflects increased appetite but can be disturbing to the patient. Decreased libido and dysphoria tend to be progestin-related side effects. Some women on triphasic pills experience increased lability of mood and will benefit from changing to monophasic OCPs.

Complications

The most common complication is hypertension in the previously normotensive woman. This usually reverses after discontinuing the pill. Vascular headaches and visual field defects reflect vascular hyper-reactivity and are cause for concern.

Signs of thrombophlebitis or pulmonary embolism must be taken very seriously, and chest pain must always be evaluated. Stroke is a very rare but serious complication of OCP use. Recent studies show slight changes in lipoproteins in women using OCPs. These changes are small and have not been linked to increased cardiovascular problems; however, it may be prudent to choose oral contraceptives with a minimum progestational effect.

Myths

The belief that the pill causes cancer is deeply held despite the fact that there is a clearly established decrease in the incidence of both endometrial and ovarian cancer in women who have used the birth control pill. Cancer of the cervix is a sexually transmitted disease related to the papillomavirus and number of sexual partners and not to OCP use per se. Linkage between OCP use and cancer of the breasts remains to be more fully evaluated; current evidence falls in both directions and is inconclusive. Although overall no increased risk of breast cancer has been demonstrated in OCP users, recent studies suggest that there may be a slightly increased number of diagnosed breast cancers in current users. These numbers gradually return to baseline after discontinuation of OCP.

Another major myth is that the use of the OCP causes infertility. There is no evidence to support this, although pregnancy may be delayed up to 2 years until ovulation resumes following the cessation of OCP use. Women using the OCP may need to be reminded that fertility decreases with advancing age.

Although it has been alleged that the OCP causes congenital abnormalities, the weight of evidence is against this.

Drug Interaction

Interactions may occur with medications that are also metabolized in the liver. Chief among these are barbiturates, antiepileptics, and antibiotics. These interactions have become more important as far as the effectiveness of the OCP is concerned as the "strength" of the contraceptive pills has been decreased and the margin of effectiveness has become very slim. It is generally held that caution is indicated if a woman is taking rifampin, but there is no solid evidence indicating that ampicillin or tetracycline decreases the effectiveness of oral contraceptive pills. As part of the overall medical history, a careful and detailed medication record is essential.

Choice

For any woman, the selection of a contraceptive method is a very personal choice. Failure of contraception represents a tragedy in any woman's life, some with far-ranging complications. The responsibility of the clinician in this important area is to provide the woman with current valid information and assist her in reaching an informed choice.

Pediatric Gynecology

Geri D. Hewitt, MD

Premenarchal girls may require gynecologic evaluation and treatment. The most common indications for gynecologic assessment are vaginal discharge, vaginal bleeding, and ovarian cysts. Physical examination of the premenarchal patient and evaluation of these common problems are reviewed.

Physical Examination

Clinicians attempting to perform gynecologic evaluations of young patients should be prepared to be patient and often spend considerable time with the patient and her parents or caregivers building trust before the actual examination is performed. Depending on the urgency of the complaints, this may include multiple visits to the office before the examination takes place. The patient should be told directly that only parents, caregivers, and doctors can examine or touch the genitals and that the examination taking place has been "sanctioned" by the parents. The patient should still be given a drape or gown for modesty purposes and to reinforce that the examination has a special meaning specific to a medical surrounding. Most gynecologic problems encountered in the prepubertal girl are vulvar and lower vaginal in origin. Unless a neoplastic process or foreign object needs to be ruled out, the upper vagina, cervix, uterus, and adnexa often do not need to be evaluated. Therefore, the extent of the examination required should be individualized to the complaints elicited while taking the patient's history.

The two different positions most useful in examining the patient are the supine position and the knee-chest position. When placing the patient in the supine position, she may sit either at the edge of the examination table or in a parent's lap on the exam table. The legs can be frog-legged, or the feet can be placed in stirrups, depending on the size of the child. The patient's head should be elevated so she can watch the examiner; also, eye contact and dialogue between the patient and the examiner can then be maintained. From this position, "lateral spread" technique can be used to visualize the vulva, clitoris, urethra, hymen, and lower aspects of the vagina. The patient or the examiner places the index and middle fingers of each hand on the lower aspects of the right and left labia and with traction gently pull downward and laterally at the same time. If the patient performs the Valsalva maneuver concurrently, either by blowing up a glove like a balloon or by blowing on the examiner's face, the lower third of the vagina can be visualized. If the upper aspect of the vagina and cervix need to be visualized, the patient can be placed in a knee-chest position with her knees and elbows on the examination table and her face turned sideways with the face and shoulder resting on the table. In this position, the buttocks can be spread, and again, with the patient blowing, the upper vagina and cervix can be visualized. An otoscope can be used as a light source and for magnification. A rectoabdominal examination should be used to assess the presence of a uterus, which will be appreciated as a small, midline mass. The ovaries, if they are enlarged, can be palpated abdominally.

If vaginal cultures or cytology are required, care should be taken in collecting them, as the vaginal mucosa is thin and atrophic and can tear easily, leading to discomfort and bleeding. Dry cotton swabs can be abrasive and painful and they should be moistened with saline before specimens are obtained. Some clinicians employ the "catheter inside catheter" technique to obtain specimens. The proximal 4 inches of an intravenous (IV) catheter can be placed inside the distal 4 inches of a red rubber catheter, which is then placed inside the vagina. The red rubber catheter will keep the walls of the vagina from collapsing on the IV catheter. A syringe is then attached to the IV catheter and 2 to 3 mL of saline is flushed into the vagina. Saline egressing from the vagina can then be sent for cytology, wet mount, and cultures. This technique may also flush out foreign objects.

Vaginoscopy may be required for patients experiencing vaginal bleeding or persistent vaginal discharge or if there is a suspicion of foreign object or neoplasm. When performing the procedure in the office, viscous lidocaine can be placed at the vaginal introitus and a pediatric endoscope can be inserted into the vagina by either the patient or the clinician. Other instruments can be used to perform vaginoscopy, including a 5 mm laparoscope, a hysteroscope, or a cystoscope. The instrument needs to be equipped with a light source and a means of irrigation.

Pediatric Vulvovaginitis

An abnormal vaginal discharge is the most common pediatric gynecologic complaint and accounts for about 50% of out-patient pediatric gynecologic visits. There are two types of vaginal discharges seen in young girls that are normal and physiologic. Leukorrhea of the newborn is a desquamation of vaginal and cervical epithelium secondary to the elimination of maternal estrogens. It may be blood-tinged and should resolve by 7 to 10 days of life. After thelarche, with increasing estrogen production by the maturing ovarian follicles, premenarchal girls may experience a homogeneous white vaginal discharge that may be irritating but should not be foul smelling. Performing a wet mount, which should reveal only squamous cells and no evidence of inflammation or infection, confirms the diagnosis.

Premenarchal girls are at risk for vulvovaginitis because of a number of factors. Obesity, diabetes, pre-existing vulvar dermatoses, or any change in immune status puts them at risk, as does poor hygiene, incorrect wiping, wearing diapers, or masturbation. The thin, atrophic vaginal mucosa is more sensitive to pathogens, and the absence of pubic hair and labial fat pads, as well as the proximity of the vagina to the rectum, are anatomic risk factors for infection.

Patients may present with discharge, dysuria, pruritus, pain, or genital irritation. The patient should be asked about the duration, quantity, consistency, and color of the discharge as well as the presence or absence of blood. Questions about hygiene and wiping, bedwetting, detergents, bubble baths, shampoos, medications, and recent infections at other sites are all important. The patient or caregiver should be asked specifically about the possibility of sexual abuse. In most patients with vulvovaginitis, evaluation of the upper vagina or cervix is not required. Initially inspection of the external genitalia and lower vagina is adequate. Diagnostic tests that are helpful include vaginal cultures for general bacterial growth, gonorrhea, and chlamydia, wet mount, cytology for maturation index, scotch tape test to rule out pinworms, urinalysis, and urine culture. Assessment of the upper genital tract is required for patients with persistent or recurrent discharge, bleeding associated with the discharge, suspicion of foreign body or neoplastic process, and with any discharge present in a diethylstilbesterol-exposed child.

The etiology of the vulvovaginitis can be either specific or nonspecific. Nonspecific vulvovaginitis is seen in up to 70% of premenarchal girls with vulvovaginitis and is a diagnosis of exclusion. The vaginal and urine cultures are negative and the wet mount usually reveals white blood cells and bacterial debris. Most commonly, nonspecific vulvovaginitis is a mixed bacterial infection caused by a disturbed bacteriologic homeostasis secondary to inadequate urinary and fecal hygiene. Treatment is focused on improving perineal hygiene and removing all offending agents. The patients should have sitz baths twice a day, and a short course of topical 0.5% hydrocortisone cream may be helpful to decrease the pruritus. If these local measures fail, a 10-day course of amoxicillin may be useful.

Specific vulvovaginitis is more often seen in older patients and can be due to a variety of organisms, which can be identified on vaginal culture. Enteric pathogens such as shigella or *Escherichia coli* may be identified, as well respiratory pathogens such as group AB hemolytic streptococcus and *Haemophilus influenzae*. Bacterial vaginosis is seen in obese patients, and candidiasis is seen in patients with diabetes or other immunocompromised states. Patients in diapers or who have recently completed a course of antibiotics may also be at increased risk for *Candida* infection. Sexually transmitted diseases

such as gonorrhea, chlamydia, or trichomoniasis can be seen in sexually active patients or those who have been abused. Treatment of specific vulvovaginitis should be directed toward the offending organism.

Vaginal Bleeding

Any vaginal bleeding, regardless of the quantity and duration, identified before the onset of menses is of clinical importance and requires evaluation. The work-up should begin with an assessment of the patient's recent growth and development, looking for any signs of puberty such as a recent growth spurt, breast bud formation, or growth of axillary or pubic hair. The patient should be asked about potential sources of bleeding such as exogenous hormones, trauma, abuse, or possible foreign objects.

When examining the patient, the clinician should try to determine whether the bleeding is vulvar, vaginal, cervical, or endometrial in origin. In most premenarchal girls, the source will be vulvar or vaginal and can usually be identified with external inspection of the vulva and vagina. Otherwise vaginoscopy is indicated to evaluate the upper vagina and cervix to rule out foreign objects and possible neoplasms.

The differential diagnosis for vaginal bleeding in the premenarchal patient includes hormonal, infectious, traumatic, and urologic causes as well as neoplasms and vulvar dermatoses. Hormonal sources of the bleeding include exogenous hormones such as oral contraceptives or estrogen cream, precocious puberty (secondary sexual characteristics in a girl less than 8 years old) or precocious menarche (menses in a girl less than 10 years old with absence of other secondary sexual characteristics), or sex hormone producing ovarian tumors. Obtaining a maturation index of vaginal cytology can identify any estrogen effect on the vagina and rule out a hormonal cause of the bleeding. Premenarchal girls should have predominantly parabasal cells on their cytology, with less than 5% of cells described being superficial cells.

Vaginal bleeding can also be present secondary to infection such as sexually transmitted diseases or parasitic infections. Bleeding can be seen with nonspecific vaginitis due to the inflammation and itching. As described earlier, these causes of bleeding can usually be diagnosed with wet mount and culture.

Genital trauma from physical activity, straddle injuries, sexual abuse, or foreign objects may cause bleeding. Clinicians evaluating girls with genital trauma need to determine the extent of the injury, if the injury can be managed nonsurgically, and if the history of the injury is compatible with the physical findings. Vulvar hematomas can be managed conservatively with ice packs, pressure, and a Foley catheter if the patient is unable to void if the hematoma is no longer expanding and the patient's hemoglobin remains stable. If these measures do not control expansion of the hematoma or if the patient's hemoglobin is dropping, the hematoma should be incised, the clots evacuated, and the bleeding points, if identifiable, should be ligated. Patients with hymenal tears should be assessed for possible upper vaginal trauma. Patients with vaginal lacerations that extend to the vaginal vault require diagnostic laparoscopy or exploratory laparotomy to exclude extension of the tear into the peritoneal cavity or broad ligament. Foreign objects lodged in the vagina can also cause bleeding and can be missed with both pelvic ultrasonography and acute abdominal series. Vaginoscopy will identify foreign objects and often the irrigation from the procedure will help flush out small foreign objects such as wads of toilet paper.

Urologic sources of presumed vaginal bleeding can include urinary tract infections or neoplasms. Urethral prolapse is identified when the urethral mucosa is seen protruding through the urethral meatus. Conservative therapy with sitz baths and estrogen cream is often therapeutic. Surgical intervention may be required if the patient is unable to void.

Vulvar lesions that may present with vaginal bleeding include hemangiomas, hymenal tags, condylomata, and molluscum contagiosum. Lichen sclerosus, which presents with flat ivory-colored papules that may coalesce into plaques, can lead to irritation and bleeding. Treatment involves improved hygiene, reduction of trauma, and topical hydrocortisone cream.

Neoplasms should be suspected with a chronic genital ulcer, atraumatic swelling of the external genitalia, or with tissue protruding from the vagina. Neoplasms that may present with vaginal bleeding include sarcoma botryoides, benign cervical tumors or polyps, and ovarian neoplasms.

Ovarian Tumors

The ovaries are never totally dormant. Autopsy studies have shown follicular activity as early as 20 weeks' gestation, which continues until menarche and beyond. Pelvic ultrasonography performed in premenarchal girls will identify ovarian cysts in approximately 70% of the ovaries visualized. Gynecologists are often asked to evaluate asymptomatic girls with ovarian cysts that are identified during renal ultrasonography. Most of these cysts are the result of low levels of gonadotropin secretion and are simple in nature without septations or calcifications. If the cyst is simple in nature and the patient is asymptomatic, she may be followed with ultrasonograms every 4 to 8 weeks. Regardless of the size of the cyst, the majority will resolve spontaneously.

Ovarian torsion is uncommonly seen in patients with ovarian cysts and is more dependent on the ovarian pedicle length and mobility than on the size of the cyst. Patients with ovarian torsion usually present with colicky abdominal pain, nausea, vomiting, a low-grade temperature, and an elevation in the white blood cell count with a left shift. Ovarian torsion requires surgical intervention, which, if possible, should be limited to ovarian cystectomy and untwisting the pedicle with preservation of ovarian function.

Patients presenting with complex ovarian masses should be evaluated for hemorrhagic cysts, ovarian torsion, tubo-ovarian abscesses, and germ cell tumors such as mature cystic teratomas or dermoids. If the ovarian tumor is solid in nature, surgical intervention is indicated to rule out malignancy.

Pelvic Inflammatory Disease

Stephanie Marie Culver, MD, MS
Mark G. Martens, MD

Pelvic inflammatory disease (PID) is a spectrum of diseases involving the cervix, uterus, fallopian tubes, ovary, and contiguous structures. Acute PID, a clinical syndrome, describes a dynamic spread of microorganisms from the vagina/endocervix (lower genital tract) to the endometrium, fallopian tubes, ovary, and contiguous structures (upper genital tract). Acute PID is often termed "acute salpingitis," but PID is not limited to tubal infections.

Acute PID is the most common and significant complication of sexually transmitted diseases (STDs). The World Health Organization estimates suggest that new cases of STDs approach 350 million per year, with up to 12 million in the United States alone. PID is the most common serious infection of women aged 16 to 25 years of age, and the morbidity produced by it exceeds that produced by all other infections for this age group. Approximately 200,000 women are hospitalized, with over 100,000 surgical procedures performed annually. Also, 2.5 million outpatients visits are made yearly in the United States.

Pelvic inflammatory disease and its sequelae affect millions of women in the United States, at substantial costs. The estimated direct costs for PID and PID-associated ectopic pregnancy and infertility were $4.2 billion in 1990. In the year 2000, costs associated with PID are projected to approach $10 billion if the current PID incidence persists.

Pelvic inflammatory disease can have significant long-term sequelae. It is estimated that at least one fourth of women who have had acute salpingitis will experience one or more sequelae of the disease. The most common is infertility. It is estimated that after one episode of PID, the risk of infertility is 12%, with two episodes the risk is 33%, and with three episodes the infertility risk climbs to over 50%. Ectopic pregnancies are 10 times more common in patients with previous episodes of acute salpingitis. Chronic pelvic pain can frequently follow resolution of salpingitis and has been documented to occur in 5% to 20% of cases. Sequelae may also include the development of tubo-ovarian abscesses, which often requires lengthened hospital stays, parenteral antibiotics, or definitive surgical treatment. Mortality has approached 10% if rupture of the tubo-ovarian abscesses occurs.

Owing to the impact PID has on women's health and the significance of its long-term sequelae, aggressive therapy initiated early and administered appropriately should be routine. Accurate diagnosis and identification of specific pathogens may warrant more liberal use of diagnostic and perhaps operative laparoscopies.

Microbiology

A common misconception is that all or most cases of PID are caused by the sexually transmitted disease resulting from infection with *Neisseria gonorrhoeae* or *Chlamydia trachomatis*. While these are important PID pathogens, their isolation from PID patients approximates 30% for *N. gonorrhoeae* and 12% for *C. trachomatis*. There is wide variation in the rates of recovery of these STDs, but it is much more common for a variety of aerobes and anaerobes to be isolated from the upper genital tract of patients diagnosed with PID. Commonly, isolated organisms include *Escherichia coli, Gardnerella vaginalis,* and *Streptococcus, Peptostreptococcus, Bacteroides, Prevotella, Mycoplasma,* and *Ureaplasma* species. One recent microbiologic association has been with bacterial vaginosis.

Etiology

Acute PID is often a polymicrobial infection caused by organisms ascending from the vagina and cervix to infect the mucosa of the endometrium, fallopian tubes, and ovaries. Eighty-five percent of PID is thought to arise in sexually active women of reproductive age. The other 15% is due to iatrogenic manipulations of the natural protective barrier of the cervix. Procedures such as endometrial sampling, dilation and currettage, and placement of intrauterine device allow vaginal flora to colonize the upper genital tract.

Debate continues as to the role of cervicovaginal flora in PID. Laparoscopic studies and direct fallopian tube cultures have demonstrated that tubal infections often consist of cervical-vaginal flora. Bacterial organisms cultured from tubal fluid include *N. gonorrhoeae, C. trachomatis,* genital *Mycoplasma* spp., *G. vaginalis,* endogenous anaerobic organisms (*Prevotella, Bacteroides, Peptococcus,* and *Peptostreptococcus*), and endogenous aerobic organisms (*Streptococcus* and *E. coli*). The type and number of organisms obtained is dependent on the method of collection as well as on the timing of collection. For instance, *N. gonorrhoeae* is frequently cultured in the first 24 to 48 hours of the disease, but anaerobes are cultured later in the course of disease. Laparoscopic tubal aspirations representing the causative organisms in the upper genital tract have shown an approximately 50% correlation to endocervical cultures.

Sweet (Sweet RL, Gibbs RS: Infectious Diseases of the Female Genital Tract. Baltimore, Williams & Wilkins, 1990, pp 241–266) has summarized the literature and concluded that in approximately one third of women with PID, *N. gonorrhoeae* is the only organism recovered by direct tubal or cul-de-sac culture. One third have a culture positive for *N. gonorrhoeae* plus a mixture of endogenous aerobic and anaerobic flora, and the remaining one third have only anaerobic and aerobic organisms. Bevan and colleagues, in the United Kingdom in 1995, identified *C. trachomatis* obtained by tubal aspirations as the causative upper genital tract organism in 39% of PID patients. *N. gonorrhoeae* was cultured in

14.4% of patients in this study, and a dual infection was present in 7.7% of the cases. These findings may represent *C. trachomatis* as the major etiologic agent of acute salpingitis, particularly in the United Kingdom. Soper and colleagues (Soper DE, et al.: Observations concerning the microbial etiology of acute salpingitis. Am J Obstet Gynecol 170:1008, 1994), in the United States in 1994, performed endometrial and fimbrial biopsies at the time of laparoscopy to confirm acute salpingitis and isolated gonococcus in 38% of the cases. Of significance in their study, bacterial vaginosis was demonstrated to be present in 61.8% of patients with acute salpingitis. All of the anaerobes isolated from the upper genital tract are common bacterial vaginosis microorganisms. The role of bacterial vaginosis as an antecedent of PID has been strengthened recently by the finding of bacterial vaginosis–associated organisms in the lower uterine segment in patients with bacterial vaginosis only, without acute PID symptoms. Bacterial vaginosis may also play a more passive role by altering cervical mucus, or by simply increasing the total inocculation of bacteria, due to the marked increase in the quantity of organisms associated with bacterial vaginosis.

The organisms *C. trachomatis* and *N. gonorrhoeae* may also act as primary pathogens by initiating acute salpingitis through tissue damage, alteration of the cervical mucus, and a change in the local genital tract environment. These changes may thus facilitate the access of lower genital tract organisms to the upper genital tract.

Risk Factors

Identification of risk factors is important for clinical diagnosis as well as prevention. There is a strong correlation between exposure to STDs and PID. Lack of barrier contraception, number of sexual partners, menstruation, vaginal douching, and geographic area (higher incidence of STDs) are all risk factors for PID development. Previous acute PID is also a risk factor for future episodes. Approximately 25% of women with a history of PID develop another acute episode.

Diagnosis

Accurate diagnosis of PID is difficult. Laparoscopy is highly specific and often recommended to rule out other surgical emergencies such as appendicitis or ectopic pregnancy. Laparoscopy should be recommended for all patients in whom

these other life-threatening surgical emergencies are strongly suspected. Laparoscopy is also helpful in obtaining microbiologic specimens and in assessing PID severity and future fertility and possible lavage, drainage, or other surgical treatment in an effort to avoid hysterectomy and adnexectomy.

Hagar and Eschenbach (Hagar WD, Eschenbach DA, et al.: Criteria for diagnosis and grading of salpingitis. Obstet Gynecol 61:113, 1983) established criteria for clinical diagnosis of acute salpingits without laparoscopy in an attempt to include patients with less obvious forms of the disease that do not fit the historic rigid criteria of the triad of lower abdominal pain, fever, and leukocytosis. Table 1 lists the most recent established criteria from the Centers for Disease Control and Prevention (CDC) for making the diagnosis of salpingitis on clinical grounds. In a 1991 review, 12 reports on the accuracy of diagnostic indicators of PID were examined. The review revealed that several laboratory tests were consistently valuable in PID diagnosis: elevated C-reactive protein, elevated erythrocyte sedimentation rate (ESR), endometrial biopsy supporting inflammation, and positive gonococcal cultures. Symptoms were generally not strong predictors of disease, however. Laparoscopy, while considered to be the gold standard, may yield normal results in patients with early disease limited to the endometrium. Endometrial cultures obtained by transcervical aspiration catheters (Pipelle) or direct culture of the fallopian tube or peritoneal fluid by laparoscopy or cul-de-sac centesis may aid in confirming the clinical diagnosis in patients with a normal-appearing pelvis by laparoscopy.

FitzHugh-Curtis syndrome (perihepatic inflammation) should be suspected if signs and symptoms of right upper quadrant tenderness and pleuritic pain develop and can be confirmed by laparoscopy.

Management

The first step in PID management is the accurate diagnosis. All patients should have cervical sampling for *N. gonorrhoeae* and *C. trachomatis*. Laparoscopy should be offered to most, if not all, patients demonstrating signs or symptoms of acute pelvic pain. Although most patients will refuse laparoscopic confirmation, it is important to give the patient full disclosure as to all her options, especially if fertility is important or the possibility of a surgical emergency exists.

It is just as important to inform the patient that nonlaparoscopic management is generally a

TABLE 1. Criteria for the Diagnosis of Acute Salpingitis

Minimum criteria

Empiric treatment of PID should be instituted on the basis of the presence of all of the following three minimum clinical criteria for pelvic inflammation and in the absence of an established cause other than PID:
- Lower abdominal tenderness
- Adnexal tenderness
- Cervical motion tenderness

Additional criteria

For women with severe clinical signs, more elaborate diagnostic evaluation is warranted because incorrect diagnosis and management may cause unnecessary morbidity. These additional criteria may be used to increase the specificity of the diagnosis.

Listed below are the routine criteria for diagnosing PID:
- Oral temperature >38.3°C
- Abnormal cervical or vaginal discharge
- Elevated erythrocyte sedimentation rate
- Elevated C-reactive protein
- Laboratory documentation of cervical infection with *Neisseria gonorrhoeae* or *Chlamydia trachomatis*

Listed below are the elaborate criteria for diagnosing PID:
- Histopathologic evidence on endometrial biopsy
- Tubo-ovarian abscess on sonography or other radiologic tests
- Laparoscopic abnormalities consistent with PID

Although initial treatment decisions can be made before bacteriologic diagnosis of *C. trachomatis* or *N. gonorrhoeae* infection, such a diagnosis emphasizes the need to treat sex partners.

PID, pelvic inflammatory disease.

safe alternative, specially in nonseptic patients with negative pregnancy tests and no signs of an acute abdomen.

As most patients will choose the nonsurgical option, we find it helpful to obtain an endometrial sampling with a thin aspiration curette such as the Pipelle. Using a multipurpose microbiologic transport tube such as the Port-a-Cult (Becton-Dickinson, Sparks, Maryland), the endometrial tissue should be layered onto the surface and then pushed into the gel using a sterile cotton-tipped swab. Part of the sample should also be placed into formalin. The gel sample can be sent to the microbiology laboratory and the formalin sample to the histology laboratory, or they can be held for 48 hours pending initial response to treatment.

Therapeutic goals in the management of acute PID are twofold. The immediate goal is to eliminate the acute infection and symptom complex. The long-term goal is to verify complete resolution of the acute disease and evaluate the patient for long-term sequelae.

After the diagnosis of PID is confirmed, antibiotic therapy should begin as soon as possible. The consensus is that broad-spectrum antimicrobial therapy is needed, owing to the polymicrobial nature of PID. The need for adequate and complete coverage for *C. trachomatis* for all cases of PID is also indisputable for long-term clinical success.

Pelvic inflammatory disease is frequently misclassified as mild to severe to arrange treatment and follow-up. Although the mild form of PID may not be as impressive clinically at the onset, consequences of the mild form of the disease may be just as devastating as the severe form in terms of long-term sequelae. The decision of committing a patient to early hospitalization and parenteral therapy may be the crucial point at which long-term sequelae and morbidity may be prevented. Currently 75% of cases of PID are managed on an out-patient basis. In Scandinavia, where reproductive health issues are of paramount social concern and a different health system exists, the vast majority of women are treated as in-patients. Recently, the Agency for Health Care Policy and Research funded a 5-year project to address the long-term efficacy and cost-effectiveness, with special attention to fertility rates with parenteral treatment.

Optimal therapeutic regimens have been debated, mainly because of the uncertainty of whether all of the many endogenous organisms play a role in PID. Out-patient protocols published by the CDC in 1993 may provide only adequate coverage of major pathogens involved in acute salpingitis. Studies have documented a

10% to 20% treatment failure rate versus a 5% to 10% failure rate with parenteral treatment, despite the supposed milder forms of disease administered out-patient therapy. Clinical follow-up within 48 to 72 hours from treatment initiation is imperative to identify women who have failed out-patient therapy and should be hospitalized.

Ideally, every women with acute PID should be hospitalized for at least 48 hours for parenteral antibiotic treatment. Although the CDC has published criteria for in-patient therapy (Table 2), more liberal criteria may reduce treatment failure rates as well as prevent the devastating long-term sequelae of PID. Women in whom the definitive diagnosis of acute PID is in question should be hospitalized, and diagnostic measures should be instituted. Other serious conditions may mimic PID and often warrant immediate intervention, such as acute appendicitis, ectopic pregnancy, adnexal torsion, and diverticular disease. Pending future definitive research on parenteral antibiotic treatment and hospitalization and their effects on long-term sequelae, all women, particularly those who desire further childbearing, should be encouraged to be hospitalized.

The two empiric protocols outlined by the CDC in 1993 for inpatient treatment are listed in Table 3. These protocols should cover a wide range of bacteria, including *N. gonorrhoeae*, *C. trachomatis*, anaerobic rods and cocci, gram-negative aerobic rods, gram-positive aerobes, and *Mycoplasma* spp. The protocols emphasize both the polymicrobial nature of PID and the need for completion of a 14-day course of oral antibiotics to eradicate slow-growing organisms, specifically *C. trachomatis*. A six-center, prospective, open-label clinical trial compared the efficacy and safety of three regimens recommended by the CDC in 1989 and are currently recommended for the in-patient treatment of PID (this

study reported on the resolution of the acute disease process and did not report on long-term follow-up). The two regimens listed in Table 3 produced almost identical cure rates, and, of the 292 women evaluated, none required alteration in therapeutic regimen. Third-generation cephalosporins such as ceftizoxime or cefotaxime may be substituted for the cefotetan or cefoxitin arms. These third-generation cephalosporins are effective against penicillinase-producing *N. gonorrhoeae*, *Peptostreptococcus* and other anaerobic species, and *E. coli* and other aerobic facultative species. The alternative regimen of clindamycin and an aminoglycoside, in contrast, provides excellent coverage against anaerobes and is historically the preferred regimen for patients with abscesses, infections related to intrauterine devices, and procedural-related pelvic infections. However, no investigation has demonstrated a statistically significant advantage. The disadvantage to clindamycin is that high doses are needed to demonstrate good activity against *Chlamydia*, while doxycycline is the preferred drug according to in vitro testing. Martens and Faro (Martens MG, Faro S, Maccato M, et al.: In-vitro susceptibility testing of clinical isolates of *Chlamydia trachomatis*. Infect Dis Obstet Gynecol 1:40, 1993), however, have documented that high doses of clindamycin at 900 mg IV q 8 hours demonstrate effectiveness against 90% of *C. trachomatis* strains.

Alternative parenteral regimens approved by the Food and Drug Administration (FDA) or CDC and within treatment guidelines include relatively new β-lactamase inhibitor combinations such as ampicillin-sulbactam and piperacillin-tazobactam. Quinolones demonstrating expanded anaerobic and chlamydial activity are under investigation, and preliminary results are promising. No single-agent therapy is currently recommended that provides sufficient coverage. The addition of anti-inflammatory drugs to anti-

---

TABLE 2. Criteria for Hospitalization of Patients with Acute Pelvic Inflammatory Disease

Hospitalization is especially recommended when the following criteria are met:
▶ The diagnosis is uncertain, and surgical emergencies such as appendicitis and ectopic pregnancy cannot be excluded
▶ Pelvic abscess is suspected
▶ The patient is pregnant
▶ The patient is an adolescent (among adolescents, compliance with therapy is unpredictable)
▶ The patient has human immunodeficiency virus infection
▶ Severe illness or nausea and vomiting preclude out-patient management
▶ The patient is unable to follow or tolerate an out-patient regimen
▶ The patient has failed to respond clinically to out-patient therapy
▶ Clinical follow-up within 72 hours of starting antibiotic treatment cannot be arranged

TABLE 3. Recommended* Treatment Regimens for In-patient Therapy of Acute Pelvic Inflammatory Disease

Regimen A

Cefoxitin 2 g IV every 6 hours

   or

Cefotetan 2 g IV every 12 hours

   or

Doxycycline 100 mg IV or orally every 12 hours

Note: This regimen should be continued for at least 48 hours after the patient demonstrates substantial clinical improvement, after which doxycycline 100 mg orally two times a day should be continued for a total of 14 days. Doxycycline administered orally has bioavailability similar to that of the IV formulation and may be administered if normal gastrointestinal function is present.

Regimen B

Clindamycin 900 mg IV every 8 hours,

   Or

Gentamicin loading dose IV or IM (2 mg/kg of body weight) followed by a maintenance dose (1.5 mg/kg) every 8 hours.

Note: This regimen should be continued for at least 48 hours after the patient demonstrates substantial clinical improvement, then followed with doxycycline 100 mg orally two times a day or clindamycin 450 mg orally four times a day to complete a total of 14 days of therapy. When tubo-ovarian abscess is present, many health care providers use clindamycin for continued therapy rather than doxycycline, because it provides more effective anaerobic coverage. Clindamycin administered intravenously appears to be effective against *Chlamydia trachomatis;* however, the effectiveness of oral clindamycin against *C. trachomatis* has not been determined.

* By the Centers for Disease Control and Prevention.

biotic treatment maybe worth considering in view of current theories of sequelae dictated by immunologic/inflammatory response.

Prevention of reinfection should include partner treatment as well as partner and patient education. Eschenbach reported that 25% of gonococcal PID patients were readmitted to the hospital within 10 weeks of initial treatment. Partners should be treated for the same causative agents as well as *C. trachomatis* and *N. gonorrhoeae*, regardless of pathogens isolated from the infected women. Treatment should include metronidazole if bacterial vaginosis or *Gardnerella* is present in the female. The CDC guidelines for management of male partners of women with PID include empiric treatment with regimens effective against both *C. trachomatis* and *N. gonorrhoeae*, regardless of the etiology of the female patient's infection. In settings where only women are treated, clinicians should make special arrangements to supply care to male sex partners of women with PID. If this is not feasible, it is important for them to ensure that sex partners are properly referred for therapy.

Surgical Management

Most women should be offered diagnostic laparoscopy to confirm diagnosis. Surgical emergencies such as appendicitis, ovarian torsion, and ruptured tubo-ovarian abscess (TOA) should be ruled out, and other inflammatory processes such as endometriosis may be excluded. Visualization of the extent of inflammatory process may aid in the decision for surgical management if medical management fails and also may serve as a prognostic indicator of long-term sequelae. Cultures taken from tubal fluid or cul de sac may aid if medical treatment is unsuccessful.

Women may also present a ruptured TOA, which is a surgical emergency and requires immediate laparotomy and definitive surgical treatment.

Unruptured TOA may initially be medically managed. Landers and Sweet (Landers DV, Sweet RL: Tubo-ovarian abscess: Contemporary approach to management. Rev Infect Dis 5:876, 1983) noted a 20% rate of early failure (after 48 to 72 hours) of antibiotic therapy. In addition,

31% required an operation several weeks to months following their acute infections for persistent disease or pain. Therefore, if no improvement or partial response is seen within 48 hours, the abscess presents for extraperitoneal drainage. If rupture is suspected or diagnosed, surgical intervention should be started. Bilateral TOA requiring definitive surgical intervention should be scheduled after the inflammation is quiescent, usually 2 to 3 months after an acute episode. Attempts at posterior colpotomy as well as percutaneous drainage under ultrasonographic or computed tomographic guidance can be attempted prior to laparoscopy or laparotomy, but the long-term success of this technique has not been well evaluated.

Conservative surgical management has been employed since the 1970s to preserve fertility in women of childbearing age. It was generally believed that in the case of obvious unilateral TOA, the contralateral ovary and tube may also be involved. Recent studies have shown, however, that in 25% to 50% of cases, the uninvolved tube and ovary are free of disease. Some surgeons may opt to leave adnexa with evidence of small hydrosalpinx or periovarian adhesions.

Ruptured TOAs are a surgical emergency. They are thought to occur in 3% to 15% of tuboovarian abscesses and carry a mortality rate of 5% to 10%. It has been observed that the longer the interval from diagnosis to surgery, the greater the increase in mortality. The surgical principle is to remove all free pus along with abscess, uterus, tubes, and ovaries. Total abdominal hysterectomy and bilateral salpingo-oophorectomy results in a 95% recovery rate. However, young patients with a clearly identified ruptured unilateral TOA should be informed that the remaining tube and ovary present an increased risk of recurrence if the uterus is left in place. Grossly contaminated incisions should be left open, to be closed by secondary intention or at a later date.

Chronic PID may be characterized by extensive adhesions, distorted anatomy, or persistent masses such as hydrosalpinx. Symptomatic and persistent masses should be removed in women who do not desire future childbearing. A "pelvic clean-out" (total abdominal hysterectomy, bilateral salpingo-oophorectomy, and lysis of adhesions) may be warranted in these patients to alleviate chronic pelvic pain and the risk of recurrence of acute PID; however, the need for the hysterectomy part of the procedure has not been proven.

Pelvic tuberculous is rare in the United States, although it is a frequent cause of sterility and chronic PID in Asia, the Middle East, Africa, and Latin America. The primary site of tuberculosis is usually the lung, and the disease is produced primarily by either *Mycobacterium tuberculosis* or *Mycobacterium bovis*. Hematogenous spread to the pelvis or the fallopian tubes, usually occurs after 1 to 2 years. Pelvic tuberculosis should be suspected when medical management fails. Laparoscopy may be necessary for diagnosis to visualize the characteristic "tobacco pouch" appearance of the distal portions of the fallopian tubes and peritoneal "studding." Treatment of pelvic tuberculosis is medical, with the combination of two or more antibiotics (isoniazid and ethambutol) for 24 months. Operative therapy is for women with resistant organisms, persistent pelvic masses, age over 40 years, and persistently positive endometrial cultures.

Pelvic Pain (Chronic)

Geri D. Hewitt, MD

Chronic pelvic pain is noncyclic pelvic pain of at least 6 months' duration. The source of the pain may be multifactorial from gynecologic, urologic, gastroenterologic, musculoskeletal, or nonsomatic causes such as a history of depression or abuse. As with other chronic pain syndromes, the cause of the pain may be difficult to determine, multiple treatment strategies may have failed, and the pain may become associated with behavioral and affective changes. Chronic pelvic pain is the principal indication for 10% of out-patient gynecologic visits, 30% of diagnostic laparoscopies, and 15% of hysterectomies performed in the United States.

Models of Pain Perception

Several models of pain have been proposed to explain patients' varying responses to painful stimuli. The Cartesian or classic medical model attributes the location and extent of the pain to the degree of local tissue destruction. Although this model may be applicable to acute pain such as a fracture, it is too limited to apply to chronic pain syndromes. The gate theory of pain describes a bidirectional transmission between peripheral nociceptive input and affective states. This model does not take into account other motivations the patient may have, such as work disability. The biopsychosocial model is the most applicable to chronic pain syndromes and integrates peripheral nociceptive stimuli, cognitive and psychological states, and the current social situation. Emphasis is placed on normalizing the patient's health-related quality of life with return to work and participation in family relationships. Symptom shifting—resolution of chronic pelvic pain only to be replaced with chronic headaches—is seen if the psychosocial issues are not resolved.

Evaluation

Somatic as well as nonsomatic causes of chronic pelvic pain should be addressed concurrently from the onset of the evaluation. Studies have shown that giving equal attention to both organic and other causative factors from the beginning of therapy, rather than reserving psychosocial evaluation only if no organic cause is found, is more likely to result in an accurate diagnosis, patient acceptance of the diagnosis, and a reduction in symptoms. A comprehensive medical and pain history should be obtained, with emphasis on urologic and gastroenterologic symptoms, as well as any precipitating events associated with the pain, or any cyclic component of the pain. Pain, menstrual, and voiding diaries can all be helpful. The physical examination should include assessment of musculoskeletal factors with emphasis on posture, flexibility, and strength as well as an evaluation of bladder, urethral, or myofascial tenderness in addition to the traditional bimanual examination. The patient should also be evaluated for any evidence of pelvic relaxation. Laboratory values that may be helpful on initial evaluation include a complete blood count with differential, stool guaiac, urine analysis, cervical cultures for gonorrhea and chlamydial infection, and cytology. Additional tests that may be helpful in select patients include sonography, cystoscopy, trigger point injections, and referral to other appropriate specialists. Pelvic ultrasonography should not be ordered routinely on all patients with chronic pelvic pain. In the absence of abnormal findings on pelvic examination, pelvic ultrasonography has not been helpful in the evaluation of these patients. Identifying a physiologic ovarian cyst on ultrasonogram may actually be detrimental to the patient if she has any psychosomatic component to her pain. Psychosocial evaluation may include interviews, questionnaires, and behavioral observation to assess the effect of the pain on the patient's life, current family and marital dynamics, work-related stressors, and possibility of concurrent or contributing

psychiatric diagnosis such as affective or psychosomatic disorders. A sexual history should be obtained, and all patients should be asked directly about any history of physical or sexual abuse.

Laparoscopy is indicated in patients with chronic pelvic pain if a suspected organic lesion is identified on physical examination or ultrasonogram, dysmenorrhea is progressive or unresponsive to oral contraceptive and nonsteroidal anti-inflammatory agents, or if the patient represents a "diagnostic dilemma" with suspected chronic pelvic inflammatory disease or endometriosis, or when the diagnosis is uncertain. Laparoscopy is more likely to identify a source of the pain when there is a suspected organic lesion or when initial medical therapy fails. Approximately 60% of the diagnostic laparoscopies performed for chronic pelvic pain will identify pathology, most commonly endometriosis and pelvic adhesions. Laparoscopy can be very useful for diagnostic confirmation, histologic documentation, and surgical treatment as well as patient reassurance. Over one half of patients undergoing a negative laparoscopy for chronic pelvic pain will be symptom-free 6 months after the procedure. If possible, pictures of the normal pelvic anatomy including the uterus, tubes, ovaries, bladder, colon, appendix, and cul-de-sac should be taken during surgery and shared with the patient for optimal reassurance. This is particularly helpful in the patient with any psychosomatic component of her pain.

Gynecologic Etiologies

Multiple gynecologic conditions have been suggested to cause pelvic pain, including endometriosis, adhesions, ovarian masses, chronic ectopic pregnancy, pelvic inflammatory disease, adenomyosis, uterine fibroids, pelvic congestion, and pelvic relaxation. Functional ovarian cysts in the absence of adnexal torsion are unlikely to be a source of pelvic pain and are more likely an incidental finding. Pelvic adhesions, particularly if they are not limiting any organ function, may or may not be the source of the pain. Adhesions are found with equal frequency in patients undergoing laparoscopy for chronic pelvic pain and in patients undergoing laparoscopy for tubal ligation. Patients with suspected pelvic adhesions should be counseled that adhesions may or may not be a cause of their pain, surgery with lysis of adhesions may or may not relieve their pain, and adhesions may re-form at old sites or form de novo.

Other Somatic Etiologies

Nongynecologic somatic pathology is found in up to 25% of patients with chronic pelvic pain and negative laparoscopy and is often from a urologic, gastroenterologic, or musculoskeletal source. Gastroenterologic causes of chronic pelvic pain include irritable bowel syndrome (IBS), inflammatory bowel disease, infectious enterocolitis, diverticular disease, neoplasia, appendicitis, hernia, ischemic bowel disease, and intestinal endometriosis. IBS is a common cause of lower abdominal pain and is seen more often in women than in men. Up to 90% of patients with IBS have psychopathology similar to that seen in patients with chronic pelvic pain, and up to 50% of patients with chronic pelvic pain undergoing diagnostic laparoscopy have symptoms consistent with IBS. Symptoms suggestive of IBS include crampy colicky pain improved after bowel movement, pain that worsens 1 to 1½ hours postprandially, constipation alternating with diarrhea, and sensation of incomplete evacuation. Physical findings include a palpable tender sigmoid colon, discomfort on rectal examination, and hard feces in the rectum. Treatment for IBS involves both medical therapy with bulk-forming agents and psychotherapy with reassurance, education, and stress reduction.

A high level of suspicion is required to diagnose a urologic problem in a patient with chronic pelvic pain. Chronic urethral syndrome, interstitial cystitis, cystitis, urethritis, urethral diverticulum, urolithiasis, radiation cystitis, neoplasm, and detrusor-sphincter dyssynergia should all be considered. Chronic urethral syndrome presents as irritative lower urinary tract symptoms for which no typical pathologic cause can be found. Symptoms include urgency, frequency, dysuria, postvoid fullness, urge or stress incontinence, vulvar irritation, dyspareunia, suprapubic tenderness, pelvic or vaginal pain, incomplete voiding, and post-coital voiding dysfunction. Findings include tenderness to palpation of the urethra and bladder base; urethroscopy shows erythema and exudate around the urethra. Therapy has included urethral dilation, bladder and voiding training, low-dose antibiotic suppression, skeletal muscle relaxants, and vaginal estrogen cream. Interstitial cystitis is a chronic inflammatory condition of the bladder wall and is most commonly seen in women 30 to 59 years of age. Symptoms include dysuria, frequency, urgency, hematuria, and dyspareunia. Physical findings include a tender bladder base and suprapubic tenderness. Urine cultures and cytology are negative; the diagnosis is made by visualization of characteristic hemorrhagic lesions on cystoscopy. Therapy involves dietary changes, hydrodistention, bladder training, tricyclic antidepressants, dimethyl sulfoxide, laser treatment, and transcutaneous electrical nerve stimulation.

Patients with chronic pelvic pain who have undergone a negative laparoscopy and psychological evaluation should be carefully evaluated for a musculoskeletal cause of their pain. The lumabar vertebrae, hip joints, and various ligaments, discs, and muscles are innervated by T12-L4 and may refer pain to the lower abdomen and anterior thigh. Frequently, musculoskeletal pain is caused by an increase in muscle tone from a variety of sources. Musculoskeletal pain typically changes in either intensity or location with variations in posture or by specific activities. Screening evaluation for gynecologists should include a careful history with questions about postural changes, low back injury, trauma, and diurnal variation; structural observations looking for unequal iliac crest height, unilateral standing habits, obesity, scoliosis, and leg length discrepancies; and assessment of mobility, palpation for tenderness, and testing for strength. Two common sources of pain are poor posture and trigger points. "Typical pelvic pain posture" with lumbar lordosis and anterior pelvic tilt has been described in up to 75% of patients evaluated for pelvic pain after a negative laparoscopy and psychological work-up. These patients respond well to physical therapy and nonsteroidal anti-inflammatory drugs. Trigger points are areas of hyperirritability within a muscle bundle that, when compressed, are tender locally and give rise to referred pain. They are both diagnosed and treated with injections of local anesthetic.

Nonsomatic Etiologies

In up to one half of patients with chronic pelvic pain who have undergone a negative laparoscopy, the etiology is psychogenic. Several studies have shown that patients with chronic pelvic pain have a higher incidence of a history of physical and sexual abuse. Depression is seen more often in women with chronic pelvic pain that in pain-free control subjects. Antidepressants have been used successfully in the management of chronic pelvic pain; they work by reducing concurrent depression and increasing pain threshold, enhancing the patient's ability to manage her pain. Many patients benefit from including psychotherapy, biofeedback, and relaxation training as part of their treatment plan. These therapeutic modalities may help the patient gain insight into the role emotional changes play on her pain, set limits on demands from others, set realistic and attainable goals, and learn appropriate assertiveness. Other psychiatric diagnoses associated with chronic pelvic pain include hypochondriasis, somatization disorders, substance abuse, anxiety, post-traumatic stress disorder, eating disorders, personality disorders, and obsessive-compulsive disorders.

Treatment

Treatment should be directed toward both correcting underlying pathology and decreasing the patient's symptoms. Analgesics are often required to reduce symptoms while the evaluation is proceeding. Nonsteroidal anti-inflammatory drugs are often helpful, particularly if the process is associated with inflammation and the release of prostaglandins. These medications should be used on a regular basis and not "as needed." Modification of the menstrual cycle with oral contraceptive pills, long-acting progestins, or gonadotropin-releasing hormone analogues can be useful if the patient has any cyclic component to her pain. Adjunctive use of antidepressants such as amitriptyline 25 to 50 mg at bedtime may also be helpful. To optimize the medical therapy, the patient should be encouraged to maintain regular office visits and medication dosages.

Several surgical procedures have been advocated in the treatment of chronic pelvic pain. Hysterectomy has been described as "definitive" surgical therapy for patients with chronic pelvic pain, but approximately 25% of patients seen in chronic pelvic pain clinics have already undergone hysterectomy. In one study, only 75% of patients who underwent hysterectomy for pain who had known pathology limited to the uterus were pain-free at 1-year follow-up. Several procedures have been described that attempt to interrupt the neural pathways of the pelvis. These include both laparoscopic and abdominal presacral neurectomy as well as laparoscopic uterosacral nerve ablation. All of the procedures have offered varying degrees of short-term success but little long-term success in relief of patients' symptoms.

Conclusions

Patients with chronic pelvic pain can present both diagnostic and therapeutic challenges for the clinician. These patients are best served with a multidisciplinary approach with equal emphasis on possible gynecologic, gastroenterologic, urologic, musculoskeletal, and psychogenic etiologies. Often the cause of the pain is multifactorial. Therapy should be aimed at correcting any identified abnormalities as well as improving the patient's symptoms. Medical therapy may include nonsteroidal anti-inflammatory drugs, oral contraceptive pills, antidepressants, counseling, and biofeedback. Surgical therapy is best suited for patients with an identifiable lesion and may include laparoscopy, adnexal surgery, hysterectomy, and various procedures designed to interrupt the neural pathways of the pelvis.

Polycystic Ovary Syndrome

Paula Amato, MD
R. Jeffrey Chang, MD

Polycystic ovary syndrome (PCOS) is an endocrine disorder that affects approximately 5% to 10% of women of reproductive age. The hallmarks of PCOS are chronic anovulation and hyperandrogenism. Clinically, chronic anovulation leads to irregular and unpredicatable uterine bleeding of varying degree as well as infertility. Hyperandrogenism stimulates excessive hair growth usually involving the face (sideburns, upper lip, chin) and neck but also sometimes including the lower abdomen (male pattern escutcheon) and chest. Evidence of severe hyperandrogenism, such as clitoromegaly, is not frequently encountered. Approximately 50% of women with PCOS exhibit obesity, and a lesser number have acne. In general, the ovaries are bilaterally enlarged and ultrasonography reveals several subcapsular follicular cysts less than 10 mm in diameter, the so-called "pearl necklace" sign, and increased ovarian stroma. It is important to note that ovarian morphology is not essential for making the diagnosis. Similarly, other hyperandrogenic states can also be associated with polycystic-like ovaries.

The association between PCOS and insulin resistance with compensatory hyperinsulinemia has been firmly established. Approximately 20% of PCOS patients are glucose intolerant and are at increased risk for the development of non–insulin-dependent diabetes mellitus. The presence of hyperinsulinemia in this disorder probably accounts for the occasional observation of acanthosis nigricans, which is a clinical marker for insulin resistance. Acanthosis nigricans is a gray-brown discoloration of the skin, usually in the neck, groin, and axillary regions of the body. The cellular and molecular mechanisms of insulin resistance in PCOS have not been clearly elucidated, and the clinical consequences of hyperinsulinemia on reproductive function are currently under investigation.

The endocrine and biochemical profile of these patients consists of (1) increased circulating androgen levels, of which the most biologically active, androstenedione and testosterone, arise primarily from the ovaries; (2) increased dehydroepiandrosterone sulfate (DHEA-S), an adrenal androgen, in about 50% of cases; (3) estrone (E_1) levels greater than those of estradiol (E_2), which represents a reversal of the normal E_1 to E_2 ratio; (4) overall increased luteinizing hormone (LH) secretion marked by elevated mean 24-hour levels, increased LH pulse frequency, and greater pulse amplitude among individual patients (however, basal concentrations of circulating LH have been found to be normal in approximately one third of patients; in contrast, follicle-stimulating hormone [FSH] secretion is normal); (5) hyperinsulinemia or evidence of insulin resistance in most patients; (6) decreased sex hormone binding globulin levels (SHBG); (7) elevated prolactin levels in 25% of cases. In the absence of ovulation, progesterone levels are consistently low.

The diagnosis of PCOS is usually made by history and physical examination. The most notable symptoms are oligomenorrhea or amenorrhea and hirsutism, which commonly become manifest during puberty or soon thereafter. In women desiring pregnancy, infertility may also be a presenting symptom. Infrequently, these symptoms may result from other similar but separate disorders. The differential diagnosis of oligomenorrhea/amenorrhea and hirsutism includes congenital adrenal hyperplasia most commonly due to a 21-hydroxylase deficiency, Cushing's syndrome, or an androgen-secreting tumor from either the ovary or the adrenal gland. A history of severe, rapidly progressive virilization, such as clitoromegaly and marked temporal balding, should alert one to the possibility of a neoplasm. Imaging studies such as ultrasonography and magnetic resonance may be required to distinguish an ovarian or adrenal tumor. Appropriate screening tests effectively eliminate many of these considerations. Measurements of serum total testosterone and DHEA-S are obtained to exclude the possibility of virilizing neoplasms. In the presence of severe hirsutism, regular cycles, or clitoromegaly, congenital adreanal hyperplasia should be considered. An early morning fasting serum 17-hydroxyprogesterone level greater than 300 ng/dL is suspicious for 21-hydroxylase deficiency, whereas some have advocated a screening value greater than 200 ng/dL. A confirmatory adrenocorticotropic hormone stimulation test is necessary to make the diagnosis. Any possibility of Cushing's syndrome may be excluded by administration of an overnight dexamethasone (1 mg) suppression test. An alternative and more expensive measure is the 24-hour urinary free cortisol, which if greater than μg per 24 hours is usually indicative of Cushing's syndrome. Ultrasonographic documentation of bilateral cystic ovaries is not necessary to making the diagnosis of PCOS. At this time, it is unclear whether assessment of insulin metabolism should be undertaken as a matter of routine in patients with PCOS. Glucose intolerance is minimal or absent and hyperinsulinemia is mild. Moreover, the newly formulated insulin-lowering drugs, such as metformin and troglitazone, have not yet been approved for use in PCOS, and their utility in this disorder is currently under clinical investigation.

The clinical and hormonal features of this disorder have an impact on three major areas of therapeutic concern. First, hirsutism and acne reflect abnormal stimulation of the pilosebaceous unit. Second, chronic anovulation predisposes to infertility. Third, persistent and uninterrupted estrogen secretion increases the risk of endometrial hyperplasia and uterine carcinoma. Fourth, longstanding hyperandrogenism and insulin resistance may predispose to cardiovascular disease and hypertension.

The development of hirsutism and acne is a result of abnormal androgen metabolism at several levels. There is excess production of androgen, primarily by the ovary and to a lesser degree by the adrenal gland. This distinction is important, since it affects consideration of therapy. When serum total testosterone is elevated, an ovarian source is implied, whereas an increase in DHEA-S suggests an adrenal source. If both hormones are elevated, treatment is directed toward reduction of ovarian androgen, since the most bioactive compounds originate from the ovary. Adrenal suppression should be considered when DHEA-S alone is increased. If extremely high androgen levels are detected, imaging of the ovary and adrenal is essential, since the likelihood of an androgen-producing neoplasm is increased, which may pose a life-threatening situation.

Another consideration is the transport of androgens in the circulation. This is particularly important for testosterone, since SHBG is reduced in hyperandrogenic and hyperinsulinemic states, resulting in increased circulating free hormone. In addition, decreased SHBG concentrations are found in obese individuals. The role of SHBG is clinically relevant, since the magnitude of excess free testosterone correlates best with the severity of hirsutism. Androstenedione is not bound by SHBG and therefore is unaffected.

A third consideration is target organ responsiveness to androgens. This is dictated to some extent by ethnic background. In some patients with hirsutism, there is increased conversion of testosterone to dihydrotestosterone, which is the intracellular hormone primarily responsible for stimulation of hair growth. Increased metabolism of androgen in target tissues may also account for the presence of excessive hair growth in patients with apparently normal circulating levels of testosterone. Thus, hair growth is ultimately controlled not only by the production of androgen and the relative biologic activity of differing types of androgens but also by the amount of free androgen presented to the hair follicle and the intracellular conversion of testosterone to dihydrotestosterone.

Reduction of ovarian androgen production has been the primary method of treating hyperandrogenism in PCOS and most commonly is achieved by administration of combination oral contraceptives. Estrogen and progesterone act in concert to suppress gonadotropin secretion and the mid-cycle gonadotropin surge, which leads to decreased ovarian steroidogenesis. In addition, estrogen increases SHBG, which results in a further reduction of serum free testosterone, while progesterone increases the metabolic clearance rate of testosterone. Since the synthetic progestins contained in these formulations are 19-nortestosterone derivatives, it seems prudent to select a formulation that has the least androgenic effect based on the relative estrogenic/androgenic ratio. Third-generation oral contraceptives contain progestins that are devoid of androgen effects and represent suitable alternative choices. Adrenal suppression by dexamethasone administration has been shown to benefit some PCOS patients with elevated DHEA-S levels and mild hirsutism. However, its effectiveness for severe hair growth is limited, since dexamethasone eliminates primarily the weak adrenal androgen, DHEA-S, and not the major ovarian androgens, androstenedione and testosterone. For patients with severe hirsutism, adjunct therapy with anti-androgens should be considered. Spironolactone is the most commonly used for this purpose in the United States and acts to block the effect of testosterone through competitive binding of its receptor on the hair follicle. It also has a direct suppressive effect on androgen synthesis and inhibits 5α-reductase activity, which is essential for conversion of testosterone to the highly potent intracellular androgen, dihydrotestosterone. As an aldosterone antagonist, spironolactone may be associated with a mild reduction in blood pressure and a mild elevation in serum potassium. Newer anti-androgens such as flutamide, a selective androgen receptor blocker, and finasteride, a selective 5α-reductase inhibitor, have been shown to be effective in the treatment of hirsutism in clinical trials. Local therapeutic regimens include electrolysis and depilatory creams. Electrolysis by experienced technicians is an effective means of removing hair follicles, but it does not alter hormone stimulation of new hair follicle recruitment and growth and may result in scarring and discomfort. The cost of this procedure may also be prohibitive. It should be understood that the duration of the hair life cycle on the beard area of the face is approximately 6 months. Thus, any drug treatment should be continued for at least this interval and likely for 1 year before therapeutic benefit derived from arresting new hair growth may become apparent. The severity of hirsutism at the initiation of treatment is also a consideration, since mild hair growth is far more easily treated than severe hirsutism.

The basic premise of therapy is directed toward improvement of hirsutism and patient satisfaction. With a successful response and nearly complete eradication of hirsutism, hormonal reassessment is probably not necessary. However, if improvement is slow or absent, and particularly if the patient's condition worsens with therapy, re-evaluation should be performed.

As previously mentioned, patients with PCOS may present with infertility as their chief complaint. In PCOS the precise mechanism for anovulation has not been determined. Decreased pituitary FSH secretion is most frequently implicated. However, evidence to support this concept is lacking, and recent studies would suggest that FSH secretion is normal in this disorder. That PCOS patients are sometimes resistant to clomiphene citrate and may require greater gonadotropin stimulation to effect follicle growth suggests an abnormality of ovarian follicle responsiveness as a mechanism for anovulation.

In patients seeking fertility, ovulation induction can generally be achieved by treatment with clomiphene citrate (CC). Clomiphene citrate is thought to exhibit anti-estrogenic properties at the level of the hypothalamus and pituitary to increase secretion of gonadotropin-releasing hormone and pituitary gonadotropins, which subsequently leads to follicle maturation and eventual ovulation. The initial dose is 50 mg/day for 5 days, commencing on day 2 or 3 of a spontaneous or progesterone-induced menses. In amenorrheic patients, vaginal bleeding induced by progesterone withdrawal provides a convenient reference point and ensures adequate estrogen levels. Indicative of a normal ovulatory response is a rise in the basal body temperature of approximately 12 to 14 days, followed by spontaneous vaginal bleeding or a serum progesterone level above 10 ng/mL in the mid-luteal phase. In the absence of ovulation, the dose of CC may be increased by 50 mg increments to 150 mg/day for 5 days until an ovulatory response is achieved. Higher doses of CC (up to 250 mg) have been recommended for resistant patients, but the success rate is minimal.

An important consideration in CC therapy is concomitant dexamethasone administration. It has been demonstrated that, in patients with a slightly increased DHEA-S, both the ovulatory and pregnancy rates following CC plus dexamethasone are significantly greater than those resulting from CC treatment alone. In the presence of coexistent mild hyperprolactinemia, use of bromocriptine alone or in combination with CC has no advantage over CC alone for ovulation induction. Therefore, it is not recommended that bromocriptine be used for ovulation induction in PCOS.

In patients resistant to clomiphene citrate, ovulation induction may be accomplished by instituting gonadotropin therapy. Formulations of gonadotropins are available as combined human FSH and LH, highly purified FSH, and, recently, recombinant human FSH. Administration of gonadotropins must be accompanied by careful clinical monitoring using ultrasonography to assess follicle growth and serial E_2 measurements to determine progressive ovarian steroid output. The dose of gonadotropins is adjusted according to the follicular response of each individual patient. Over an entire course of therapy, PCOS patients appear to be exquisitely sensitive to gonadotropin administration and thus have a greater predisposition for developing hyperstimulation syndrome with its attendant complications. A so-called "low-slow protocol" is often employed to avoid this potentially serious consequence.

In cases in which all medical therapy fails, it is not unreasonable to consider an ovarian drilling as a method of restoring spontaneous ovulation. This procedure involves penetrating the ovarian capsule with either electrocautery or laser and puncturing identifiable follicular cysts.

This procedure is usually performed during laparoscopy, thereby reducing operative risk. Studies have shown improvement in the hormone profile, and resumption of spontaneous ovulation is common. However, permanent resolution of ovulation is not guaranteed and may be temporary in some cases. In addition, the risk of adhesion formation following this procedure is of theoretical concern.

Beyond the immediate concerns of hair growth and infertility in PCOS, persistent stimulation of the endometrium by chronic unopposed estrogen may lead to endometrial hyperplasia or even frank carcinoma in some women. This problem is compounded by the presence of obesity. It is not surprising that in young women with endometrial cancer there commonly is a history of menstrual irregularities consistent with the diagnosis of PCOS. For this reason, endometrial sampling is mandatory in patients with a long history of chronic anovulation, and therapy must be directed toward prevention of endometrial proliferation. Reduction of the risk of endometrial hyperplasia may be provided by the administration of progesterone, either alone or in combination with estrogen as in oral contraceptives. If prevention of endometrial hyperplasia is the primary goal of therapy, medroxyprogesterone acetate may be given at a dose of 10 mg a day for 12 days each month. Oral contraceptives are similarly effective and have the advantage of regulating menstrual cyclicity. It is noteworthy that progestin therapy significantly reduces but does not exclude the risk of endometrial abnormalities. Therefore, in the presence of abnormal bleeding, office endometrial biopsy or formal dilatation and curettage should be performed to rule out significant endometrial pathology.

Mention of other long-term health consequences associated with PCOS is warranted given the growing body of evidence that demonstrates dyslipidemias in these patients and the potential greater risk for vascular and cardiac disease. In addition, the hyperinsulinemia that accompanies glucose intolerance and non–insulin-dependent diabetes mellitus not only increases these risks, but also places PCOS patients at increased risk for hypertension and stroke.

In summary, PCOS is a common endocrine disorder of women of reproductive age characterized by chronic anovulation and hyperandrogenism. Therapeutic considerations include addressing immediate concerns such as infertility and hirsutism as well as potential long-term problems such as endometrial cancer, dyslipidemias, and cardiovascular disease. The recognition of insulin resistance and hyperinsulinemia in

PCOS extends these concerns to include hypertension, stroke, and diabetes mellitus. Active interventional treatments are available to deal with the reproductive endocrine difficulties, whereas preliminary investigations have demonstrated that insulin-lowering agents show promise as potential therapeutic agents for both short-term and long-term health issues.

Precocious Puberty

Elizabeth Kennard, MD

The appearance of any signs of sexual maturation before the age of 8 years, or of menarche before age 9, constitutes precocious puberty. In about 10% of cases, a female with precocious puberty has a life-threatening central nervous system disease. Consequently, when first confronted with this problem, the clinician must rule out neoplastic causes. However, most cases of precocious puberty are idiopathic. In these cases, the two concerns are the eventual final height of the child and her psychological well-being.

In an effort to determine what has caused precocious puberty, it is categorized according to presenting complaint. There are two types of precocious puberty: the early occurring, normal process of maturation and an abnormal process occurring independent of the hypothalamic-pituitary-ovarian axis.

Isosexual precocious puberty, also called complete or true precocious puberty, involves early activation of the hypothalamic-pituitary-gonadal axis. It results in completely normal reproductive functioning and is the most common cause of precocious puberty. Maturation of the hypothalamic-pituitary-ovarian axis can be stimulated by idiopathic causes, tumors, infections, trauma, hypothyroidism, and other causes.

Isosexual pseudoprecocious puberty, or incomplete precocious puberty, is diagnosed when premature pubertal changes occur due to estrogen stimulation independent of the hypothalamic-pituitary-ovarian axis. The source of the estrogen can be iatrogenic or can be from ovarian or adrenal tumors or functioning ovarian cysts.

Heterosexual pseudoprecocious puberty is found when virilization occurs in a female child at an early age. This can occur secondary to iatrogenic causes, ovarian and adrenal tumors, and adrenal enzyme defects in the steroid pathway.

Sexual maturation normally occurs as a progression through maturation of different tissues. Children can also present with *premature thelarche, premature adrenarche,* or *premature pubarche,* representing isolated early maturation of the breasts, axillary hair, or pubic hair, respectively. These conditions are generally benign and do not have long-term consequences. Premature adrenarche and pubarche need to be investigated for adrenal enzyme defects and carefully watched for further progression into possible precocious puberty.

Evaluation

As mentioned earlier, the clinician must rule out any life-threatening condition prior to making a diagnosis of idiopathic precocious puberty. Once this most common diagnosis is made, attention can be turned to improving the final height and psychological development of the child. Careful follow-up is mandatory.

A thorough history and physical examination must be performed. The history should document the progression of the pubertal changes, the past medical history of the child, any head trauma or central nervous system (CNS) infections, and history of exposure to iatrogenic sources of estrogen (such as lotions or creams). The height and weight are measured and plotted on standard growth tables. Physical examination results should note any dermatologic findings, Tanner staging of breast and pubic hair, clitoral enlargement, and presence of an abdominal mass. A careful neurologic examination should be performed.

A large number of tests are performed. Bone age should be determined by hand-wrist films and repeated at 6-month intervals. The presence of a bone age less than chronologic age is highly suspicious for hypothyroidism. All other precocious puberty patients will likely have advanced bone age. Disorders of the CNS are diagnosed with magnetic resonance imaging, and electroencephalography. Ultrasonography of the abdomen and pelvis will assess ovarian volume and adrenal mass. Blood tests for levels of thyroid-stimulating hormone, thyroxine, luteinizing hormone, follicle-stimulating hormone, estradiol, dehydroepiandrosterone, and human chorionic gonadotropin are performed. If heterosexual changes are occurring, 17α-hydroxyprogesterone and testosterone levels should also be determined.

Diagnosis

A large number of neoplastic, degenerative, or inflammatory processes of the CNS can result in precocious puberty, including tuberculosis, encephalitis, trauma, hydrocephalus, neurofibromatosis, granulomas, and other conditions. Most will be diagnosed by neurologic examination or brain imaging.

Iatrogenic causes are diagnosed by elucidating a history of exposure to hormone-containing medications or creams.

McCune-Albright syndrome (polyostotic fibrous dysplasia) is a rare cause of precocious puberty. Patients with this condition have a chronically activated G protein system and precocious puberty that results from end-organ activation. About 40% of children with McCune-Albright syndrome will have precocious puberty. This syndrome is diagnosed by the presence of a triad of café-au-lait spots, fibrous dysplasia, and cysts of the skull and long bones.

Blood tests will help diagnose hypothyroidism and congenital adrenal hyperplasia. As discussed earlier, the presence of a bone age less than chronologic age is also highly suggestive of hypothyroidism.

The presence of a functioning ovarian or adrenal tumor is usually determined by abdominal examination and ultrasonogram, combined with serum hormone levels. Most commonly, the ovarian tumor is palpable abdominally. These tumors are usually greater than 8 cm when precocious puberty occurs.

The diagnosis of idiopathic or constitutional precocious puberty is a diagnosis of exclusion. Patients should be carefully followed to ensure that another process has not been overlooked.

Treatment

Treatment of precocious puberty is obviously dependent on the cause. Adrenal and ovarian tumors as well as several CNS processes require surgical intervention. Hypothyroidism and congenital adrenal hyperplasia require hormone therapy. Most patients have idiopathic precocious puberty and require treatment with gonadotropin-releasing hormone (GnRH) agonist therapy.

Therapy of precocious puberty is aimed at arresting the progress of pubertal development for improvement of final adult height and for psychological reasons. Children with precocious puberty have premature closure of their epiphyseal plates. Consequently, although tall for their age as children, over half will be less than 5 feet tall as adults. These children also may be exposed to isolation and ridicule from peers and may be subjected to sexual abuse. Counseling is recommended for these girls and their families.

The treatment of choice for idiopathic precocious puberty is GnRH agonist therapy, either intranasally or by injection of a "depot" form. These agents create a hypogonadotropic hypogonadal state by down-regulation of the pituitary gland. The results thus far are excellent, with a large decrease in growth velocity, an increase in final predicted adult height, and return of steroid hormone levels to the prepubertal range. Often, secondary sexual characteristics such as breast development and pubic hair regress.

Because McCune-Albright syndrome represents end-organ activation, the use of GnRH agonist therapy is ineffective in this disease. Medroxyprogesterone acetate (Depo-Provera) at 100 to 200 mg/m² or testolactone can be used to decrease breast development and interval between menses.

With any treatment of precocious puberty, the removal of the medication will result in return of the progression of puberty. Many clinicians stop treatment when the patient reaches 11 years of age, although this is a matter for individualization.

Premenstrual Syndrome

David A. Baram, MD

Definition

Premenstrual dysphoric disorder (PDD) is a distressing constellation of physical, behavioral, and emotional symptoms occurring with a regular, cyclic pattern in the 7 to 10 days prior to the onset of menstruation during an ovulatory menstrual cycle. While many women, perhaps 80% of the adult population, notice minor physical and emotional changes in the week prior to menstruation, only 3% to 5% of women experience symptoms severe enough to cause marked impairment of their ability to function socially, with their family, or in their occupation.

The myriad symptoms of PDD may include (1) depressed mood and feelings of hopelessness; (2) marked anxiety; (3) emotional labilty; (4) persistent irritability and anger; (5) decreased interest in activities of daily living; (6) difficulty concentrating; (7) fatigue and lethargy; (8) changes in appetite that may be associated with binge eating or with cravings for certain foods; (9) hypersomnia or insomnia; (10) feelings of being overwhelmed or out of control; and (11) a host of physical symptoms including headaches, bloating, breast tenderness, hot flashes, and muscle and joint pain. Symptoms of PDD usually begin to remit within a few days of the onset of menses and are always absent in the week following menstruation.

Three temporal patterns of PDD have been described. These include (1) symptoms beginning at ovulation, with gradual worsening of symptoms during the luteal phase; (2) symptoms that begin during the second week of the luteal phase; (3) a brief time-limited episode of symptoms at ovulation, followed by symptom-free days and a recurrence of symptoms late in the luteal phase.

While PDD can occur at any time after menarche, women usually seek evaluation and treatment for these symptoms during the third and fourth decade of life. Symptoms usually remit during times of amenorrhea such as pregnancy, lactation, and menopause.

Etiology

Despite decades of research, the etiology of PDD has not been identified. Epidemiologic studies indicate that PDD is often associated with a prior affective disorder like major depression or postpartum depression. Several genetic studies looking at identical twins show increased concordance for heritability of PDD.

Numerous studies looking at titers of ovarian steroids have failed to consistently identify any hormonal etiology for PDD. When compared with women without PDD, women who meet the research criteria for PDD do not demonstrate any consistent dysfunction at any point in the hypothalamic-pituitary-ovarian axis. Theories proposed as possible etiologies for PDD but never proven include alterations in the secretion of prolactin and thyroid hormone, vitamin deficiencies, increased aldosterone activity, endogenous endorphin withdrawal, increased adrenal activity, increased renin-angiotensin activity, and hypoglycemia. Therefore, an extensive hormonal evaluation of women with symptoms of PDD is not warranted unless there is a suspicion of a specific endocrinopathy such as hypothyroidism.

Ovarian steroid hormones do affect the synthesis, release, and reuptake of neurotransmitters and can also act directly on nerve membranes in the central nervous system. Several authors have suggested that the etiology of PDD may be explained by the effect of ovarian steroids on the central nervous system neurotransmitters, particularly serotonin, that affect behavior, mood, and cognition. Perhaps women with PDD are more sensitive than women who do not have PDD to the alterations in central nervous system neuro-

transmitters caused by the monthly fluctuations in ovarian hormones and are more likely to have their mood changed or destabilized during the luteal phase of the menstrual cycle.

Many authors believe that PDD is a learned or conditioned response. In our culture, many women expect to experience symptoms such as bloating, cramping, irritability, and mood changes premenstrually, and many myths exist about how women are expected to behave premenstrually. If a woman grows up in a house where her mother or older sister became symptomatic during the luteal phase of the menstrual cycle, perhaps she too will become symptomatic. Men often reinforce the stereotype of how women are expected to behave premenstrually. However, when carefully controlled prospective studies of large groups of women in the general population are carried out, no significant changes in motor skills, cognition, or social behavior can be demonstrated during the various stages of the menstrual cycle.

Diagnosis

The diagnosis of PDD is made by exclusion. Before the diagnosis of PDD can be made, other physical and psychiatric diagnoses, especially depression, must be ruled out. Only about 25% of all patients presenting with premenstrual symptoms will meet the criteria for PDD. The other 75% of patients are either depressed (about 50%) or do not have symptoms that can consistently be related to the menstrual cycle.

A careful medical and psychiatric history and thorough physical examination must be carried out in every patient presenting with symptoms of PDD. Since PDD only occurs in women who ovulate, those women who are on oral contraceptives, experience chronic amenorrhea, or have undergone oophorectomy or menopause do not meet the criteria for the diagnosis of PDD. A search should be made for other medical disorders that may explain the patient's symptoms. Several medical conditions, including chronic headaches, recurrent herpes outbreaks, irritable bowel syndrome, and seizure disorders may become exacerbated premenstrually. These conditions should be treated appropriately.

As noted earlier, no exact diagnostic test exists for the diagnosis of PDD. The most accurate way to make the diagnosis of PDD is to have the patient keep a prospective record of symptoms during the entire menstrual cycle for at least 3 consecutive months. Forms for recording menstrual symptoms are readily available. Since a myriad of physical, emotional, and cognitive symptoms may be present in any individual, it is often best to ask the patient to pick her five worst symptoms and to record the occurrence and severity of these symptoms (on a scale of 1 to 10) daily. It is important to document the recurring nature of symptoms during the luteal phase and the disappearance of symptoms once menstruation begins. For the diagnosis of PDD to be made, symptoms must be severe enough to interfere with work, family obligations, or lifestyle. The diagnosis of PDD can be made when (1) no other disorder can be found that can account for the woman's symptoms; (2) prospective daily charting of symptoms over 3 months demonstrates a luteal pattern of symptomatology; and (3) a symptom-free interval can be consistently demonstrated during the follicular phase of the menstrual cycle.

Through symptom charting, many women are able to gain a sense of control over their condition. Being able to visualize the severity, timing, and type of symptoms may make the condition more manageable for them. About one half of all patients who present with premenstrual symptoms are significantly depressed. These patients may have vegetative symptoms of depression such as sleep disturbance, difficulty concentrating, loss of libido, loss of appetite, feelings of hopelessness and helplessness, crying episodes, and suicidal ideation. Depression can be diagnosed both clinically and with the aid of the Beck Depression Inventory, a brief, accurate self-administered depression test easily administered and scored in the office. Chronically depressed patients often notice a premenstrual exacerbation of their existing depression that can be confused with PDD.

After an initial office assessment, including a complete medical and psychiatric history and thorough physical examination, the patient's prospective daily symptom rating charts should be reviewed. Based on the daily rating charts, several patterns emerge. Patients with PDD will exhibit the typical pattern of premenstrual symptomatology followed by a symptom-free interval during the menstrual and follicular stage of the menstrual cycle. Other patients may exhibit the cyclic recurrence of another disorder like migraine headaches, depression, or dysmenorrhea. It is also possible for PDD to coexist with another chronic condition like depression. Once the diagnosis of PDD has been made, several treatment options are available.

Treatment Options

Treatment options for patients who meet the criteria for PDD can be divided into three broad categories: (1) education, emotional support, psychosocial treatment, and healthy lifestyle changes; (2) medications that target specific symptoms; and (3) syndromal therapy with antidepressants or ovulation suppression or both. Patients should have realistic goals for treatment, understand that no treatment regimen is likely to abolish all of their symptoms, and realize that they will have a bad month from time to time.

Healthy Lifestyle Changes

Although lifestyle modifications may benefit women with PDD, few controlled trials have been done to evaluate the effectiveness of dietary changes, exercise, or relaxation techniques on symptoms of PDD. Self-help therapy for PDD includes modification of tobacco, alcohol, and illicit drug use, dietary changes, exercise, stress reduction, and vitamin and mineral supplements. In addition, some patients may benefit from an alteration in their circadian rhythm (achieved by staying up all night early in the luteal phase), which may help by reducing the symptoms of depression.

Women should become aware of what makes their symptoms better or worse and make an effort to avoid anything that aggravates their symptoms. In addition, family members can be brought into the treatment plan. Increased household help and understanding from the patient's children and spouse during her symptomatic period may be useful in coping with symptoms. Some women find PDD support groups helpful. In addition, some women may want to delay undertaking especially difficult work or new projects during their symptomatic time.

Anecdotally, many women report symptom improvement after dietary modification. The usual guidelines for dietary modification include decreasing salt, sugar, and caffeine, increasing complex carbohydrates, and eating more frequent, smaller meals instead of three large meals a day. One recent double-blind, placebo-controlled, crossover study demonstrated that luteal phase consumption of an experimental carbohydrate-rich beverage known to increase serum tryptophan blood titers relieved the psychological and appetitive symptoms of PDD. Decreasing salt may help with fluid retention. Alcohol may exacerbate symptoms of depression and should be decreased or avoided.

Women who exercise regularly have fewer luteal phase symptoms than women who do not exercise. Exercise has also been shown to relieve symptoms of depression, possibly through increased endorphin secretion and improved self-esteem. Women should be encouraged to start an exercise program by walking briskly 1 to 2 miles a day, 5 days a week, eventually working up to a moderate, regular, aerobic exercise.

Stress reduction through meditation has been shown to improve symptoms of PDD more effectively than an unstructured quiet activity like reading. Women who experience anxiety as a major component of PDD should be encouraged to learn how to elicit the relaxation response through biofeedback or self-hypnosis. Some women may also benefit from short-term counseling to learn more effective ways to cope with stress in everyday life. A recent randomized controlled study of foot, hand, and ear reflexology was shown to be helpful in relieving the symptoms of PDD.

For many years, over-the-counter nonprescription drugs, as well as vitamin, mineral, and nutritional supplements, have been used to treat PDD. Vitamin B6 (pyridoxine) has often been cited as effective for symptom reduction in PDD. However, research does not support its effectiveness, and large doses of B6 (>100 mg/day) can cause peripheral neuropathy. In recent clinical trials, both calcium (1000 mg daily) and magnesium (360 mg daily) have been shown to improve mood, water retention, and pelvic pain during the luteal phase. Commonly used supplements like evening primrose oil have never been scientifically proven to be of benefit in the treatment of PDD.

Treatment of Specific Symptoms

Specific physical symptoms commonly occur as part of the symptom complex of PDD, and each can be targeted for treatment. *Fluid retention* symptoms can be treated by decreasing salt intake and with the use of a mild potassium-sparing diuretic, such as spironolactone (50–100 mg daily) during the luteal phase. *Mastalgia* can be treated by reducing caffeine consumption and with the use of bromocriptine (2.5–5 mg daily) or vitamin E (400 mg daily) during the luteal phase. *Sleep disturbance* often responds to sleep hygiene measures, including establishing a regular time to go to sleep and avoiding caffeine late in the day. Physicians should be careful about prescribing sedatives for sleep owing to their addiction potential. Doxepin, a tricyclic antidepressant, is effective in low doses (25–50 mg) as a nighttime sedative. *Menstrual migraines* occur during the late luteal phase of the cycle and should first be treated with nonsteroidal anti-

inflammatory drugs. Migraines can also be treated prophylactically with a beta blocker like propranolol. Some patients with menstrual migraines respond to ovulation suppression with danazol (see subsequent discussion). *Food cravings* may respond to behavior modification techniques and nutritional counseling. Fenfluramine and clomipramine, anorectic drugs with serotonergic activity, will reduce food cravings and may improve mood in patients with PDD.

Syndromal Treatment

Women with a mixture of physical, emotional, and cognitive symptoms respond well to treatment with either psychotrophic medication, especially serotonin reuptake inhibitors (SRIs), or hormonal treatment that suppresses ovulation. The antidepressant SRIs are the drug of first choice for women who meet the criteria for the diagnosis of PDD. If patients do not experience relief of symptoms after 2 to 3 months of treatment with SRIs, they are given a trial of ovulation suppression. Occasionally, SRIs and medication for ovulation suppression are given simultaneously. Surgery (oophorectomy) is rarely used for treatment of PDD and only as a last resort.

Psychotrophic Medication

The SRIs (fluoxetine 20 mg/day, sertraline 50 mg/day, paroxetine 20 mg/day) have been shown in several double-blind, placebo-controlled trials to be highly effective in the treatment of PDD. SRIs, used to treat depression, reduce the tension, irritability, and dysphoria of PDD and should be used as first-line treatment. Although SRIs are remarkably well tolerated by most patients, some patients discontinue their use because of insomnia, nausea, shakiness, fatigue, or decreased sexual desire. Most practitioners prefer to give antidepressants like the SRIs throughout the entire month, but some studies describe the successful use of SRIs taken only during the luteal, or symptomatic, phase of the cycle.

Other antidepressants like the tricyclic antidepressants (nortriptyline, amitriptyline (50–150 mg/day) may be useful in the treatment of PDD and should be considered if patients cannot tolerate treatment with the SRIs. Tricyclic antidepressants must be given throughout the entire menstrual cycle and have numerous bothersome anticholingeric side effects, including dry mouth, blurred vision, urinary retention, constipation, and palpitations.

Antianxiety medications (buspirone 30 mg/day

and alprazolam 0.25 mg tid) are effective in reducing irritability and anxiety during the luteal phase in women with severe PDD. In one double-blind study comparing alprazolam with placebo and oral micronized progesterone, alprazolam was significantly better than placebo and progesterone for reducing total premenstrual symptoms. In this study, progesterone was no more effective than placebo. Antianxiety medications, especially the benzodiazepines, should be used sparingly and cautiously because of their addiction potential.

Hormonal Treatment

If first-line therapy with psychotrophic medication is ineffective, hormonal therapy to suppress ovulation should be considered. Hormonal therapy can be used either alone or in combination with psychotrophic medication. Despite years of use, progesterone has been shown to be no better than placebo for treatment of PDD. Oral contraceptives interrupt ovulation but have never been demonstrated in controlled trials to significantly decrease the psychological symptoms of PDD.

Danazol, a synthetic androgen, suppresses the hypothalamic-pituitary-ovarian axis by inhibiting the release of gonadotropins. Even in relatively small doses (100–400 mg/day) danazol can inhibit ovulation and provide symptomatic relief to patients with PDD. In small doses, danazol has minimal side effects. Danazol can also be used intermittently during the symptomatic luteal phase of the menstrual cycle. Long-term adverse effects of low-dose danazol include reduction of high-density lipoproteins.

Gonadotropin-releasing hormone (GnRH) agonists have also been used to treat PDD and reduce symptomatology by blocking ovulation and creating a "medical oophorectomy." However, GnRH agonists, while highly effective, severely reduce estrogen titers and expose the patient to the symptoms of hypoestrogenism and the risks of cardiovascular disease and osteoporosis. Some researchers have advocated the use of "add back" estrogen and progesterone to reduce these risks and side effects when GnRH agonists are used.

Surgery (bilateral oophorectomy) should be used only as a last resort and only when all other measures have been ineffective. Surgery may be appropriate in older, severely symptomatic women who have completed childbearing and have not responded to treatment with nonmedical regimens and psychotrophic medication. Some women with severe and incapacitating PDD who respond to treatment with danazol or a GnRH agonist may be candidates for oophorectomy and continuous estrogen replacement therapy.

Other hormonal treatments, including treatment with estradiol implants and levothyroxine, have never been demonstrated to be superior to placebo for the treatment of PDD.

Conclusion

Medical treatment of PDD with psychotrophic medication or ovulation suppression should be undertaken only when the diagnosis has been confirmed with prospective daily symptom rating charts and all other physical and psychological diagnoses have been excluded. Treatment should always begin with education, support, psychological treatment, and healthy lifestyle changes. If medication is indicated, begin with treatment targeted to specific symptoms. If syndromal treatment is warranted, begin with a serotonergic antidepressant or the careful luteal phase administration of an antianxiety medication. When psychotrophic medications are not effective, ovulation suppression with danazol or a GnRH agonist should be tried. Oophorectomy should be used only as a last resort.

Primary Amenorrhea

Daniel H. Riddick, MD, PhD

Primary amenorrhea is the failure to begin uterine bleeding when expected in relation to the onset of sexual development. In general, menses should begin within 2 years of the onset of breast budding (thelarche). The earliest and latest ages based on normative data for thelarche are ages 8 and 14, respectively. Thus, menses should begin between ages 10 and 16, but the specific age will be directly related to when thelarche began in a given individual.

The clinical approach to the patient presenting with failure to begin menses (primary amenorrhea) will be a systems approach. The evaluation of patients with primary amenorrhea derives directly from the history and physical examinations. It is based on logic rather than memorization of flow charts, and it limits laboratory testing to specific selected tests. The approach combines an assessment of the history of the patient relating to sexual development and the determination by physical examination of the extent and normalcy of sexual development.

Failure to Initiate or Achieve Complete Sexual Development

When the history and the physical examination reveal that by age 16 either no secondary sexual development has begun or some mild degree of sexual development began but has not progressed, either the hypothalamic-pituitary system has not stimulated the ovarian response necessary for the onset of puberty and its continued progression, or the ovary has been unable to respond to that stimulation with estrogen production.

The most common hypothalamic dysfunction is that associated with inadequate body weight for the physical structure of the individual or the physiologic stress of excessive exercise, or a combination of the two. Careful history of body image and eating habits will reveal those patients who have inadequate caloric intake or who, having consumed appropriate food, utilize vomiting or laxatives to avoid the effects of weight gain. Similarly, a history of excessive physical training in young athletes such as gymnasts and long-distance runners or ballerinas will often indicate the source of the problem. The timing of the caloric restriction or exercise program will determine whether any sexual development occurs or whether sexual development is arrested partway through its completion.

Hypothalamic dysfunction can be the result of destructive lesions in the hypothalamus, such as hamartomas, craniopharyngiomas, or infiltrative or infective lesions such as sarcoidosis or encephalitis. Genetic and developmental abnormalities can also result in hypothalamic dysfunction. The most common developmental abnormality of the hypothalamus is Kallmann's syndrome, which is failure of development of the rhinencephalon and its accompanying anosmia. The genetic autosomal recessive disorders of Prader-Willi and the Laurence-Moon-Biedl syndromes have associated physical findings and mental retardation. Constitutional delay of normal puberty is a diagnosis of exclusion and will occasionally have an associated family history.

Diagnosis of abnormalities of the hypothalamus begins with the finding of low follicle-stimulating hormone (FSH) levels. This excludes the ovary as the source of the amenorrhea. When a destructive lesion or Kallmann's syndrome is suspected, further evaluation is best achieved with magnetic resonance imaging (MRI).

The pituitary gland itself may cease to function normally either because of the presence of a tumor, the most common of which is a prolactinoma, or because of pituitary failure secondary to an invasive lesion, the most common of which is a craniopharyngioma. Again, the timing of the appearance of the lesion will determine whether complete sexual development is inhibited or sexual development began and then ceased before its completion. FSH will be low in pituitary disorders similar to hypothalamic disorders. A prolactin determination should be obtained in patients suspected of pituitary dysfunction. Although other hormone-producing tumors occur in the pituitary gland, they are, relatively speaking, very uncommon, and many of those will have an elevation of prolactin as well. MRI will confirm the diagnosis.

Ovarian failure will also produce primary amenorrhea. Ovarian failure that results from developmental abnormalities such as Turner's syndrome or Swyer's syndrome will have failure of onset of sexual development. Premature ovarian failure, either idiopathic or secondary to radiation and chemotherapy, will result in either failure to develop any secondary sexual characteristics or early development with inhibition of progress, depending on when the failure occurs. Patients suspected by history and physical examination of having ovarian failure will have this diagnosis confirmed by an elevated level of FSH. Additional considerations include the need for removal of the gonads or gonadal streaks only in patients who have a Y chromosome on karyotyping. Clearly, chromosomal analysis is only indicated in those patients with established ovarian failure. It is currently unclear whether radiation or chemotherapy resulting in ovarian failure is permanent.

Once the diagnosis has been made, all patients with primary amenorrhea should be given estrogen and progesterone to induce and maintain secondary sexual development. I begin therapy at a higher dose of estrogen such as 5 mg of Premarin daily for the first 3 or 4 months of treatment before beginning Provera withdrawal on a monthly basis. Subsequently, I reduce the Premarin to 1.25 mg daily and then to 0.625 mg as a maintenance dose daily and 5 mg Provera for the first 12 calendar days of each month. Once satisfactory pubertal development has been achieved, an oral contraceptive is also acceptable for maintenance therapy.

In summary, patients with failure to begin the onset of secondary sexual development or who have initial onset with failure to progress require a careful history and physical examination to point to the most likely area of system failure. An FSH determination will separate patients with ovarian failure from those with hypothalamic-pituitary dysfunction. Additional laboratory testing and imaging studies are dictated by the specific findings in the history and physical examination.

Normal Secondary Sexual Development Without Menses

Patients who have normal onset and progression of puberty but fail to begin menses at the expected time interval following the onset of puberty may suffer from disorders that overlap those seen in patients with no secondary sexual development. Destructive lesions of the hypothalamus, pituitary dysfunction, premature ovarian failure, and radiation and chemotherapy damage to the ovary can occur in such a time-related fashion that normal puberty occurs but no menstrual function begins. Clearly, the clinical history is of great importance in this regard.

The other major clinical indicator of this group of disorders will be found in the pelvic examination. Müllerian abnormalities are found in a majority of patients in this category. The patient with normal secondary sexual characteristics and a blind vaginal pouch will have one degree or another of müllerian dysgenesis, from an imperforate hymen to complete müllerian failure with the absence of other than rudimentary uterine structures. A low FSH level confirms the presence of normally functioning ovaries in these patients, and vaginal ultrasonography or laparoscopy will confirm the extent and degree of the abnormality.

Appropriate surgical treatment depends entirely on a determination of the degree of the abnormality. If a normal uterus is present, the possibility for childbearing exists and should be preserved if possible. A basal body temperature curve can be helpful in determining whether cyclic pain is secondary to ovulation or to an obstructed menstrual outflow tract. Occasionally, a small amount of endometrial tissue will reside in a rudimentary structure in what is otherwise complete müllerian dysgenesis, producing cyclic pelvic pain. This is the only indication for removal of rudimentary müllerian structures. Vaginal reconstruction in the patient with müllerian dysgenesis above the level of the hymen will usually require split thickness skin grafting and prolonged use of a vaginal stent. This operation should be delayed until regular coitus is soon expected and the patient's level of maturity can tolerate the compulsive vaginal dilating necessary for a successful result. This operation is extremely difficult to attempt a second time and everything possible should be done to ensure its success on the first operative procedure.

Abnormal Secondary Sexual Development or Sequence

A history of isolated development of one or another of the secondary sexual characteristics points to a primary abnormal hormone production. This group of abnormalities is also suspected from the history and physical examination.

Breast development without the presence of significant pubic and axillary hair can be the result of either an estrogen-producing neoplasm or of androgen insensitivity syndrome. The androgen insensitivity syndrome is confirmed by the presence of a blind vaginal pouch, male levels of testosterone, and a 46,XY karyotype. Hormonally active neoplasia producing estrogen can occur either from an ovarian or an adrenal source and vaginal ultrasonography and MRI evaluation will confirm the diagnosis, along with extremely high levels of circulating estrogen.

When the only secondary sexual development of consequence is that of pubic or axillary hair, this is usually associated with other signs of masculinization and points toward an androgen-producing tumor or adult-onset congenital adrenal hyperplasia. Androgen-producing tumors can occur in either the adrenal gland or the ovary. Testosterone, dehydroepiandrosterone sulfate, and 17-hydroxyprogesterone levels and appropriate imaging will confirm the diagnosis.

If a neoplasm is present, appropriate surgical therapy is indicated. Cortisol replacement reverses the abnormal hormonal dynamics of congenital adrenal hyperplasia.

The androgen insensitivity syndrome is the only abnormality of the gonads containing a Y chromosome in which gonadectomy is not performed as soon as the diagnosis is made. In patients with this syndrome, the gonads are left in place until the late teenage years, after sexual maturity has been completed. The gonads are then surgically removed to avoid the development of a dysgerminoma associated with intra-abdominal testes. Appropriate sex hormone replacement is indicated along with vaginal dilation exercises, which are usually successful, avoiding the need for surgical plastic reconstruction of the vagina. One should expect this progressive dilation to take 6 months to 1 year, however. Surgical therapy will be indicated in only a few individuals.

As important as the medical therapy to the success of treatment is the sensitive education of the patient and her family about the condition. Inflammatory terms such as testes, testicular feminization, male genes, and so on are not only unhelpful but also destructive. The terms androgen insensitivity, abnormal ovarian or gonadal development, and genetic abnormality should be substituted. Long-term or intermittent counseling will be helpful to many patients. The patient should be progressively educated about her condition, that is, given direct answers to the questions she raises without providing information in advance of her readiness to accept it. In today's world of higher education, one can expect that patients with this disorder will discover themselves in textbooks of biology; they should be properly educated and prepared long before such discovery.

In summary, the detailed history and physical examination will point to disorders in this group of patients, and limited laboratory and selected imaging studies will be necessary to confirm a suspected diagnosis.

Secondary Amenorrhea

Moon H. Kim, MD

Secondary amenorrhea is a symptom associated with endocrine and structural disorders of the hypothalamic-pituitary-ovarian-uterine axis. Therefore, an understanding of the anatomic and functional requirements of a normal menstrual cycle is essential in evaluating secondary amenorrhea. It is usually defined as the absence of menses for 6 months or for three cycle intervals. The prevalence of secondary amenorrhea varies depending on the age group; 8.5% in women aged 13 to 18 years, and 3% in women aged 25 to 34 years.

Initial Evaluation

Considering the prevalence of various causes, one must start with excluding pregnancy, the most common cause of secondary amenorrhea,

by a pregnancy test. Once pregnancy is excluded, evidence of endogenous estrogen secretion, hyperprolactinemia, androgen excess, and endometrial status must be evaluated. Clinically, it is helpful to group patients with secondary amenorrhea into several categories according to the presence or absence of endogenous estrogen effect, hyperprolactinemia, and hyperandrogenism. A careful history should also include weight changes, the use of drugs such as oral contraceptives or antidepressants, any history of trauma on the endometrium, and stress in life or vigorous exercise.

Evaluation of Estrogen Effects

Evidence of endogenous estrogen effects suggests an intact hypothalamic-pituitary-ovarian axis. Well-stimulated vaginal mucosa and cervical mucus with good ferning suggest the ovarian estrogen secretion, which indirectly reflects adequate gonadotropin secretion. Progestin administration such as medroxyprogesterone acetate (10 mg daily for 5 to 7 days) will result in uterine bleeding, which is evidence of the presence of intact endometrium previously primed by estrogens. In the absence of these findings, a hypoestrogenic condition must be considered. The determination of serum estradiol confirms the state of ovarian estrogen production. Levels less than 35 pg/mL suggest a severe hypoestrogenic state. In these women, serum level of follicle-stimulating hormone (FSH) is the most sensitive test to further evaluate the ovarian function. If serum FSH level is elevated over 40 mlU/mL, it indicates primary ovarian failure (Table 1).

Progestin Challenge Test

The progestin challenge test is based on the fact that the endometrium responds to a progestin only when it is adequately primed by estrogens. Thus, the test allows assessment of endometrial status and, indirectly, ovarian function. In normal women with anovulation, the administration of a progestin (intramuscular progesterone 100 to 150 mg or oral medroxyprogesterone acetate 10 mg/day for 5 to 7 days) should result in withdrawal bleeding 2 to 7 days following therapy.

Withdrawal bleeding following progestin administration establishes the diagnosis of euestrogenic amenorrhea. It rules out ovarian failure and end-organ failure such as Asherman's syndrome. On the other hand, the absence of withdrawal bleeding suggests either hypoestrogenic

TABLE 1. Causes of Secondary Amenorrhea According to Hormonal Status

	Normal or Low FSH/LH Levels	High FSH/LH Levels	Elevated PRL Levels
Euestrogenic	Hypothalamic-pituitary dysfunction (stress, weight changes, exercise, psychogenic) Estrogen-secreting tumor of ovaries Systemic illnesses	Rare FSH/LH–secreting tumor of the pituitary	Idiopathic Pituitary tumor Primary hypothyroidism Iatrogenic (psychotropic drugs, OCs)
Hypoestrogenic	Hypothalamic/pituitary failure (neoplasm, severe dysfunction, anorexia nervosa, trauma, Kallmann's syndrome, severe weight loss, exercise)	Ovarian failure Gonadotropin-resistant ovary syndrome	Idiopathic, pituitary tumor Iatrogenic hyperprolactinemia
Hyperandrogenic	PCO Masculinizing tumor Congenital adrenal hyperplasia Cushing's syndrome		PCO

FSH, follicle-stimulating hormone; LH, luteinizing hormone; PRL, prolactin; OC, oral contraceptive; PCO, polycystic ovary syndrome.

amenorrhea or end-organ failure (ie, Asherman's syndrome) including outflow obstruction such as cervical stenosis. When the progestin challenge fails to induce withdrawal bleeding, the sequential administration of estrogen and progestin (conjugated estrogen 1.25 to 2.5 mg/day for 28 days and medroxyprogesterone acetate 5 to 10 mg/day for the final 7 days) should be tried. In the absence of intrauterine synechiae or outflow obstruction, this sequential approach should result in withdrawal bleeding, confirming hypoestrogenic amenorrhea. All women with hypoestrogenic amenorrhea should be further investigated by measuring serum FSH levels to rule out a hypergonadotropic state, namely primary ovarian failure.

In the setting of normal FSH levels, failure to respond to the sequential estrogen and progestin therapy strongly suggests end-organ failure. Intrauterine synechiae, partial or complete (Asherman's syndrome), is the most common cause of such amenorrhea. The diagnosis is established by hysterosalpingography, sonohysterography, or hysteroscopy. Women with Asherman's syndrome usually present with a history of endometrial curettage. An endocrine evaluation is rarely necessary. Other potential causes of endometrial failure include tuberculosis and radiation exposure.

Evaluation of Hyperprolactinemia

Hyperprolactinemia is associated with amenorrhea in approximately 20% to 30% of cases. It can be a cause of hypoestrogenic or euestrogenic amenorrhea. Therefore, serum prolactin measurements should be performed in all amenorrheic patients. Underlying causes of the hyperprolactinemia include drug use (eg, dopamine antagonists, psychotropic medications), hypothalamic or pituitary lesions (eg, neoplasm), elevated thyroid-stimulating hormone levels as in primary hypothyroidism, and chest wall injury, among others. When an underlying cause is not found, imaging evaluation of the sella turcica by cone-down view with radiography, computed tomography, or magnetic resonance imaging is recommended in all women. However, an evaluation by a simple cone-down view radiography is cost-effective in excluding macroadenoma unless prolactin levels are greater than 60 ng/mL or neurologic signs and symptoms are present. In such cases, computed tomography or magnetic resonance imaging must be done to rule out a pituitary tumor.

Further Investigation

The patient with hypoestrogenism should be further evaluated by the determination of serum gonadotropins. When FSH levels are greater than 40 mlU/mL, a diagnosis of ovarian failure is certain. If the patient is young (less than 30 years of age) and nulliparous, chromosome analysis is also indicated to exclude the possibility of gonadal dysgenesis. On the other hand, if the gonadotropin levels are low, one must consider various pituitary or hypothalamic conditions such as neoplasms and hypothalamic dysfunction associated with exercise and weight loss.

An evaluation of androgen excess is indicated

in the patient with clinical signs of hyperandrogenism such as hirsutism, acne, oily skin, and obesity. When virilization (eg, balding, clitoral enlargement, deepening of voice) is present, especially with an acute onset and increasing severity, an androgen-secreting neoplasm of the ovary or the adrenal must be considered, although it is rare. In women, androgens are secreted by the ovary or the adrenal. Therefore, the evaluation is confined to these two organs. The determination of serum levels of dehydroepiandrosterone sulfate (DHAS) and testosterone is a good screening test. Normal levels of serum DHAS usually rule out an adrenal cause of hyperandrogenism. When serum levels of DHAS and testosterone are mildly elevated, a 17-hydroxyprogesterone level may be of help in determining whether the patient has late-onset congenital adrenal hyperplasia. Further evaluation by an adrenocorticotropic hormone stimulation test can be helpful in testing for the condition.

The most common form of secondary amenorrhea (non-pregnancy related), however, is polycystic ovary syndrome (PCO) in which serum testosterone levels are mildly elevated and DHAS levels are often normal. No other diagnostic tests, such as ratios of luteinizing hormone to FSH or ultrasonography, are warranted as they are not helpful for the diagnosis or clinical management. The patient with hyperandrogenic amenorrhea will bleed after progestin therapy. Because of a significantly increased risk of endometrial hyperplasia and adenocarcinoma if untreated, the patient with PCO should be monitored closely and treated appropriately with cyclic progestational therapy if she is not desirous of conceiving. In addition, the patient with PCO may have an insulin resistance, which should be investigated if suspected.

Therapeutic Approaches to Secondary Amenorrhea

Because amenorrhea represents a symptom of various functional or organic disorders of the hypothalamic-pituitary-ovarian-uterine axis, its management varies greatly and should be individualized. Therapeutic approaches depend on the diagnosis, associated conditions, age of the patient, and the patient's desire for conception. The treatment may be mainly for symptomatic relief but should be directed to eliminate any etiologic factors (Fig. 1).

Euestrogenic Amenorrhea (Anovulation)

For the patient wishing to conceive, an induction of ovulation with clomiphene citrate is indicated as the first line of treatment. For the patient not responding to clomiphene citrate, human menopausal gonadotropin therapy or other adjuvant therapy should be considered. As chronic anovulation represents a condition of persistent unopposed estrogen effects on the endometrium, those not desiring conception must be treated with cyclic progestin (medroxyprogesterone acetate 10 mg daily for 5 to 10 days) or oral contraceptives to prevent endometrial hyperplasia or dysfunctional uterine bleeding.

When a diagnosis of hyperandrogenemia is established in a patient with anovulation (ie, PCO), the use of oral contraceptives may be considered to suppress ovarian androgen production and to prevent endometrial hyperplasia. The administration of corticosteroids (eg, dexamethasone 0.25 to 0.5 mg daily) should be considered when adrenal hyperandrogenism is diagnosed. Often a combination of oral contraceptives and corticosteroids is effective in managing patients with both an ovarian and an adrenal contribution to hyperandrogenism.

The patient with Asherman's syndrome presents with euestrogenic secondary amenorrhea. As it is caused by synechiae of the endometrial cavity, the management consists of hysteroscopic lysis followed by postoperative high-dose estrogen administration (conjugated estrogen 2.5 mg daily for 4 weeks followed by a 7-day course of progestin) to stimulate regeneration of the endometrium. Menses can be restored in most cases.

Hypoestrogenic Amenorrhea

One must differentiate hypergonadotropic amenorrhea from hypogonadotropic states before considering therapeutic options for the patient presenting with hypoestrogenic amenorrhea. For the patient with hypogonadotropic amenorrhea, ovulation and menses can be restored with the administration of human menopausal gonadotropins. Pulsatile infusion of gonadotropin-releasing hormone is also effective in cases of hypothalamic dysfunction causing hypogonadotropinemia. Generally, the patient with hypoestrogenemia will not respond to clomiphene citrate. When fertility is not a concern, cyclic estrogen-progestin therapy, as in estrogen replacement therapy, may be recommended to prevent long-term effects of estrogen deficiency on bone density, atrophic changes of the reproductive tract, and lipid metabolism. The treatment of psycho-emotional conditions such as anorexia nervosa or stress should be carefully coordinated with men-

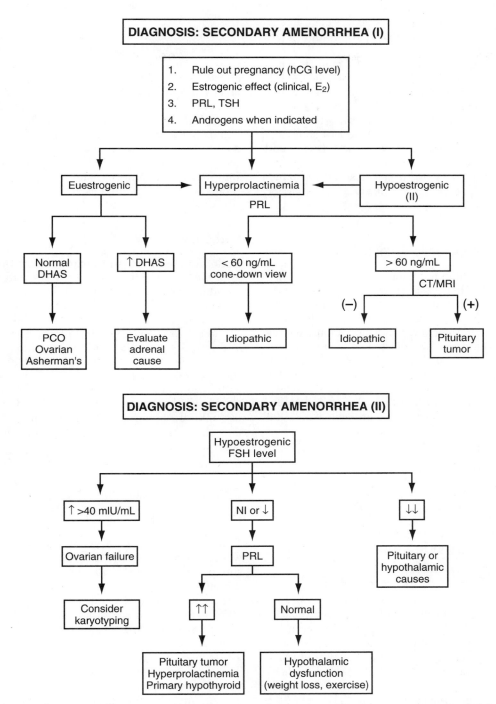

Figure 1. Algorithms for the evaluation of secondary amenorrhea. CT, computed tomography; DHAS, dehydroepiandrosterone sulfate; E_2, estradiol; FSH, follicle-stimulating hormone; hCG, human chorionic gonadotropin; MRI, magnetic resonance imaging; NI, not isolated; PCO, polycystic ovary; PRL, prolactin; TSH, thyroid-stimulating hormone.

tal health providers. Likewise, the patient with hypoestrogenic amenorrhea due to weight loss or strenuous exercise will benefit from appropriate counseling.

The diagnosis of ovarian failure is made when hypergonadotropinemia is confirmed in the patient with secondary amenorrhea. All patients with premature ovarian failure have increased risks for coronary heart disease and osteoporosis. Therefore, they should be advised to start hormonal replacement therapy (cyclic estrogen and progestin). For the patient desiring fertility, the use of donor oocytes through assisted reproductive technology (in vitro fertilization) may be considered.

Hyperprolactinemic Amenorrhea

Hyperprolactinemic amenorrhea can be associated with either a euestrogenic or a hyperestrogenic state. Bromocriptine, a dopamine agonist, is very effective in suppressing prolactin secretion and restoring ovulation and menstruation. The dosage must be adjusted to achieve a normalization of serum prolactin levels. Bromocriptine therapy is also effective in reducing the tumor size in patients with micro- or macroadenoma of the pituitary. Although rare, when suprasella extension causes neurologic manifestations not responsive to bromocriptine therapy, neurosurgical therapy is indicated.

Septic Shock

Denis Cavanagh, MD
Papineni S. Rao, PhD

Shock is a life-threatening condition in which the circulating blood volume is less than the capacity of the vascular bed. This disparity results in hypotension, reduced perfusion of vital organs, metabolic acidosis, cellular hypoxia, and ultimate cell dysfunction and death. Septic shock is shock associated with infection and is most commonly caused by gram-negative bacilli. The condition has become increasingly important over the past 20 years among hospitalized patients, and the reported mortality from septic shock has ranged from 11% to 82%. The Centers for Disease Control and Prevention reported a dramatic increase in the rate of septicemia in hospitalized patients, from 73.6 per 100,000 population (164,000 cases) in 1979 to 176 per 100,000 (425,000 cases) in 1987.

Gynecologic patients at particular risk for septic shock include those with infected abortions, tubo-ovarian abscesses, and severe postoperative infections and those taking immunosuppressive or myelosuppressive drugs. The organisms most commonly isolated in these patients are *Escherichia coli*, *Klebsiella* and *Enterobacter* species, *Pseudomonas*, *Proteus*, and *Serratia*. There is no doubt, however, that gram-negative anaerobes, such as *Prevotella* species (formerly *Bacteroides* spp) may be causative in many cases of so called "gram-positive" septic shock.

Pathophysiology

Endotoxins are released from gram-negative bacteria after the death of the organism, and these agents elicit a variety of biologic responses. Chemically, endotoxins are lipopolysaccharides, and the lipid A component has been identified as the active component for toxicity. Endotoxins and certain exotoxins are responsible for the most serious clinical manifestations seen in septic shock through activation of the coagulation cascade, the complement pathway, and cytokine production by macrophages. In endotoxic shock, multiple organs are affected, particularly in the late phase, making the treatment more difficult and the mortality rate very high.

Clinical Classification
Primary Shock

Primary shock has two phases. In the early or warm hypotensive phase of primary septic shock, the patient is alert and apprehensive, with flushed face and warm skin. Usually her temperature is between 38.4°C and 40.6°C (101°F and 105°F). Profuse sweating and shaking chills are not uncommon. Most patients have moderate tachycardia (100 to 110 per minute), but in our experience about 20% have a relative bradycardia with a pulse rate of less than 72 per minute. The pulse pressure remains satisfactory in this phase, and urinary output is good. In the late or cold hypotensive phase, the patient is pale and her skin is clammy. The temperature may be subnormal. Gradually she becomes less alert and less apprehensive. As pulse pressure drops, oliguria may ensue. The triad of hypotension, tachycardia, and oliguria is typical of this phase of septic shock.

Secondary or Irreversible Shock

Prolonged cellular hypoxia and anaerobic metabolism are manifested by metabolic acidosis and elevated blood lactate levels, which should arouse strong suspicion of irreversible shock. Anuria, cardiac or respiratory distress, and coma are grave signs.

Laboratory Investigations

Minimal laboratory studies should include a complete blood count with differential leukocyte count. The leukocyte count is usually high but leukopenia is a bad prognostic sign. Urinalysis should include a gram-stained smear, cultures, and antibiotic sensitivity testing. Cultures should be done on blood samples drawn at admission and at times of shaking chills. Blood determinations should include electrolytes, blood urea nitrogen, creatinine, uric acid, pH, and arterial blood gases. A coagulation profile should include prothrombin time, partial thromboplastin time, fibrinogen, platelet count, and testing for fibrin split products. Evaluation of intrinsic and extrinsic coagulation factors is best left to the discretion of the attending physician. In early shock, the patient may display a transient respiratory alkalosis, probably as a result of endotoxin-induced hyperventilation. Later, metabolic acidosis develops as anaerobic metabolism increases and plasma levels of lactic acid rise. Respiratory failure also contributes to severe metabolic derangements in shock, and patients with irreversible shock are in a state of metabolic and respiratory acidosis and a decrease in arterial pH, HCO_3, and oxygen partial pressure.

Radiographic studies should be obtained. Pulmonary changes consistent with the adult respiratory distress syndrome can have a severe, adverse effect on a patient's prognosis, and early diagnosis is essential for optimal results.

Plain radiographs of the abdomen are useful if bowel obstruction, perforated viscus, or abdominopelvic abscess is likely to be the septic focus. In selected cases, computed tomography and ultrasonography may be helpful to detect a pelvic abscess. Likewise, excretory or retrograde urography may be useful to diagnose a perinephric abscess, or ureteral damage with urinary ascites or retroperitoneal urinoma formation.

An electrocardiogram is obtained, but echocardiography should also be considered to evaluate possible valvular dysfunction. A Swan-Ganz catheter should be inserted to assess pulmonary artery wedge pressure (PAWP), left arterial filling pressure, and cardiac output.

Medical Treatment

Blood pressure, pulse, and respirations should be monitored. If a Swan-Ganz catheter is available, the PAWP should be obtained. The PAWP, being a reflection of left ventricular end-diastolic pressure, is a much more helpful guide to volume replacement than central venous pressure.

The urinary output and specific gravity, urine, and serum osmolality should be recorded.

The essentials of treatment are as follows:

1. The patient should be in an *intensive care unit* and a pulmonary medicine consultation should be obtained. Make sure that the patient has an adequate airway. If necessary, insert an endotracheal tube or perform a tracheostomy. If there is documented hypoxemia, oxygen therapy should be started while oxygen saturation is being monitored.

2. *Replace fluid and blood loss,* using as guides the central venous pressure, or preferably PAWP, urinary output, and serum osmolality. The main aim of fluid replacement is to convert the hypodynamic state to a hyperdynamic state by the use of fluid challenge. Suppose that a patient has a PAWP of 7 mm Hg and 200 mL of isotonic saline is infused over a 10-minute period with the effect of the PAWP being observed. When the pressure rises by 7 mm Hg, the infusion is stopped, and later if the PAWP falls to less than 3 mm Hg the infusion is restarted.

   The normal cardiac output is about 5 L per minute, but in the early warm hypotensive phase of septic shock it may be as high as 10 to 15 L per minute. In the cold hypotensive phase, however, hypodynamic shock occurs, and it is essential to use the fluid challenge mechanism with crystalloids to obtain the maximum cardiac output. It should be noted that this is not always achieved with a high PAWP. Colloid solutions do not appear to have a significant advantage over crystalloid solutions. Metabolic acidosis is common in patients with septic shock and is progressive if not corrected, and 0.45% saline solution with one or two ampules of sodium bicarbonate added is useful for correction.

3. Select *antibiotics* based on what the most likely infecting organisms are, keeping in mind the antibiotic sensitivities of those organisms in your hospital. Give the appropriate agents in massive doses by the intravenous route. A logical regimen is

ampicillin/sulbactam 3 g every 6 hours, aztreonam 2 g every 8 hours, and metronidazole 500 mg every 8 hours for the average adult. If possible, try to avoid the use of nephrotoxic drugs such as aminoglycosides.

4. Give *vasomotor drugs* as indicated by the patient's clinical condition. In septic shock, the primary aim of therapy is to improve tissue perfusion rather than obtain a normal blood pressure. The choice depends largely on a patient's clinical state and so consideration of the choice between drugs designated as "vasopressors" and "vasodilators" is more practical. Furthermore, despite what has been written to the contrary, it is our conviction that in the *warm hypotensive phase* of septic shock, the use of a vasopressor rather then a vasodilator is indicated. We have found metaraminol to be the most useful vasopressor in this situation. We give only enough to maintain the systolic blood pressure at the lower limit that ensures adequate urinary output. The dosage of metaraminol required varies from 10 mg to 300 mg, with the infusion rate adjusted to maintain the blood pressure at the desired level.

In the *cold hypotensive phase* of septic shock, marked by general vasoconstriction, an element of hypovolemia is also present. Volume replacement together with administration of a vasodilator drug in small doses is indicated. The agent that we have found to be best is chlorpromazine (5 to 10 mg every ½ hour IV). If the PAWP or central venous pressure is elevated and the pulse rate is in the normal range, isoproterenol may be used for its inotropic and vasodilator (β-receptor) effects. A patient with a pulse rate exceeding 120 per minute should not be given isoproterenol because it tends to produce cardiac arrhythmia.

Dopamine hydrochloride (Intropin) is usually the drug of choice to improve myocardial function, but it must be used with care. Dopamine (200 mg) is administered in 500 mL of 5% dextrose in water at an infusion rate adjusted according to the desired blood pressure. This drug must be given with care because different dosages have opposite effects in the same patient. Thus a dose of 2 μg/kg/min augments renal and mesenteric perfusion via dopaminergic receptor activity with no significant change in cardiovascular dynamics, whereas when the dose is raised to 20 μg/kg/min, the heart rate increases, there is increased

vasoconstriction, and renal perfusion continues to improve. In general, however, it may be said that when dopamine is used, its β-adrenergic action predominates except in large doses. The drug has a direct vasodilator action on resistance vessels and can be used to increase renal and mesenteric blood flow. It is therefore particularly useful in patients who have a reduced urinary output. It is superior to isoproterenol because it has less effect on myocardial oxygen consumption and heart rate.

5. *Digitalize* patients who have tachycardia and whose PAWP exceeds 16 mm Hg or whose central venous pressure exceeds 15 cm H_2O. If the serum potassium is in the normal range, digoxin 0.5 mg IV and then 0.25 mg every 6 hours IV up to 1.0 mg total daily dose is given.

6. Consider giving *heparin* if clotting studies indicate disseminated intravascular coagulation. If a full coagulation profile is not available and the patient is not responding to standard treatment, heparin may be given (10,000 units IV with a maintenance dose of approximately 1,000 units per hour). However, heparin should not be used routinely in cases of septic shock.

7. In the past 25 years, studies have focused on the use of high dose *steroids*. Dexamethasone (6 mg/kg/day) or methylprednisolone sodium succinate (30 mg/kg/day) was recommended as a continuous intravenous infusion after an intravenous injection of a loading dose of 20 mg of dexamethasone or 125 mg of methylprednisolone. We have found steroids to be useful when given at an early stage in septic shock. In late shock they are of no avail, however, and in 1987 two prospective, randomized, double-blind clinical trials of high-dose methylprednisolone were reported, showing no decrease in mortality or morbidity.

8. *Other therapies,* such as immunotherapy using either human or murine monoclonal antibodies, in sepsis do not reduce the overall mortality rate. Recent studies suggest that nitric oxide (endothelium-derived relaxing factor) produced in response to endotoxin may be responsible in part for the hypotensive effect in sepsis, and isolated clinical reports show some promise in the treatment of sepsis when specific nitric oxide synthase blockers are used, but large-scale studies will be necessary before this regimen can be adopted. There is no evidence that *hypothermia* or *hyperbaric*

oxygen is of value in the treatment of endotoxic shock.

Surgical Treatment

If the nidus of infection can be extirpated surgically, this method is the keystone in the treatment of septic shock. In septic abortion or postpartum endometritis with shock, the nidus should be removed within 6 hours after antibiotic and adequate supportive therapy begins. Oxytocic agents may expedite the expulsion of infected products of conception. Usually, dilatation of the cervix and evacuation of the uterine contents with ring forceps, followed by suction and sharp curettage, are adequate surgical treatments in such patients. However, if the disease has advanced to myometrial microabscess formation, hysterectomy is the only logical surgical treatment. A hysterectomy should be considered (1) if shock persists after curettage and adequate supportive therapy, (2) if the uterus is larger than a 16-week gestation, (3) if the uterus is perforated, (4) if the patient is oliguric, or (5) if intrauterine infection with *Clostridium welchii* is diagnosed.

Septic pelvic thrombophlebitis, with involvement of both the ovarian and hypogastric vessels, is not too uncommon in patients with long-standing infected abortions, severe postpartum endometritis, or severe postoperative pelvic infections. Septic pulmonary embolization and fatal lung abscesses may ensue. Some observers have suggested that this condition can be treated successfully with heparin, but in the cases described, the diagnosis has been presumptive. When septic pelvic thrombophlebitis is suspected, it is reasonable to give heparin in therapeutic dosage, and, in most cases, improvement occurs. When the diagnosis is established, however and the problem is unresolved, the treatment of choice is ligation of the inferior vena cava and ovarian veins with postoperative heparin therapy. The surgical approach must be transperitoneal to gain access to the ovarian veins.

Persistence of oliguria or anuria may necessitate dialysis and is an indication for consultation with a nephrologist. Acute tubular necrosis and acute cortical necrosis carry a mortality of 50% and 90%, respectively. Anuria in a normovolemic patient suggests the possibility of acute bilateral cortical necrosis.

Gynecologic Cancer and Septic Shock

The cancer patient taking chemotherapy and the transplant patient taking immunosuppressive agents have reduced defenses against infection. Myelosuppression may give rise to an acute problem associated with neutropenia (granulocytopenia). The course of infection may be rapid, with septicemia and shock developing in 4 to 8 hours. The physician must be aware that, when the granulocyte level falls below 1000/mm^3, immediate preventive action should be taken and a careful search made for any septic focus. Appropriate ancillary investigations, such as radiographs of the abdomen, intravenous urograms, ultrasonography, and computed tomography, should be done. Aspiration of an abscess under computed tomographic guidance may save a patient a laparotomy, but if with appropriate antibiotics there is no improvement within 24 hours, laparotomy is indicated.

When the granulocyte level falls below 1000/mm^3, preventive measures should be taken immediately, as follows:

1. Preventive isolation techniques, using a "life island" or even reverse isolation, are worthwhile.
2. Prophylactic antibiotics should be given, and clindamycin and aztreonam are effective with ampicillin/sulbactam (Unasyn) or piperacillin/tazobactam (Zosyn) combinations.

In the management of these myelosuppressed patients, the general plan is as follows:

1. Granulocyte colony stimulating factor (Neupogen) 5 mg/kg subcutaneously until the absolute neutrophil count is over 10,000/mm^3.
2. Platelet transfusions are given if the platelet count is under 50,000/mm^3, otherwise the patient may die of hemorrhage.
3. Intravenous antibiotics ampicillin/sulbactam (Unasyn) 3 g or piperacillin/tazobactam (Zosyn) 4.5 g every 6 hours, with aztreonam 2 g every 8 hours, and metronidazole 500 mg every 8 hours.
4. General supportive measures for shock are instituted as previously outlined.
5. If a septic focus is found, it is dealt with promptly if a surgical approach is appropriate.

Summary

Septic shock still remains one of the leading causes of morbidity and mortality in the gynecologic and obstetric population. Our overall mortality rate in a series of 86 patients was 14%

using the regimen described. Early diagnosis, careful monitoring, prompt removal of any septic focus, and appropriate antibiotic and supportive treatment are the most important factors influencing prognosis.

Sexual Abuse and Rape

Diane Blake Brashear, PhD

Sexual assault is one of the fastest growing violent crimes in America. It is estimated that each year over 700,000 women are sexually assaulted. One in five females is assaulted by the age of 21 years, and 61% of those female victims are under the age of 18 years.

The term *rape* is defined as forced carnal knowledge of a woman. Some states have not made the term gender-neutral. States vary as to the age and ability to give consent.

Physicians are the most likely professionals to care for the sexual assault victim. Many victims do not seek medical care in the critical 72 hours after sexual assault. A small percentage, about 17%, come to an emergency department for immediate medical attention. Treatment in the acute phase differs from later care in a primary care setting.

Acute Care and Management of Sexual Assault Victims

The rape experience creates physical and emotional disorganization. Victims may present in a variety of ways, from being calm and in control to disorganized and agitated. Presentation at this time should be interpreted as the victim's way of coping and attempting to regain medical and emotional balance.

As in any acute care, the sexual assault victim's medical status must first be assessed. The next priority is to provide a safe environment so that the physician may obtain informed consent, gather necessary medical and sexual history, and perform a physical and evidence examination. A safe environment should ideally have a quiet and private area for the patient to be examined. She should not be left alone, and the physician should address her quietly and ask permission for each step of the examination as it proceeds. By being provided a safe environment, the patient can reestablish emotional and physical boundaries. The

physician should always inform the patient of what is happening and what procedures need to be done.

The physician's role is to provide medical care and gather evidence. Most emergency departments have protocols for gathering evidence related to sexual assault. Materials related to this are often part of "rape kits." Physicians working in this setting need to become familiar with protocol for rape. Some evidence rapidly decays, so quick examination may be important.

Empathy and support are essential at the time of examination. It is not the physician's role to determine whether a rape occurred; rather, it is important for the physician to establish rapport and gather data. The physician must also be clear about the legal role. In some states, reporting of sexual assault is required. In all states, report of sexual abuse and assault is required for individuals under the age of 18 years.

Medical History

When obtaining a history from a rape victim, the physician should prepare the victim for questions that may be very personal in nature. It may be helpful in obtaining information to use street or conversational language rather than medical terms. Questions should be simple and direct and allow for brief answers. The physician should be nonjudgmental in every way, either by voice tone or manner, and should avoid making the patient give an elaborate detail of the assault. Some victims report that post-rape treatment was very traumatic because of the way in which the treatment was delivered. Extensive questioning with a cognitively disorganized patient can serve as a disadvantage to the patient and to later legal remedies. Some individuals in emotional crisis do not benefit from expressing detailed emotions and memories, which can stimulate agitated responses rather than improving mood.

The medical history should include basic questions such as recent illnesses and surgeries, current medications, allergies, tetanus immunization, sexually transmitted disease history, contraception, last consensual sexual experience, and drug or alcohol use. It is most important to know what steps the patient has taken since the assault, such as douches, baths, dietary intake, and medications.

The patient should be gently questioned about the sexual assault, including where and when the assault occurred, how many attackers had physical contact, and how many had sexual contact. Then, a history specific to the sexual acts should be obtained, including whether the perpetrator used a condom or lubricant, threatened violence, or used objects and how. It is important to get as precise a history of the sexual assault as possible.

Evidence Examination

In keeping with the rape protocol, physicians should be prepared to document injuries and medical treatment and collect legally mandated specimens and laboratory samples in a competent manner so as not to jeopardize the patient's option to pursue criminal charges. Rape kits commonly include receptacles to collect the patient's clothing, blood samples for typing and DNA analysis, oral examination samples for injuries and saliva, fingernail scrapings, findings of genital examination, samples of the patient's body, head, and pubic hair, vaginal and anal swabbings, and a urine sample, and forms for documentation of the patient's injuries. Many emergency departments use a Wood's light, which can locate dried ejaculate. Such a finding should be recorded in the medical record; however, samples of ejaculate can be a false-positive finding and thus collection is controversial.

Sexually Transmitted Diseases and Pregnancy

The Centers for Disease Control and Prevention recommend that acute care patients be tested for trichomoniasis, chlamydiosis, gonorrhea, and bacterial vaginosis as well as gastrointestinal infections such as with anal *Giardia lamblia* and *Entamoeba histolytica*. Acute care includes therapy for these as well as immunization against hepatitis B and postexposure prophylaxis using hepatitis B immunoglobulin. Human immunodeficiency virus transmission has been reported from sexual assault but its incidence is low. Female patients should be tested for pregnancy, and prophylactic regimens are recommended when needed. Should the individual physician have moral conflicts about this, the patient should be referred to someone who can counsel and treat her.

Support System

The availability and presence of the patient's family and friends are most important at this time. Professional services by a rape crisis counselor can assist in following the patient after acute care. Often family members, particularly sexual partners, are themselves traumatized by the patient's experience and are not as supportive as they could be. Thus, professional help may be most important.

Treatment in the Primary Care Setting

Patients who seek medical care in later phases after sexual assault often present with symptoms that meet the category of post-traumatic stress syndrome or acute stress disorder. Symptoms may include intrusive memories, awake or asleep, avoidance of discussing the attack, and other symptoms relative to trauma. Often victims feel ashamed and responsible for the attack and are reluctant to deal directly with their experience. Some victims, such as those who have been "date-raped," fail to report the rape or to seek help because they are embarrassed and blame themselves. A victim of rape, no matter what the conditions, often feels that she is the only one with this experience and may not understand that she also requires psychological help.

Women in the later phase of the rape trauma may present with physical symptoms that indirectly express their concern and anxiety. Common symptoms after assault may be headaches, gastrointestinal distress, and back or pelvic pain. It may be through careful history and a supportive approach in such a case that the patient will offer the information that she has been raped. Then, she has to understand that these symptoms may represent her anxiety. Some patients have difficulty in understanding how physical symptoms may be related to the stress of the rape.

Clearly, physicians should maintain a supportive, nonjudgmental response and be prepared to help the patient get appropriate counseling. Physicians who provide primary care to women should already have available resources for women who have been sexually assaulted and be prepared to help them transfer to these resources. If the patient requires psychotropic medication, she should be followed by the physician or office staff to monitor use and results. The use of tranquilizers is particularly risky with the patient who has been raped, since she could be vulnerable to drug dependency.

Physicians and their staff should have information available in their offices about preventing sexual assault. The presence of information often supports the patient in revealing her experience and getting appropriate assistance.

Post-Childhood Sexual Abuse

The prevalence of child sexual abuse is undetermined but known to be quite high. In 1994, 345,000 child sexual abuse incidents were reported to Child Protective Services in the United States. At least 20% of adult women, 15% of college women, and 12% of adolescent women have experienced some form of sexual abuse or assault during their lifetime. It is estimated that about 90% of all child sexual abuse goes unreported. There is increasing evidence suggesting that childhood sexual abuse has long-term effects, and the physician is apt to find some of these incidents in the process of taking a history. Some women who experience sexual abuse in their childhood find that it is an unpleasant memory but that the experience has not had a significant negative impact on their later adjustment; other women, particularly those who are exposed to repeated abuse, have significant psychological problems. Sexual dysfunction, particularly sexual aversion, eating disorders, pseudoseizures, and depression are common in these cases. It is important to understand that the total life experience for these individuals is complicated and often psychologically damaging. Thus, the sexual abuse is harmful, but so are many other parallel psychological experiences of the patient. Sexual abuse and the response to learning about the abuse does not occur in a vacuum. Women who have been victims of childhood sexual abuse are often victimized in many ways. When physicians are presented with a patient who has a history of sexual abuse and physical symptoms that apparently have no physiologic basis, it is tempting to attribute these symptoms to the childhood sexual abuse. This is a simplistic interpretation, however, believing that if the patient works out her negative feelings about the sexual abuse, her physical symptoms will abate. Most patients in this situation require comprehensive evaluation by mental health specialists who are experienced in working with women about their history and their current psychological functioning. A referral by the physician often supports and permits the patient to get psychological help; however, the physician should continue to follow the patient's medical status as well.

Sexual Dysfunction

Stephen F. Pariser, MD

Elizabeth Patnoe, RN, MA

Christopher M. de Groot, MD

As obstetrician-gynecologists routinely address sex education, contraceptive counseling, sexually transmitted diseases, (in)fertility, pregnancy, reproductive tract surgery (including cancer), and the life cycle, issues of women's sexual health and dysfunction also emerge. While most obstetrician-gynecologists are not trained as sex therapists, all should have a fundamental and modern understanding of healthy and unhealthy human sexuality.

Professional Behavior

The physician's charge in the Hippocratic oath is to refrain "from all wrong doing or corruption, and especially from any act of seduction, of male or female, of bond or free." However, reports of physicians becoming sexually involved with their patients indicate that deviations from the oath do occur. Naturally, no physician or patient—regardless of gender—is immune to or protected from sexual attraction. But acting on this attraction is a clear abuse of vulnerability and power. Its repercussions are self-evident: psychological trauma, usually for the patient but perhaps also for the doctor, and professional sanctions and/or allegations of negligence. In the event that both patient and physician wish to develop an intimate relationship together, their professional relationship should cease; the patient can then seek medical service elsewhere.

In this area, while intentions are important, perceptions are perhaps more so. Even the most honorably intentioned physicians need to conduct themselves to avoid being misperceived. They may be assisted by the following guidelines:

1. All physicians are advised to familiarize themselves with, and avoid the use of, sexist or misogynistic language and should take care to speak to their patients with respect. For example, they should avoid patronizing patients, not assume the gender of patients' partners (especially that the partners are male), try not to interrupt during an interview (if it is necessary to do so, explain why), avoid using terms such as "honey" or "girl," honor how patients wish to be addressed (especially regarding mari-

tal status and first names), and encourage patients to ask questions (if time does not permit on one visit, schedule another).

2. As soon as physicians have concerns about the propriety of a relationship with a patient, they should consult with a mentor or psychiatrist.

3. Even if the physician is not interested in a personal relationship with a solicitous patient, it may be necessary to resign as the patient's physician and to refer the patient elsewhere for care. This situation should be handled sensitively and professionally, with a witness present. Although a physician may not need to document the reason for the change of care provider in the patient's record, it is wise to document how the situation was handled in a separate document.

4. All physicians should have a nurse or attendant present during examinations. Documentation may prevent serious medical-legal problems.

5. Although it is essential that physicians conduct thorough examinations, hand-genital contact must not be prolonged beyond what is necessary to ensure complete assessment. Before and throughout all examinations, but especially those that involve genital contact, physicians should tell patients what they are doing and why they are doing it, and they should encourage patients to ask questions and express discomfort. This helps patients maintain a sense of control. If, at any time, the patient experiences somatic or psychological discomfort from the examination, the physician should pause and discuss it with the patient; in some cases, the examination may need to be terminated.

6. Personal revelations about the physician's intimate life should be avoided.

Taking a Sexual History

When a patient raises a sexual concern, it is useful to gather information with the following considerations in mind:

1. If a patient uses the term "frigidity," the physician should explain that this term is used in various ways—for instance, to refer to the loss of sexual desire or the inability to experience orgasm. It may also be inappropriately applied to the patient by the partner. The patient should be asked to specify what she means by this word. Since the term is pejorative and imprecise, physicians should not use it except when they are clarifying patients' usage.

2. The physician should identify the onset and duration of the problems, to plan a treatment approach. If loss of desire occurs following childbirth, for example, it may be an early symptom of depression, a reflection of stress, or a result of dyspareunia.

3. The physician should determine whether the problem is primary (lifelong) or secondary (following a period free of dysfunction). Primary sexual dysfunctions often have poorer prognoses and may be the consequence of deeply ingrained conflict or performance anxiety. Understanding that a problem is secondary may help clarify its cause. For example, secondary loss of sexual desire may follow apprehension and worry associated with an abnormal pap smear or a diagnosis of a sexually transmitted disease. In a menopausal woman, cessation of coital activity may reflect dyspareunia resulting from inadequate estrogen support for lower tract genitalia.

4. The physician should determine whether the problem is partner-specific. If it is, and there is, or has been, another relationship free of difficulty, individual or dyadic therapy may be necessary before beginning focused treatment of the dysfunction.

5. The physician should gather information about factors that improve or worsen the symptoms. A woman concerned about the loss of sexual excitement in her marriage following the birth of a child may note that on vacations she and her husband have a vibrant intimate relationship. Useful suggestions might address planning, time management, and perhaps more support at home from her spouse.

6. The physician should ask the patient what she thinks is causing the problem and, if appropriate, determine what the partner believes is causing the problem by asking the patient directly or asking the partner (only after obtaining the patient's permission to do this). Identifying discrepancies and similarities is often fruitful. For instance, a patient may complain of general uninterest, while her partner may note that the disinterest worsens when the partner drinks.

The Life Cycle

Sexual interest or activity frequently decreases during pregnancy. This change may continue postpartum and be aggravated by sleep deprivation, stress, and, in some cases, depression. Support and good dyadic communication may help restore patterns of intimacy. When postpartum depression presents, treatment with supportive psychotherapy and antidepressants is indicated.

Perimenopausal women do not appear to experience difficulties with desire for, responsiveness to, or satisfaction with sex as a result of their life cycle. However, postmenopausal women with low estradiol levels are very likely to experience coital discomfort secondary to atrophic lower genital changes. Estrogen replacement therapy can prevent the reduction in coital frequency that commonly ensues.

As men age, they experience more sexual dysfunction (in desire, arousal, and potency), which often affects their partners. However, aging does not necessarily lead to loss of sexual enjoyment. Naturally, poor health and the loss of one's intimate partner can be sexually disruptive.

Other Factors Interfering with Healthy Sexual Function

A complete drug history is important, since a variety of prescribed and nonprescribed agents can interfere with sexual well-being. These include some antihypertensive agents, H_2 receptor antagonists, psychotropic agents (which can be helpful in cases of low desire or can lead to dysfunction and loss of desire), anticancer agents, alcohol, cocaine, narcotics, and prescribed hormones. Surgery such as radical vulvectomy, head trauma or spinal cord damage, and illnesses such as diabetes and multiple sclerosis are also sources of difficulty. Chronic pain syndromes and clinical depression commonly result in poor libido. Bipolar illness often results in exaggerated sexual desire and what might be interpreted as promiscuous behavior during manic or hypomanic episodes. When mood disorders present as a component of dysfunction, appropriate medical and psychological intervention are often extremely helpful.

The Sexual Dysfunctions

One of the significant advances in the treatment of sexual dysfunction is the development of inclusion-exclusion diagnostic criteria by the American Psychiatric Association. The following discussion of the diagnoses of psychosexual dysfunction relies on the general schema in *Diagnostic and Statistical Manual of Mental Disorders, Third Edition, Revised*, 1987.

When sexual dysfunction occurs, it affects the sexual response cycle in one or more of its phases. These include the following:

Desire
1. Hypoactive Sexual Desire Disorder
2. Sexual Aversion Disorder

Arousal
1. Female Sexual Arousal Disorder
2. Male Erectile Disorder

Orgasm
1. Inhibited Female Orgasm
2. Inhibited Male Orgasm
3. Premature Ejaculation

Resolution (not associated with a specific dysfunction)

Another category of sexual dysfunction not specifically tied to a cycle phase is

Sexual Pain Disorders
1. Dyspareunia (men and women)
2. Vaginismus

For a condition to be classified as a psychosexual dysfunction, it must not be caused by either traditional medical illness or other psychiatric disorder (eg, major depression). Hence, these syndromes, while having clear physiologic changes, are considered psychosomatic. Sexual dysfunctions resulting from traditional medical illness (eg, diabetes), surgery (eg, radical prostatectomy), trauma, or medication can be described using similar descriptive nomenclature, but are considered either psychogenic-biogenic or purely biogenic.

The prevalence of the psychogenic sexual dysfunctions according to S. G. Nathan are as shown in Table 1.

TABLE 1. Prevalence of Psychogenic Sexual Dysfunctions

Women	
Hypoactive sexual desire	1–35%
Sexual arousal disorder	Unclear
Inhibited orgasm	5–30%
Men	
Hypoactive sexual desire	1–15%
Male erectile disorder	10–20%
Premature ejaculation	35%
Inhibited orgasm	5%

From Nathan SG: The epidemiology of the DSM-III psychosexual dysfunctions. J Sex Marital Ther 12(4):267–281, 1986.

Hypoactive Sexual Desire Disorder

With hypoactive sexual desire, there are deficient or absent fantasies and desire for sexual activity (taking into account age, gender, and other contextual issues). A number of other diagnoses should also be considered: major depression (including dysthymia), endocrine disorders (eg, hyperprolactinemia), hypogonadal states, or chronic illness (eg, diabetes).

A lifetime history of depression is often common in patients with low sexual drive, and loss of libido is often symptomatic of depression. While antidepressants may be part of a successful treatment regimen, they can cause sexual side effects in up to 20% of cases. However, the newer serotonin-specific antidepressants appear to cause sexual side effects with lower frequency. There appears to be an association between low sexual desire and premenstrual depression, and there is growing support for the use of antidepressants in its treatment. Behavioral issues in psychogenic low sexual desire can include history of sexual abuse or trauma, relationship conflict, strict religious upbringing, poor self-image, poor self-esteem, and negative prior experience with sex.

The treatment of low sexual desire focuses on enhancing self-esteem, reducing performance anxiety, increasing knowledge, and resolving relationship issues. Directed reading or even the use of educational professional video material may also be employed to augment psychotherapy.

Sexual Aversion Disorder

This disorder refers to the persistent or recurrent severe aversion to and avoidance of all or almost all genital sexual contact with a partner. It is not to be confused with obsessive-compulsive disorder, where treatment with antiobsessional agents and behavioral therapy would be the treatment of choice. When it occurs in a hostile relationship, relationship therapy is the most important dimension to treatment.

Female Sexual Arousal Disorder

This disorder occurs when women experience difficulty attaining the lubrication-swelling response associated with sexual excitement or maintaining this response until the completion of a sexual activity, or when they have persistent or recurrent lack of sexual excitement and pleasure during sex. Relationship issues, fear of loss of control, fear of pregnancy, poor dyadic sexual

communication, and even the fear of disturbing nearby children can all contribute to this disorder. Sometimes this dysfunction is absent with self-stimulation or is partner-specific. Supportive psychotherapy with the affected woman or with the couple is often helpful. Sensate-focus behavioral therapy may reduce performance anxiety because it is graduated and re-establishes control. It may also facilitate open constructive discussion between partners about their love-making preferences.

Male Erectile Disorder

This term refers to men who experience difficulty obtaining an erection and/or maintaining it until completion of the sexual activity, or who experience a significant lack of subjective excitement and pleasure during sexual activity. This disorder is of interest to obstetrician-gynecologists because patients may present concerns about their partners' potency or because it is an issue during infertility evaluations. The differential diagnoses of impotence include diabetes, other endocrine disorders, vascular disease, multiple sclerosis and other neuralgic syndromes, trauma, radical surgery, and medication-induced impotence.

Features suggestive of psychogenic impotence include spontaneous erections, morning erections, sporadic erections, and healthy erections with masturbation.

Performance anxiety is a frequent cause of psychogenic impotence. This can result from an episode of loss of erection associated with alcohol use, leading to anxiety about future erectile functioning significant enough to cause persistent impotence. Frustration and anger—on the part of the man or his partner—over early ejaculation can also lead to psychogenic potency difficulties. Depressive illness has also been found to impair potency. In such cases, antidepressant therapy with appropriate psychological treatment can be helpful.

Inhibited Female Orgasm

Inhibited female orgasm refers to the delay in or inability to attain orgasm following sexual excitement. This diagnosis should not be applied simply because a woman fails to achieve orgasm during intercourse without manual stimulation. It is common for women to experience orgasm during manual stimulation with much more ease than during coitus without direct manual stimulation. This is not necessarily abnormal, but, when it is a concern to the patient, it may represent some inhibition and may benefit from treatment. This diagnosis appears to be less common today, perhaps the result of increased awareness about sexual health and function disseminated through the media.

Depression, medication, and pain (eg, from arthritis or endometriosis) can also impair the ability to achieve orgasm. Psychological factors that can raise the orgasmic threshold include relationship conflict, fear of loss of control, performance anxiety, inadequate intimacy and foreplay, premature ejaculation, religious prohibition, and fear of pregnancy.

Treatment strategies vary, depending on the level of inhibition. A graduated hierarchy of behavioral assignments for nonorgasmic women can include graduated self-exploration, self-stimulation, graduated sensate focus, coitus combined with manual clitoral stimulation, and coitus. Bibliotherapy can also be helpful for both partners.

Clearly, the most important ingredients to ensure success are self-comfort, education, and supportive, open relationship dialogue. The focus of discussion between partners should include issues of personal affection and intimacy and requests about mutual pleasuring.

Inhibited Male Orgasm

The delay or absence of orgasm following a "normal sexual excitement phase" (and considering factors such as age) is known as inhibited male orgasm. Usually the inability to experience orgasm for men is problematic during coitus, but not so with masturbation or extravaginal penile stimulation. This is a relatively rare dysfunction, but it is important to the obstetrician-gynecologist because of its relationship to infertility. The absence of sperm in a postcoital test is very suggestive of inhibited male orgasm. Inhibited male orgasm should not be confused with retrograde ejaculation. Rarely is a medical illness causative, although medication can be a factor. Psychological factors associated with inhibited male orgasm can include strict religious upbringing, unresolved oedipal issues, anger, partner ambivalence, and fear of pregnancy.

Treatment strategies employ dyadic therapy, conflict resolution, performance anxiety reduction, and the progressive use of sensate-focus techniques.

Premature Ejaculation

Premature ejaculation is the most common male sexual dysfunction. It refers to ejaculation oc-

curring with minimal sexual stimulation before or in close proximity to penetration, or before the male would like to ejaculate. In making this diagnosis, one must consider factors such as age, situation, and frequency of ejaculation. Unfortunately, voluntary control of ejaculation is not a natural skill, but it can be learned. Sex therapy is directed at increasing the patient's sensitivity to arousal so that coital activity can be paced without premature arrival at ejaculatory inevitability. Sensate-focus and "stop-start" techniques are often useful in assisting the male in gaining control.

While premature ejaculation may cause a variety of negative reactions in the male, the obstetrician-gynecologist may also witness negative reactions in his female patients. Women partners may feel troubled, frustrated, angered, and even guilty about the condition—and those negative reactions, like the male's, may exacerbate the problem and damage the relationship. In some cases premature ejaculation can lead to male erectile disorder. During couples therapy, instruction regarding behavioral treatment with the stop-start technique can be given along with attention to relationship issues.

Dyspareunia

Recurrent, persistent genital pain before, during, or following coitus is referred to as dyspareunia. It occurs in women and, rarely, in men. In women, if the discomfort is caused by a lack of vaginal transudate or is exclusively the result of vaginismus, the diagnosis is not psychogenic dyspareunia, but may be female sexual arousal disorder. Gynecologic causes of painful coitus that need to be excluded include endometriosis, atrophic vulvovaginitis, sexually transmitted diseases, and Bartholin's gland infection.

Once gynecologic causes have been excluded, treatment can employ both a dyadic and a behavioral approach. Sensate focus is often utilized in the treatment process. On occasion, dyspareunia may be associated with major depression or obsessive-compulsive disorder. If present, those disorders require appropriate psychopharmacologic and behavioral treatment to resolve the sexual problem.

Vaginismus

Vaginismus occurs when there is recurrent or persistent involuntary spasm of the perivaginal muscles at the outlet, interfering with coitus. The diagnosis may be confirmed during gentle pelvic examination. In some cases, however, the spasm may not occur in the gynecologic setting, yet be problematic in love-making. Dyspareunia, psychogenic or gynecologic in etiology, may lead to vaginismus. Treatment involves progressive desensitization using fingers. In years past, some gynecologic texts recommended the use of glass dilators; for obvious reasons, this is to be avoided. In some cases, vaginismus is associated with phobic avoidance of sex.

Summary

The obstetrician-gynecologist must be comfortable addressing sexual concerns and dysfunctions. Approaching patients with sensitivity and nonjudgmental professionalism is the first step in assuring positive outcomes. In addition, the physician should be knowledgeable about related problems that are associated with sexual dysfunction and that often are successfully addressed with the assistance of other professionals: mood disorders, relationship conflict, difficulties with self-esteem, and traditional medical and gynecologic concerns. An integrated approach is necessary if sexual problems are to be successfully defined and managed.

Sexually Transmitted Diseases

Sebastian Faro, MD, PhD

Herpes Genitalis

Herpes simplex is the most common cause of genital ulcerative sexually transmitted disease in the United States. The increased incidence of genital herpes in the past 20 years may be attributed to a decrease in the use of barrier contraception, an increased use of oral contraceptive pills, and sexual promiscuity. Herpes simplex virus (HSV) types 1 and 2 are DNA viruses that possess common and type-specific antigens. HSV 1 preferentially infects the oral-pharyngeal mucosa, and HSV 2 is responsible for genital infection. However, HSV 1 may cause genital infection as well (10–15% of cases) and HSV 2 can infect the oral-pharyngeal mucosa. The disease is most prevalent in patients aged 15 to 30 years. Patients infected with HSV 1 develop antibodies

that often reduce the severity of disease when the patient is exposed to HSV 2.

Patients exposed to HSV 2 may develop either a primary infection or an initial infection. A primary infection occurs in those individuals who have never been exposed to the herpesvirus, and therefore, do not have antibodies to this virus. It is characterized in female patients by numerous ulcerative lesions distributed over the vulva. The vagina, cervix, and bladder may be involved. The lesions appear within 2 to 12 days after inoculation has occurred and are usually preceded by a flu-like syndrome. Patients commonly develop bilateral inguinal adenopathy. Coincident with development of ulcerations may be dysuria and urinary retention.

Patients with initial herpetic genital infection have had previous exposure to the virus and have developed antibodies. The lesions are few in number and painful. Their development is not usually preceded by a flu-like syndrome.

Herpes infection is characterized by the recurrence of genital lesions. Approximately 60% to 80% of patients with HSV 2 infection experience recurrent outbreaks within 1 year, compared with 15% to 16% of patients with genital HSV 1 infection. Patients with recurrent infections usually report prodromes of itching, pain, or discomfort at the site of recurrence. Recurrent outbreaks are not usually associated with inguinal lymphadenopathy, and the ulcer usually resolves within 3 to 7 days.

Typically, the diagnosis is made on clinical appearance but should be confirmed by culture or fluorescent viral antigen detection. When any sexually transmitted disease is suspected, it is important that its presence be confirmed. Pap smears or other stained preparations are not reliable. It is also important to remember that the presence of one sexually transmitted disease is usually indicative of other sexually transmitted diseases. Therefore, patients with primary or initial HSV 2 infection should be screened for *Neisseria gonorrhoeae, Chlamydia trachomatis, Trichomonas vaginalis,* and human papillomavirus.

Treatment for primary herpes with topical acyclovir (Zovirax) has not been very effective. If administered very early in the course of primary herpes, acyclovir, 200 mg administered orally five times daily for 7–10 days, may result in rapid healing, thus shortening the duration of lesions. Patients who develop severe genital infection, disseminated herpes, or herpetic hepatitis should be hospitalized and administered 5 to 10 mg/kg of acyclovir, intravenously over 1 hour, every 8 hours. When acyclovir is administered in high doses, the patient should be kept well hydrated (Table 1).

Patients with frequent recurrences of genital herpes can be treated with oral acyclovir, 200 mg, five times a day for 5 days. To be effective, the medication should be started as soon as the patient notes the prodrome or development of a lesion. Suppressive acyclovir therapy using various dosing regimens has also been shown to be effective. For example, a regimen of acyclovir, 200 mg taken twice daily for 1 year, has been effective in suppressing recurrent outbreaks. Patients on long-term suppression have not been shown to develop resistance to acyclovir, nor have there been adverse effects on bone marrow or renal or hepatic function.

The pregnant patient with genital herpes should be treated with acyclovir only if severe disease occurs. In the absence of significant infection, the pregnant patient can be treated with topical anesthetics, local hygiene, and sitz baths. There are no data to support the use of acyclovir administered prophylactically to prevent recurrent infection in the pregnant patient.

The risk that a pregnant patient with a history of recurrent disease will shed virus asymptomatically on the day of delivery is about 1.4%. In one study 34 infants born to women who were asymptomatically shedding herpesvirus, no neonatal infection occurred.

Pregnant women with a history of genital herpes or with partners who have herpes should be educated about the potential risks of infection in the absence of lesions. If a patient experiences an outbreak within 2 weeks of the onset of labor, her infant should be delivered by cesarean section. A patient admitted in labor with no history of recent lesions should have vulvar and cervical specimens obtained for the isolation of herpesvirus to determine whether the neonate has been exposed to the virus. The patient should then be allowed to labor and deliver vaginally.

Patients with genital lesions and ruptured membranes should be delivered by cesarean section if no more than 6 hours have elapsed. No good data are available on the management of patients whose membranes have been ruptured more than 6 hours with respect to mode of delivery. Perhaps these patients should be given acyclovir, 5 to 10 mg/kg intravenously, and allowed to attempt vaginal delivery.

Patients who develop primary herpes in pregnancy, especially in the last trimester, have a 50% to 60% chance of having an affected neonate. The pregnant patient with primary disease has a 10% chance of having recurrent disease.

Vaginal Trichomoniasis

Trichomonas vaginalis is a flagellated protozoan that attaches to epithelial cells. In the United States, 2.5 to 3 million women are estimated to be infected annually. The prevalence of infection correlates with the degree of sexual activity. For example, in family planning clinics, approximately 5% of women are found to have trichomoniasis; in gynecology clinics, up to 25%; in sexually transmitted disease clinics, approximately 35%; and, among prostitutes, up to 75%.

The individual infected with *T. vaginalis* may be asymptomatic or may complain of urinary frequency, dysuria, dyspareunia, lower abdominal pain, or a foul-smelling vaginal discharge. Asymptomatic carriers usually become symptomatic within 6 months. Vaginal discharge, usually described as dirty-gray and purulent, is reported in 50% to 75% of women diagnosed with trichomoniasis. Around 10% of women with trichomoniasis complain of a foul odor. Symptoms of acute infection are usually noted at the time of or following menstruation.

Physical characteristics of infection depend on the severity of disease. Patients with a low inoculum tend to be asympomatic but also tend to have a dirty-gray discharge. The pH of the vaginal discharge is usually greater than 4.5. Microscopic examination of the discharge reveals white blood cells, larger numbers of bacteria, and flag-

---

TABLE 1. Rcommendation for the Treatment of Herpesvirus Infection°

First episode—oral regimens
    Acyclovir 400 mg tid × 7–10 days,
    Acyclovir 200 mg five times a day × 7–10 days,
    Famciclovir 250 mg tid × 7–10 days, or
    Valacyclovir 1 g bid × 7–10 days
Recurrent disease—oral regimens
    Acyclovir 400 mg tid × 5 days,
    Acyclovir 200 mg five times a day × 5 days,
    Acyclovir 800 mg bid × 5 days,
    Famciclovir 125 mg bid × 5 days, or
    Valacyclovir 500 mg bid × 5 days
Suppressive therapy—oral regimens
    Acyclovir 400 mg bid,
    Famciclovir 250 mg bid,
    Valacyclovir 500 mg qd, or
    Valacyclovir 1000 mg qd
Severe disease—administer intravenously
    Acyclovir 5–10 mg/kg body weight q 8 hrs

°1998 recommendations by the Centers for Disease Control and Prevention.

ellated protozoa. Increasing inoculum size is associated with various physical findings: frothy discharge, which tends to be more commonly associated with bacterial vaginosis; punctate hemorrhages of the cervix; erythematous vaginal walls; and vulvar edema.

The disease can be diagnosed by examining the vaginal discharge microscopically and identifying the mobile, flagellated trichomonads. Cultures of these organisms can easily be obtained by using Diamond's medium, incubating at 38°C, and examining the medium microscopically within 48 to 72 hours. Trichomonads can be seen on microscopic examinations of vaginal discharge in 40% to 80% of cases. Obtaining cultures raises the diagnosis to 90%. *T. vaginalis* can also be identified on Pap smear, which has a 60% to 70% sensitivity when compared with microscopic examination of the vaginal discharge.

Metronidazole continues to be the agent of choice in the treatment of trichomoniasis. Related agents, tinidazole and ornidazole, have similar efficacy, but are not available in the United States. When used alone, topical or vaginal preparations are not well suited for the treatment of trichomoniasis because concomitant infection of the urethra and periurethral glands will not absorb adequate levels of metronidazole.

Oral metronidazole in a dosage of 250 mg given three times daily for 7 days, or 500 mg twice daily for 7 days, cures 95% of cases. An alternative regimen is 2 g of metronidazole as a single dose, which will cure 82% of cases, or, if the partner is treated simultaneously, 90% of cases. Patients failing to respond to either of these regimens should be treated with 250 to 500 mg, given three times daily for 10 to 14 days. During the treatment period, they should be advised to refrain from sexual intercourse until a cure has been established. If this therapeutic regimen fails, the oral regimen can be repeated with the addition of intravaginal metronidazole gel, one applicatorful daily for 10 to 14 days. If the patient fails to respond to this therapeutic regimen, metronidazole, 2 to 4 g daily, can be administered intravenously.

High-dose metronidazole may be associated with adverse side effects, so patients receiving higher doses should be closely monitored. Most patients complain of an unpleasant or metallic taste. Nausea occurs in 10% and transient neutropenia in 7.5%. Patients should be warned not to imbibe any alcohol-containing liquids because a disulfiram-like reaction could occur. Repeated long-term use may be associated with neutropenia and peripheral neuropathy. Vaginitis secondary to *Candida* infection has been reported in 16% of patients taking metronidazole.

Metronidazole has been found to be mutagenic in bacteria and carcinogenic in animals. However, no data are available with regard to humans. Metronidazole crosses the placenta; therefore, its use in the first trimester should be reserved for severe cases. Although alternative treatments, such as topical clotrimazole or Betadine gel, can be offered, these agents have not been demonstrated to be efficacious.

Vaginal Candidiasis

Vaginitis due to yeast is most commonly caused by *Candida albicans,* which is also a commonly found inhabitant of the healthy vagina, the oral cavity, and the gastrointestinal tract. *Candida* appears to be the second most common cause of vaginal infections. It is estimated that 7% of all women will experience at least one episode of vulvovaginal candidiasis during their reproductive period and approximately 50% of these women will have a second episode. Approximately 5% of these women will be subject to repeated episodes. Patients with recurrent or intractable candidiasis should be screened for diabetes and HIV.

The most common symptom of vulvovaginal candidiasis is pruritus vulvae, which may be associated with edema or erythema of the vulva or both. Characteristically, the patient with vulvovaginal candidiasis will have white patches on the infected areas and what typically is referred to as a cottage cheese–like vaginal discharge. However, some patients may have a milky-white liquid discharge. The pH is typically within the normal range (3.8–4.2) because the fungi prefer an acid environment. An aliquot of vaginal discharge can be mixed with a drop or two of 10% KOH and examined microscopically. The cell walls of the fungi or yeast are made up of chitin, which is resistant to alkali and therefore remains intact. Budding yeast forms or pseudohyphae can easily be identified. Vaginal yeast cultures should be obtained in patients whose symptoms suggest a yeast infection but in whom none can be identified on microscopic examination of vaginal discharge and in patients failing to respond to therapy. Once the yeast has been isolated, it should be identified. Sensitivities to antifungal agents are not routinely done in general laboratories but can be requested from research laboratories, if needed.

A variety of antifungal creams for intravaginal use are available, including two over-the-counter preparations: miconazole (Monistat) and clotrimazole (Gyne-Lotrimin). Patients who experience their first episode of yeast vulvovaginitis should not be treated over the telephone. The infection should be confirmed by examination and the patient educated as to signs and symptoms of the disease. Individuals who undergo self-treatment should be advised, if their symptoms do not resolve within 3 days, to discontinue the medication and wait 5 to 7 days before being examined. Table 2 lists antifungal vaginal preparations.

The agents listed in item A of Table 2 can be used either for short courses (3 days) or for longer periods (7 to 10 days). Treatment can usually be repeated without much concern for adverse side effects, the most common being a local allergic response to the carrier agent or active ingredient. Ketoconazole (Nizoral) and fluconazole (Diflucan) have been approved for use in the treatment of vulvovaginal candidiasis. These agents are usually reserved for individuals with chronic or intractable disease. Ketoconazole is associated with gastrointestinal disturbances, hepatotoxicity, and, rarely, anaphylaxis. Fluconazole may cause similar adverse effects, but much less frequently.

Individuals with chronic or intractable disease require long-term maintenance and suppressive prophylaxis. Oral agents offer better compliance because of ease of administration. The patient with an acute exacerbation can be treated with ketoconazole, 400 mg daily for 5 days, followed by 100 mg daily for 6 months. Fluconazole can be administered as follows: 200 mg for 1 day,

followed by 100 mg daily for 3 days, and a 500 mg Mycelex-G vaginal tablet weekly for 6 weeks (author's personal regimen). There are no published data for fluconazole.

Chronic or intractable yeast infections may be due to infection by a resistant strain or selection for a resistant strain secondary to chronic use of antifungal agents. The typical yeast encountered in this situation are *Saccharomyces cerevisiae*, *Candida glabrata*, and *Candida tropicalis*. These yeasts are typically resistant to the "azoles," but tend to be sensitive to the oral imidazoles, topical flucytosine (Ancobon), or topical boric acid. Topical flucytosine should be limited in its use because of the selection of resistant strains.

Bacterial Vaginosis

Bacterial vaginosis is considered by some investigators to be the most prevalent cause of vaginitis in women of childbearing age. The prevalence of this disease appears to be related to the frequency of sexual intercourse and the number of partners involved. This complex infection is polymicrobial in make-up and dominated by anaerobes and an absence of *Lactobacillus*. *Gardnerella vaginalis* and *Mycoplasma* are characteristically associated with anaerobes, such as *Peptostreptococcus*, *Bacteroides*, and *Mobiluncus*.

This condition can easily be diagnosed by the characteristic homogenous, liquid, dirty-gray, frothy, malodorous discharge. The pH of the vaginal discharge is usually greater than 4.5, and a whiff test is positive (10% KOH mixed with vaginal discharge liberates amine, fish-like odor). Microscopic examination of the discharge reveals numerous clue cells, numerous individual free-floating bacteria, and a noticeable absence of white blood cells.

Treatment of this condition can be carried out with the various antimicrobial agents listed in Table 3. Patients being treated for this condition tend to relapse frequently. The reason for these frequent relapses is not understood, but may be due to reinfection via sexual intercourse or failure of the vagina to restore a normal flora characterized by *Lactobacillus*. However, it seems logical that, during the treatment period, the patient should refrain from sexual intercourse or should advise her partner to use a condom. It may even be prudent to treat her partner at the time she is being treated.

Gonorrhea

Neisseria gonorrhoeae continues to be an important cause of disease among sexually active

---

TABLE 2. Antifungal Vaginal Preparations

A. Initial treatment
   1. Imidazoles
      a. Clotrimazole (Lotrimin, Gyne-Lotrimin, Mycelex, Mycelex-G)
      b. Miconazole (Monistat)
      c. Butoconazole (Femstat)
      d. Terconazole (Terazol)
      e. Tioconazole (Vagistat-1)
   2. Polyenes
      a. Candicidin (Vanobid)
      b. Nystatin (Candep, Mycostatin, Nilstat, O-V Statin, Mycolog°)
      c. Amphotericin B
B. Chronic or intractable disease
   1. Ketoconazole (Nizoral)
   2. Fluconazole (Diflucan)

°Mycolog is a combination of triamcinolone acetonide 0.1%, neomycin sulfate, gramicidin, and nystatin.

TABLE 3. Treatment of Bacterial Vaginosis

1. Metronidazole, 500 mg, orally bid × 7 days
2. Metronidazole gel, one applicatorful bid × 5 days
3. Clindamycin cream, 2%, one applicatorful qd × 7 days
4. Amoxicillin/clavulanate, 500 mg, orally tid × 7 days
5. Clindamycin, 300 mg orally, bid × 7 days
6. Metronidazole, 2 g orally, in a single dose
7. Metronidazole gel, 0.75% once daily × 5 days
8. Metronidazole, 750 mg extended release tablets once daily for 7 days

individuals. The number of cases rose steadily from 1966 until 1976, at which time the number of cases plateaued at approximately 1 million cases annually until 1981. A decline in the number of cases occurred from 1981 until 1989, at which time an increase was again noted.

The most common site of infection in women is the endocervix. Infection tends to be asymptomatic but can mark the beginning stage of pelvic inflammatory disease. A second important characteristic of this asymptomatic state is that the endocervix constitutes a large reservoir for the gonococcus. Gonococcal infection of the cervix may serve as the gateway to upper genital tract infection, especially during menstruation. Progression of the infection upward leads to endometritis and may eventually result in salpingitis.

Presence of the gonococcus in the endocervix should lead the physician to check for other sites of infection, such as urethra, Skene's and Bartholin's glands, rectum, and oral pharynx. Pharyngeal infection is common in patients who develop gonococcal septicemia. Disseminated gonococcemia develops in approximately 25% of patients with pharyngeal infection. Disseminated gonococcal infection is characterized by tenosynovitis, arthralgia, septic arthritis, and rash.

Patients with trichomoniasis who are sexually active should have cultures for *N. gonorrhoeae* and *Chlamydia trachomatis*. Women at greatest risk for acquisition of a sexually transmitted disease are those in the early reproductive age group (15 to 25 years of age); those with multiple sex partners; those whose sexual partners have multiple partners; those with previous exposure to a sexually transmitted disease; those with an intrauterine device; those using oral contraception who are unmarried; and those with a history of pelvic inflammatory disease. Patients with any risk factors should be screened for gonorrhea

and chlamydia, since these infections tend to be asymptomatic.

Endocervical infection can be diagnosed by isolation and identification or other specific tests (DNA probe), which must be done prior to informing the patient that she has gonorrhea. Gram stain may be performed on an endocervical specimen for the presence of intracellular gram-negative diplococci. During examination of the patient, if a purulent exudate is noted issuing forth from the urethra or orifices of Skene's or Bartholin's glands, the physician should obtain specimens for culture of *N. gonorrhoea* and *C. trachomatis*. A positive Gram stain from these sites is indicative of infection. If the patient participates in oral-genital sex, specimens should also be obtained from the pharynx.

If there is a strong clinical evidence of infection, treatment should not be delayed until culture data are available. Recommended treatment for gonococcal cervicitis, urethritis, or anorectal or pharyngeal infection is ceftriaxone (Rocephin), 125 mg intramuscularly once, plus doxycycline, 100 mg orally bid for 7 days. Ceftriaxone is effective against penicillinase-producing strains and penicillin- and tetracycline-resistant strains. Doxycycline is administered in the event the patient has a coincident *C. trachomatis* infection. Patients who are allergic to ceftriaxone should be given spectinomycin, 2 g intramuscularly in a single dose. Alternatives to these regimens are oflaxacin, 400 mg given orally in a single dose, or azithromycin 1 g orally in a single dose, or doxycycline 100 mg bid for 7 days, or trovofloxacin 200 mg in a single dose.

Chlamydia

Chlamydia trachomatis, an obligate intracellular parasite, is considered the most common sexually transmitted bacterium. It most commonly causes endocervicitis but is also associated with pelvic inflammatory disease, urethritis, and infection of Skene's and Bartholin's glands. Like *N. gonorrhoeae*, *C. trachomatis* has been linked to septic abortion, premature rupture of membranes, chorioamnionitis, postpartum endometritis, neonatal conjunctivitis, and pneumonia.

Endocervicitis caused by *C. trachomatis* or *N. gonorrhoeae*, or both, is often asymptomatic, with only a scant endocervical mucopurulent discharge. However, infection can often be detected by noting edema and hypertrophy of the endocervical epithelium as well as friability of this tissue. In 20% to 60% of cases, *N. gonorrhoeae* and *C. trachomatis* are found to be coinfecting the cervix. The fact that these infections are usually present for a period of time prior to their discovery and that their discovery is often accidental should raise caution when short-term therapy is considered. No available data address the consequences or efficacy of short-term (single dose or 3-day) therapy in relation to tubal damage. Therefore, long-term therapy should be administered when treating either of these diseases. The recommendation by the Centers for Disease Control and Prevention (CDC) of adding doxycycline to a cephalosporin addresses this concern.

The diagnosis of chlamydial infection can be made by isolating the organism by tissue culture, enzyme-linked immunosorbent assay, or direct fluorescent monoclonal antibody. The prevalence of C. trachomatis varies, depending on the population. In high-risk populations (15- to 25-year-olds who are sexually promiscuous), the prevalence is 25% to 40%; in moderate-risk groups, the prevalence is 10% to 20%; and in low-risk groups the prevalence is about 5%. In evaluation of a patient known to be at risk, a dacron-tipped applicator can be inserted deep into the endocervical canal and rotated for 30 to 40 seconds. The presence of mucopus is an indication of infection. The specimen should be processed for the isolation of N. gonorrhoeae and C. trachomatis. Prior to obtaining the specimen, the portion of the cervix should be cleansed of all vaginal discharge because it may contain toxic substances that inhibit the detection of C. trachomatis. Next, a wet prep can be made of the endocervical discharge by placing the swab in 2 mL of normal saline and examining a drop or two microscopically. The specimen can be considered valid if fewer than 20 squamous epithelial cells are noted. If white blood cells are present, but no bacteria, yeast, or trichomonads, the presence of C. trachomatis and N. gonorrhoeae can be suspected. If a Gram stain is performed and gram-negative intracellular diplococci are observed, N. gonorrhoeae can be suspected, but C. trachomatis cannot be ruled out, nor can Mycoplasma and Ureaplasma bacteria.

Treatment should be directed against both C. trachomatis and N. gonorrhoeae. Therefore, ceftriaxone, 125 g, as a single intramuscular dose, should be given for N. gonorrhoeae. Doxycycline, 100 mg orally twice daily for 7 days, will be adequate for chlamydial infection of the lower genital tract. Doxycycline is even effective against 85% of the strains of N. gonorrhoeae and 100% of the strains of C. trachomatis. The patient's partner should be treated with the same antibiotic regimen. Again, the partner should be advised to use condoms until a cure has been established in both partners. Pregnant patients can be treated with erythromycin base, 500 mg orally qid for 10 days.

Alternative regimens for the nonpregnant patient are ofloxacin, 300 mg bid for 7 days, or trovafloxacin, 200 mg for 7 days, which is effective against both C. trachomatis and N. gonorrhoeae; ampicillin, 500 mg orally qid for 10 days; or amoxicillin or amoxicillin/clavulanate acid, 500 mg orally tid for 10 days, azithromycin 1 g orally in a single dose, or trovofloxacin 200 mg for 7 days. However, a test-of-cure culture should be obtained. If N. gonorrhoeae is present, it should be tested for penicillin resistance. Clindamycin, 300 mg orally tid for 10 days, should be effective against C. trachomatis. Azithromycin, 1 g orally as a single dose, is effective for the treatment of both acute chlamydial and gonococcal urethritis and cervicitis. However, caution should be taken because of the impossibility of knowing how long the chlamydial infection has been present or whether or not there has been progression of the disease process. No data are available with regard to sequelae of infection, such as tubal damage, with a single-day treatment regimen.

In treating both N. gonorrhoeae and C. trachomatis endocervicitis, the physician should remember the goals: (1) eradication of the organism; (2) prevention of tubal damage (infertility, ectopic pregnancy); (3) treatment of patient's contacts; and (4) patient education, including transmission, prevention, and long-term sequelae. Remember, sexually transmitted diseases are not solely a problem of individual patient management, but are a public health issue with significant impact on the community, both medically and economically.

Pelvic Inflammatory Disease

Pelvic inflammatory disease (PID) is not only a national problem, but also a worldwide health issue. In the United States, it is estimated that there are 1,000,000 patient visits annually for PID. This population base results in 250,000 hospital admissions annually and generates approximately 100,000 surgical cases. The most common causes for PID are N. gonorrhoeae and C. trachomatis. The former tends to cause a more symptomatic disease. The latter has been designated the most common cause of "silent PID." Its more subtle signs are frequently overlooked by both physician and patient. The disease is suspected only when the patient presents with an ectopic pregnancy or for an infertility evaluation.

Presenting signs and symptoms of gonococcal PID are lower abdominal pain; purulent vaginal discharge; fever (may or may not be present); elevated white blood cell count; and tender cervix, uterus, and adnexa. The patient may or may not have adnexal masses, raising the suspicion of tubo-ovarian abscesses or inflammatory mucosa. Patients with chlamydial PID may note any of the following signs: vague lower abdominal pain, recent onset of dysmenorrhea, breakthrough bleeding while taking oral contraception, intermenstrual spotting if not utilizing oral contraceptive pills, and recent onset of postcoital bleeding. The physician may note during the pelvic examination hypertrophy of the endocervical epithelium; friability of the endocervical epithelium, which bleeds briskly when gently touched; or cervical, uterine, or adnexal tenderness on bimanual examination. Another possible sign of chlamydial infection is noted in the individual who previously has had no difficulty in conceiving and delivering but now presents with unexplained infertility.

Another major concern is when to hospitalize a patient for treatment. Ambulatory treatment can be instituted if the patient meets the following criteria:

- Temperature less than 38°C (100.4°F)
- Tolerance of oral liquids and solids
- No evidence of pelvic or abdominal peritonitis
- No evidence of a pelvic mass

Patients on ambulatory management should be seen any time their condition worsens or within 72 hours for re-evaluation. This approach is necessary because patients with acute uncomplicated PID typically respond to antibiotic therapy within 48 to 72 hours. However, ambulatory treatment for PID has not been well studied, and the current CDC recommendation is not well supported. Patients should be hospitalized if any of the following conditions apply:

- The diagnosis is uncertain.
- The pelvic abscess or inflammatory mass is suspected.
- The patient is unresponsive to the out-patient regimen.
- The patient cannot tolerate the out-patient regimen.
- Follow-up cannot be arranged within 72 hours.
- A pregnancy has been documented.

The following antibiotic regimens are recommended:

1. Ceftriaxone, 125 mg intramuscularly for 1 day, plus doxycycline, 200 mg bid for 10 to 14 days (CDC recommendation).
2. Augmentin, 500 mg orally tid for 10 days.
3. Ofloxacin, 400 mg orally bid for 14 days plus metronidazole, 500 mg orally bid for 14 days.

All these regimens are effective against *N. gonorrhoeae* and *C. trachomatis*. Regimen 3 also provides activity against gram-positive and gram-negative aerobic, facultative, and obligate anaerobic bacteria. Ofloxacin's obligate anaerobic activity is weak; therefore, until more data are available, patients who have had their disease for a prolonged period should also receive an anaerobic agent, such as clindamycin or metronidazole (Table 4).

Patients who have failed to respond to outpatient therapy should be considered for other diagnostic tests. Laparoscopy should be performed in those patients who have not responded to either an out-patient or in-patient regimen. Although patients may have had classic symptoms and signs of PID, studies have shown that one third of these patients will not have PID. Ultrasound may be helpful in detecting a mass or abscess. Ultrasonography or computed tomography scan may assist in draining the abscess percutaneously.

Laparoscopy should not be attempted on patients who have peritonitis or markedly distended abdomens. Patients who have had their disease for an extended period also should not undergo laparoscopy. These individuals should have exploratory laparotomy because they often have markedly distended loops of bowel, fibrous adhesions, and free pus in the intraperitoneal cavity. These individuals must have a thorough abdomi-

---

TABLE 4. Treatment of Pelvic Inflammatory Disease

Alternative Parenteral Regimens

1. Cefotetan 2 g q 12 hrs plus doxycycline 100 mg orally q 12 hrs.
2. Cefoxitin 2 g q 6 hrs plus doxycycline 100 mg orally q 12 hrs.
3. Clindamycin 900 mg q 8 hrs plus gentamicin 2 mg/kg of body weight, followed by a maintenance dose of 1.5 mg/kg q 8 hrs.
4. Ofloxacin 400 mg q 12 hrs plus metronidazole 500 mg q 8 hrs.
5. Ampicillin/sulbactam 3 g q 6 hrs.
6. Piperacillin/tazobactam 3.375 g q 6 hrs.
7. Trovafloxacin 200 mg q 24 hrs.

nal exploration, including the subdiaphragmatic and subhepatic spaces. The bowel must be inspected, checking for intraloop abscesses. Once the abdomen has been entered, fluid should be obtained for culture of aerobic and anaerobic bacteria. Biopsies should be taken of infected and inflammed tissue and placed in an anaerobic transport vial for processing for isolation of aerobic and anaerobic bacteria. The extent of surgical removal of tissue is dependent on the condition of the infected tissue and the patient's desire to maintain reproductive capabilities. Conservative surgical approaches, such as incision and drainage of tubo-ovarian abscess, may necessitate additional operative procedures, and the patient should be made well aware of these possibilities.

Syphilis

Treponema pallidum is the causative agent of syphilis, which has been on the rise over the last 5 years. This disease in women is rarely diagnosed in the primary stage but more commonly found in the secondary stage. The surge in the number of cases of syphilis has been directly related to human immunodeficiency virus (HIV) infection. The incidence of syphilis in the United States in 1988 was 16.8 cases per 100,000. However, more recently the incidence of primary and secondary syphilis in the United States decreased to 4.3 cases per 100,000. Risk factors for the contraction of syphilis associated with sexual activity are socioeconomic class, illicit drug use, availability of health care, and residence in high endemic areas.

Syphilis is divided into stages: primary, secondary, and tertiary. The incubation period is related to inoculum size. It is thought to be 10 to 90 days from exposure to onset of chancre development. The chancre usually heals spontaneously in 3 to 6 weeks. Dissemination of spirochetes occurs during the primary stage, and 60% to 90% of patients develop secondary syphilis. This stage of syphilis develops within 4 to 10 weeks following the development of primary syphilis. In one-third of these cases, the patient still has the chancre of primary syphilis. Secondary syphilis is divided into early and late secondary syphilis. Early secondary syphilis will resolve spontaneously in 3 to 12 weeks. This stage can be marked with recurrent lesions and is known as early latent syphilis (the disease has been present for less than 1 year) versus late latent syphilis (the disease has been present for more than 1 year). This distinction is important because during early latent syphilis, the patient can experience lesions characteristic of secondary syphilis, whereas in the later latent phase, no lesions recur.

Early latent syphilis is characterized by flu-like symptoms consisting of myalgia, arthralgia, malaise, and low-grade fever; generalized lymphadenopathy; nonpruritic maculopapular rash on trunk, limbs, palms, and soles, which may be pustular, nodular, eczematous, or plaque-like; condylomata lata; patchy alopecia; hepatitis; nephritic syndrome; aseptic meningitis; and cranial neuropathies.

Late latent syphilis is not associated with clinical manifestations but is detected by reactive syphilis serologic tests. Patients with early latent syphilis are to be considered infectious, whereas late latent syphilitics are not infectious. This difference is also important in treatment. During primary and early latent syphilis, the inoculum is larger and the treponemes are reproducing rapidly, making a single dose of a long-acting penicillin adequate. During late latent and tertiary syphilis, the inoculum is low and reproduction is slower, requiring multiple doses of antibiotic.

Tertiary syphilis is characterized by the manifestations of disease; for example, gummatous disease may occur within 1 year of initial infection. Typically, about one third of patients who go untreated will develop tertiary disease, which occurs within 10 to 30 years of the time of acquisition. This stage is characterized by gummatous lesions, cardiovascular syphilis, or neurosyphilis. It is important to note that central nervous system involvement can occur at all stages and is not restricted to tertiary syphilis.

Tertiary syphilis is diagnosed by serologic tests. However, specimens obtained from chancres, condylomata lata, or mucous patches can be examined by dark-field microscopy for the presence of treponemes. Specimens obtained from the oral cavity and rectum must be considered less reliable than specimens from the genitalia because treponemes are present in the former. Two broad serologic tests, nontreponemal for screening and treponemal, are used.

Nontreponemal tests detect the presence of antibody to reagin, a cholesterol-lecithin-cardiolipin antigen that cross-reacts with antibodies found in sera of syphilitics. The two most common tests used are the Venereal Disease Research Laboratory (VDRL) and the rapid plasma reagin (RPR) tests. These tests become positive in 4 to 7 days following the appearance of the chancre. However, the tests may be nonreactive in up to 40% of individuals with primary syphilis. These tests are usually positive in patients with advanced syphilis, such as secondary syphilis. All patients with a reactive VDRL or RPR should have a confirmatory test with a specific treponemal test, such as the fluorescent-treponemal antibody-absorbed test or microhemagglutination-*T. pallidum* test.

Treatment is most successful when patients are administered penicillin. Agents such as ceftriaxone should be efficacious in treating incubating syphilis.

Primary, secondary, and early latent syphilis can be treated with benzathine penicillin, 2.4 million units intramuscularly (1.2 million in each buttock). Penicillin-allergic patients who are not pregnant can be given doxycycline, 100 mg orally bid for 14 days, or tetracycline, 500 mg orally qid for 14 days. Pregnant patients who are allergic to penicillin should be admitted to the hospital, desensitized, and administered penicillin under close observation. Late latent and syphilis of unknown duration should be treated with benzathine penicillin, 7.2 million units, divided into weekly doses of 2.4 million units. The penicillin-allergic patient can be treated with doxycycline, 100 mg orally bid for 28 days, or tetracycline, 500 mg orally qid for 28 days.

Patients with neurosyphilis should be treated with aqueous crystalline penicillin G, 12 to 24 million units IV daily (2 to 4 million units every 4 hours) for 10 to 14 days; procaine penicillin G, 2 to 4 million units intramuscularly daily; or probenecid 500 mg orally qid for 10 to 14 days.

All patients should be followed by serology for VDRL or RPR at 3, 6, and 12 months following the completion of therapy. An appropriate response is defined as a fourfold or greater sustained increase in titer. Patients failing to demonstrate appropriate serologic responses should be retreated with 7.2 million units of benzathine penicillin. These patients should undergo serologic testing at 3, 6, and 12 months after therapy.

Thyrotoxicosis

Ernest L. Mazzaferri, MD, FACP

Thyrotoxicosis develops in about 2 of every 1000 pregnancies. Untreated, it results in spontaneous abortion, premature labor, and fetal death. Thyrotoxicosis is a clinical syndrome that results when tissues are exposed to abnormally high concentrations of *free* (unbound) thyroid hormone. It has several causes (Table 1), but its laboratory hallmark is a suppressed serum thyrotropin (thy-

TABLE 1. Causes of Abnormal Thyroid Activity

Condition	Cause
Thyrotoxicosis during or immediately after pregnancy	Graves' disease
	Autonomously hyperfunctioning nodule ("hot" nodule)
	Multinodular goiter
	Silent thyroiditis
	Thyroid hormone replacement
Hyperthyroidism during and after pregnancy	Hyperemesis gravidarum (uncommon)
	Trophoblastic disease (rare)
	Postpartum thyroiditis (common)
Thyroid-stimulating hormone suppression unrelated to thyrotoxicosis	Nonthyroidal illness
	Pituitary or hypothalamic hypothyroidism
	Recovery from hyperthyroidism
	Drugs (glucocorticoids, dopamine agonists)

roid-stimulating hormone [TI TSH]) concentration, which occurs before serum thyroid hormone levels are perceptibly elevated, a condition termed *subclinical thyrotoxicosis.*

Hyperthyroidism, which is simply the term for an overactive thyroid gland, is caused by several disorders and is characterized by an abnormally high thyroidal radioiodine uptake (RAIU). Although thyrotoxicosis and hyperthyroidism often coexist, there are instances when thyrotoxicosis is not associated with an overactive thyroid gland, as occurs with ingestion of thyroid hormone or thyroiditis. The RAIU normally plays an important role in defining the etiology of thyrotoxicosis, but it is *absolutely contraindicated* during pregnancy because it crosses the placental barrier and may destroy the fetal thyroid gland. The cause of thyrotoxicosis thus may be difficult to identify during pregnancy.

Clinical Syndrome

Goiter does not occur during normal pregnancy and its presence should prompt a search for thyroid disease. Severe thyrotoxicosis is usually easy to recognize. Recognizing mild or moderate thyrotoxicosis during pregnancy is another matter, however. Severely thyrotoxic patients tend to have multiple symptoms, including weight loss with a normal or increased appetite, dyspnea, palpitations, profuse sweating, anxiety, nervousness, emotional lability, and muscle weakness. Some features of thyrotoxicosis occur during normal pregnancy, but the disorder should be suspected when a pregnant woman fails to gain weight normally, develops a goiter, has muscle weakness, or experiences severe dyspnea. The main physical signs of thyrotoxicosis are a flushed appearance, goiter, hyperkinetic behavior, fine tremor of the fingers, upper eyelid retraction, a pulse over 100 beats per minute, muscle weakness, and a forceful precordial pulsation. Diffuse goiter, infiltrative eye signs, and pretibial myxedema are characteristic of Graves' disease.

Thyroid Physiology

An appreciation of the normal changes in thyroid physiology that occur during pregnancy is critical to the interpretation of the laboratory diagnosis of thyrotoxicosis during pregnancy. Basal meta-

bolic rate increases about 20%, causing a degree of heat intolerance. Estrogen stimulates the hepatic production of thyroid-binding globulin—the main transport protein for thyroid hormone—and its serum concentration doubles early in pregnancy (Fig. 1A). Because thyroid-binding globulin binds more thyroxine (T_4) and triiodothyronine (T_3) than normal, the *total* serum T_3 and T_4 concentrations nearly double, rising well above normal (Fig. 1B). However, *free* (unbound) serum thyroid hormone concentrations fall because of the increased binding but remain within the normal range (Fig. 1C). The thyroid gland becomes overactive, showing histologic features of stimulation, and radioiodine uptake increases; however, during this time, serum TSH declines to the lower limits of normal (Fig. 1D). Thyroid stimulation appears to be due to beta-human chorionic gonadotropin (β-hCG): its serum levels are highest when those of TSH are

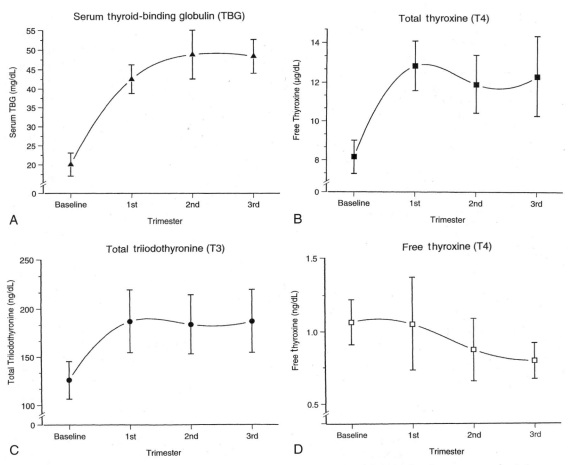

Figure 1. Thyroid function during pregnancy. **A,** Serum thyroid-binding globulin levels; **B,** serum total thyroxine (T_4) concentration; **C,** serum total triiodothyronine (T_3) concentrations; **D,** serum free thyroxine (T_4) concentrations.

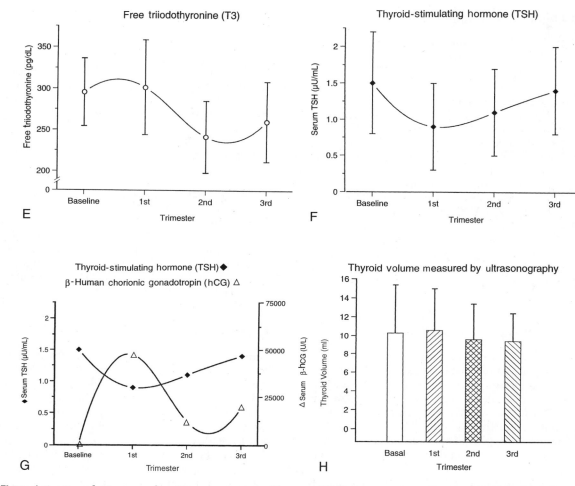

Figure 1 *Continued.* **E,** serum free T_3 concentrations; **F,** serum TSH concentrations; **G,** serum TSH and β-hCG concentrations; **H,** thyroid volume measured by ultrasound. (Data from Berghout A et al: Thyroid function and thyroid size in normal pregnant women living in an iodine replete area. Clin Endocrinol 1994;41:375–379.)

the lowest (Fig. 1E). A serum β-hCG concentration of 50,000 mIU/L is estimated to be equivalent to a TSH level of 35 μU/mL, which accounts for the intense thyroid stimulation caused by trophoblastic tumors.

Maternal Thyroid Function and the Fetus

The fetal thyroid begins functioning after 10 to 12 weeks' gestation and is under pituitary TSH control by about 20 weeks. Prior to 10 weeks, fetal thyroid hormone requirements appear to be met by placental transfer of maternal thyroid hormone (T_3 more than T_4), but its role in early fetal development remains debatable. Because iodide is actively transported across the placenta, the fetus is susceptible to iodine-induced goiter and hypothyroidism when the mother is given pharmacologic amounts of iodine. This may occur with many intravenous, oral, mucosal, or topical iodine compounds, including those used in amniography. Radioiodine and anti-thyroid drugs cross the placenta and have a profound effect on fetal thyroid function. Fetal hypothyroidism may be suspected when a goiter is seen by ultrasonography or when delayed distal femoral or proximal tibial epiphyses are seen by radiography. Hypothyroidism is most reliably identified by measuring serum T_4 and TSH concentrations in fetal blood from percutaneous umbilical cord sampling, which is more reliable than measuring them in amniotic fluid. A fetus can absorb thyroid hormone that has been injected into amniotic fluid, which can be used to treat hypothyroidism and goiter in utero.

Laboratory Diagnosis

Pituitary TSH secretion is exquisitely sensitive to small changes in serum free thyroid hormone concentrations, changing well before alterations in serum thyroid hormone levels are detectable. Thus, measurement of the serum TSH concentration is the most sensitive test for the diagnosis of thyrotoxicosis. It is between about 0.5 and 5.0 μU/mL in euthyroid women and is suppressed to undetectable levels (<0.01 μU/mL) in thyrotoxic women (Table 2) and in other conditions (see Table 1). The rare exceptions to this are thyrotoxicosis with a normal or high serum TSH concentration caused by a TSH-secreting pituitary tumor or pituitary resistance to thyroid hormone. Serum T_4 concentrations above 15 μg/dL suggest thyrotoxicosis and elevated serum free thyroid hormone levels confirm the diagnosis (see Table 2; Fig. 1).

Thyrotoxicosis Classification

There are several important causes of thyrotoxicosis during pregnancy (see Table 1). Therapy is directed to the thyroid gland when thyrotoxicosis (with an undetectable TSH) is associated with hyperthyroidism. When thyrotoxicosis is not due to an overactive thyroid gland, as occurs for example with thyroid hormone ingestion, therapy is directed to the underlying cause of thyrotoxicosis.

Thyrotoxicosis associated with pregnancy may be due to several disorders (see Table 1), some of which are associated with hyperthyroidism (Graves' disease, an autonomously hyperfunctioning nodule, or a multinodular goiter) or it may not be due to hyperthyroidism (silent thyroiditis or postpartum thyroiditis). Normally, the RAIU differentiates thyrotoxicosis with and without hyperthyroidism; however, this test is absolutely contraindicated in pregnancy and one must rely on the clinical presentation to make this differentiation.

Thyrotropin-Induced Hyperthyroidism

This unusual category includes patients with a TSH-secreting pituitary tumor and others with selective pituitary resistance to thyroid hormone. Both have thyrotoxicosis with diffuse thyroid enlargement and *elevated* serum TSH concentrations. This is a rare cause of thyrotoxicosis.

Graves' Disease

Graves' disease is the major cause of thyrotoxicosis in women of childbearing age. It is an autoimmune disorder in which thyroid-stimulating and blocking antibodies react with TSH receptors in the thyroid gland, causing autonomous thyroid dysfunction independent of pituitary TSH. The antibodies are IgG immunoglobulins that cross the placenta to stimulate or block fetal thyroid function, which may cause fetal thyrotoxicosis or goiter even in euthyroid mothers.

TABLE 2. Laboratory Diagnosis of Thyrotoxicosis During Pregnancy

Test	Normal Pregnancy	Hyperthyroidism and Pregnancy*	Hyperemesis Gravidarum	Postpartum Thyroiditis with Hyperthyroidism†
TSH	Normal	Undetectable‡	Normal or Low	Undetectable
TBG	Increased	Increased	Increased	Increased
Total T_4	Increased	Increased	Normal or Increased	Increased
Free T_4‡	Normal	Increased	Normal or Increased	Increased
Total T_3	Increased	Increased	Normal or Increased	Increased
Free T_3‡	Normal	Increased	Normal or Increased	Increased
Thyroid RAIU (contraindicated in pregnancy)	Increased	Increased	Increased	Low

*Tests for overt hyperthyroidism are shown; serum TSH is undetectable and free T_4 and T_3 levels are normal in patients with subclinical thyrotoxicosis.

†In patients with a pituitary tumor or pituitary resistance to TSH, serum TSH levels are inappropriately high.

‡Free thyroid hormone levels may be measured by radioimmunoassay using T_4 or T_3 analogues or may be calculated from the total T_4 and a test that estimates serum hormone binding (such as the T_3 resin uptake) termed the free T_4 index (a similar calculation can be made for free T_3).

RAIU = radioiodine uptake; T_3 = triiodothyronine; T_4 = thyroxine; TSH = thyroid-stimulating hormone.

The main features of Graves' disease are diffuse goiter, infiltrative ophthalmopathy, and infiltrative dermopathy (pretibial myxedema). Its peak occurrence is in middle-aged women, in whom it has an insidious onset. Thyrotoxicosis is the most common manifestation. It is caused by a diffuse, non-tender, firm goiter that is small to medium in size. Infiltrative ophthalmopathy occurs at some time in nearly half the patients but is usually mild. More advanced stages are characterized by proptosis, periorbital edema, and extraocular muscle dysfunction. Sometimes, however, ophthalmopathy is the only manifestation of the disorder.

Graves' disease is recognized by its clinically distinct features. During pregnancy it is usually verified by detecting thyroid-simulating immunoglobulin or thyrotropin-binding inhibiting immunoglobulin in the mother's blood. High titers of these maternal antibodies increase the likelihood of neonatal thyrotoxicosis.

Graves' disease typically undergoes spontaneous exacerbation and remission, usually remitting during pregnancy and exacerbating in the postpartum period, perhaps as the result of changes in the maternal immune system that occur during pregnancy. Nonetheless, Graves' disease is the most likely cause of thyrotoxicosis during pregnancy.

Trophoblastic Tumors

Trophoblastic disease affects about 1 in 1500 pregnancies and causes mild hyperthyroidism with a small goiter. High serum β-hCG concentrations stimulates the thyroid gland. Although hCG has only a small fraction of the biologic activity of TSH, patients with trophoblastic tumors have serum hCG concentrations from 300 to 2000 mIU/L by 10 to 12 weeks' gestation, which is well within the range to stimulate thyroid function. Thyroid dysfunction ranges from minimal hyperthyroxinemia without clinically obvious thyrotoxicosis to striking hyperthyroidism with severe thyrotoxicosis. Removal of the source of β-hCG results in quick amelioration of the syndrome.

Multinodular Goiter

Long-standing colloid goiters tend to develop autonomously hyperfunctioning nodules that eventually cause thyrotoxicosis. Although predominantly a disorder of older women, it may occur during the childbearing years. The thyroid contains multiple palpable nodules that concentrate most or all of the ^{123}I on scan. However, since radioactive iodine cannot be used during pregnancy, a presumptive diagnosis of multinodular goiter can be verified by thyroid ultrasonography. Thyrotoxicosis can be managed by antithyroid drugs during pregnancy but, unlike Graves' disease, does not undergo spontaneous remission and ablation of the goiter with ^{131}I or surgery is eventually necessary.

Toxic Adenoma (Autonomously Hyperfunctioning Thyroid Nodule)

The autonomously hyperfunctioning ("hot") nodule is usually an isolated benign follicular adenoma or adenomatoid nodule that secretes thyroid hormone independent of TSH. It may predominantly secrete T_3. Thyrotoxicosis is usually caused by nodules larger than 3 or 4 cm that concentrate all or most of the ^{123}I on scan, leaving the surrounding thyroid tissue with little or no ^{123}I uptake. Since radioiodine cannot be used during pregnancy, a presumptive diagnosis can be made by palpating a large single nodule in a thyroid gland that is otherwise barely palpable and verifying this observation by thyroid ultrasonography. The thyrotoxicosis is usually mild, but does not remit spontaneously unless the nodule undergoes infarction, which requires no treatment. Infarction causes transient neck pain radiating to the jaw and ear, and nodular tenderness. In pregnant women, the thyrotoxicosis can be controlled by anti-thyroid drugs, but ablation of the nodule is eventually necessary.

Subacute Thyroiditis

There are two distinct forms of thyroid inflammation with similar clinical courses. One is a painful and somewhat uncommon form of viral thyroiditis usually termed de Quervain's or pseudogranulomatous thyroiditis. The other is painless thyroiditis, a variant of Hashimoto's disease that has a particularly high prevalence during the postpartum period.

Painful (de Quervain's) thyroiditis is attributed to a viral infection, although different viruses have been found in carefully studied patients. It usually begins with malaise, myalgia, fatigue, and fever, often with an upper respiratory infection. The fever may be as high as 40°C (104°F), and the systemic manifestations may be severe. The thyroid becomes exquisitely tender, with pain radiating to one or both ears or the jaw. The thyrotoxicosis is typically mild, requiring no treatment, and is usually associated with slight to moderate enlargement of one or both thyroid lobes, or a discrete nodule may develop in the thyroid gland. The problem tends to last for 2 to 5 months and classically goes through three distinct phases: thyrotoxicosis, hypothyroidism, and finally sustained normal thyroid function.

During the initial thyrotoxic phase, which generally lasts for less than 1 month, the painfully inflamed thyroid gland leaks its hormonal contents. The sedimentation rate is often above 100 mm/hr, but serum thyroid antibodies are usually not present. This is followed by a period of transient hypothyroidism that may last for months. Although a full recovery usually ensues, about 20% of patients experience recurrences.

Painless or silent thyroiditis is a variant of Hashimoto's disease with a clinical course similar to that of painful subacute thyroiditis. It accounts for 15% to 20% of all cases of thyrotoxicosis, including the large number of cases that occur in the postpartum period. The thyroid gland is painless and in about half the patients is diffusely enlarged, yielding lymphocytes on fine-needle aspiration biopsy. There are no prodromal symptoms, fever, or thyroid pain, and the sedimentation rate is not high. Most patients have detectable antiperoxidase antibodies detectable by radioimmunoassay and some develop thyroid nodularity. Thyroid function evolves in the same way as it does in painful subacute thyroiditis, except up to half the patients develop goiter, and persistent hypothyroidism is more common, especially in those with goiter.

Postpartum thyroiditis is silent thyroiditis that affects about 5% of pregnant women during the first year after parturition and occurs at an even greater frequency in type 1 diabetic patients. Thyroid antibodies are present in over 75% of the patients. Thyrotoxicosis occurs a few months after delivery, lasts less than 2 months, and is distinguished from relapsing Graves' disease by a low RAIU. Hypothyroidism develops about 3 to 6 months after delivery, occasionally without clinically apparent preceding thyrotoxicosis. The symptoms are typically quite mild, with fatigue being most prominent in both phases; however, painless goiter is almost always present. Postpartum depression is more common in women with postpartum thyroiditis. Although most patients are euthyroid within 1 year after parturition, some develop permanent hypothyroidism.

Thyroid Hormone Ingestion

Thyroid hormone taken either as medicine or in food can cause thyrotoxicosis. Most often this is due to thyroid hormone taken as prescribed, a condition termed *iatrogenic thyrotoxicosis.* It is typically asymptomatic but may cause osteoporosis or atrial fibrillation in postmenopausal women who have had subclinical thyrotoxicosis for many years. Therefore, it should be avoided.

Rarely, thyroid hormone is ingested in food, which can cause severe thyrotoxicosis and even death. *Factitious thyrotoxicosis* is a less common problem caused by surreptitious thyroid hormone ingestion. Thyrotoxicosis undergoes wide and often abrupt changes in severity. Serum T_4 and T_3 are elevated if levothyroxine is ingested, but only serum T_3 is high if liothyronine sodium (triiodothyronine) is ingested. The diagnosis is suspected in a patient with easy access to thyroid hormone, such as a health care provider who has thyrotoxicosis *without* a palpable goiter. The serum thyroglobulin is undetectable. Patients with this disorder deserve careful psychiatric treatment.

Treatment of Thyrotoxicosis During Pregnancy

Anti-Thyroid Drugs. Anti-thyroid drugs, either propylthiouracil or methimazole, are the treatment drugs of choice during pregnancy. They should be administered in the lowest possible dose (<300 mg/day of propylthiouracil or <20 mg/day of methimazole) that keeps the mother's serum free T_4 concentrations in the upper limit of normal, because both drugs cross the placenta and can cause goiter and fetal hypothyroidism. After the thyrotoxicosis is controlled, the dose should be lowered to 50 to 100 mg of propylthiouracil or 5 to 10 mg of methimazole daily. Propylthiouracil is the drug of choice: less of it crosses the placenta, only small amounts appear in mother's milk, and it does not affect thyroid function of the breast-feeding infant. However, methimazole may also be used during pregnancy or breast feeding. *Aplasia cutis congenita*—a rare congenital absence of skin that usually involves the scalp—is associated with methimazole but not propylthiouracil therapy during pregnancy.

Serious side effects of the anti-thyroid drugs (Table 3) occur in about 3 of every 1000 patients, regardless of which drug is given; although low doses of methimazole (<30 mg/day) may be safer in regard to agranulocytosis than either propylthiouracil or higher doses of methimazole. Agranulocytosis is an idiosyncratic reaction that is more common during the first several months of therapy and in patients older than 40 years. Patients should be instructed to stop the drug

TABLE 3. Side Effects of Anti-Thyroid Drugs

Serious and rare complications°
  Agranulocytosis
  Hepatitis (propylthiouracil)
  Cholestatic jaundice (methimazole and
    propylthiouracil)
  Aplastic anemia
  Thrombocytopenia
  Lupus-like vasculitis
Minor complications
  Fever
  Pruritus
  Urticaria
  Arthralgia
  Gastrointestinal distress
  Hypoglycemia due to insulin antibodies
  Metallic taste

°Serious side effects that require immediate cessation of anti-thyroid drug therapy.

and contact a physician immediately if sore throat or fever occurs. Although it develops so rapidly that routine blood counts are often not helpful, one study found this usually detected agranulocytosis before symptoms occurred. Accordingly, it may be useful to do routine blood counts during the first 3 months of therapy. Patients with neutropenia usually recover within 2 to 3 weeks after the drug is stopped, but some die despite appropriate therapy. Therapy with recombinant human granulocyte colony-stimulating factor shortens the recovery time. This and the other serious complications (see Table 3) are an absolute contraindication to further therapy with anti-thyroid drugs.

About half the women with Graves' disease have a recurrence of thyrotoxicosis after delivery.

β-Adrenergic Blocking Drugs. The adrenergic manifestations of thyrotoxicosis such as tachycardia and tremor, muscle weakness, and other symptoms are controlled by β-blockers. Propranolol LA 80 mg every 12 hours or atenolol 50 to 100 mg daily will usually maintain the maternal heart rate around 80 beats per minute. While the use of β-blockers is generally considered to be safe during pregnancy, intrauterine growth retardation, impaired response to anoxic stress, postnatal bradycardia, and hypoglycemia can occur.

Iodides. Used briefly in preparation for thyroidectomy or in the treatment of thyroid storm, iodides may be safe, but maternal exposure to pharmacologic doses for more than a few weeks

may cause fetal hypothyroidism and goiter, which in the most extreme cases result in tracheal obstruction.

Surgery for Hyperthyroidism. Thyroidectomy is reserved for patients who cannot take anti-thyroid drugs or when compliance is a problem. Surgery is usually performed during the second trimester, but in an urgent situation can be done earlier when the risk of spontaneous abortion is higher. Thyrotoxicosis must be controlled before surgery, which is customarily done with anti-thyroid drugs and β-blockers. When anti-thyroid drugs are contraindicated, β-blockers can be given alone preoperatively. Postoperative hypocalcemia can precipitate premature delivery.

Thyroid Storm

This is a rare, life-threatening complication of thyrotoxicosis in which the signs and symptoms of thyrotoxicosis are greatly intensified. The patient often experiences vomiting and diarrhea, jaundice, manic behavior, and marked tachycardia. Rarely, older patients may have an apathetic affect. Within hours, fever to 41.1°C (106°F), prostration, lethargy, dehydration, and striking tachycardia develop. Heart failure, usually with atrial fibrillation, is typically present. Within a day or two, cardiovascular collapse and death occurs in the untreated patient.

The patient usually requires admission to an intensive care unit where treatment is immediately started without laboratory confirmation of the diagnosis, because of the serious nature and rapid progression of this complication. Serum T_4 and T_3 concentrations are usually very high, and TSH is suppressed. The patient should be carefully monitored while appropriate therapy is started and consultation with an endocrinologist is obtained. Patients should be given fluids, and the fever should be treated with antipyretic drugs but not aspirin, which raises free thyroid hormone levels. Specific therapy should be directed to the precipitating cause of the thyroid storm. About half the patients have a serious infection that has precipitated the problem.

Propylthiouracil has a theoretical advantage over methimazole because it also blocks peripheral tissue conversion of T_4 to T_3. Up to 1200 mg/day of propylthiouracil is given orally or by nasogastric tube in divided doses every 4 hours, or methimazole 120 mg daily is given in divided doses. Organic iodine (Lugol's solution, eight drops every 6 hours) or the contrast compounds ipodate (Oragrafin) or iopanoic acid (Telepaque) are given to block the release of thyroid hormone and to block peripheral conversion of T_4 to T_3. Ipodate, 3 g orally, is given on a daily basis. These drugs may be given intravenously and should be administered an hour or two after propylthiouracil or methimazole has been given. Hydrocortisone or dexamethasone are given in large doses to block peripheral conversion of T_4 to T_3. A β-adrenergic blocking drug is usually given to control the heart rate; however, β-blockers must be used judiciously and under careful cardiovascular monitoring. Propranolol is usually given orally at a dose of 60 to 120 mg every 6 hours, or 1 mg is given intravenously while the patient's cardiac rhythm and cardiac status are carefully monitored. Propranolol is contraindicated in patients with asthma and must be used cautiously in diabetic patients because it obscures the symptoms of hypoglycemia. Other selective $β_1$-adrenergic blocking drugs or short-acting intravenous β-blockers may be used.

The mortality rate of thyroid storm remains about 10% and is closely related to the underlying precipitating event and the patient's age.

Urinary Incontinence

W. Glenn Hurt, MD

Every patient with primary, persistent, or recurrent urinary incontinence deserves an in-depth evaluation to determine the cause of and the best way to manage the disorder. Physicians must classify the disorder according to its type (Table 1) to determine its cause. This will serve as the basis for managing the problem. For example, some causes of urinary incontinence are more likely to respond to nonsurgical therapy than to surgical therapy. When surgical therapy is indicated, the first surgical procedure is the one that is most likely to succeed, and with fewest complications. No woman with urinary incontinence should resort to the long-term use of pro-

TABLE 1. Types of Urinary Incontinence

> Stress incontinence
> Urge incontinence
> Overflow incontinence
> Functional incontinence
> Other types of incontinence

tective pads or diapers until she has had a diagnostic evaluation and therapy.

Clinical Evaluation

History

An incisive urogynecologic history is used to document the patient's complaint of urinary incontinence, its duration, and the degree to which it interferes with her life. For completeness, the history should be supplemented with a standardized questionnaire. It is important to realize, however, that the history alone cannot be used to precisely diagnose the types and causes of a patient's urinary incontinence.

Urinary Diary

A urinary diary provides important pretreatment information on fluid intake, voiding frequency, and incontinence episodes. It is most helpful if the patient records these activities around the clock for a minimum of 3, and preferably 7, consecutive days while she goes about her daily routine. A urinary diary can be repeated to assess the results of nonsurgical or surgical therapy.

Physical Examination

The physical examination should be complete. It must focus on the patient's general health and functional status, her hormonal status, the condition of her respiratory system, any evidence of a neurologic disorder, and abdominal and pelvic findings.

Demonstration of Incontinence

A trained observer should document the individual's urinary leakage and the characteristics of that leakage. Attempts to demonstrate urinary incontinence are referred to as stress testing, which is performed when the patient has at least 250 mL of urine or an appropriate sterile fluid in the bladder. She is asked to perform Valsalva's maneuvers (eg, coughing and bearing down) and gravitational maneuvers (eg, heel bouncing) to produce sudden increases in intra-abdominal pressure that might result in urinary leakage. If leakage is not demonstrated in the lithotomy position, the patient should be tested in the erect position.

The involuntary loss of a spurt of urine from an anatomically and neurologically intact lower urinary tract, coincident with a sudden increase in intra-abdominal pressure, such as may result from a Valsalva effort (eg, coughing), is documentary evidence of *stress incontinence*. On the other hand, the involuntary loss of a stream of urine from an anatomically and neurologically intact lower urinary tract, whether spontaneous or as a result of a Valsalva effort, is evidence of an *unstable bladder* (detrusor instability) until proven otherwise. When a patient shows evidence of both stress incontinence and incontinence due to an unstable bladder, she is referred to as having *mixed incontinence*.

If a patient suffers from urinary incontinence, yet the involuntary loss of urine cannot be demonstrated, she is a candidate for further urodynamic investigation. Even though the patient's history and other findings are compatible with a diagnosis of stress incontinence, surgery is not recommended unless the characteristic urinary leakage of stress incontinence is clinically demonstrable.

Uroflowmetry

Uroflowmetry may be performed by having the patient void into a toilet that has a commode insert as a urine collection container and by using a stopwatch to measure the time from the onset to the completion of micturition. Normally, the mean flow rate (volume/time) should exceed 10 mL/second. Voided volumes of less than 200 mL often give unreliable results; when this occurs, uroflowmetry should be repeated. Mean flow rates of less than 10 mL/second may indicate bladder outlet obstruction or detrusor dysfunction and require further urodynamic evaluation.

Urinary Residual

Urethral catheterization is performed after the patient voids to determine the urinary residual. Measurement of the postvoid urinary residual is an important method of determining the efficiency of the bladder in emptying itself. Repeated urinary residuals in excess of 100 mL should be considered abnormal, even in patients with significant pelvic organ prolapse. Large urinary residuals indicate the presence of urethral or bladder outlet obstruction or a neurologic disorder and require further investigation. If surgery on the lower urinary tract is indicated, pre-operative large urinary residuals may predict postoperative voiding dysfunction.

Infection Screen

The catheterized urinary residual should be tested for infection. When urine testing strips show the presence of leukocyte esterase or nitrites, immediate treatment and bacterial cultures are indicated. With rare exception, further invasive diagnostic testing or operative procedures are contraindicated until the urine is proven to be sterile by subsequent urine culture.

Urethral Mobility

Urethral mobility can be documented by performing a "Q-tip" test. With the patient in the lithotomy position, the lubricated cotton swab of a Q-tip is placed transurethrally until it is located just within the urethrovesical junction. Measurements are taken of the arc through which the distal end of the Q-tip moves with the patient at rest and when she is performing a maximum Valsalva effort. Patients with limited excursion of the distal end of the Q-tip (<25 degrees) are less likely to have anatomic stress incontinence and, based on this finding, require further investigation.

Screening Cystometry

A balloon (14F or 16F Foley) catheter, the barrel of an irrigation syringe, and sterile water or normal saline can be used to determine gross bladder capacity and neurologic control in the majority of patients whose history and examination indicate that they have uncomplicated stress incontinence and have had no prior continence surgery. The catheter is inserted transurethrally into the bladder and the balloon is inflated. The patient is asked to assume the erect position, and the barrel of the irrigation syringe is connected to the catheter. With the barrel of the syringe held at the level of the symphysis pubis, it is slowly filled with sterile water or normal saline. The patient is asked to tell the observer when she feels the first urge to void (normally 150 to 200 mL) and when she feels her bladder has reached its capacity (normally 400 to 600 mL). There should be no evidence of spontaneous or provoked detrusor contractions as might be suggested by the bladder not readily accepting the fluid or by the fluid backing up in the barrel of the irrigation syringe. When the patient's first urge to void or her bladder capacity is outside of the normal ranges or if her bladder does not readily accept the fluid, this is taken as evidence of abnormal neuromuscular control or capacity and requires further urodynamic investigations (eg, multichannel urethrocystometry).

I prefer a complete urodynamic investigation of women over 60 years of age; those with urinary urgency, frequency, nocturia, and enuresis; those who complain of urinary incontinence but whose stress test does not document stress urinary incontinence; those with low urine flow rates, high urinary residuals, or urinary retention; those with limited urethral mobility; those with an unusual sense of urgency or evidence of an unstable bladder; and those who have been unsuccessful in having their incontinence corrected by surgery. In these women, multichannel subtracted urethrocystometry, leak point pressures, urethrocystoscopy, radiologic and ultrasonographic imaging, videourodynamics, and consultation are often of benefit.

Treatment

Stress incontinence is characterized by the involuntary loss of a spurt of urine from the external urethral meatus coincident with an increase in intra-abdominal pressure, in the absence of a detrusor contraction or overdistension of the bladder. Stress incontinence may be caused by an anatomic factor or by intrinsic urethral sphincter deficiency. The anatomic origin of most cases of stress incontinence is damage to tissues that normally support the proximal urethra and bladder neck and thus determine the anatomic urethrovesical relationships. Damage to the supporting tissues usually results in hypermobility of the urethrovesical junction with its downward displacement during stress. Intrinsic urethral sphincter deficiency may be the result of congenital sphincter weakness (eg, myelomeningocele) or acquired sphincter damage (eg, surgical trauma, radiation). In such cases, the anatomic urethrovesical relationships may be reasonable, but the urethra may be serving as no more than a functionless drainpipe without sphincteric function.

Anatomic stress urinary incontinence may be managed by nonsurgical or surgical therapy. Nonsurgical therapy is most effective in premenopausal women who have lesser grades of urinary incontinence. Their condition may be improved or cured by performing pelvic muscle exercises (Kegel's exercises, retaining vaginal cones), by electrical stimulation of the pelvic muscles, or by using a vaginal tampon or pessary as a urethral occlusive device. Hypoestrogenic women are more likely to respond to these forms of nonsurgical therapy if given long-term estrogen replacement therapy (oral, vaginal, or both), provided there is no contraindication to its use. Progesterone therapy should be added if the patient has a uterus.

The goals of surgical therapy for anatomic stress incontinence are (1) retropubic elevation and stabilization of the urethrovesical junction; (2) preservation of posterior rotational descent of the trigone and base of the bladder to provide urethral compression; (3) preservation of the compressibility and pliability of the urethra; and (4) protection of the integrity of the urethral sphincter mechanism. These goals are best accomplished by performing an abdominal retropubic (Marshall-Marchetti-Krantz or Burch type) urethropexy/colposuspension procedure if there is mobility of the urethrovesical junction. In the surgical literature, these procedures are recognized as the "gold standard" for the treatment of primary, persistent, and recurrent cases of pure anatomic stress incontinence. They are relatively easy to learn and to perform, and, for most surgeons, they are associated with the least number of complications and the best long-term rate of cure. The Burch procedure has the advantage of correcting a minor coexistent cystourethrocele, whereas the Marshall-Marchetti-Krantz procedure may not. The development of an enterocele is an infrequent (10–15%) but recognized potential complication of all urethropexy/colposuspension procedures. Therefore, when the peritoneal cavity is entered as a part of the operative procedure, it is recommended that a prophylactic obliteration of the cul-de-sac (Moschcowitz or Halban type) be performed. When performing an abdominal retropubic urethropexy/colposuspension, the surgeon may still find it is necessary to operate vaginally to repair a coexisting rectocele.

Although many surgeons use vaginal "needle" procedures (Pereyra or Raz type) to treat most cases of anatomic stress incontinence, I use them primarily in women who have significant degrees of pelvic organ prolapse. In these cases, a needle procedure will enable the surgeon to perform the entire combination of procedures vaginally, except for the placement and typing of the suspending sutures. Needle procedures do not appear to have as good a long-term cure rate as do retropubic urethropexy/colposuspension procedures. Needle procedures may contribute to the development of postoperative apical vaginal support defects.

Complications of surgical therapy may be classified as immediate (hemorrhage, infection, urinary retention, nerve and organ injury) and delayed (urgency and frequency of urination, voiding dysfunction, unstable bladder, persistent or recurrent incontinence, pelvic organ prolapse). However, a properly selected and performed continence procedure can be expected to provide a long-term (>10 years) cure in over 90% of cases of pure anatomic stress incontinence.

I use an anterior colporrhaphy or a paravaginal repair to correct a cystourethrocele or cystocele. These procedures may correct stress incontinence if it is due to this specific anatomic defect; however, they are usually not used to treat persistent or recurrent postoperative stress incontinence.

Stress incontinence due to intrinsic urethral sphincter deficiency does not respond well to nonsurgical therapy, and the response to many surgical procedures is often unsatisfactory. If there is coexistent hypermobility of the urethrovesical junction, an abdominal retropubic urethropexy/colposuspension may successfully restore continence. If there is little or no hypermobility of the urethrovesical junction, periurethral bulk injections of bovine collagen implant, a suburethral sling procedure, or an artificial urinary sphincter might be preferable.

Women with mixed urinary incontinence combining stress incontinence and unstable bladders (detrusor instability) incontinence should have their bladders treated with a maximum nonsurgical effort prior to having surgery. In a patient with mixed incontinence due to anatomic causes and an unstable bladder (detrusor instability), it is important to know to what extent pharmacologic therapy will control that component of their incontinence caused by the unstable bladder, in case it persists postoperatively and requires pharmacologic therapy.

Urge incontinence is characterized by the involuntary loss of urine in the presence of an abrupt and strong desire to void (urgency). It is usually associated with urodynamic evidence of uninhibited detrusor contractions (detrusor overactivity). It may be caused by an irritant or associated with a neurologic disorder, or it may be idiopathic. If the condition is caused by an irritant (infection, stones, neoplasm, or a foreign body) and the source of the irritation is eliminated, it is likely that the urge incontinence will disappear. Therefore it is important to prove that there is no urinary tract infection prior to performing diagnostic urodynamic or endoscopic procedures.

If a neurologic disorder (eg, stroke) is the cause of urge incontinence, its accompanying involuntary detrusor contraction is referred to as detrusor hyperreflexia. Some patients with multiple sclerosis and suprasacral spinal cord lesions will also have urodynamically proven external sphincter dyssynergia. Women with neurologic bladders are best managed by specialists trained in caring for patient who are neurologically impaired.

Idiopathic urge incontinence, which is the result of an unstable bladder contraction (detrusor instability), by definition, has no detectable irritative or neurologic cause and accounts for 10% to 15% of cases of female urinary incontinence. Its prevalence increases with age and it is the most common cause of urinary incontinence in older women. Women with unstable bladders are best managed by nonsurgical therapy consisting of bladder retraining drills, pharmacologic therapy (eg, parasympatholytics), biofeedback protocols, and electrical stimulation of the pelvic muscles. Only as a last resort should the surgeon consider subvesical nerve resections, sacral nerve root resections, bladder augmentation by clam cystoplasty, or urinary diversion for intractable incontinence due to an unstable bladder.

Overflow incontinence is caused by overdistension of the bladder due to urethral or bladder outlet obstruction, a hypocontractile or acontractile detrusor, or some idiopathic cause. In women, it is most often a surgical complication of a continence procedure that obstructs the urethrovesical junction or of a radical surgical procedure that denervates the bladder; the result of significant degrees of pelvic organ prolapse (ie, cystocele, procidentia, or vaginal vault prolapse); a possible consequence of drug therapy; or the result of a neurologic disorder (eg, diabetes mellitus). Following continence procedures and radical pelvic surgery, overdistension of the bladder is best prevented by indwelling suprapubic or transurethral bladder catheter drainage. Chronic cases of overflow incontinence are best managed by clean intermittent self-catheterization.

Functional incontinence is caused by factors unrelated to the lower urinary tract that may be the result of chronic impairments of physical or cognitive functions. Frequently leakage of this description results from patients' inability to toilet themselves. The condition is best managed by improving the patient's functional status, adjusting fluid intake, controlling the use of certain types of medications, and reducing environmental barriers to toileting.

Other forms of urinary incontinence are managed according to their causes. Among the causes are urethral diverticula, genitourinary fistulas, and ectopic ureters. For each of these causes there are one or more operative procedures that can be expected to cure the condition. The management of other rare forms of urinary incontinence is beyond the scope of this chapter.

The reader is encouraged to obtain publications from the U.S. Department of Health and Human Services' Agency for Health Care Policy and Research entitled *Clinical Practice Guideline: Urinary Incontinence in Adults* (AHCPR 92–0038) and the reference guide for clinicians entitled *Managing Acute and Chronic Urinary Incontinence, No. 2, 1996 Update* (AHCPR 96–0686). To order single copies, call the AHCPR Publications Clearinghouse at 800–358–9295, or write to AHCPR Publications Clearinghouse, P.O. Box 8547, Silver Spring, MD 20907. These publications were used as the basis for much of the terminology in this chapter.

Urinary Tract Infections

Sebastian Faro, MD, PhD

Urinary tract infection (UTI) is one of the most common bacterial infections, with an estimated 8 million ambulatory cases and 1.5 million hospital cases per year in the United States. It is estimated that there are approximately 100,000 cases of pyelonephritis per year. The significance of UTI is reflected in the costs associated not only with direct morbidity but also with the time lost from work and with physician, hospital, and treatment charges. It should be pointed out that UTI is the most common cause of bacteremia; this must also be factored into the economics of the cost of UTIs.

The majority of UTIs are caused by bacteria ascending through the urethra to the bladder. The bacteria involved are derived from microorganisms colonizing the periurethral area. Once bacteria colonize or infect the bladder, they can ascend via the ureters to the kidney, resulting in pyelonephritis. A small number of UTIs may occur via hematogenous dissemination, resulting in bilateral kidney infection. Hematogenously derived kidney infection is usually caused by *Staphylococcus aureus*, *Salmonella* spp., or *Candida* spp.

UTIs can be classified as uncomplicated (usually occurring in healthy individuals) or complicated. The latter occur in individuals with an abnormal urinary tract, such as those with anatomical irregularities, functional defects, or the presence of a foreign body, or in individuals who are highly susceptible to infection. *Escherichia coli* accounts for approximately 80% of uncomplicated UTIs. The remainder, 20%, are commonly caused by *Proteus mirabilis*, *Klebsiella pneumoniae*, and, in younger women, *Staphylococcus saprophyticus*. Complicated UTIs are caused by a broader spectrum of microorganisms.

UTIs are divided into lower urinary tract infections (urethritis and cystitis) and upper urinary tract infections (pyelonephritis). The bladder may also be colonized by bacteria and the individual can be completely asymptomatic. Asymptomatic bacteriuria is found in approximately 5% of school-aged females, 1% to 3% of young nonpregnant women, and 20% to 50% of elderly women. Asymptomatic bacteriuria is found in 2% to 10% of pregnant women, and the incidence rises as the individual's parity increases. It has also been found that women who have had asymptomatic bacteriuria in childhood are more likely to experience this syndrome when pregnant. Asymptomatic bacteriuria in pregnancy, left untreated, is associated with a 25% to 50% risk of pyelonephritis. The presence of asymptomatic bacteriuria has also been linked to a higher incidence of premature delivery and low birth weight. A meta-analysis of the published data also showed that if the condition is treated appropriately, the incidence of low birth weight infants is significantly reduced. Thus, all pregnant patients should be screened for asymptomatic bacteriuria during the first prenatal visit, and, if it is present, the patient should be treated with an antibiotic for 10 days. The antibiotic should have a limited distribution that is restricted to the urinary tract, such as nitrofurantoin, 100 mg orally, twice daily. A reculture should be done 1 week after the patient completes therapy to determine whether eradication of the bacteria has occurred. Patients with a negative culture result should be screened in each trimester.

Asymptomatic bacteriuria is defined as the presence of the same bacterium in a concentration of 10^5 or more bacteria per milliliter of urine (commonly referred to as colony forming units, CFU/mL), obtained as a clean catch specimen on two occasions at least 1 week apart. It is important when obtaining a clean catch urine specimen that vaginal discharge be kept out of the specimen. Therefore, the patient's vagina should be examined, and, if there is a significant amount of vaginal discharge, a tampon can be inserted immediately prior to cleansing the vestibule and periurethral area. Following collection of the urine specimen, the tampon should be removed.

Although it has been shown that no significant association exists between the presence of asymptomatic bacteriuria in the elderly patient and mortality, the question of the significance of asymptomatic bacteriuria and morbidity following pelvic surgery has not been addressed. During pelvic surgery, the bladder is repeatedly manipulated, as with catheterization, and mobilized to some degree, which may result in bacteria gaining entrance to the vascular system. Once in the vascular system, bacteremia and bacterial dissemination can occur and may result in metastatic infection, such as pneumonia or renal infection. Therefore, it may be prudent to screen the patient for bacteriuria prior to surgery.

Approximately 20% of all women will experience at least one UTI in their lifetime. Acute UTI is often associated with frequency of urination, dysuria, pyuria, and bacteriuria. The diagnosis of pyuria requires, at least, that the urine be examined microscopically. This is not routinely performed in the office, if at all, however, which has led to the development of rapid tests that can be performed in the office and yield results within minutes, thereby avoiding delay in treatment of the patient.

The white blood cell esterase test, a dipstick test, is performed, in which one end of the dipstick is impregnated with indoxyl carboxylic acid ester and diazonium salt, which, when immersed in urine containing at least 10 white blood cells per high power microscopic field or more than 10^5 bacteria per milliliter of urine, will turn the impregnated end of the dipstick an indigo blue color. A false-positive test result can occur when *Trichomonas vaginalis* is present, the patient is on nitrofurantoin or gentamicin, or there is a high concentration of albumin, detergents, and preservatives. False-negative results occur when the white blood cell count is less than 10 cells per high power field or if the urine specific gravity is high.

The nitrite test is dependent on the fact that most UTIs are caused by one of the Enterobacteriaceae, such as *E. coli*, which are capable of reducing nitrates to nitrite. Nitrates are obtained from dietary sources that are converted by these bacteria to nitrite. Streptococci, staphylococci, enterococci, *Acinetobacter* spp., and other non-fermenting organisms are not capable of converting nitrates to nitrite. In this test, the nitrite reacts with *p*-arsanilic acid to form 1,2,3,4-tetrahydro-benzo-(h)quinolin-3-ol, which is pink in color. This reaction forms the basis of this test and therefore can detect the presence of Enterobacteriaceae. The test is more likely to be positive when a first morning specimen is utilized. Urine that has been in the bladder for less than 6 hours has not allowed the bacteria sufficient time to metabolize nitrate to nitrite. Other factors that may yield a false-negative test result are a vegetable-free diet; use of diuretics, which creates a washout phenomenon, not allowing enough time for the bacteria to achieve a significant inoculum; high concentrations of urobilinogen; a pH less than 6; and high daily intake of vitamin C. The presence of hematuria may yield a false-positive result.

Another test, which has not enjoyed popularity but may prove to be useful in the office, is the catalase test. Catalase is an enzyme that is typically produced by Enterobacteriaceae but not found in gram-positive organisms such as streptococci, enterococci, and *Aerococcus* spp. The test is performed by mixing 2 mL of urine with reagent powder and adding 4 drops of 10% hydrogen peroxide. Within 2 minutes, a layer of foam will appear on the surface of the urine, indicating a positive result. The test is available commercially. False-positive results occur when a significant number of somatic cells are present. This raises an important point: when collecting a urine specimen, especially a clean catch specimen, the patient should be examined for vaginal discharge in terms of quantity as well as quality. If there is a significant amount of discharge present and it is highly likely that this discharge will contaminate the urine specimen, the patient should insert a tampon in the vagina prior to collecting the urine specimen. The tampon should be removed after the specimen has been collected.

Utilization of a rapid urine screening test has become more popular, especially since the current recommendation is to initiate treatment for uncomplicated cystitis without obtaining a urine specimen for culture. The key to treatment is the presence of pyuria, but most obstetricians and gynecologists do not perform a microscopic examination of urine. Therefore, the recommendation to treat empirically has evolved because uncomplicated cystitis is usually caused by relatively few bacteria, usually one of the Enterobacteriaceae, predominantly *E. coli*. These bacteria are usually sensitive to the antibiotics usually employed to treat uncomplicated cystitis. Three-day treatment regimens have proven to be as successful as longer treatment regimens.

Urine culture should be performed for the following:

1. Failed empiric therapy
2. Hospitalized patients who develop sepsis
3. Acutely ill patients
4. Hospitalized patients who subsequently develop symptoms and signs of a UTI
5. A specimen that is not appropriate for screening
6. Short-course therapy not likely to be successful because of:
   a. complicated UTI
   b. suspected pyelonephritis
   c. pregnancy
   d. immunosuppression
   e. neutropenia
   f. presence of fever and a Foley catheter
   g. fever following manipulation of the genitourinary tract

If more than one organism is present and it is a valid specimen, then one organism should be dominant. If two organisms are present and they are both contributing to the patient's UTI, they should both be present in a concentration of more than 10^3 CFU/mL of urine. If there are more than two different genera present, then the dominant genus should be present in a concentration of more than 10^4 CFU/mL of urine. If all genera are present at this concentration or greater, then all organisms should be considered significant.

Treatment of UTI depends on the stage of disease: lower UTI, asymptomatic or symptomatic (cystitis); or upper UTI, pyelonephritis. In addition, treatment regimens must be tailored to the patient's medical status, whether a pregnancy exists, and the trimester of pregnancy.

The treatment of acute uncomplicated cystitis in the nonpregnant patient can be adequately accomplished by administering a 3-day course of antibiotic, such as nitrofurantoin, trimethoprim, or trimethoprim-sulfamethoxazole. Nitrofurantoin is a suitable choice, especially for the postoperative patient in whom a clear-cut diagnosis of cystitis cannot be differentiated from an early pelvic cellulitis. Nitrofurantoin will achieve high urine levels, while tissue levels will be relatively low. Therefore, nitrofurantoin will not affect the bacteriology of a soft tissue infection and mask a developing pelvic infection such as pelvic cellulitis. A disadvantage of nitrofurantoin is that it will have a limited effect, if at all, on the vaginal and periurethral flora. This makes nitrofurantoin not a particularly good choice for those individuals

with a history of recurrent cystitis. An alternative choice is the fluoroquinolones, which have been shown to be as effective as those agents listed earlier. The quinolones should not be used as first-line agents. They should be reserved for those patients who have failed empiric therapy, have a history of recurrent infection, or cannot tolerate the initial choice, or for those in whom the resistance pattern of the organism dictates a specific choice of antibiotic.

Treatment of acute cystitis in pregnancy can be effectively accomplished with nitrofurantoin. During the second trimester, trimethoprim or trimethoprim-sulfamethoxazole can be utilized. Quinolones should not be administered to pregnant or breast-feeding women. Ampicillin or related agents should not be administered empirically to treat acute cystitis because up to 40% of the strains of *E. coli* are resistant to this antibiotic. Administration of ampicillin is likely to result in failure and to place the patient at risk for the development of pyelonephritis. Treatment of asymptomatic and symptomatic bacteriuria should be treated with a 10-day course of antibiotics because of the significant risk of pyelonephritis and the seriousness of this disease in pregnancy. It is also advisable to obtain a urine culture when administering antibiotic therapy to the pregnant patient to determine whether *Streptococcus agalactiae* (group B streptococcus) is present because of the potential increased risk associated with maternal colonization for the fetus. Following treatment, the patient's urine should be recultured to determine whether there has been bacterial eradication, and the urine should be screened at least once in each trimester to determine whether bacteriuria is present.

Pyelonephritis in the nonpregnant patient is typically treated with the combination of ampicillin plus gentamicin or imipenem-cilastatin. These agents provide coverage for gram-negative bacilli and enterococci. An alternative would be the intravenous administration of a fluoroquinolone followed by the oral form when the patient's signs and symptoms have resolved. Perhaps it would be more economical and logical to perform a Gram stain of the patient's urine to determine whether the offending organism is gram-positive or gram-negative. If the bacterium is gram-positive, a penicillin-type agent should be administered. If bacteremia is suspected, then ampicillin plus gentamicin should be administered. If the bacterium is gram-negative, then a second- or third-generation cephalosporin, depending on the medical parameters present, should be given.

Pyelonephritis in pregnancy is typically caused

by *E. coli* infection, and therefore initial treatment is empirically begun with a first-generation cephalosporin. Once the patient has improved, the antibiotic can be changed to an oral form of the same agent that was administered intravenously. The patient should receive a total of 10 days of antibiotic therapy. Shortly after completion of antibiotic therapy, a repeat urine culture should be performed. If the urine culture result is negative, the patient could be placed on a daily maintenance dose (100 mg) of nitrofurantoin for the remainder of the pregnancy.

A particular problem is management of the patient with recurrent infection. First it must be established that this is a recurrent infection, not a failure of treatment or a new infection. Recurrent infection is caused by the same organism found in the previous episode. This should lead to an investigation of a precipitating cause, such as frequent intercourse, use of a diaphragm, or an atrophic genital tract. Individuals developing postcoital cystitis ("honeymoon cystitis") can be treated with a maintenance course of nitrofurantoin, 100 mg orally, nightly. If a diaphragm is being used, a smaller size may relieve obstruction of the urethra. Patients with atrophic vaginitis may have resolution of their cystitis by applying intravaginal estrogen cream.

Obstetricians and gynecologists must become familiar with diagnosing UTI in each age group, beginning with the adolescent through the geriatric patient. Bacterial colonization, whether asymptomatic or symptomatic, may result in significant morbidity and mortality.

Vaginosis (Bacterial)

David A. Eschenbach, MD

Bacterial vaginosis (BV) is a syndrome in which a complex alteration of vaginal bacterial flora occurs. In about half of patients, BV causes an odorous discharge. *Gardnerella vaginalis* is present at high concentrations in virtually all women with BV, but it is the anaerobic bacteria that produce the characteristic fishy odor and appear responsible for upper genital tract infections.

Patients with BV have a distinct alteration in vaginal flora with an overgrowth of the normal lactobacilli by high concentrations of *G. vaginalis*, anaerobes, and *Mycoplasma hominis*. This syndrome differs from other causes of vaginitis because inflammation is generally absent while the propensity for upper genital tract infection is present.

Factors that predispose to BV include those associated with sexual activity, such as longer history of coital experience, greater number of sexual partners, a new partner, and presence of *Trichomonas vaginalis*. Intrauterine device use is also associated with BV. Recent antibiotic administration, use of a diaphragm or spermicidal cream, age, and smoking have not been confirmed as risk factors; however, direct evidence of the sexual transmission of BV is limited. *G. vaginalis*, *M. hominis*, and *Mobiluncus* species can be isolated from the urethras of male partners of women with BV, but these organisms probably do not persist in the male genital tract. Evidence against sexual transmission is the failure to reduce recurrences by the treatment of male partners. On the other hand, inoculation of whole vaginal material from women with BV to other women produced the syndrome.

Bacterial vaginosis accounts for about 45% of symptomatic vaginitis. The prevalence of symptomatic and asymptomatic BV in nonpregnant patients is quite variable, ranging from 4% in an asymptomatic student population to 15% to 25% in patients attending gynecology clinics, and 30% to 60% in sexually transmitted disease populations. From 12% to 22% of pregnant patients have BV (Table 1), and it represents one of the more common lower genital tract infections.

Bacteriology

Normal vaginal flora consists predominantly of *Lactobacillus* species, which make up about 95% of the total bacterial count at concentrations of 10^5 to 10^8 *Lactobacillus* per milliliter of vaginal secretion. *Lactobacillus* not only helps maintain a low vaginal pH, but strains in normal women produce hydrogen peroxide, which inhibits the growth of many other bacteria. The net result of a *Lactobacillus*-dominant flora is the suppression of the remaining vaginal flora and a reduced

TABLE 1. Upper Genital Tract Infection Associated with Bacterial Vaginosis

Pregnant women
    Amniotic fluid infection
    Chorioamnionitis
Nonpregnant women
    Postpartum endometritis
    Postabortion pelvic inflammatory disease
    Posthysterectomy cuff cellulitis

prevalence and concentration of bacteria such as *G. vaginalis, Bacteroides* species, peptostreptococci, and *M. hominis*, which are associated with BV. The remainder of vaginal flora among women with a *Lactobacillus*-dominant flora consists of about 10 to 15 types of bacteria per patient, usually in concentrations at or below 10^4 bacteria per milliliter of vaginal fluid. These other bacteria usually account for only 5% of the total count of bacteria.

In contrast, patients with BV have a reversal in the ratio of *Lactobacillus* to other bacteria. One third to one half of women with BV have no lactobacilli; the remainder have a reduced concentration of *Lactobacillus*, and these lactobacilli when present usually do not produce hydrogen peroxide. Women with BV have an increased prevalence of *G. vaginalis*, anaerobic bacteria, *Mobiluncus* species, and *M. hominis*. More importantly, women with BV have a 20- to 100-fold increase in the concentration of *G. vaginalis*, a 20- to 1,000-fold increase in the concentration of anaerobic bacteria and a 20- to 1,000-fold increase in the concentration of *M. hominis*, as compared with those with a *Lactobacillus*-dominant flora. The large increase in the concentration of potentially virulent bacteria in the vagina of women explains the relationship between BV and upper genital tract infection.

Clinical Diagnosis

Symptoms make poor criteria to define any type of vaginitis. Only symptoms of a vaginal odor and increase in vaginal discharge correlated with BV. Patients also often complain of fishy odor with intercourse when alkaline seminal fluid causes volatilization of amines. A yellow vaginal discharge, vulvar pruritus, and abnormal vaginal bleeding do not correlate with BV.

Rather, four clinical criteria have been used to diagnose BV: a homogeneous (skim milk) appearance, a pH greater than 4.5, a fishy amine odor after the addition of 10% KOH, and clue cells by microscopy. The presence of three of these four criteria identifies BV. The homogenous appearance is the most subjective criterion, while an elevated pH has a very high negative predictive value, since only 3% of patients with BV have a pH less than 4.7. Thus, a normal pH is a very useful finding to exclude BV. An amine odor is not sensitive but is highly specific. The presence of clue cells has both a high sensitivity and positive predictive value for BV. The appearance of clue cells in patients without the other of the criteria usually represents a false-positive

finding. If large *Lactobacillus* rod morphotypes are identified between epithelial cells together with clue cells, it probably represents a false-positive test for clue cells. In contrast, a predominance of small non-*Lactobacillus* morphotypes is seen in the wet mount of patients with BV. Gram stain can also be used to diagnose BV when increased counts of gram-negative rods and gram-positive cocci and decreased counts of gram-positive *Lactobacillus* rod morphotypes are present.

Laboratory Methods for Diagnosis

Because BV is caused by replacement of the normal *Lactobacillus*-dominant flora with *G. vaginalis*, anaerobes, and *M. hominis*, no single microorganism defines the syndrome. A positive culture for *G. vaginalis* should not be used to direct therapy, or for "test of cure" following treatment, since about one half of women with normal vaginal flora are colonized by *G. vaginalis*. This means that the majority of women who are colonized by *G. vaginalis* do not have BV. Even high concentrations of *G. vaginalis*, present in 3 to 4+ quantities on the agar plate, are not predictive of BV.

Complications
Preterm Labor, Low Birth Weight, and PROM

A large number of upper genital tract infections have been associated with BV (see Table 1). Preterm delivery represents one of the most serious consequences. BV is roughly twice as common as the combination of infections commonly sought in pregnancy: gonorrhea, chlamydia, and urinary tract infection. BV can account for a substantial population attributable risk of preterm delivery, up to 6% of all preterm or low birth weight infants. BV was consistently related to preterm/low birth weight delivery in virtually all of the studies where the presence of BV was determined prior to delivery. The association between BV and preterm/low birth weight delivery is very consistent; the only two reported studies in which BV was not related to preterm delivery and low birth weight were either small or originated from among patients who delivered infants less than 2500 g and had vaginal swabs taken for Gram stain after delivery when postpartum blood would hinder diagnosis. BV has generally been present in 25% to 35% of those who deliver preterm and in 10% to 20% of those who deliver at term. The largest of these studies is noteworthy in that potential confounding variables in the association between BV and premature delivery and low birth weight such as demographic factors, smoking, prior preterm delivery, and the recovery of other microbes were adjusted by logistic regression analysis.

In addition, the presence of *Lactobacillus* in concentrations of 10^7 or more microorganisms per milliliter of vaginal fluid was associated with a reduced rate of preterm delivery. By contrast, the presence of the anaerobic bacteria associated with BV, particularly *Bacteroides* species *(prevotella)* was associated with an increased rate of preterm delivery.

If BV causes preterm delivery, one would expect an association between BV and upper genital tract infection because upper genital tract infection has been highly associated with preterm delivery. Indeed, BV is associated with upper genital tract infections in pregnancy. A 2.7- to 4.9-fold increased risk of amniotic fluid infection occurs in patients with BV. Additionally, about 55% of patients with amniotic fluid infection have the anaerobic bacteria associated with BV isolated from amniotic fluid. A 3.2-fold increased risk of chorioamnion infection and a 2.6-fold increased risk of histologic chorioamnionitis occurs among patients with BV in preterm labor.

A significant reduction in preterm births occurred in two randomized metronidazole treatment trials conducted in the second trimester among patients at high risk for preterm delivery. The birth rate in the treated group was reduced to the level present in patients without BV. Thus, patients at high risk for preterm delivery should be screened and treated for BV in pregnancy.

Patients with BV diagnosed by Gram stain had 5.1 times (95% CI, 2.6–9.9) the risk of postpartum endometritis following cesarean section compared with those with a *Lactobacillus*-dominant flora. After adjustment for possible confounding factors (maternal age, length of labor, duration of membrane rupture), patients with BV remained with a 5.8-fold (95% CI, 3.0–10.9) risk of postpartum endometritis compared with those with a *Lactobacillus*-dominant flora. BV was also associated with abdominal wound infection. These postpartum and wound infections developed despite the widespread use of prophylactic antibiotics for cesarean delivery. Additionally, the endometrial aspirates of 61% of patients with postpartum endometritis contained the anaerobes associated with BV, *G. vaginalis*, or both at the time of postpartum endometritis. Among patients who delivered vaginally, anaerobes (most commonly *Bacteroides bivius*), *G. vaginalis*, and *M. hominis* in the amniotic fluid resulted in a 14-fold increased risk of postpartum endometritis.

In two separate studies, postabdominal hysterectomy cuff cellulitis occurred about four times more commonly among patients with BV than among patients with a normal *Lactobacillus*-dominant flora. Prophylactic antibiotics were not used in these studies, but about one third of the women with BV developed infection following hysterectomy. The attributable risk of BV for cuff cellulitis was 69%. Although a randomized treatment trial has not been done for patients with BV prior to hysterectomy, a single 2 g tinidazole dose 12 hours before surgery significantly reduced postoperative vaginal cuff cellulitis following both vaginal and abdominal hysterectomy. The effectiveness of tinidazole suggests that treatment prior to surgery may significantly reduce postoperative infection.

Postabortion pelvic inflammatory disease (PID) occurred 2.4 times (95% CI, 1.1–5.3) more commonly among patients with BV than in those with a *Lactobacillus*-dominant flora. *Chlamydia trachomatis* was also weakly related to postabortion PID ($p = 0.06$) in this study.[53] However, more than twice as many patients had BV as had *C. trachomatis* infection, and postabortion PID occurred in eight patients with preoperative BV, two patients with preoperative *C. trachomatis* infection, and 18 patients with neither. In a follow-up double-blinded trial, placebo-treated patients had three times (95% CI, 1–11.8) the rate of postabortion PID as patients treated with metronidazole, suggesting that treatment of BV significantly decreased infectious morbidity following termination of pregnancy.

The role of BV in spontaneous PID not associated with abortion is less clear. Many of the bacteria recovered from the endometrium and fallopian tubes of patients with pelvic inflammatory disease are those bacteria present in the vagina in high numbers among women with BV. However, the attack rate of BV in causing PID may be relatively low compared with that of *Neisseria gonorrhoeae* or *C. trachomatis*.

Treatment

Symptomatic nonpregnant patients deserve treatment of BV to alleviate symptoms. Thus, patients with BV and a fishy vaginal odor, a fishy vaginal odor during intercourse, or an increased vaginal discharge deserve treatment. More controversial is whether treatment should be given to the estimated 50% of asymptomatic patients with BV.

Regression of BV to normal vaginal flora over several months suggests that treatment may be unnecessary for some asymptomatic individuals, and treatment of nonpregnant asymptomatic patients is not advocated at present. However, as a word of caution, many "asymptomatic" women report a fishy odor upon direct questioning, and the concern over various upper genital tract infections in the pregnant woman and the nonpregnant woman undergoing surgery places probably even asymptomatic patients in a high-risk category. In addition, other invasive procedures could potentially be associated with an increased rate of infection, including intrauterine device insertion, hysteroscopy, hysterosalpingography, and dilatation and curettage. Double-blinded, randomized, placebo-controlled studies are needed before routine treatment is advocated for the low-risk pregnant patient, but individualized treatment of symptomatic or high-risk patients should be considered.

The increased rate of postpartum endometritis among patients with BV undergoing cesarean section occurs despite the use of currently recommended doses of cephalosporin prophylaxis. These data suggest that patients with BV are either infected prior to surgery or have such high bacterial concentrations or antibiotic-resistant bacteria that currently used prophylactic agents are ineffective. Either BV needs to be treated prior to delivery, or more prolonged dosing or different antibiotics could be considered for the prophylaxis of patients with BV to prevent postpartum endometritis. An increased duration of the antibiotic prophylaxis would constitute treatment rather than true prophylaxis. Given this apparent weakness of the present prophylactic regimens against BV-derived postpartum infection, radical changes in thinking are required and further research is clearly needed.

Antibiotic regimens

Several antibiotic regimens successfully treat BV. First-line regimens include three antimicrobials with excellent activity against anaerobic bacteria: metronidazole, clindamycin, and tinidazole (Table 2). Initial success rates range from 90% to 100% 1 to 2 weeks following therapy and decrease to 70% to 90% 4 weeks or more after the onset of therapy.

Oral regimens tend to produce more systemic side effects such as nausea, vomiting, and a metallic taste than the intravaginal regimens do. Since intravaginal preparations contain only 38 mg of metronidazole and 100 mg of clindamycin per dose, limited levels of the antibiotic are systemically absorbed and systemic side effects from the intravaginal regimens are low.

Second-line regimens with less efficacy include the 2 g single dose oral metronidazole

TABLE 2. Antimicrobial Regimens for Bacterial Vaginosis

Antimicrobial	Route	Dose	Duration (days)
First Line			
Metronidazole	Oral	500 mg bid	7
Metronidazole	Intravaginal	0.75% gel bid	5
Clindamycin	Oral	300 mg bid	7
Clindamycin	Intravaginal	2% cream nightly	7
Tinidazole	Oral	500 mg bid	5
Second Line			
Metronidazole	Oral	2 g	Single dose
Amoxicillin/clavulanic acid	Oral	500 mg tid	7
Third Line			
Ampicillin/amoxicillin			
Ciprofloxacin			
Triple sulfa cream			
Ineffective Antimicrobials			
Erythromycin			
Tetracycline			
Doxycycline			
Povidone-iodine			
Acetic acid			
Dinestrinol			
Lactobacillus			

regimen, which is generally 5% to 10% less efficacious than the 7-day dose. Other regimens less well studied but with reasonable efficacy against BV include amoxicillin and clavulanic acid. Third-line regimens that have minimal efficacy in treating BV include ampicillin, amoxicillin, ciprofloxacin, and intravaginal triple sulfa cream. Cure rates using these regimens have generally ranged from 20% to 50%. Ineffective regimens with poor to no efficacy against BV should not be used; these are erythromycin, tetracycline, doxycycline, intravaginal povidone-iodine, acetic acid gel, and dinestrinol cream and *Lactobacillus*.

Patient Follow-Up After Antibiotic Treatment of Bacterial Vaginosis

The best evidence of therapeutic efficacy is the absence of three or more of the clinical signs. Vaginal pH remains elevated for several weeks following successful therapy in a large number of patients, and persistent pH elevation is not a good indicator of a poor response.

In patients who fail to respond to the first-line regimens, my first recommendation is to switch to a different class of an intravaginal antimicrobial agent. Thus, patients not responding to oral metronidazole would be treated with intravaginal clindamycin and vice versa, or patients not responding to intravaginal clindamycin would receive intravaginal metronidazole. Patients with a rapid recurrence of symptoms within a few days of completing therapy possibly have resistant bacteria. Most commonly, patients will develop recurrent symptoms several weeks after the completion of therapy and the cause or causes of the late developing failures require further study. Among patients with two or more of these late recurrences, I recommend a longer 3-week therapy with either metronidazole or clindamycin and that the prolonged intensive treatment be followed with intravaginal therapy every third day for 3 additional weeks. The intent is to inhibit the bacteria associated with BV in the initial 3 weeks of therapy and to then provide therapy to intermittently inhibit these bacteria, while allowing *Lactobacillus* to re-establish itself in the vagina.

Treatment of males with oral metronidazole has been advocated to reduce recurrent BV in their female partners. Unfortunately, treatment of males has not prevented recurrent BV. This is perhaps related to the fact that BV is a complex infection involving the overgrowth of multiple bacteria in the vaginal flora and not the result of simple sexual transmission. At present, it is not necessary to administer antibiotic treatment to male sexual partners of women with BV.

Adjunct Therapy

Adjunct therapy should be considered only as an addition to antibiotic therapy, since adjunct therapy alone does not appear to cure BV and more information is needed from controlled studies. Since the goal of therapy is to establish a normal *Lactobacillus*-dominant vaginal flora, intravaginal *Lactobacillus* could help establish the return of *Lactobacillus* dominance to the vaginal flora.

Vesicovaginal Fistulas

Walter B. Hull, MD

The vesicovaginal fistula (VVF) is an abnormal communication between the urinary bladder and the vagina, resulting in the uncontrolled and constant loss of urine per vaginam. Although the VVF has been recognized since antiquity and a variety of procedures have been used to correct it, it was J. Marion Sims (1813–83) in the United States who developed the first effective surgical technique for its repair. In 1855, Sims opened the first fistula hospital in New York where the Waldorf Astoria Hotel now stands. Great strides in the repair of the VVFs have been made by surgeons like Kelly, Martius, Mahfouz, Mackenrodt, Lawson, and others. Drs. Hamlin and Nicholson of Australia opened the second fistula hospital in Addis Ababa, Ethiopia, in the 1960s, which today repairs between 500 and 600 VVFs per year, achieving a 90% success rate at first attempt.

Successful repair of the VVF yields one of the most grateful patients in gynecologic surgery. Sims said, "The accident is never fatal; but it might well be imagined that a lady of keen sensibility so afflicted and excluded from all social enjoyment might prefer death." To quote the Hamlins of Ethiopia, "The women with the VVF come with only faith, hope and urine-soaked clothes." Thus, a failed attempt to repair a VVF yields one of the most demoralized patients.

Frequency

The VVF, along with the occasional ureterovaginal fistula (UVF), occurs in between 0.05% and

0.5% of women undergoing pelvic surgery in the United States and in other developed countries.

The frequency of the obstetrically induced VVF is a reflection of the quality and primarily the accessibility of basic obstetric care. Hence it has rightly become a rarity in developed countries. It remains a major feature of gynecologic surgery in underdeveloped countries because of widely unavailable basic obstetric care, especially in rural areas. The author's hospital in central Congo is representative: in 1988, 30 of 692 (4.3%) obstetric and gynecologic operations performed were for VVFs; several were associated with a rectovaginal fistula. The Hamlins in Addis Ababa have operated on some 15,000 VVFs over their more than 25 years of experience there. Elkins and colleagues estimate that in West Africa the incidence of VVFs is 3 to 6 per 1000 deliveries; of those, 50% will be greater than 4 cm in diameter, and nearly 100% of those will subsequently have degrees of vaginal stenosis or atresia after standard repair.

Causes

There are four basic causes of VVF:

Obstetric. Obstetric trauma is the cause of 90% of VVFs in underdeveloped countries, although rare in developed countries. The most important contributing factor is prolonged neglected labor causing pressure necrosis of the bladder floor as it becomes entrapped between the pubic bone and the fetal head; the level at which the head becomes impacted determines the level of the subsequent fistula along the anterior vaginal wall. Other factors include careless manipulations of all sorts to achieve vaginal delivery; an ill-applied vacuum extractor catching a piece of the anterior vaginal wall; a symphysiotomy causing urethral trauma; a cesarean section with damage to the bladder fundus; or a uterine rupture and its subsequent surgical care. Associated local infection in many of these situations aggravates the risk of fistula formation.

Surgical. Surgical trauma to the bladder and ureters is the leading cause of VVF in developed countries. Abdominal hysterectomy is the procedure most often complicated by a VVF; vaginal hysterectomy is a less frequent cause. If one suspects intraoperative damage to the bladder or ureter, intravenous indigo carmine (5 mL), intravesical sterile milk or methylene blue, and transvesical ureteral catheterization are all useful maneuvers to identify such damage. Prompt and appropriate repair of that damage almost always prevents the formation of the onerous fistula.

Radiation. Radiation therapy, especially for treating cervical cancer, is an important cause of VVF in developed countries. It is rare in the underdeveloped world because radiation therapy is generally unavailable. It should be noted that these fistulas are most difficult to repair because of radiation damage to the local tissue microcirculation. Repair usually requires flap grafts for success.

Neoplasm. Neoplasms, such as cervical cancer, occasionally cause a VVF. Repair is impossible short of removing the cancer.

The remainder of the discussion is limited to the fistulas caused by obstetric and surgical trauma. Surgical fistulas are generally small and associated with healthy tissues; obstetric fistulas are often large with much loss of tissue and more infection and fibrosis. Surgical fistulas are generally easier to repair because the tissues are healthier.

Anatomic Classification

It is helpful to group VVFs according to their anatomic location. This is important in the selection of the route of surgical approach, the technique of repair, the risk of complication during repair, and the prognosis.

VVF may be classified as follows (Fig. 1):

1. Urethrovaginal fistula
2. Juxtaurethrovaginal fistula involving the bladder sphincter zone
3. Midvaginal fistula located above the bladder neck and below or in the interureteric ridge
4. Juxtacervical VVF
5. Vesicocervicovaginal fistula
6. UVF, which must be distinguished from VVF
7. The large VVF that encompasses two or more of these anatomic sites, often with much scarring and fixation to the pubic rami and with partial or total destruction of the urethra

Diagnosis

The diagnosis of a urinary fistula is suggested by the uncontrollable and incessant flow of urine per vaginam. This is in contradistinction to stress

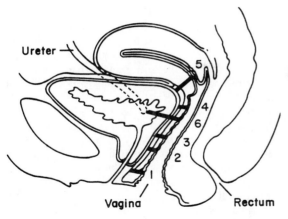

Figure 1. The anatomic location of vesicovaginal fistulas. 1, Urethrovaginal; 2, juxtaurethrovaginal; 3, midvaginal; 4, juxtacervical; 5, vesicocervicovaginal; 6, ureterovaginal.

incontinence in which loss of urine is dependent on position and effort. Perineal odor is offensive and is caused by the ammonia liberated by urea-splitting vaginal microorganisms. The constant wetting of the vulva by urine also causes a vulvar dermatitis manifested by white papules and tenderness.

Speculum examination reveals the velvety bladder mucosa through a large VVF. Digital vaginal examination enables one to delineate fistula size and borders. It is imperative to locate the VVF anatomically to determine surgical approach. Inspection may reveal concretions from the precipitation of urinary salts in the fistula tract or calculi in the bladder. They must be removed before surgical therapy. Sutures from previous attempts at repair must likewise be removed.

It is occasionally necessary to distinguish between a tiny VVF and a UVF. The simplest technique is the methylene blue test in the office. A French catheter is placed in the bladder, and 50 to 100 mL of a dilute solution of methylene blue in saline is instilled in the bladder. If blue liquid appears in the vagina, it indicates at least a VVF; if no blue liquid appears, one must presume a UVF. One then can give an ampule of indigo carmine intravenously; one should see blue liquid collect in the vagina within 10 minutes, confirming the presence of a UVF (Fig. 2). An intravenous pyelogram is appropriate to further delineate the UVF and on which side it is located.

Air or liquid cystoscopic examination is helpful in the event of a small fistula to more precisely localize the VVF in relation to the ureteral orifices. This can often be bypassed with high fistulas, however.

Treatment

A discussion of the treatment of the VVF must consider when to operate, the preoperative preparation of the patient, the route of repair, the position of the patient on the operating table, necessary instruments and materials, fistula exposure, techniques of the repair itself, postoperative care and complications, when not to attempt a repair and the alternative treatment, and attention to an associated rectovaginal fistula.

Timing

Timing of the repair of the VVF is critical. The first attempt offers the best chance for success. One must have healthy, noninflamed, nonedematous, and supple tissues for success in the repair. The traditional waiting period of 4 to 6 months between the occurrence of the fistula and the repair is questioned by many. Small VVFs consequent to surgical injury can often be repaired 1 to 3 months after their occurrence. Drs. Hamlin and Nicholson of Addis Ababa often attempt repair of the obstetrically caused VVF at 2 to 4 months. The obvious reason to attempt earlier repair is to shorten the socially compromising "wet" period that causes such embarrassment, depression, and restricted social and marital ac-

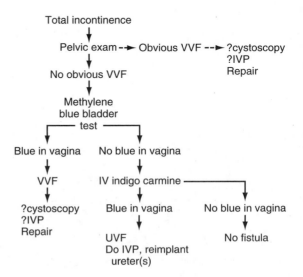

Figure 2. Algorithm to distinguish between a vesicovaginal fistula and a ureterovaginal fistula.

tivities of the patient. Nevertheless, one must hasten to add that premature attempts at repair are doomed to failure and thus prolong the unpleasantness of a VVF. The critical factor is the healthiness of the tissues around the VVF. When they are well healed, one can proceed with repair, be it 1 month or 6 months after the injury.

Preparation

Any malnutrition and anemia should be corrected before surgery. Any local infection should be cleared up with antibiotics. Concretions, calculi, and old suture material should be removed from the fistula tract.

Some authors use corticosteroids for 2 to 3 weeks preoperatively to reduce local inflammation. I have used chloroquine, 100 mg/day for a month, for its anti-inflammatory effect. There are no studies evaluating the efficacy of such measures. If the patient is estrogen-deprived, systemically or locally applied estrogens should be offered during the waiting period to soften and vascularize local tissues.

An intravenous pyelogram and cystoscopy are often recommended but are not essential in most cases. One must be careful to look for ureteral orifices during the repair. If one suspects a UVF, an intravenous pyelogram should be done.

Because of perineal tenderness or fistula location and size, it may be necessary to examine the patient under anesthesia in the operating room to evaluate the fistula adequately and to plan surgical therapy.

Route of Approach

Urologists usually prefer the transabdominal route of surgery, and gynecologists prefer the vaginal route. Both routes should be available to the surgeon. The choice is based on which route provides the best exposure and the easiest dissection and which avoids damage to ureters. The level of the fistula and pelvic shape are also determining factors. The vaginal approach is preferred for most VVFs. It is the only approach for the juxtaurethral fistula. The transabdominal approach is preferred for very high fistulas, a fistula in the face of a very anthropoid pelvis, or a vesicocervicovaginal fistula; or if the ureters cannot otherwise be safely avoided by the vaginal approach. The transabdominal approach allows for a ureteral reimplantation in the event that adequate fistula repair means catching the ureter.

It is of interest that the greatly experienced Hamlins of Addis Ababa almost never use the abdominal approach and have excellent results with difficult fistulas. The author uses both routes selectively.

Patient Position

For the transvaginal approach, the knee-elbow position provides excellent operative access to the fistula. The patient is prone with the thighs flexed over the end of the table and the feet suspended in the stirrups of the lithotomy poles (Fig. 3). Sandbags or pillows under the chest and the pubis are essential to allow adequate abdominal excursion for adequate ventilation. This position allows the surgeon to look down onto the bladder floor and to work more easily. To avoid fecal soiling of the field, the anus is temporarily closed with a circumferential suture to be removed at the end of the operation.

Some surgeons (the Hamlins of Addis Ababa) prefer only the dorsal lithotomy position for the

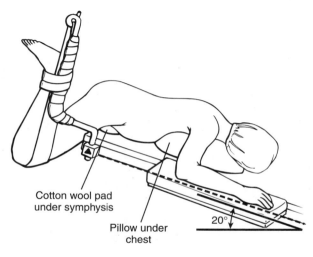

Cotton wool pad under symphysis

Pillow under chest

20°

Figure 3. The knee-elbow position. The pillows or sandbags under the chest and pubis allow abdominal respiratory excursion. The flexed thighs keep the patient from sliding up the table.

vaginal approach. It is the best position if one anticipates doing a Martius fat graft.

Instruments

An operating headlight is highly recommended. Overhead lamps are not adequate to work in the deep recesses. One needs to see well the extremities of the fistula in order to dissect and to place the sutures. Good suction with a long, narrow tip is ideal. Sharp pointed dissecting scissors and a curved pointed knife blade (no. 12) should be available. Sutures may be 2-0 or 3-0 chromic or polyglycolic (Dexon) or polyglactin (Vicryl). The 5/8 circle urologic needle is excellent for placing sutures in deep recesses.

Fistula Exposure

Ordinary vaginal retraction suffices for adequate exposure. In the presence of a scarred introitus, a narrow pubic arch, or a deep VVF, a perineotomy in the form of a Schuchardt incision can be made to facilitate exposure.

Repair

The fundamental principles of repair of the VVF are (1) adequate exposure, (2) wide dissection and mobilization of the bladder, (3) nonexcision of the fistula tract, (4) a tension-free closure of bladder without obstructing the ureters, and (5) grafting as necessary. Injecting the tissues around the fistula with a solution of 1:100,000 epinephrine does two things: it provides a degree of hemostasis, and it helps create tissue planes that can be more easily dissected.

For a small posthysterectomy VVF in the apex of the vaginal pouch the Latzko repair is effective. It consists of a circular incision of the fistula tract, wide dissection of vaginal mucosa from the bladder wall, closure of the fistula tract with 3-0 delayed absorbable suture, one or two additional imbricating layers of bladder wall, and then closure of the vaginal mucosa.

In the event of large VVFs, the ureteral orifices will likely be on or near the fistula margin. They should each be catheterized and the two ureteral catheters brought out through the urethra. If the ureteral orifices are hard to identify, one of two maneuvers will help: either inject 5 mL of indigo carmine intravenously, which will appear from the ureteral orifices within 10 minutes, or inject 10 to 20 mg of furosemide

(Lasix) intravenously, which will cause a rapid diuresis and thus reveal the ureteral orifices.

Using a no. 12 curved hooked scalpel, one incises circumferentially the fistula margin. Then using sharp pointed scissors, one dissects 2 to 3 cm laterally from the margin in all directions. This maneuver usually well mobilizes the bladder wall, allowing closure of the bladder defect without tension. A wide dissection is imperative, with care taken to preserve bladder muscularis intact and yet not render the vaginal mucosa too thin.

Although most textbooks advise excision of the fistula borders, experts like the Hamlins of Addis Ababa advise categorically against it. They insist that former teaching is based on no real study of the issue, and that, moreover, one needs to preserve all the tissue possible in large fistulas.

A three-layer closure is ideal although not always possible. The bladder edges are approximated with interrupted 2-0 or 3-0 delayed absorbable sutures using the 5/8 circle needle for placement at intervals of 3 to 5 mm. One attempts to invert but not to traverse the bladder mucosa. A second layer of bladder wall, if possible, is imbricated over the first layer using the same interrupted sutures. That the repair is watertight should be verified by instilling methylene blue solution in the bladder and checking for leaks along the repair line. Any leaks must be closed. Then the vaginal layer is closed with similar interrupted sutures.

In the case of a large VVF, and especially with fistulas involving the bladder neck area, success of repair is greatly enhanced by use of the Martius bulbocavernosus fat graft. This is a remarkably easy procedure with great benefit. The graft is developed by making a vertical incision along the labia majora up to the mons pubis. The band of fibrofatty tissue deep to the labia majora skin is dissected out. The extremity of the fat pad toward the mons is divided high. The posterior extremity of the fat pad is left attached so as to preserve its pudendal artery blood supply. A tunnel is made from the graft site, under the skin and mucosal bridge of the labia minora and lateral vaginal wall, and into the dissected space around the fistula. The fat graft is anchored around the fistula site with four absorbable sutures. The vaginal mucosa is then closed over it. The vulvar skin incision is closed in two layers. Elkins and colleagues describe a useful modification of the Martius fat graft to gain skin to allow closure of the compromised vaginal mucosa over the fistula. They excise an island of skin in the groin, leaving it attached to the upper extremity of the bulbocavernosus fat pad, and swing this over the fistula site. This compensates for vaginal mucosal deficit.

When the transabdominal approach is used, a vertical skin incision is used, the space of Retzius is developed, and the dome of the bladder is entered. The fistula can be exposed well and repaired in layers as with the vaginal approach, although in reverse order. If a ureter cannot be avoided and a good fistula border apposition still achieved, the ureter can be reimplanted into the fundus of the bladder. It is often helpful to catheterize the ureters during the closure of the fistula.

It is beyond the scope of this chapter to discuss the repair of more complicated fistulas such as those associated with the loss of the urethra, severe adhesions to the pubic rami, marked gynatresia, and so on.

Postoperative Care

The most critical element is catheter drainage. Urethral or suprapubic catheters, or both, can be used. Ureteral catheters may also be left in place in case of a repair in which the ureteral orifices were very close to the fistula margin or in the event of ureteral reimplantation. One must be sure that the urethral catheter works. If ever one suspects urethral catheter blockage, one should not hesitate to change it. Several hours of a blocked catheter can destroy a meticulous repair.

The catheter drainage is continued for 12 to 14 days postoperatively. Some leakage may occur around the catheter and be mistaken for breakdown; the catheter should be kept in place. One is often surprised that healing finally occurs. Antibiotics are continued for 2 to 3 weeks.

Complications of Surgery

The most immediate complication is that of ureteral ligation. One ureter can be ligated and the incident can pass silently and unrecognized. Usually, however, severe flank pain, costovertebral tenderness, and vomiting announce the problem. If both ureters are ligated, anuria will be evident. If ureteral ligation is recognized in the first 48 hours postoperatively, the ureter or ureters should be promptly reimplanted into the bladder transabdominally.

Intravesical hemorrhage is occasionally a serious problem. Frequent irrigations with sterile saline are required to remove clots and prevent catheter obstruction. Rarely it is necessary to do a suprapubic cystotomy to evacuate the clots and suture the bleeding points.

Fistula breakdown, if it occurs, usually takes place during the second week postoperatively. Catheter drainage should be continued for the usual 2 weeks in the hope that at least partial closure of the fistula will occur. The patient requires a great amount of encouragement at that point. A second attempt at closure can be made 2 to 3 months later when tissues are healed.

A late complication of repairing a juxtaurethral fistula is loss of urethral sphincter and urethral support. The patient remains incontinent even though the fistula has been successfully closed. This can be corrected eventually by the Goebel-Frangenheim-Stoeckel sling operation using a vertical band of abdominal rectus fascia. The patient subsequently can urinate only in the squatting position. More recently the technique of periurethral injection of silicone gives great promise for correcting this unstable urethral syndrome.

Pregnancy can occur after the repair of even a very large fistula. Delivery probably should be by cesarean section to avoid damage to a difficult fistula repair.

When Not to Repair a Vesicovaginal Fistula

There are several situations in which it is wisest not to attempt a VVF repair because failure is quite certain. A large VVF with dense scarring of the borders to the pubic rami, total destruction of the urethra, severe vaginal stenosis (gynatresia), and repeated failed attempts at repair are such situations. Urinary diversion should be considered. An ileal or a sigmoid urinary conduit would be the choice in the developed world, where materials exist for chronic conduit care. However, for lack of such materials in the underdeveloped world, a conduit would be no better than the fistula itself.

Another option is to transplant the ureters into the functioning rectum. Urinary reflux and therefore upper tract urinary infection are major concerns with this technique. Kashiwai and colleagues described a seromuscular folding technique for the ureterosigmoid anastomosis that minimizes reflux and also minimizes the stenosis at the anastomosis site often associated with the Ledbetter or Coffey technique of transplantation. It must be underscored that an intact anal sphincter without any rectovaginal fistula is necessary before such an implantation can be undertaken.

Another option for urinary diversion requiring minimal equipment for ostomy care is the Florida pouch. It uses the isolated, extended, detubularized right colonic segment as a urinary reservoir and the plicated terminal ileum as the skin stoma. The patient must catheterize the stoma frequently to empty the reservoir. There is no leakage of urine otherwise and thus no collecting equipment is needed. This pouch avoids the infectious complication inherent with the ureterosigmoid anastomosis.

Associated Rectovaginal Fistulas

If a high rectovaginal fistula exists with a VVF, a diverting colostomy usually is necessary before an attempted repair. Low and small rectovaginal fistulas can usually be closed without a diverting colostomy. When the VVF is associated with a rectovaginal fistula, the VVF usually is closed first as a separate operation. The reason is that closure of the rectovaginal fistula first may reduce the vaginal lumen such that it would compromise exposure for repair of the VVF.

Success Rate

Repairs of small fistulas secondary to surgical trauma should be successful in 95% to 100% of first attempts. However, one is content with an 80% to 90% success rate in primary repair of large obstetric fistulas secondary to pressure necrosis. Remember, the first effort at repair gives one the best opportunity for success. One must be judicious in timing the operation and preparing the patient and be meticulous in executing the repair. There is no happier patient than one who has undergone a successful repair of a VVF.

Vulvodynia

Stanley C. Marinoff, MD, MPH

Vulvodynia simply means *vulvar pain*: *vulv-* referring to the vulva plus *-odynia* from the Greek meaning pain. It is similar to scrotodynia in the male or glossodynia. When doing a literature search or using the Internet, be sure that you use the term vulv*o*dynia, not vulv*a*dynia. Vulvodynia was defined by the International Society for the Study of Vulvovaginal Disease in 1983 as "chronic vulvar discomfort especially that characterized by the patient's complaint of burning (and sometimes stinging, irritation or rawness)." It is a symptom that may have multiple causes. The chronicity of the problem is important to differentiate this entity from other acute causes of vulvar pain, such as vaginitis. There are no prevalence data available at the present time, so one can only guess at the magnitude of this problem. A rough estimation is that about 7% of the population suffers from some sort of dyspareunia, with 2% to 3% having vulvodynia. Because vulvar pain constitutes such a large category, it is helpful for treatment purposes to divide it into subsets. McKay suggested the following categories:

- Vulvar dermatoses
- Cyclic vulvovaginitis
- Vulvar vestibulitis syndrome
- Dysesthetic (essential) vulvodynia
- Pudendal neuralgia

Etiology and Diagnosis

Determining a specific etiology when possible is useful in prescribing the proper treatment.

The patient presents with the symptom of burning, which can be intermittent or constant and is described sometimes as rawness or irritation. The first diagnostic step is a good history and physical. In the history, I specifically look for the nature, location, and duration of the symptoms. Here we must differentiate burning from pruritus and determine the chronicity of the problem. Previous treatments and medications used and their results must be ascertained. It is not unusual for a patient to present with a large bag of medications she has been prescribed. It is important to take the time to review these and the results of their use, either positive or negative. A careful sexual history must be explored, especially changes in sexual practices or contraceptive methods. Hygienic patterns are important. Many women feel "unclean" in this area and respond by excessive washing and douching, which may lead to a vicious circle of irritation and burning.

A pertinent medical history of trauma or metabolic disorders such as diabetes mellitus may be the clue as to the origin of this disorder. There is a high incidence of relationship between vulvodynia and other disorders such as interstitial cystitis, fibromyalgia and irritable bowel syndrome. The cause of this commonality is not known.

Physical examination will lead to important diagnostic aids. One must carefully inspect the entire vulva, especially the area termed the *vesti-*

bule, which extends from the frenulum of the clitoris anteriorly to the forchette posteriorly. The inner borders are the hymenal ring, and the lateral border is Hart's line, marking the beginning of the mucosal membrane, on the inner aspect of the labia minora. Into this space open the major vestibular glands (Bartholin's, Skene's, and periurethral) and the minor vestibular glands. Adequate lighting and magnification are important, and the use of the colposcope is helpful. Carefully inspect for erythema, dermatoses, condylomata, and excoriations. To localize areas of tenderness in the vestibule, I use a moistened applicator stick. Vaginitis must be ruled out, so appropriate cultures are obtained and wet mounts with both saline and potassium hydroxide inspected. Vulvar colposcopy identifies condylomata accuminata and may be helpful in pinpointing areas of hypertrophic lesions that could harbor vulvar interepithelial neoplasia.

Abnormal areas should be biopsied. Biopsies are not generally useful in those areas that show only erythema, the most common finding being chronic inflammation.

After the physical examination, I use the schemata shown in Figure 1 to separate patients into categories for treatment purposes.

The first leg of the schemata constitutes essentially dermatologic problems, such as inflammatory dermatoses, which are discussed in other chapters. Vulvar vestibulitis syndrome is also described elsewhere. This article dwells on what has been called *essential* or *dysesthetic* vulvodynia or *pudendal neuralgia*. The difference between these two entities is ill defined, but I separate them on the basis of whether definitive neurologic findings can be demonstrated. In that case I prefer the term *pudendal neuralgia.*

The chief complaint of patients with this condition is of a constant or intermittent vulvar burning in a diffuse pattern over the entire vulvar area. With pudendal neuralgia, the pain follows the distribution of the pudendal nerve (S2, S3, S4) so the localization of the pain may include a combination of any of these areas: clitoris, vestibule, urethra, labia minora with or without labia majora, perineum with or without the perirectal area, the mons and upper thighs, and even the posterior thighs and legs. Objective sensory findings include allodynia (pain due to a stimulus that does not usually provoke pain), dysesthesia (a spontaneous or evoked disagreeable sensation present with ordinary stimuli), and hyperalgesia (increased response to a stimulus that is normally painful). The symptoms are worse as the day progresses and especially with long periods of sitting.

Understanding the physiology of the burning sensation helps to explain one theory of the causation of this disease. It involves

1. Nerves
2. Mediators
3. Perception

Nociceptors transmit "pain" and "touch" sensations along unmyelinated C fibers. Sensitization of these fibers from prolonged inflammation allows the sensation to remain even after the original stimulus has been removed. Mediators are present in inflamed tissue and consist of biogenic amines such as prostaglandins and histamine and polypeptides like bradykinin and serotonin. The mechanism by which the brain receives these signals may result in the alteration of the perception so that all sensations are perceived as pain.

There is no doubt that there is a psychological aspect to this disease. Any patient with chronic pain that interferes with life for more than 3 months is by definition depressed. A few psychological studies have shown that in general these patients do not differ significantly in many psychological parameters from control patients. Given my personal experience, these patients at

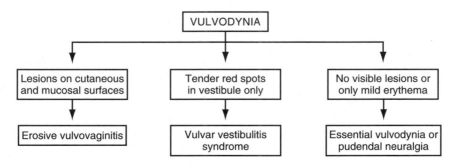

Figure 1. Diagnosis of vulvovaginitis.

the onset of their disease are no different from similar patients once the diagnosis has been made. The major problem is their being shifted from one physician to another with the repeated diagnosis of "yeast" infections. The neurologic theory seems to explain why many varied therapies seem to help, although no *one* therapy works all the time in every patient.

Reid first suggested that this syndrome is associated with the chronic irritation of the vulva, which has many sensory nerves. Anything that would cause chronic irritation could be the initiating factor, such as chronic yeast infections or the irritation of the many topical treatments used in their treatment, herpesvirus infections and a pseudo-postherpetic neuralgia syndrome, trauma either by accident or from prolonged stretching of the pudendal nerve due to childbirth or the use of the dorsal lithotomy position for long periods of time, or chemical or laser destruction of "subclinical" human papillomavirus. Certain metabolites in the urine or many other factors could initiate this cycle. Mediators released by these events activate the nociceptors, causing prolonged firing of the nerves and sensitizing the neurons in the dorsal horn, which then respond abnormally to the "touch" and "pain" fibers so that stimulation of either is reported as pain.

The causes of pudendal neuralgia may range from trauma, neoplasms of the spinal cord, infection, and neurologic disorders to muscle spasm or stress. Recent articles have suggested that pelvic floor adjustment by physical therapy and biofeedback have worked in some patients. Unfortunately, no specific cause is found in most cases and the etiology must be termed idiopathic.

Race is an interesting issue that needs to be addressed. Many case control studies have shown this to be a disease of the white middle-class female. In my practice, there are few patients of either African-American or Hispanic origin with this condition. This finding does not seem to be a function of social or economic factors, since my practice includes many middle-class, well-educated African-Americans. In fact, a fellow African-American obstetrician-gynecologist friend who has an almost complete African-American practice has not seen a single patient with vulvodynia or vulvar vestibulitis. I do not believe this is an issue of communication, but may represent a difference in tissue factors. Attempts to show differences in tissue factors by using vital stains are now under investigation.

Treatment

The treatment for dysesthetic vulvodynia or pudendal neuralgia is the use of tricyclic antide-pressants such as amitriptyline or desipramine. These are neuronal norepinephrine reuptake inhibitors and have been shown to be effective in pain management such as post-herpes zoster neuralgia and diabetic neuropathy, even if no clinical depression is present. I start with the smallest dose and increase the dosage until I get results or the patient complains of significant side effects. With amitriptyline, the most common side effects are drowsiness, constipation, and an increased appetite. This drug should be taken 1 to 2 hours before bedtime. If the side effects are too bothersome, then other similar drugs can be tried, such as desipramine or nortriptyline. Each has its own side effects and must be titrated accordingly. These drugs should not be discontinued abruptly, as severe reactions can occur. The pure serotonin reuptake inhibitors have not been found to be as useful. Sometimes anticonvulsants can be used, such as phenytoin and carbamazepine. These drugs are especially helpful in those patients with paroxysmal or shooting pains in addition to the constant burning pain. Their method of action deals with increasing the threshold at which nerve transmission occurs. Monitoring of blood levels is necessary to obtain therapeutic levels. Liver function tests and blood counts must also be monitored. A careful history of other medications the patient is using is important, as drug interactions are common.

Prophylaxis with acyclovir, 400 mg twice a day, should be reserved for those patients who can be demonstrated to have active lesions associated with flare-ups of their symptoms, and they should be on tricyclic antidepressants.

Measures that decrease irritation of the sensitive vulvar mucosa, such as the use of loose-fitting clothes, hypoallergenic soaps, cold soaks, and the elimination of bubble baths and feminine deodorant sprays, are helpful. Protection of the mucosa with a protective layer of an emollient like plain petroleum jelly or vegetable shortening is helpful in conjunction with the tricyclic antidepressants.

Surgical procedures should be limited to those patients whose symptoms are limited to touch in the vulvar vestibule (see Chapter 56). Many alternative therapies have been tried with some success in some patients. Biofeedback, acupuncture, and transepidermal nerve stimulation (TENS) have been used with varying results.

Although I believe this is not a psychosomatic disorder, psychological support is often necessary to help the patient cope with what may be a severely disabling disorder. There have been sporadic reports of suicide in patients with vulvodynia. There are consumer organizations that offer support groups and are devoted to educating affected women as well encouraging further research to find more effective treatment and eventual cures for vulvodynia. The National Vulvodynia Association is one of these that has a medical advisory board to monitor their newsletter and advice to be sure that a comprehensive picture is presented. It is a nonprofit organization funded through private donations and membership dues.

The key to treatment is early diagnosis. Potential vulvodynia therapies include

1. Vigorously treating the initiating event
2. Stabilizing the dorsal horn with tricyclic antidepressant therapy
3. Breaking the mucosal "pain loops" with symptomatic treatment and removal of all irritants
4. Breaking the deeper "pain loops" with biofeedback or physical therapy
5. Supporting the patient with emotional and psychological help as needed

Symptomatic treatment to improve the mucosal membrane with soaks, hygiene, removal of irritants, and use of an emollient coupled with tricyclic antidepressant medication is the treatment of choice in pure vulvodynia, but many other remedies may need to be tried before a cure for this potentially devastating disease can be accomplished.

Vulvar Vestibulitis

Raymond H. Kaufman, MD

Vulvar vestibulitis has been defined by Friedrich as "severe pain on vestibular touch or vaginal entry; tenderness to pressure localized within the vulvar vestibule; and physical findings confined to vestibular erythema of varying degrees." In addition to the findings, there is a subset of patients demonstrating acetowhite change after washing the vulva with 1% to 5% acetic acid. It has been suggested that this group of individuals may have a human papillomavirus (HPV)–related vestibulitis.

Clinical Presentation

The majority of patients presenting in the physician's office complain about persistent vulvar burning, irritation, and entrance dyspareunia.

Very often there is a complaint of associated mild vulvar pruritus, but more often the patient will indicate that there is a persistent burning that is exacerbated with intercourse. At times, however, the only symptom is that of dyspareunia. Often the patient has been to numerous physicians, repeatedly diagnosed as having vaginitis, especially candidiasis, and treated with a variety of topical medications to the vagina and vulva. These treatment modalities invariably have not relieved the patient's symptoms.

In reviewing the characteristics of patients with vulvar vestibulitis, Mann and colleagues found three factors that appeared to be associated with this problem. In comparing a group of patients with control subjects, they found the patients had a significantly greater frequency of a history of recurrent candidiasis, condyloma acuminata, and allergies. Several other authors have also noted an association between candidiasis and vulvar vestibulitis. However, the occurrence of candidiasis in the patient with vulvar vestibulitis may in fact be somewhat misleading, since many of these patients have been treated for candidiasis on the basis of symptoms alone, when in fact candidal infection may not have been present.

In taking a careful history regarding dyspareunia, the most common complaint consists of pain associated with insertion that lasts through intercourse and for a variable period of time following intercourse, from minutes to days. In many cases the patient finds it necessary to discontinue intercourse because of the pain, or often avoids intercourse because of the fear of pain. This pain is often described as the sensation of rubbing against a raw area, or of sandpaper rubbing against the vulvar vestibule. It is frequently described as a burning, searing type of discomfort. On physical examination, the vulvar vestibule often has a diffuse or localized erythematous appearance. In 77% of the patients reported by Mann, the erythema was diffuse. Often, the areas around the openings of the Bartholin's ducts and Skene's ducts demonstrate an accentuated hyperemia. Occasionally, small micropapillomas may be distributed throughout the vestibule. However, this should not be considered indicative of an HPV infection, since in fact the presence of these small micropapillomas in most instances is not HPV related. Using a moist cotton-tip applicator, the vestibule should be gently palpated. It usually is not necessary to ask the patient if this causes discomfort, since the immediate response on the part of the patient will convey this information to the examining physician. The area between the clitoris and urethra should also be palpated since, occasionally, the changes of vestibulitis extend to this area as well.

Evaluation of the Patient

Following a detailed history and physical examination, KOH and saline wet mount preparations should be obtained from the vagina, looking for the presence of pathogens. A culture for candida, which should be plated on Sabouraud's medium, should also be obtained. The vaginal pH should be measured; this can easily be done with colorpHast indicator strips (EM Science; Cherry Hill, NJ). A pH in the range of 4 is indicative of either a healthy vaginal ecosystem or may be associated with the presence of a vaginal candidal infection. Following these tests, the vulvar vestibule should be washed with 4% to 5% acetic acid and sufficient time allowed for an acetowhite change to develop. The development of a distinct acetowhite change may be indicative of the presence of an HPV infection. This has been demonstrated by Umpierre and colleagues, who found a correlation between the presence of acetowhite change and the finding of HPV DNA in biopsy specimens from the vulvar vestibule. The development of an acetowhite appearance may be diffuse or patchy. The borders of this change are somewhat irregular, and small acetowhite islands are frequently noticed distant from the central area of change.

In most instances, it is not necessary to obtain a biopsy from the vulvar vestibule. In the overwhelming majority of cases, nonspecific chronic inflammatory changes will be seen. Although the finding of distinct acetowhite change is probably adequate to presume that the vestibulitis is HPV related, the demonstration of koilocytosis within the biopsy specimen lends credence to this diagnosis.

Treatment

For patients with mild signs and symptoms, or with recent onset of symptoms (less than 6 months), conservative therapy may be instituted. This therapy consists of warm sitz baths several times daily, lubrication with intercourse, and the use of a 1% hydrocortisone cream applied topically to the vestibule several times a day. Patients use a wide variety of lubricants for intercourse; however, the use of plain vegetable shortening has proven to be as effective as any of the commercially available lubricants. If a candidal infection is found, this should be appropriately treated with one of the antifungal agents instilled into the vagina or with a 150 mg fluconazole (D flucan) tablet taken orally. A follow-up culture should be obtained 1 month after completion of therapy to be sure that the candidal organisms are no longer present on culture.

It is only the occasional patient who is able to tolerate the discomfort following these measures, and in whom no additional management is required. In the overwhelming majority of cases, conservative therapy proves to be inadequate, and patients return with the same complaints they had prior to institution of such treatment. In such cases further management is necessary.

Further therapy in our clinic has consisted either of the use of intralesional interferon biofeedback, or perineoplasty. Initially, it was believed that interferon, would be of value in managing patients with vulvar vestibulitis that was HPV related. Early studies certainly suggested this. More recent experience suggests, however, that the response to interferon is in no way related to the presence or absence of HPV DNA within biopsy specimens taken from patients with vulvar vestibulitis. Those patients without evidence of HPV DNA appear to respond equally to those in whom this is found. It can only be presumed that the interlesional interferon acts in some way in modulating the local immune response of the tissues and, in this fashion, brings about a resolution of the vestibular inflammation. When this approach to therapy is followed, a total of 12 injections into the vestibule in an "around-the-clock" fashion is carried out (Fig. 1). The injections are given three times a week for a period of 4 weeks. In some cases, however, when the reaction to the interferon has been minimal, we have injected two sites at each visit, thus cutting the number of office visits almost in half. Each injection consists of 1 million units of recombinant alpha-2A -interferon, diluted to 0.5 mL with saline. A different site (or two sites) is injected at each visit. A 30-gauge needle is used and inserted just outside the hymenal ring beneath the vestibular mucosa. As the interferon is injected, the needle is slowly withdrawn and inserted in a different direction, "fanning out" the distribution of the solution. In most instances, the patients develop flu-like symptoms following the first, and sometimes the second, injection of interferon. Following this, however, adverse responses to the medication rarely occur. Patients are given a 500 mg capsule of Tylenol at the time of each injection to minimize these symptoms. We have had success in alleviating the symptoms of vestibulitis in 50% of the patients treated with interferon. Marinoff and

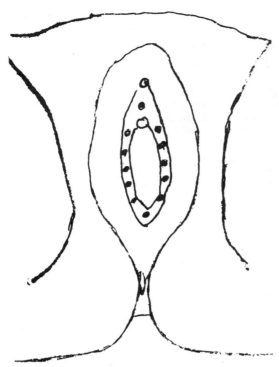

Figure 1. Sites for submucosal injection of alpha interferon. (From Kaufman RH, Friedrich EG, Gardner HL: Benign Diseases of the Vulva and Vagina. Chicago: Mosby-Yearbook Medical Publishers, 1989.)

Turner have had similar results and have suggested that, on the basis of cost-effectiveness, it may pay to arbitrarily first treat with alpha interferon all patients with vulvar vestibulitis, thus avoiding a surgical procedure in those who respond.

Recently, Glazer and colleagues proposed the use of biofeedback in managing patients with vulvar vestibulitis. If this approach is utilized, it is important that the patient be referred to a facility that is familiar with biofeedback involving the pelvic musculature. Generally, a physical therapist trained in this area or a pain clinic with specific knowledge related to biofeedback training of the pelvic outlet musculature is recommended. Patients are given a computerized electromyographic evaluation of the pelvic floor muscles and then given portable electromyographic biofeedback instrumentation with instructions on how to perform at home daily biofeedback-assisted pelvic floor muscle rehabilitation exercises. Patients are then seen on a regular basis to be sure that they are complying with instructions and are using the instruments correctly. Their progress and symptomatology are evaluated at each visit. Glazer observed that after

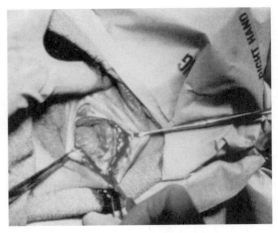

Figure 2. A U-shaped incision is made beginning in the region of Skene's ducts and carried down along Hart's line to the midperineum.

an average of 16 weeks, pelvic floor muscle contractions increased 95% and the resting muscle tension levels decreased by almost 70%. Muscle instability decreased by 62%. They reported subjective decrease in pain in 83% of 33 women studied. Twenty-two of 28 women who had abstained from intercourse for an average of 13 months were able to resume intercourse. A 6-month follow-up of these patients revealed maintenance of therapeutic benefits.

When symptoms persist following conservative therapy, the use of intralesional interferon or

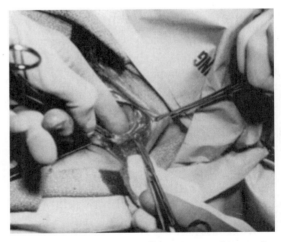

Figure 3. The vestibule and vagina are then undermined so that vaginal mucosa can be attached to the adjacent skin without tension.(From Kaufman RH, Friedrich EG, Gardner HL. Benign Diseases of the Vulva and Vagina. Chicago: Mosby-Yearbook Medical Publishers, 1989, p 343.)

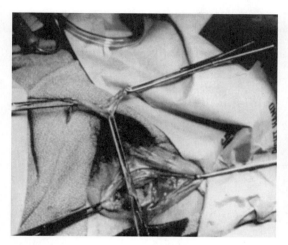

Figure 4. The specimen includes the vulvar vestibule and portions of the upper perineal skin. The hymenal ring is also removed. (From Kaufman RH, Friedrich EG, Gardner HL: Benign Diseases of the Vulva and Vagina. Chicago: Mosby-Yearbook Medical Publishers, 1989.)

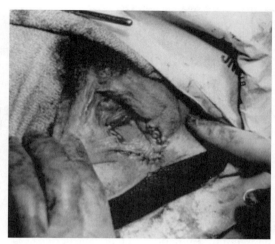

Figure 5. The vaginal mucosa is approximated to the skin edges. (From Kaufman RH, Friedrich EG, Gardner HL. Benign Diseases of the Vulva and Vagina. Chicago: Mosby-Yearbook Medical Publishers, 1989, p 343.)

biofeedback, perineoplasty is often the definitive therapy. Perineoplasty is also frequently recommended as primary treatment to older patients and to patients living outside the city. This operation is carried out in the hospital under general anesthesia with the patient in the lithotomy position. A scalpel blade is used to outline the incision, which should begin in the region of the Skene's ducts, and continue out laterally and superiorly for approximately 0.5 to 1 cm. The incision should then continue inferiorly along Hart's line to the midportion of the perineal skin (Fig. 2). Using a scissor, the entire strip of mucosa and skin is then undermined up beyond the hymenal ring, both laterally and inferiorly (Fig. 3). A Y-shaped portion of tissue is then excised (Fig. 4), with the inner incision running just inside the hymenal ring. In other words, almost the entire hymenal ring should be removed. The vagina is

then further mobilized so that it can be pulled down and out to the edges of the incision without tension. Frequently, there is a brisk and constant oozing of blood from the operative bed. These bleeding points should be controlled with ligatures or electrodesiccation. Once adequate hemostasis has been obtained, the deeper layer of tissue is approximated using 3-0 interrupted Dexon sutures. This accomplishes further hemostasis and also takes tension off the line of closure of the vaginal mucosa to the lateral and perineal skin. Once the deeper layer of sutures has been placed, an outer layer of interrupted 3-0 Dexon sutures is then placed, coapting the vaginal mucosa to the skin edges (Fig. 5). This closure should be without tension; otherwise the edges may pull apart during the postoperative period, resulting in scarring and further discomfort. During the dissection, care must be taken

TABLE 1. Dyspareunia 6 Months After Treatment Compared with Control Subjects°

Dyspareunia	Perineoplasty (*n* = 56)	Interferon (*n* = 13)	Both (*n* = 2)	Controls (*n* = 69)
None	19 (36%)	3 (25%)	1 (50%)	33 (48%)
Sometimes	22 (42%)	3 (25%)	1 (50%)	34 (49%)
Often	6 (11%)	1 (8%)		2 (3%)
Always	6 (11%)	5 (42%)		
No response to question	3	1		

°From Mann M, Kaufman RH, Brown D. Vulvar vestibulitis: Significant clinical variables and treatment outcome. Am J Obstet Gynecol 1992; 79:122–125.

TABLE 2. Degree of Vulvar Pain 6 Months After Treatment[*]

Vulvar Pain	Perineoplasty (n = 56)	Interferon (n = 13)	Both (n = 2)
100 % improved	16 (29%)		
Much improved	21 (37%)	5 (38%)	1 (50%)
Somewhat improved	12 (21%)	7 (54%)	
No change	5 (9%)	1 (8%)	1 (50%)
Worse	1 (2%)		
No response to question	1 (2%)		

[*]From Mann M, Kaufman RH, Brown D. Vulvar vestibulitis: Significant clinical variables and treatment outcome. Am J Obstet Gynecol 1992; 79:122–125.

to identify and avoid injury to the urethra and the rectum. Immediately following surgery, an ice pack is placed on the perineum. No perioperative antibiotics are used. The patient is encouraged to void and, once she does so spontaneously, she is discharged from the hospital and instructed to begin warm sitz baths three times daily until she is seen for a postoperative visit, scheduled 4 to 6 weeks following the surgery.

During the first week following surgery, the patients will frequently complain of significant discomfort, swelling, discharge, and slight bleeding. Analgesics by mouth will usually alleviate the pain, and warm sitz baths will aid in the subsidence of the edema and discharge. Once the operative site is well healed, the patient is encouraged to resume intercourse, using a lubricant, approximately 6 to 8 weeks following surgery. In our experience, approximately 78% of patients had significant relief of dyspareunia following surgery (Table 1). Sixty-six percent of the patients indicated that there was a significant decrease in the vulvar pain following treatment, and another 2% indicated that the vulvar burning and pain had decreased, but was still present to a minor degree (Table 2).

In those patients who continue to have symptoms following perineoplasty, it is occasionally necessary to excise residual areas of vestibulitis that were not removed during the first procedure. Probably the most common cause for failure is an inadequate operation; that is, insufficient vestibular tissue has been removed. The hymonal ring should be routinely removed as part of the procedure; when this is not done, it frequently does not result in relief of symptoms for the patient. I suspect that the procedure of perineoplasty, including excision and mobilization of the vestibular tissue, causes considerable relaxation of the vaginal outlet, which may be the reason so many of these patients have significant improvement in the symptom of entrance dyspareunia.

In the occasional patient who has residual pain and tenderness around the opening of the Bartholin's or Skene's ducts, spot lasering of these areas may relieve residual symptoms. As a rule, however, the use of the carbon dioxide laser to treat diffuse areas of the vulvar vestibule is to be discouraged, since in many instances the patient's symptoms have been increased by this approach.

Gynecologic Malignancies

Cancer Screening

Robert E. Rogers, MD

Screening for cancer should be a role for every primary care physician. The annual health maintenance examination provides an excellent opportunity to search for early cancer in several areas. All women should begin an annual health checkup, to include a pelvic and breast examination, at age 18 or with the onset of sexual activity.

Not every neoplastic condition is suitable for screening. A suitable condition should have a high prevalence, a significant mortality, a preclinical phase, and improved outcome if found early. The neoplastic condition that has been the model for other conditions is cervical cancer. Cervical cancer fits all of the requirements of an ideal condition for screening. Tests for other neoplastic conditions in women are being sought, and several are being evaluated for their suitability in terms of cost-effective screening strategies.

Cervical Cancer

At one time cervical cancer was a leading cause of death in young women. Mortality rates have decreased considerably in the past 30 years. The reason for this decrease is not fully explained, but the availability of cancer screening techniques is certainly a factor. Cervical cytology (the Papanicolaou smear) is of primary importance in the diagnosis of preinvasive lesions of the cervix. When cancer is recognized and treated effectively in its developmental phase, there is a marked decrease in the incidence of invasive cancer and subsequent death.

The American College of Obstetricians and Gynecologists, in agreement with a number of other medical organizations, has suggested that cervical cytology and pelvic examination should be obtained starting at age 18 or with the onset of sexual activity and repeated annually. After three or more consecutive, satisfactory, normal examinations, the cervical smear might be performed less frequently at the discretion of the physician. Smears should be performed at 1- to 3-year intervals, depending on the presence of risk factors for cervical cancer. Some of the risk factors for cervical cancer include genital infec-

tion with human papillomavirus, infection with human immunodeficiency virus, multiple sex partners, cigarette smoking, and having high-risk partners.

A cervical cytologic sample is easily obtained by scraping the external cervix with a wood or plastic device to include the entire transformation zone. The endocervix should be sampled with a cotton-tipped applicator or preferably with an endocervical brush. The material is then spread on a glass slide, properly fixed, and sent to a laboratory for evaluation. Most modern cytology laboratories are reporting their results using the Bethesda system for reporting cervical/vaginal cytologic diagnoses.

The Bethesda system allows the laboratory to report their findings in a more precise manner than previous systems allowed. Squamous cell abnormalities are reported as

1. atypical squamous cells of undetermined significance
2. low-grade squamous intraepithelial lesion (human papillomavirus or mild dysplasia/cervical intraepithelial neoplasia [CIN] I)
3. high-grade squamous intraepithelial lesion (moderate or severe dysplasia, carcinoma in situ/CIN II and CIN III)
4. squamous cell carcinoma

Glandular cell abnormalities are reported as

1. atypical glandular cells of uncertain significance
2. adenocarcinoma, site specified if possible

Following an abnormal cytology report, the cervix should be carefully evaluated. All suspicious cervical lesions should be biopsied in the office. Most low-grade and high-grade intraepithelial lesions should be evaluated colposcopically and abnormalities biopsied. An endocervical curettage is usually performed unless the patient is pregnant. Persistent atypical squamous cells of undetermined significance should be evaluated colposcopically if the smear remains abnormal after a 3- to 6-month interval.

Management of Abnormal Cervical Cytology (Fig. 1)
Breast Cancer

Over 180,000 women in the United States develop breast cancer on an annual basis, and

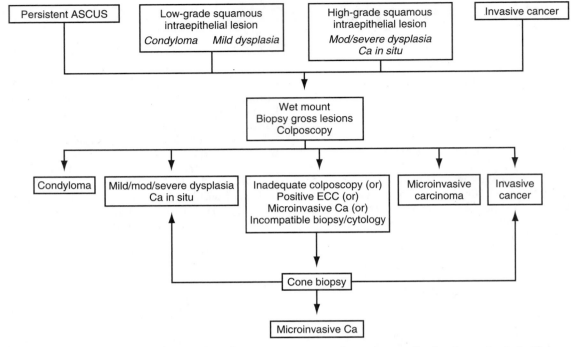

Figure 1. Diagnosis of abnormal cervical condition. ASCUS, atypical squamous cells of undetermined significance; Ca, carcinoma; ECC, endocervical curettage; Mod, moderate.

46,000 die of the disease each year. It appears that the disease is being diagnosed earlier with the aid of mammography, and there is hope that this will be reflected in a decrease in mortality in the near future. Several screening strategies are important to the patient.

Self breast examination must be taught to every young woman and its use on a monthly basis reinforced. Self breast examination is best performed just after each menstrual period. Many pamphlets and other teaching devices are available for patient education.

An annual breast assessment that is meticulously and methodically performed is important. Mammography is an important tool that has been recognized as effective and beneficial. Periodic mammography should begin sometime between 35 and 45 years of age, depending on the patient's breast findings and history of family breast disease. Annual mammography should begin at age 50 and be continued for life. The technique is known to be safe, although unfortunately it is costly.

The recent isolation of the *BRCA1* gene provides an opportunity for screening women from families with a history of early-onset breast or ovarian cancer that appears to be inherited in an autosomal dominant pattern. Women who have the *BRCA1* gene mutation have an 80% to 90%

lifetime risk of breast cancer, a 40% to 65% lifetime risk of ovarian cancer, and an increased risk of colon cancer. The place of *BRCA1* gene testing is still under study. Many questions remain regarding the use of the test and the counseling and follow-up strategies that must accompany the test.

Endometrial Cancer

Endometrial cancer is the most common genital cancer in older women. Approximately 32,000 new cases of endometrial cancer appear each year, and approximately 8000 women die of this disease annually. There is no cost-effective screening tool available for asymptomatic women. The most common symptom in patients with endometrial cancer is postmenopausal uterine bleeding. Women with abnormal bleeding in the perimenopausal time frame should be evaluated with endometrial biopsy. While routine endometrial biopsy and routine pelvic ultrasonographic examination in asymptomatic patients has been advocated by some, it does not appear to be cost-effective.

Ovarian Cancer

Approximately 21,000 new cases of ovarian cancer occur each year, and approximately 13,000 of these women die. One woman in every 70 will develop ovarian cancer during her lifetime. This neoplasm is the leading cause of death from gynecologic cancer. Because of the deadly nature of this cancer, the search for a sensitive, specific, and cost-effective screening procedure carries a high priority. The availability of such a test would be important because most ovarian cancers are diagnosed in an advanced stage. Research into a number of techniques continues, among them serum CA 125, *BRCA1* gene evaluation, and pelvic and transvaginal ultrasonography. Although these techniques might be useful in women with a history of familial ovarian cancer, they are not suitable for mass screening.

Colorectal Cancer

There were approximately 77,000 new cases of colorectal cancer in women in 1996, and approximately 29,000 of these women are likely to die. Most colorectal cancer patients may be identified in a high-risk group. Physicians should be particularly vigilant in their surveillance of patients who have a history of colon polyps. Inflammatory bowel disease and a number of genetic disorders, such as familial adenomatous polyposis, familial colorectal cancer syndrome, and Lynch II syndrome, commonly precede colorectal cancer. Since the majority of the cancers of the colorectum occur within reach of the examining finger, a digital rectal examination should be performed at the time of each pelvic examination, particularly after the age of 50. Fecal examination for occult blood is not a particularly specific indicator of colorectal cancer but is important in that it leads to other diagnostic studies. Colorectal endoscopy is possibly one of the most effective tools for screening. Over 50% of cancers should be visible with flexible sigmoidoscopy. All cancers should be visible with colonoscopy. The American Cancer Society has recommended sigmoidoscopy every 3 to 5 years after the age of 50 years. The screening interval depends on the patient's risk factors.

Lung Cancer

Lung cancer is the most common cause of death secondary to malignant disease in the United States in both men and women. Approximately 66,000 cases of lung cancer were diagnosed in women last year, and the incidence continues to increase; 53,000 of those women affected will die. The majority of lung cancer occurs in women who smoke; therefore the practitioner should be especially sensitive to symptoms in this group. There are no accepted guidelines for lung cancer screening. Regular screening with chest radiography or sputum cytology has had no effect on mortality. An annual chest radiograph in smoking women after the age of 50 is supported in some areas.

Vulvar Cancer

The vulva is an organ that, like the breast, is available for self-examination. Self-examination should be taught to patients and should be performed on a monthly basis at the time of her self breast examination. Examination is easily performed by palpating the vulva and inspecting it with a mirror. Any abnormalities or changes in vulvar skin should be reported to the physician.

Examination of the vulva should be routinely performed at the time of the annual examination. There is no absolutely characteristic finding in preinvasive disease of the vulva; any suspicious area should be biopsied. Raised white lesions are particularly suspect. Itching and the presence of a vulvar mass are common complaints.

One of the most significant services that a physician can provide to the female patient is to make her aware of the importance of the annual health assessment. While cancer screening techniques are not available or cost-efficient for all of the common neoplastic conditions in the female patient, the opportunity to evaluate her pelvis and breasts and to educate her in regard to personal health strategies may save her life.

Cervical Carcinoma

Matthew F. Kohler, MD

Philip J. DiSaia, MD

Both the incidence and mortality rate of invasive cervical cancer have declined dramatically in the United States since the introduction of widespread Pap smear screening. Nonetheless, in 1998, there were 13,700 cases of invasive cervical cancer registered in the United States, with 4900 deaths. Invasive cervical cancer remains the leading cancer-related cause of death in developing countries.

In concert with the decline in invasive cervical cancer in countries where Pap smear screening programs have been instituted, there has been a dramatic increase in the frequency of preinvasive cervical intraepithelial neoplasia. Therefore the clinician must remain familiarized with the diagnosis and management of a full spectrum of cervical neoplasia.

Epidemiology

A variety of factors have been associated with an increased risk of developing invasive cervical cancer, including a young age at first intercourse, multiple sexual partners, intercourse with males who have had multiple sexual partners, and cigarette smoking. In many respects, the epidemiology of cervical cancer mimics that of a sexually transmitted disease, which has prompted a search for a responsible infectious agent. While a number of infectious agents have been implicated, the association of human papillomavirus (HPV) infection with both invasive cervical cancer and cervical intraepithelial neoplasia appears particularly strong. HPV is a DNA virus with more than 60 subtypes. Certain "high-risk" HPV subtypes (16 and 18 in particular, but also 31, 33, and 35) can be demonstrated in the great majority of invasive cervical cancers and high-grade cervical intraepithelial neoplasias, which are known to have a significant premalignant potential. In contrast, "low-risk" HPV subtypes (6, 11) are more commonly associated with benign genital condyloma and low-grade cervical intraepithelial neoplasias, which are far less likely to progress to invasive cervical cancer. In invasive cervical cancers, HPV is usually found integrated into the host cell DNA, whereas in cervical intraepithelial neoplasia (CIN), the HPV DNA is usually present in episomal (nonintegrated) form. Within the infected cervical tissues, HPV gener-ates the E6 and E7 viral proteins, which are capable of binding to, and inactivating, the products of the critical $p53$ and Rb tumor suppressor genes, respectively.

Pap Smear Screening

In countries that have adopted the widespread use of exfoliative cytology (Pap smear) to screen for cervical neoplasia, the incidence and mortality rate of invasive cervical cancer have declined substantially. The prevention of cervical cancer by means of mass screening programs is possible because most cervical carcinomas are preceded by well-defined premalignant lesions that progress only after a relatively long latency period. Nonetheless, the success of Pap smear screening depends on the quality of the specimen and accurate cytologic interpretation. Approximately 10% of smears are reported to be technically inadequate, due to sampling errors or air-drying artifacts. Moreover, technically adequate but falsely negative Pap smears are not uncommon; 15% to 25% of cervical intraepithelial lesions are associated with a normal Pap smear, and grossly obvious invasive cervical cancers are occasionally found in patients whose Pap smear show only necrotic debris or inflammation. Finally, the potential for laboratory error in the interpretation of Pap smears, while probably uncommon, has been well publicized in recent media headlines.

In 1988, the Bethesda system was introduced for the interpretation of cervical cytology and has gradually supplanted older classification systems. In the Bethesda system, two designations describe cytologic abnormalities suggestive of underlying cervical intraepithelial neoplasia. A Pap smear reporting low-grade squamous intraepithelial lesion refers to cytologic abnormalities that on biopsy usually correspond to HPV effect only or CIN 1 (mild dysplasia), although low-grade squamous intraepithelial lesion is occasionally found in association with histologic evidence of CIN 2 or 3. A Pap smear reporting a high-grade squamous intraepithelial lesion demonstrates cytologic abnormalities that usually correspond to CIN 2 or 3 on biopsy but may be found in association with invasive cancer as well. The Bethesda system also has a third category for epithelial cell abnormalities termed atypical squamous cells of uncertain significance (AS-CUS). Although the clinical significance and management of Pap smears demonstrating AS-CUS is controversial, consideration must be given to the fact that 20% of ASCUS will be found in association with underlying cervical dysplasia. The American College of Obstetricians and Gynecologists and the American Cancer Society currently recommend that all women receive annual Pap smears beginning at age 18 or when they become sexually active. If three consecutive annual Pap smears have been normal, subsequent screening examinations may be obtained at less frequent intervals in women who are considered to be at low risk for cervical neoplasia.

Management of the Abnormal Pap Smear and Cervical Intraepithelial Neoplasia

Because it represents a screening test and not a tissue diagnosis, the Pap smear must not be used to direct definitive therapy. In the absence of a gross cervical lesion, the finding of intraepithelial neoplasia or carcinoma on Pap smear should prompt colposcopic examination of the cervix. During colposcopy, the cervix is painted with 3% to 5% acetic acid (which accentuates areas of high nuclear to cytoplasmic ratio found in dysplastic cells) and examined with a low-power (16×) microscope. To be deemed adequate, the colposcopic examination must include inspection of the entire squamocolumnar junction (transformation zone). Areas of abnormal-appearing epithelium are biopsied and a gentle endocervical curettage is performed, unless the patient is pregnant, in which case biopsies and endocervical curettage are deferred unless colposcopy suggests invasive carcinoma.

Definitive treatment may proceed if (1) an adequate colposcopic examination has been performed that visualizes the extent of the lesion, (2) cervical intraepithelial neoplasia has been documented by biopsy that can account for the Pap smear findings, (3) the endocervical curettage is negative, and (4) microinvasion has not been demonstrated. If any of these criteria are not met, additional diagnostic evaluation, such as cold knife or loop electrosurgical excision procedure (LEEP) cervical conization may be indicated.

Since the regression rate for low-grade squamous intraepithelial lesions is significant, many clinicians elect to follow this lesion without specific treatment, but patient expectations and reliability of follow-up are usually taken into consideration. Given their well-defined premalignant potential, high-grade cervical intraepithelial neoplasias (CIN 2 or CIN 3) should be treated definitively. Some clinicians prefer ablative meth-

ods such as cryotherapy and laser, and others excisional techniques such as LEEP, but the clinical efficacy of these modalities is very similar. Since it provides a tissue specimen that is often diagnostic and therapeutic, some clinicians employ LEEP at the initial evaluation of patients with Pap smear and colposcopic evidence of high-grade dysplasia (who are likely to require definitive treatment), thereby eliminating redundant cervical biopsies and treatment delays. With this approach, however, there is a significant potential for overtreatment of patients with minimal lesions. Moreover, while generally safe, LEEP is associated with delayed hemorrhage (5%) and cervical stenosis (1–3%) and should not be regarded as a benign procedure.

Management of Invasive Cervical Carcinoma

Microinvasion

A diagnosis of invasive cervical cancer is rendered with the demonstration of malignant squamous epithelium below the basement membrane. However, lesions that demonstrate minimal stromal invasion (termed microinvasive) have generally a low risk of lymph node metastasis and recurrence. While a number of definitions of microinvasive cervical cancers have been proposed, it is clear that cancers with less than 3 mm of stromal invasion and no vascular space invasion or tumor confluency are associated with a very small risk (1%) of lymph node metastases. As a result, most clinicians believe that cervical conization (if further childbearing is desired) or simple extrafascial hysterectomy (if childbearing has been completed) are adequate treatment for such lesions. If hysterectomy is contemplated and the diagnosis of microinvasion has been arrived at by punch biopsy alone, however, cervical conization is always indicated first to exclude a more deeply invasive cervical cancer, the therapy of which is necessarily more radical (see later).

Somewhat more controversial is the treatment of cervical cancers with 3 to 5 mm of stromal invasion (FIGO stage 1A2). However, since review of the literature indicates that approximately 7% of stage 1A2 cancers are associated with pelvic lymph node metastases, we believe that management of these lesions should be similar to that of stage 1B cancers.

Stage 1B/Stage 2A

By FIGO definition, cervical cancers with more than 5 mm of stromal invasion or 7 mm of horizontal spread are classified as stage 1B cancers. Moreover, the finding of **any** degree of stromal invasion in a cervical lesion that is grossly visible designates at least stage 1B disease. Extension to the upper one third of the vagina but with no evidence of parametrial or sidewall disease, or ureteral obstruction, designates a stage 2A cancer.

The patient who presents with a grossly apparent cervical tumor should undergo a biopsy under direct visualization to establish a tissue diagnosis. Monsel's solution or vaginal packing can be employed if necessary to control troublesome bleeding after biopsy. Cervical conization or dilatation and curettage are unnecessary in the evaluation of grossly visible cervical cancers and may cause severe hemorrhage.

Stage 1B and 2A cervical cancers may be treated with either a radical hysterectomy and pelvic lymphadenectomy or with radiotherapy. Numerous studies have demonstrated essentially identical survival rates for these two treatment modalities, although their potential treatment-related complications differ considerably. Radical hysterectomy with pelvic lymphadenectomy is a 3- to 5-hour procedure and should be considered only in patients who are reasonable surgical candidates. The procedure differs greatly from a simple extrafascial hysterectomy insofar as the retroperitoneal spaces are extensively developed, the uterine artery is taken at its origin from the hypogastric, the cardinal and uterosacral ligaments are divided at their lateral origins, the ureter is dissected out completely from its attachments to the vesicouterine ligament, and the upper one third of the vagina is taken with the specimen. In addition, all visible lymph node–bearing tissue is removed from the pelvic vessels. As such, hemorrhage, bladder dysfunction (caused by interruption of bladder parasympathetic nerves) and a 1% to 2% incidence of genitourinary fistulae are all potential surgical complications. Infection and pulmonary emboli have decreased with the routine use of antibiotics and thromboembolism prophylaxis.

Pelvic radiotherapy generally involves the initial administration of out-patient external beam radiation over 4 to 6 weeks followed by one or two intracavitary or interstitial implants. While the morbidity of a major abdominal operation is avoided, most patients will experience some degree of acute radiation cystitis or proctitis, and 5% to 10% may develop serious late sequelae including radiation-induced bowel obstruction and gastrointestinal fistulae. Moreover, it should be remembered that placement of the radiation implants requires hospitalization with at least one

(usually more) anesthetics, with prolonged immobility and attendant risks of thromboembolism.

We tend to favor radical hysterectomy in patients with stage 1B/2A cervical cancer who are good surgical candidates, believing that it offers particular advantages for young patients. Since squamous cancers of the cervix almost never metastasize to the ovaries, radical hysterectomy allows for ovarian preservation, which is not possible with radiotherapy. Radical hysterectomy also provides for better preservation of vaginal length and function, an important consideration in sexually active women. Finally, radical hysterectomy allows for a direct histopathologic assessment of the pelvic lymph nodes, supplying important prognostic information. On the other hand, radiotherapy should be offered as an option to all patients and may be particularly appropriate for patients who are poor surgical candidates, very elderly, or morbidly obese.

The management of bulky (>4 cm) or barrel-shaped (endophytic growth pattern) early-stage cervical cancers remains controversial. Some centers favor primary radiotherapy alone while others prefer preoperative radiotherapy followed by extrafascial hysterectomy. We have tended to employ radical hysterectomy and pelvic lymphadenectomy with adjuvant postoperative external beam radiotherapy and have reported patient survival rates similar to those achieved with other treatment modalities, with acceptable morbidity. We and others have reported that neoadjuvant chemotherapy can often reduce tumor volume dramatically prior to radical hysterectomy, although the extent to which this may contribute to improved survival remains to be determined. Regardless of treatment, bulky cervical cancers are associated with a worse outcome, a fact now implicit in the subdivision of stage 1B cancers into stage 1B1 (<4 cm) and stage 1B2 (>4 cm) lesions in the updated FIGO staging system.

Stage 2B and Above

Patients with suspected advanced-stage cervical cancer should undergo an examination under anesthesia with cystoscopy and proctoscopy prior to initiation of therapy, as this provides the optimal setting to assess tumor volume, to detect extension of disease into the parametrium (stage 2B) or sidewall (stage 3B), and to exclude bladder or rectal invasion (stage 4A). At a minimum, patients should also undergo a metastatic survey consisting of chest radiograph, intravenous pyelogram, and routine hematologic and chemistry profiles. Abdominal and pelvic CT scanning is frequently used to aid in treatment planning, as it may allow the detection of extrapelvic nodal and distant metastatic disease, but the findings of computed tomographic scanning cannot be considered when assigning FIGO stage.

In the past, pretreatment staging laparotomy was performed routinely prior to initiating treatment for patients with advanced-stage cervical cancers, to detect occult para-aortic lymph node metastases requiring extension of standard radiation portals. Serious bowel complications were common, however, particularly when a transperitoneal approach to periaortic lymphadenectomy was utilized in patients who then underwent aortic radiation. More recently, a retroperitoneal approach to para-aortic lymphadenectomy has been emphasized, leading to a reduction in morbidity. However, since only a minority of patients are expected to benefit from the information gained from pretreatment staging laparotomy, we believe that this procedure should be offered only in the setting of research protocols. Pelvic radiotherapy remains the mainstay of treatment for patients with advanced-stage cervical cancer in the United States. Five-year survival rates for patients with stage 2B and stage 3B cancers average 60% and 30%, respectively. There is evidence from a randomized Gynecologic Oncology Group study that oral hydroxyurea, acting as a radiosensitizer, can improve outcome in patients with advanced cervical cancer undergoing radiation therapy. Ongoing Gynecologic Oncology Group studies are currently investigating the activity of various systemic chemotherapy agents as radiosensitizers in advanced cervical cancers.

Recurrent Disease

Most patients who are destined to develop disease progression or recurrence following treatment for invasive cervical cancer will do so within 2 years of diagnosis, and frequent follow-up visits (every 3 months) with pelvic examination and Pap smears should be performed during this time. Complaints of vaginal bleeding, weight loss, unilateral leg edema, and sciatic pain are worrisome, although not pathognomonic of disease recurrence, and should be investigated with thorough pelvic examination, biopsies, and appropriate radiographic surveys. Patients with recurrent disease confined to the central pelvis can be considered for pelvic exenteration, which offers a realistic possibility of cure (30–50%) to highly selected patients. Advances in techniques of surgical reconstruction, including the use of low

rectal anastomosis, continent urinary diversion, myocutaneous and omental flaps for neovagina creation, and pelvic revascularization have improved the quality of life in patients undergoing exenteration. Unfortunately, only a tiny percentage of patients with recurrent cervical cancer will be candidates for exenteration, with most patients manifesting unresectable disease beyond the pelvis, for which palliative chemotherapy may be offered. Response rates to even the most active agents remain modest, however, so quality of life must be considered prior to initiating treatment.

The Future

Novel strategies continue to evolve for the treatment of invasive cervical cancer, such as high dose rate afterloading brachytherapy and the use of neoadjuvant and radiosensitizing chemotherapy, but may ultimately yield only modest improvements in patient outcome. Perhaps more promising is research currently directed toward additional preventative measures, such as the development of anti-HPV cervical cancer vaccines, which may be particularly relevant to the Third World, where screening is often unavailable, and the use of protein biomarkers and computer-assisted Pap smear analysis, which ultimately may improve the accuracy of cytologic screening. Nonetheless, since cervical cancer is largely preventable using currently available technology, efforts must continue to educate the public, physicians, and managed-care providers about the importance of regular Pap smear screening.

Endometrial Carcinoma

Andrew Berchuck, MD
Frank D. Cirisano, MD

More than 30,000 new cases of endometrial cancer are diagnosed in the United States each year, and the median age at presentation is 60 years. Most women who develop this condition consult a physician because of abnormal uterine bleeding. Endometrial biopsy is the cornerstone of proper diagnosis. The vast majority of endometrial cancers are adenocarcinomas, whereas uterine sarcomas constitute only 3% to 5% of cases. Most endometrial adenocarcinomas resemble normal endometrium and are called endometrioid adenocarcinomas. In contrast, there are three histologic variants that are associated with advanced stage disease and poor survival, namely adenosquamous cancer, clear cell adenocarcinoma, and papillary serous adenocarcinoma. Fortunately, the majority of endometrial cancers are still confined to the uterus at diagnosis, and 70% to 80% of patients are cured.

Primary Therapy

Once the diagnosis of uterine cancer is confirmed histologically, the patient should be prepared to undergo surgical therapy. Since many of these patients are elderly, however, a careful preoperative medical evaluation should be performed. Women with endometrial cancer frequently are obese and have accompanying medical conditions such as diabetes mellitus and hypertension. These medical problems should be addressed prior to surgery in hopes of avoiding perioperative complications. In addition to a complete history and physical examination and routine preoperative blood tests, a chest radiograph should be performed to exclude the presence of lung metastases. Additional radiographic studies and other diagnostic procedures should be employed selectively in the minority of patients who have signs or symptoms of metastatic disease.

Following the initial evaluation, almost all patients are found to be suitable candidates for primary surgical therapy. In occasional cases in which surgical risk is considered unacceptably high, curative treatment often can be accomplished with radiation therapy. For patients with cancer confined to the uterus, the cure rate with radiation therapy is only 50% to 60%, compared with 80% to 90% with surgery. Patients in whom neither surgery nor radiation can be accomplished are best treated with progestin therapy. Many patients respond well to progestin therapy, as evidenced by cessation of bleeding, and in some cases progestin therapy may be curative.

Women with endometrial cancer often are at increased risk for the development of postoperative deep venous thrombophlebitis due to risk factors such as old age and obesity. Thrombophlebitis leading to pulmonary embolus is the most common cause of postoperative death following surgery for endometrial cancer. Therefore, either minidose heparin or intermittent pneumatic compression devices are used for prophylaxis. In addition, since the vagina is heavily colonized with bacteria, prophylactic antibiotics (cefazolin [Ancef]) are administered periopera-

tively to decrease the incidence of pelvic infection. Finally, prior to surgery, the patient's bowel is prepared with oral magnesium citrate and enemas.

The cornerstone of therapy for the vast majority of patients with endometrial cancer is surgical exploration with removal of the uterus, fallopian tubes, and ovaries. Laparotomy is performed through a midline lower abdominal incision to allow exploration of the upper abdomen. The abdominal organs are carefully palpated, with special attention paid to the omentum and peritoneal surfaces. Following exploration, a self-retaining retractor is placed in the incision and the bowel is packed into the upper abdomen. Approximately 100 mL of normal saline then is instilled into the pelvis, aspirated, and submitted for cytology. Extrafascial hysterectomy and bilateral salpingo-oophorectomy are then performed. After the specimen has been extirpated, the uterus is opened and the cavity is inspected. The location of the cancer and gross depth of invasion into the uterine wall are noted. In many cases frozen section is performed to define the depth of invasion intraoperatively. In addition, a sample of tumor is submitted for determination of estrogen and progesterone receptor levels.

The majority of endometrial adenocarcinomas are either well or moderately differentiated, and these cancers usually are confined to the inner part of the uterine wall. Since these cancers have a low incidence of occult metastases, further staging beyond gross inspection and palpation usually is not productive. If the cancer is poorly differentiated or is noted to invade into the outer one half of the uterine wall, however, surgical staging is performed. This involves sampling of the regional lymph nodes, which are the most common site of occult metastases. Since the lymphatic drainage of the uterus is both to the pelvic sidewall via the cardinal ligaments and to the aortic area via the infundibulopelvic ligaments, lymph nodes in both of these areas are sampled. Occult lymph node metastases are found in 10% of apparent stage I cases.

Approximately 5% to 10% of patients with endometrial cancer will be found to have gross extrauterine disease at surgical exploration. The most common sites of visible metastases are the ovaries, peritoneal surfaces, and lymph nodes. In these cases, attempts usually are made to remove the extrauterine metastases. In addition, although uterine papillary serous cancer frequently is only superficially invasive, it has a propensity to spread throughout the peritoneal cavity, similar to epithelial ovarian cancer. Even when these cancers appear to be confined to the uterus, we routinely biopsy the omentum and peritoneal surfaces in addition to lymph node sampling.

Recently, several groups began to employ a laparascopic approach to the surgical treatment of endometrial cancer. Laparascopically assisted removal of the uterus, fallopian tubes, and ovaries through the vagina is a well-accepted technique. In addition, it has been shown that adequate exploration of the abdominal cavity and pelvic/periaortic lymph node sampling also can be performed laparascopically. The most significant limitation of this approach in treating endometrial cancer is that it is technically difficult in obese women, who represent a significant portion of cases. In addition, if the uterus is enlarged due to cancer it may be impossible to deliver it intact through the vagina. Although we have begun to use the laparoscopic approach in selected cases, the precise indications for this technique still are not well defined.

Most patients with endometrial cancer have stage I or II disease that appears to be confined to the uterus (Table 1), and survival rates for this group are excellent with surgery alone. Since 10% to 20% of patients will develop recurrent cancer, adjuvant therapy often is given to patients at high risk for recurrence. External pelvic radiation has been employed frequently as adjuvant therapy for patients with endometrial cancer, but an unequivocal survival benefit has not been demonstrated. In the past, 30% to 40% of patients with early stage disease have been considered candidates for adjuvant pelvic radiation on the basis of prognostic factors such as poor histologic grade, deep myometrial invasion, or cervical involvement. More recently, selective lymph node sampling has been used to identify patients who actually have evidence of early metastatic disease and are most likely to benefit from adjuvant radiation. Using this selection process, only 10% to 20% of patients receive pelvic radiation. In addition, if aortic lymph nodes are involved, the radiation field can be tailored to include this area, which is not part of the standard pelvic field. Thus, with surgical staging, more patients are spared the potential morbidity of radiation while radiation fields can be planned accurately for patients who are most likely to benefit from adjuvant therapy.

Approximately 10% to 15% of patients with early stage endometrial cancer are found to have malignant cells in pelvic peritoneal washings obtained at laparotomy. Most reports have suggested that positive cytology is associated with an increased risk of recurrence even when there is no other evidence of metastatic disease. When positive cytology is the only evidence of extrauterine spread, we have instilled radioactive ^{32}P intraperitoneally 5 to 7 days postoperatively using a small plastic catheter that is inserted at the time of surgery. Survival of these patients has been better than that of a historical control group. When positive cytology and lymph node metastases are found we do not combine ^{32}P and external radiation, however, since an unacceptably high proportion of patients treated in this fashion subsequently developed small bowel obstruction.

Postsurgical Surveillance and Treatment of Recurrent Disease

Four weeks after surgery the patient is seen back in clinic to assess healing of the abdominal incision and vaginal cuff. Although postsurgical surveillance has not been proven to improve outcome in patients who have undergone treatment for early stage endometrial cancer, we continue to encourage patients to return for periodic examinations. Eighty-five percent of patients who develop recurrence do so within 3 years of primary therapy. Patients are seen every 6 months for the first 3 years and annually the third through fifth years. Detection of vaginal recurrence is the primary focus of our examination, since approximately one half of patients with localized vaginal recurrence can be salvaged with radiation or surgery, or both. A chest radiograph may be ordered on a yearly basis to detect recurrent disease in the lungs, but the utility of this

TABLE 1. FIGO Staging of Endometrial Carcinoma

Stage I	Confined to the uterus
IA	No myometrial invasion
IB	Inner one half myometrial invasion
IC	Outer one half myometrial invasion
Stage II	Cervical involvement
IIA	Endocervical gland involvement
IIB	Cervical stromal invasion
Stage III	
IIIA	Positive peritoneal cytology, adnexal metastases, uterine serosal involvement
IIIB	Vaginal metastases
IIIC	Pelvic or aortic lymph node metastases
Stage IV	
IVA	Bladder or rectal involvement
IVB	Distant metastases

Note: Within each stage, the histologic grade also is recorded: G1, well differentiated; G2, moderately differentiated; G3, poorly differentiated.

FIGO, International Federation of Gynecology and Obstetrics.

practice is dubious since pulmonary metastases cannot be treated effectively.

Endometrial cancer initially recurs locally in the pelvis in 50% of patients, at distant sites in 25% of patients, and at both local and distant sites in 25% of patients. A significant proportion of pelvic recurrences are confined to the vagina and can be cured with radiation therapy. Other pelvic recurrences also usually are treated with radiation, but salvage rates are much poorer. Treatment of distant metastases is with either progestin therapy or cytotoxic chemotherapy. Approximately 25% of patients with metastatic disease will have a significant response to progestins (Megace, Provera), and some of these responses are prolonged. A favorable response to progestins usually occurs in well-differentiated cancers that express steroid receptors. Unfortunately, most cancers that recur are poorly differentiated and do not express steroid receptors. We use the receptor status of the tumor to determine whether progestin therapy is appropriate. If tumor from the site of recurrence cannot be obtained to measure estrogen and progesterone receptor levels, we use the receptor status of the primary tumor to guide therapy.

Patients with metastatic or recurrent cancers that do not express steroid receptors are treated with cytotoxic chemotherapy. The most frequent regimen employed includes adriamycin and cisplatin administered every 3 weeks. Although a substantial proportion of patients have objective responses, few are cured. The overall survival rate for all patients with recurrent endometrial cancer is less than 20%. Thus, although survival rates are excellent following surgery in patients with early stage disease, further improvement in survival for patients with endometrial cancer awaits the development of effective treatment for metastatic disease.

Gestational Trophoblastic Disease

Donald Peter Goldstein, MD
Ross Stuart Berkowitz, MD

A presumptive diagnosis of gestational trophoblastic disease (GTD) is made in any postmenarchal woman with an elevated serum (or urine) human chorionic gonadotropin (hCG) level in the absence of pregnancy. For practical purposes, the only other consideration is the rare ovarian germ cell tumor containing trophoblastic elements.

The majority of cases of GTD follow molar pregnancy. They are detected by careful post-evacuation monitoring with serial serum hCG levels utilizing a quantitative radioimmunoassay for the β-subunit of hCG. Patients are followed with weekly hCG tests until the levels are normal (undetectable) for 3 weeks and then monthly for 6 months. A diagnosis of postmolar GTD is made when the hCG level plateaus for 3 or more consecutive weeks or re-elevates. This finding occurs in 15% to 20% of patients with a complete hydatidiform mole and 5% to 10% of patients with a partial hydatidiform mole.

Postmolar GTD may have the histologic pattern of either invasive mole, placental site trophoblastic tumor (PSTT), or choriocarcinoma. Choriocarcinoma differs from invasive mole in that it does not contain chorionic villus structures but is composed entirely of sheets of anaplastic cytotrophoblast and syncytiotrophoblast. GTD after a nonmolar pregnancy is either PSST or choriocarcinoma (CR). The presence of metastases does not differentiate between the three histologic types of GTD because invasive mole can be deported to sites beyond the confines of the uterus.

PSTTs represent an uncommon variant of choriocarcinoma. PSTTs do not contain chorionic villi but are composed almost entirely of cytotrophoblast with very minimal syncytiotrophoblast. PSTTs secrete very limited amounts of hCG and are generally resistant to chemotherapy. There are few, if any, long-term survivors with metastatic PSTTs, despite intensive multimodal therapy. Because of their poor response to chemotherapy, a diagnosis of nonmetastatic PSTTs should be followed by prompt hysterectomy, although in rare instances cures have been reported following curettage.

Patients with nonmetastatic disease (locally invasive) present with irregular vaginal bleeding, uterine subinvolution, and elevated hCG values. The trophoblastic tumor may perforate the myometrium, producing intraperitoneal bleeding, or may erode into uterine vessels, causing vaginal hemorrhage.

Metastatic GTD suggests the presence of choriocarcinoma because of its propensity for early vascular invasion with widespread dissemination. The most common metastatic sites are lung (80%), vagina (30%), liver (10%), and brain (10%). Because trophoblastic tumors are supplied by many fragile vessels, metastatic lesions are often hemorrhagic, and patients commonly present with signs and symptoms of bleeding from metastases.

Staging System

The International Federation of Gynecology and Obstetrics has begun reporting data on GTD using an anatomic staging system. *Stage I* includes all patients with persistently elevated hCG values and tumor confined to the uterine corpus. *Stage II* comprises all patients with tumor outside the uterus but localized to the vagina and/or pelvis. *Stage III* includes all patients with pulmonary metastases with or without uterine, vaginal, or pelvic involvement. *Stage IV* patients have far-advanced disease with involvement of the brain, liver, kidneys, or gastrointestinal tract. Patients with stage IV disease are at highest risk of becoming resistant to chemotherapy. Stage IV tumors generally have the histologic pattern of choriocarcinoma and almost always follow a nonmolar pregnancy.

In addition to anatomic staging, it is helpful to employ other prognostic variables to predict the likelihood of drug resistance and to aid the clinician in selecting appropriate chemotherapeutic protocols. The World Health Organization has proposed a prognostic scoring system, based on one developed by Bagshawe, which reliably predicts the potential for resistance to chemotherapy (Table 1). When the prognostic score is 8 or greater, the patient is placed in a high-risk category and requires intensive combination chemotherapy to achieve remission. Patients with stage I disease generally have a low-risk score, and patients with stage IV disease have a high-risk score. Patients in stage II and III may fall into either the low-risk or the high-risk group.

Diagnostic Evaluation

The optimal management of GTD requires a thorough assessment of the extent of disease prior to the initiation of treatment. The staging work-up should include a careful physical examination, chest radiograph, abdominal and pelvic sonograms, computed tomographic scan or magnetic resonance image of the brain, and baseline β-hCG assay. All of the available pathology should be reviewed. Uterine curettage should be reserved for patients with a subinvoluted uterus, significant bleeding, or ultrasonographic evidence of intrauterine tumor.

Management

The protocols used for the treatment of patients with GTD depend on the extent of disease and on prognostic factors (e.g., risk of resistance). In general, patients with low-risk disease, either metastatic or nonmetastatic, can be treated with single-agent therapy with excellent results, whereas patients with high-risk disease (always metastatic) should be treated with combination drug protocols. In addition to chemotherapy, surgery and radiation therapy may play a role in selected cases.

Nonmetastatic Disease (Stage I)

Patients with nonmetastatic disease who no longer wish to preserve fertility are candidates for primary hysterectomy with adjuvant single-agent chemotherapy. Adjuvant chemotherapy is administered for three reasons: (1) to reduce the likelihood of disseminating viable tumor at surgery, (2) to maintain a cytotoxic level of che-

TABLE 1. Scoring System Based on Prognostic Factors

	Score			
Prognostic Factors	0	1	2	4
Age (years)	<39	>39		
Antecedent pregnancy	HM	Abortion	Term	
Interval (months)	<4	4–6	7–12	>12
hCG (IU/L)	<10^3	10^3–10^4	10^4–10^5	>10^5
Largest tumor (including uterine)		3–5 cm	>5 cm	
Site of metastases		Spleen, kidney	GI, liver	Brain
Number of metastases identified		1–4	4–8	>8
Prior chemotherapy			Single drug	Two or more drugs

hCG, human chorionic gonadotropin; HM, hydatidiform mole; GI, gastrointestinal.

TABLE 2. MTX-CF Protocols

1. MTX	1.0–1.5 mg/kg	IM	Days 1, 3, 5, 7
CF	0.1–0.15 mg/kg	IM	Days 2, 4, 6, 8
2. MTX	100 mg/m^2	IV	30-min infusion
	200 mg/m^2	IV	12-hr infusion
CF	15 mg	IM or	Every 12 hr × 4
		PO	doses (days 2–4)

CF, citrovorum factor; MTX, methotrexate.

motherapy in the blood stream and tissues in case viable tumor cells are disseminated, and (3) to treat any occult metastases that may already be present.

The preferred treatment of patients with nonmetastatic disease who desire to preserve fertility is primary single-agent chemotherapy with either methotrexate (MTX) or actinomycin D (ACT-D).

Methotrexate with citrovorum factor (CF) rescue has been the preferred single-agent regimen in our facility since 1974. Two regimens have been used with comparable effectiveness: (1) intramuscular MTX alternating with intramuscular CF and (2) intravenous MTX infusion followed by oral CF (Table 2). The use of CF rescue reduces toxicity without impairing therapeutic effectiveness. ACT-D administered intravenously at a dosage of 10 to 12 µg/kg/day for 5 days is reserved for patients with hepatic toxicity (increased serum glutamic-oxaloacetic transaminase [SGOT] or those with MTX resistance. Single-agent chemotherapy is administered at our center on the basis of the hCG regression curve. If the hCG level fails to fall 1 log (10-fold) following the use of one drug, resistance to that drug is suspected, and the protocol should be changed. Following the first course of single-agent chemotherapy, further treatment is withheld as long as the hCG level falls progressively. If the hCG plateaus for 3 consecutive weeks or rises, additional chemotherapy is indicated. No chemotherapy courses are administered after the first normal titer unless relapse occurs. An alternative treatment program utilizes regularly scheduled courses of chemotherapy at 2-week intervals (toxicity permitting) until one course has been completed after the first normal titer. Either MTX or ACT-D will induce permanent remission in 80% to 90% of patients when used primarily. The 10% to 20% of patients who prove resistant to one drug will usually respond to the other. Occasionally, hysterectomy, local resection, or combination chemotherapy will be required, but virtually all of these cases are curable. Follow-up hCG titers are required for 1 year before pregnancy is permitted.

Metastatic Disease

All patients with metastases should be referred to a center with experience in the treatment of trophoblastic tumors, since only 90% will be cured even in an optimal environment. This is particularly true of patients with high-risk disease, for which the cure rate in most centers is still only 80%.

For patients with low-risk metastatic disease, such as those diagnosed shortly after molar evacuation and those with vaginal or pulmonary metastases (stage II or III), single-agent chemotherapy using MTX with CF rescue or ACT-D is usually adequate. Combination chemotherapy using MTX with CF rescue, ACT-D, and etoposide (VP-16) may also be employed to shorten treatment time and reduce the likelihood of resistance, although there is a significant increase in toxicity (Table 3). When these patients have considerable myometrial invasion, hysterectomy may be indicated because of hemorrhage, infection, or perforation. In spite of the presence of metastases, the cure rate in patients with low-risk metastatic disease still approaches 100% when adequate therapy is utilized.

Patients with high-risk metastatic disease almost invariably have choriocarcinoma and are at serious risk of dying. For these patients, combination chemotherapy utilizing etoposide (VP-16), MTX with CF rescue, and ACT-D is employed. Treatment is administered every 2 to 3 weeks, depending on toxicity, and is continued for two to three courses after hCG remission is achieved. Patients with brain metastases require wholehead radiation therapy (3000 rads in 10 days). This therapy should be initiated as soon as the diagnosis is confirmed by computed tomographic scan, magnetic resonance imaging, or cerebrospinal fluid hCG determination to reduce the risk of life-threatening hemorrhage. Intrathecal highdose MTX therapy has also been shown to pre-

TABLE 3. EMA Protocol

Etoposide (VP-16) Days 1–2	100 mg/m^2	IV
ACT-D Days 1–5	12–15 µg/kg	IV
MTX Day 1	300 mg/m^2	IV
CF Days 2–4	15–30 mg q12 hr × 4	IM or PO

ACT-D, actinomycin D; CF, citrovorum factor; MTX, methotrexate.

vent hemorrhage and facilitate tumor shrinkage. On occasion, craniotomy should be performed, particularly when the tumor is peripheral or bleeding is present.

The use of radiation therapy in patients with hepatic metastases is less well defined. Surgical intervention may be necessary for hepatic metastases in the presence of hepatic hemorrhage or rupture.

Local resection of vaginal metastases is risky because of the extreme vascularity of the tumor and should be reserved for those cases in which chemotherapy has failed and acute hemorrhage is present. Similarly, thoracotomy is reserved for the treatment of resistant pulmonary nodules.

In our experience, failure to cure patients with high-risk GTD is usually due to drug resistance complicated by toxicity. For this reason, it is unwise to continue treatment with a regimen that fails to decrease the hCG titer after each course. When resistance is documented, other therapeutic modalities should be utilized as second-line treatment.

Pregnancies After Gestational Trophoblastic Disease

Data from the New England Trophoblastic Disease Center, National Cancer Institute, and Charing Cross Hospital demonstrate that patients with GTD who are successfully treated with chemotherapy can anticipate normal reproductive potential. The incidence of full-term live births, premature deliveries, ectopic pregnancies, stillbirths, first-trimester abortions, and congenital malformations is comparable with incidences in the general population. It is particularly reassuring that the incidence of congenital anomalies is not increased. The subsequent pregnancies have no increased risk of complication during either the prenatal or the postpartum period.

However, all patients who have had prior trophoblastic tumors and who have completed a subsequent pregnancy should be screened at the time of the 6-week postpartum or postabortion check-up with a serum hCG level to exclude recurrent disease.

Hydatidiform Mole

Donald Peter Goldstein, MD
Ross Stuart Berkowitz, MD

Although hydatidiform mole (or molar pregnancy) has been known since antiquity, it is only during the past 40 years that we have come to understand its epidemiology, pathology, genetics, and clinical spectrum. Technologic advances in hormone measurement, sonography, cytogenetics, surgery, anesthesia, and chemotherapy have all contributed to the vast improvements that have been achieved in the management of this condition.

Pathology and Cytogenetics

Hydatidiform mole is characterized as either partial or complete on the basis of histopathology and karyotype. Its distinguishing morphologic characteristics are hydropic swelling of the chorionic villi and trophoblastic hyperplasia. It is the presence of hyperplastic trophoblast that distinguishes molar pregnancy from the hydatidiform changes that may be associated with spontaneous abortion. In complete moles, the villous swelling and trophoblastic proliferation are generally diffuse and the villi are avascular. Embryonic and fetal tissues are not present. In contrast, partial moles contain two populations of chorionic villi, normal and molar. The molar villi in partial moles differ from the villi in complete moles in that they commonly contain fetal vessels and exhibit focal trophoblastic hyperplasia as well as villous scalloping and stromal inclusions. Another important morphologic feature that distinguishes partial from complete mole is the presence of embryonic and fetal tissues.

Chromosomal banding and enzyme analysis have demonstrated that in complete moles all chromosomes are paternally derived and the mitochondrial DNA is maternal in origin. The mechanism for loss of maternal chromosomes from the ovum is unknown. Most complete moles develop from fertilization of an anuclear ovum by a haploid (23,X) sperm that then duplicates its own chromosomes, resulting in a 46,XX chromosomal pattern. Ten percent of complete moles have a 46,XY karyotype that is caused by dispermy.

Partial moles usually have a triploid chromosomal pattern resulting from fertilization of an apparently normal ovum by two sperm. When fetuses are identified with partial moles they usually have the stigmata of triploidy, including growth retardation and multiple congenital anomalies such as syndactyly, cleft palate, microphthalmia, omphalocele, and hydrocephaly.

Epidemiology

The reported incidence of hydatidiform mole varies widely in different regions of the world. Some of this variation in the incidence rate may be explained by differences in the method of reporting data as hospital-based or population-based. The incidence of molar pregnancy in Europe and North America is approximately 0.6 to 1.1 per 1000 pregnancies. In Asian countries, the rate is 3 to 10 times higher. A recent study from Ireland based on the pathologic review of all products of conception showed that the incidence of partial mole and complete mole was 1 in 695 and 1 in 1945 pregnancies, respectively.

The high incidence of molar pregnancy in some countries may be due to nutritional and socioeconomic factors. Patients with complete moles have been shown to have decreased consumption of dietary betacarotene (vitamin A precursor) and animal fat. Other risk factors for complete molar pregnancy include a history of previous miscarriages and advanced maternal age. In contrast to complete moles, maternal age and nutrition do not appear to influence the incidence of partial moles, whereas the long-term (>4 years) use of oral contraceptives and a history of irregular menstrual cycles are significant.

Clinical Presentation and Diagnosis of Complete Hydatidiform Mole

The presentation and diagnosis of molar pregnancy has changed significantly over the past 20 years because of the widespread use of ultrasonography during the first trimester of pregnancy and the availability of sensitive and specific quantitative methods for measuring human chorionic gonadotropin (hCG). Most published descriptions of the clinical presentations of complete molar pregnancy through the 1980s commonly listed vaginal bleeding, anemia, rapid and excessive uterine enlargement, theca lutein ovarian cysts, pre-eclampsia, hyperthyroidism, and acute respiratory insufficiency. The diagnosis of complete molar pregnancy in the pre-ultrasonography era was based primarily on these clinical findings, which even now are associated with an increased risk of post-mole tumor. Since the ad-

vent of ultrasonography and radioimmunoassay measurement of hCG, the diagnosis is being made earlier by the characteristic sonographic findings of a vesicular pattern and absent fetal sac together with an elevated hCG level. Ultrasonographic diagnosis on occasion can be misleading if a large amount of blood is present in the uterus, since clots may be mistaken for fetal sacs. In the past, a high percentage of patients with complete molar pregnancy presented with the classic syndrome while spontaneously aborting at 16 to 18 weeks. The diagnosis of molar pregnancy is now usually suggested by the sonogram performed during the first trimester because of vaginal bleeding or an absent fetal heart beat, or both. In some cases, the diagnosis is made by the pathologist after the patient undergoes a curettage for what appeared on ultrasonogram to be a missed or incomplete abortion. The finding of an inappropriately high level of hCG should alert the clinician to the possibility of a mole.

Earlier diagnosis has also changed the clinical presentation of complete mole at our Center. Although vaginal bleeding continues to be the most common presenting symptom, we now infrequently encounter patients who develop other classic clinical stigmata. Although early diagnosis reduces the incidence of pre-eclampsia, hyperthyroidism, and other medical complications, it does not reduce the likelihood that the patient will develop postmolar trophoblastic tumor. For that reason it is important to have tissue from patients undergoing termination of pregnancy and miscarriages examined whenever possible.

Clinical Presentation and Diagnosis of Partial Hydatidiform Mole

The clinical presentation of partial mole is quite different from the dramatic clinical syndrome that in the past characterized patients with complete molar pregnancy. Typically, patients with partial mole present with signs and symptoms of incomplete or missed abortion. In fact, in most instances the diagnosis is made by the pathologist on reviewing the curettages rather than by the clinician. The main presenting sign of partial mole is vaginal bleeding, which occurs in approximately three quarters of patients. Excessive uterine enlargement and pre-eclampsia are present in only 10% and 2% of patients, respectively. Furthermore, patients infrequently develop theca lutein ovarian cysts, hyperemesis, or hyperthyroidism, and pre-evacuation hCG levels rarely exceed 100,000 mIU/mL. In fact, the clinical

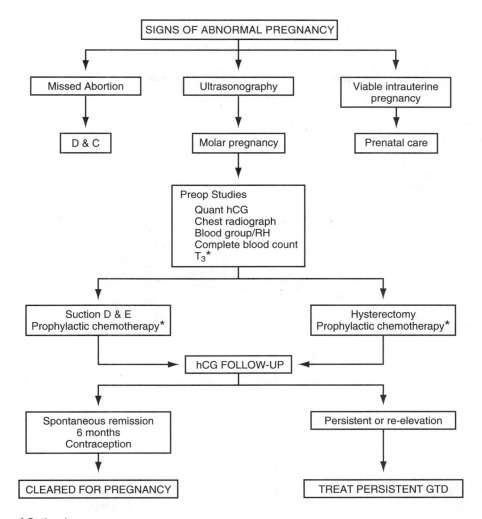

Figure 1. Molar pregnancy algorithm. D & C, dilatation and curettage; D & E, dilatation and evacuation; GTD, gestational trophoblastic disease; hCG, human chorionic gonadotropin; T₃, triiodothyronine.

features of partial mole are not unlike those seen currently in early complete mole.

Ultrasonographic diagnosis of partial mole may be possible if the sonographer can demonstrate focal cystic spaces in the placental tissues and an increase in the transverse diameter of the gestational sac. In most instances, however, the sonographic picture is consistent with missed or incomplete abortion.

Molar Evacuation

Once the diagnosis of molar pregnancy has been made, the patient should be evaluated and treated for any associated medical complications such as pre-eclampsia, hyperthyroidism, electrolyte imbalance due to hyperemesis, and anemia. Each patient should have a blood type and Rh, chest radiograph, and quantitative hCG level. The presence of large theca lutein cysts rarely interferes with evacuation but if they are sufficiently large, they might compromise respiratory function. Transabdominal decompression with ultrasonographic guidance may be performed as an interim measure if indicated, since it takes many weeks for these cysts to resolve spontaneously.

Suction curettage is the preferred method of evacuation regardless of uterine size in women who desire to preserve fertility. Laminaria are generally not required preoperatively unless the patient has a late second trimester partial mole or coexisting fetus. In fact, the use of laminaria may be associated with hemorrhage and the induction of spontaneous evacuation. Evacuation of all complete and most partial moles can safely be accomplished using a #12 cannula. Oxytocin (Pitocin) is usually administered at the start of cervical dilatation. When evacuating a molar pregnancy larger than 14 weeks' size it is advisable to keep one hand on the fundus during the initial phase to reduce the likelihood of perforation and to massage the uterus to facilitate involution. Although bleeding may start during evacuation, it is best to proceed expeditiously since significant bleeding usually stops when the uterus has been emptied. After completion of the suction evacuation, a gentle sharp curettage is recommended to remove any residual molar tissue. Since trophoblast cells express Rho(D) factor, Rho(D)-negative patients should receive Rh immune globulin.

Patients with larger-than-dates uteri are at increased risk of developing acute respiratory distress post evacuation due to molar embolization. This sudden development can usually be anticipated if the anesthesiologist notices that the patient has unexplained decreasing blood oxygen saturation levels during the evacuation procedure. Prompt initiation of therapy including cardiorespiratory support generally facilitates spontaneous resolution in 48 to 72 hours.

If the patient desires sterilization, a gravid hysterectomy with ovarian preservation may be performed. When the uterus is excessively enlarged, it may be prudent to evacuate the contents before undertaking its removal. Large theca lutein ovarian cysts can be safely decompressed by needle aspiration at the time of surgery. This may reduce the likelihood of rupture and torsion postoperatively. Although hysterectomy removes the risk of locally invasive mole, it does not prevent metastases from developing subsequently. Therefore, patients still require fastidious gonadotropin monitoring.

Prophylactic Chemotherapy

The use of prophylactic chemotherapy at the time of evacuation of a complete mole has been shown to reduce the incidence of postmolar tumor. However, the availability of excellent hCG monitoring makes the use of this technique superfluous except in cases in which the patient may be unreliable or gonadotropin follow-up is not possible.

Postevacuation Follow-Up

Early Complications

The most common immediate complications after molar evacuation are bleeding and infection. These rarely occur if evacuation has been properly performed and in the absence of perforation. A repeat curettage is indicated only for bleeding or other signs of retained tissue. A repeat dilatation and curettage is not indicated routinely after evacuation because of the risk of perforation and uterine synechia.

Another early complication is respiratory difficulty and abdominal pain from sudden enlargement of theca lutein ovarian cysts. This can be dealt with expeditiously by transabdominal depression under ultrasonographic guidance. The sudden onset of lower abdominal pain with nausea and vomiting may also indicate torsion of a theca lutein cyst and should be treated on an emergent basis if the ovary is to be saved.

Late Complications

The most important late complication after molar evacuation is persistent trophoblastic disease, which develops after complete mole in 18% to 29% of patients and in 2% to 4% of patients after partial mole. Most centers in the United States define postmolar trophoblastic disease by a re-elevation or persistent plateau of hCG for at least 3 consecutive weeks. Since early detection and intervention is associated with the least morbidity and best outcome, fastidious hCG follow-up is essential. After molar evacuation, patients should be followed with weekly hCG levels until these are nondetectable for 3 consecutive weeks, then by monthly levels until nondetectable for 6 consecutive months. In patients with partal mole in whom the hCG level has reached normal within 7 weeks from the time of evacuation, follow-up can be discontinued after 3 months of undetectable hCG values. The average time to achieve the first normal hCG level after evacuation of either a complete or partial mole is 9 to 11 weeks.

At the completion of follow-up, pregnancy may be undertaken at any time. Patients should use contraception during follow-up to prevent an intercurrent pregnancy, which would confuse monitoring. Either hormonal or barrier contraception is usually recommended. Intrauterine devices should not be inserted until the hCG level is normal because of the potential of bleeding, perforation, or infection due to the presence of tumor.

Subsequent Pregnancy

Patients who have been treated for molar pregnancy can anticipate normal future reproductive outcomes with no increased incidence of miscarriage, major or minor congenital abnormalities, prematurity, or cesarean section rate. However, patients with molar disease are at increased risk of developing either a complete or a partial mole in subsequent conceptions. After one molar pregnancy, the risk of having molar disease in a future pregnancy increases 10-fold to 1%. Following two episodes of molar pregnancy, that risk increases to 20%. For this reason, these patients should be advised to undergo ultrasonographic examination routinely during the late first trimester or if vaginal bleeding or other signs of molar pregnancy develop. Patients with a history of molar pregnancy are also at increased risk of developing choriocarcinoma following a term pregnancy or miscarriage. Therefore it is advisable to obtain an hCG test at the 6-week examination, at which time the hormone level should be undetectable.

Ovarian Cancer*

Robert R. Taylor, MD
Michael J. Birrer, MD, PhD

Ovarian carcinoma affects nearly 26,000 American women annually. This disease is the fourth leading cause of cancer mortality in women and accounts for approximately 15,000 deaths annually. An American woman has a 1.4% lifetime risk of developing ovarian carcinoma. With the exception of the uncommon germ cell tumors, which are extremely sensitive to intense short courses of combination cytotoxic chemotherapy, the 5-year survival rate of patients diagnosed with ovarian cancer is approximately 40% and has not changed appreciably over the past 30 years, despite important advances in surgery, chemotherapy, and radiation therapy. Despite this lack of improvement in long-term survival, there has been a significant extension of the progression-free survival of patients treated with aggressive surgery and combination chemotherapy.

*The views expressed herein are those of the authors and are not intended to reflect the opinion or official policy of the US Government, by whom MJB is professionally employed.

Biology, Etiology, and Genetics

Ovarian cancer results from the malignant transformation of one of the three basic histologic components of the ovary. The most common type of malignancy arises from the ovarian epithelium and represents 80% of the ovarian malignancies. Less common are malignancies that arise from germ cells or stromal elements. Lastly, the ovary may be a site of metastatic carcinoma from an adjacent gynecologic or distant primary tumor (breast and gastrointestinal cancers are the most common of these).

Epithelial ovarian cancer is most prevalent in industrialized countries, with the exception of Japan. It remains a disease of elderly women, with the mean age of epithelial ovarian cancer diagnosis being 61 years. In contrast, malignant germ cell tumors and stromal tumors are most prevalent in the prepubertal or early reproductive years.

Recent investigation has identified cases of epithelial ovarian carcinoma in related women. In these families, cases of ovarian cancer may be observed as an isolated finding or in conjunction with other cancers, usually of the breast or bowel. Pedigree analysis of these patients has revealed their family members to be cancer prone, and subsequent molecular biologic analysis has confirmed vertical or hereditary transmission of genotypic abnormalities that appear to lead to an increased cancer susceptibility. Fortunately, these hereditary cancer families are uncommon and constitute less than 5% of the total of patients with ovarian malignancies. Thus, the vast majority of ovarian cancer arises sporadically in the population.

Diagnosis

Ovarian cancer patients are found at the time of diagnosis to have advanced disease in approximately 70% to 80% of cases. This finding is one of the most important reasons for the poor survival associated with ovarian cancer. In an attempt to diagnose more stage I cases, early detection strategies have been developed and evaluated for epithelial ovarian cancers. These strategies include noninvasive imaging modalities such as transabdominal or transvaginal ultrasonography and color flow Doppler, and biochemical markers such as tumor-associated antigenic markers (CA-125).

Results from screening studies utilizing these modalities have not proven them to be beneficial, even when limited to a high-risk patient population (those with a family or hereditary predisposition). Unfortunately, ultrasonographic techniques lack the specificity to be of clinical value, while serum tests suffer from lack of sensitivity to detect early-stage disease. Furthermore, a defined premalignant lesion for ovarian cancer has yet to be identified that would serve as the target of an appropriate screening test. Despite these problems, current clinical practice still offers some program of screening to high-risk patients. Certainly, high-risk patients should be counseled for an increased risk of developing ovarian cancer. They can then be followed with a combination of the aforementioned tests. In addition, although controversial, prophylactic bilateral salpingo-oophorectomy should be offered to these patients at the completion of childbearing, as this will eliminate the risk for ovarian cancer, although it will not remove the risk for developing an epithelial nonovarian peritoneal cancer.

Symptoms of ovarian carcinoma are generally vague, particularly those noted in early epithelial carcinoma. Nonspecific dietary, bowel, or bladder changes, or a sense of pelvic fullness should be fully evaluated to include pelvic examination and, most importantly, a rectovaginal examination. If a pelvic mass is palpable, an endovaginal ultrasonogram may be obtained that can further describe the adnexal process and assist in management recommendations. Ultrasonography can reliably comment on physical characteristics such as size, architecture of adnexal masses, capsule thickness, presence of excrescences, and abnormalities in vascular flow, all of which have been shown to have some measurable association with malignancy. When, in the premenopausal woman, endovaginal ultrasonography reveals an 8 cm or smaller simple ovarian cyst, it is likely to be a functional ovarian cyst that will resolve over a menstrual cycle, particularly if ovarian suppression is prescribed. If the clinical examination reveals a nodular or fixed pelvic mass, ultrasonography will not likely provide any additional information to refute the suspicion of malignancy.

In contrast to the more common epithelial carcinomas, germ cell and some stromal neoplasms often present in the pediatric or adolescent patient. Having a rapid growth rate, the presenting symptoms may be the result of hemoperitoneum, an acute surgical abdomen, or a hormonal imbalance leading to either virilization or isosexual precocious puberty. These young women should have assays for beta-human chorionic gonadotropin and alpha-fetoprotien. In the presence of virilization, one should assay for testosterone and dehydroepiandrosterone. A karyotype should be obtained to resolve any suspicion of dysgenic gonads (those carrying a Y chromosome).

Surgical Therapy

The cornerstone of ovarian cancer therapy is surgery. Prior to surgery, however, a detailed preoperative assessment is mandatory. Appropriate consultation with medical specialists and optimization of the patient's medical condition will certainly improve her tolerance of surgery and subsequent adjuvant therapy. We routinely obtain a CA-125 level and provide appropriate cancer screening tests according to the American Cancer Society Guidelines with respect to Pap smear, mammogram, and flexible sigmoidoscopy. As symptoms and clinical findings dictate, a barium enema and upper gastrointestinal examination are recommended. A computed tomographic scan of the abdomen and pelvis offers visualization of possible mass effect on the ureters, retroperitoneal lymph node enlargement, and parenchymal hepatic or splenic metastasis. Following preoperative assessment, some patients may be deemed poor surgical candidates. Standard recommended therapy for these patients (with epithelial ovarian cancer) is biopsy proof of malignancy and three cycles of neoadjuvant combination chemotherapy. An interval cytoreductive procedure can be offered to those responders (presuming an improved medical condition) followed by the completion of the prescribed chemotherapy. For surgical treatment, preoperative management usually includes a bowel preparation of magnesium citrate or Go-Lytely, deep venous thrombosis prophylaxis, and antibiotic prophylaxis for cases likely to be long or in which the vagina or bowel will be entered.

With the increasing experience of laparoscopic surgical techniques, one may consider this route for the diagnosis and treatment of nonsuspicious adnexal masses (absent tumor markers, simple mass by ultrasonography). Frozen section diagnosis must be available intraoperatively on the cystectomy or oophorectomy specimen, and the patient should be counseled preoperatively for the potential of laparoscopic surgical staging or formal laparotomy, should malignancy be discovered. Laparoscopic surgery for adnexal masses often results in capsular rupture, and this occurrence will upstage ovarian cancer patients. Although controversial, it appears that such rupture has no measurable effect on survival, provided appropriate staging surgery and adjuvant chemotherapy is not delayed.

In most cases of suspected ovarian cancer,

surgery begins with a midline or paramedian incision, as this affords the best exposure to the upper abdomen and pelvis and, furthermore, can be easily extended cephalad as the operation dictates. Ascitic fluid or, in its absence, cell washings from the cul de sac, bilateral paracolic gutters, and right diaphragm are submitted with 1 mm of heparin, which decreases cell aggregation and improves the quality of cytologic assessment. When faced with a suspicious ovarian neoplasm, an adnexectomy is performed and a frozen section diagnosis is obtained. If a pathologic diagnosis of malignancy is returned, a staging procedure is performed, which generally consists of a total abdominal hysterectomy, bilateral salpingoophorectomy, and infracolic omentectomy. Sampling of bilateral pelvic and para-aortic lymph node spaces and multiple peritoneal biopsies from the pelvis and abdomen, one of which should be from the right diaphragm, is required only if there is no evidence of spread, or if any spread of disease or metastasis has been fully reduced. A thorough inspection of all peritoneal surfaces is performed, noting the location and size of metastatic disease. The importance of comprehensive staging procedures is certain given the finding of a 30% upstaging of ovarian carcinoma patients having lesser procedures. Sadly, it is common to encounter bulky metastatic disease. In this situation, cytoreductive efforts are added to the surgical procedures just named, with the goal of reducing the volume of residual disease. Optimal cytoreduction generally means that the largest residual metastatic tumor is less than 1 cm. Historically and in current practice, the value of successful cytoreductive surgery is measured by its correlation to the patient's progression-free survival. It is important to note that there are no prospective randomized studies to prove the survival benefits for cytoreductive surgery. Not all ovarian cancer surgery need be inclusive of hysterectomy or bilateral salpingoophorectomy. Patients with unilateral stromal or well-differentiated epithelial tumors, having no obvious metastatic disease and a desire to preserve childbearing potential, can undergo a unilateral salpingoophorectomy and staging biopsies. Patients with unilateral germ cell tumors can undergo a unilateral procedure even in the presence of bulky disease, owing to the exquisite sensitivity of this disease to chemotherapy. Advances in assisted reproductive technologies are certainly applicable to these patients.

Formal review of the surgical pathology and operative findings are required to assign a surgical stage and grade. Epithelial ovarian cancer treatment is predicated on stage, grade, and tumor volume as follows:

1. Low malignant potential tumors, formerly known as borderline ovarian cancer, are diagnosed as stage I disease in 85% of cases and treated with observation only. This recommendation is based on the known excellent 5-year survival rate of greater than 95% in stage I patients. Curiously, those patients with advanced disease, or with bulky residual, have more guarded prognosis but still have 5-year survival rates ranging from 60% to 80%. In addition, adjuvant chemotherapy has not been conclusively shown to be effective in extending the survival of patients with low malignant potential tumors. If staging biopsies reveal invasive metastatic implants, adjuvant combination chemotherapy is recommended, as these patients have been shown to have a poor survival with a clinical course that reproduces that of true ovarian carcinoma.

2. Stage I grade 1 or 2 invasive tumors are considered low risk for recurrent disease and are treated with observation. These patients have a 5-year survival rate of 90%, and adjuvant therapy has been shown to offer no increase in survival.

3. Stage I grade 3 and advanced stages of invasive ovarian cancer obviously represent high risk for recurrence or persistence of disease and patients should be offered further therapy. Standard therapy for stage I grade 3 patients consists of intraperitoneal p32 therapy, although ongoing studies are evaluating the effectiveness of short courses (three cycles) of combination cytotoxic chemotherapy. Stage II, III, and IV disease requires combination chemotherapy, although the mode of administration depends on the amount of residual disease. A recent study has suggested that optimally debulked disease (<1 cm) is best treated with intraperitoneal combination chemotherapy, while bulky disease is treated with systematic therapy.

Combination Chemotherapy

Standard combination chemotherapy consists of a platinin-containing regimen for six cycles. Multiple studies have demonstrated superior results with platinin-containing regimens. In addition, there is no evidence that prolonged therapy (more than six cycles) affords any advantage. Recently, a prospective randomized study demonstrated that paclitaxel and cisplatinin was superior to cisplatin/cyclophosphamide in terms of response and disease-free survival. This regimen has rapidly become standard therapy for advanced bulky disease. One can anticipate a 70% to 80% response rate to these agents and a progression-free survival that is proportional to the volume of disease at initial treatment (approximately 18 months). Unfortunately, the vast majority of these patients relapse with drug-resistant tumors. For these patients, the therapy options are limited. If the response interval has been long (>12 months), retreatment with the original induction drugs would be a reasonable choice. If the response interval has been short (<6 months) treatment with other second-line chemotherapy agents would be more reasonable. These agents include etoposide, altretamine [Hexalen], ifosamide, or investigational agents such as topoisomerase inhibitors. Unfortunately, the response rate in these patients is quite low and the duration of response remains short.

Controversies

Controversy persists regarding the treatment recommendations for patients with advanced stage disease. Optimal upfront chemotherapy is still being defined. While taxol/cisplatin has been demonstrated to be superior to cytoxan/cisplatin, the optimal dose and schedule for taxol has not been determined and is presently under investigation. Further, the value of carboplatinin in the treatment of advanced disease remains to be determined. While clearly less toxic and easier to administer, carboplatinin remains more expensive and less studied compared with cisplatin. Finally, the role of dose intensity in the treatment of ovarian cancer remains undefined. Several randomized trials have provided conflicting information concerning any survival benefit to dose intensification. However, these trials have suffered from minimal dose escalations and moderately severe toxicity. With the availability of colony-stimulating factors, neuroprotectors, and bone marrow transplants, trials can now be conducted to more accurately address this issue.

The patients who have a complete clinical response (as evidenced by physical examination imaging studies, and normalization of CA-125) to chemotherapy can be offered a second-look laparotomy procedure. A second-look or response laparotomy involves a generous abdominal incision and careful inspection of all peritoneal surfaces with multiple peritoneal biopsies. Of the 50% of patients having a complete clinical response to primary chemotherapy, approximately half of these patients will have a complete pathologic response at second-look laparotomy (all biopsies negative for tumor). Detractors of the second-look laparotomy cite that disease in at least 50% of those patients with a negative second-look finding will recur and that, furthermore, no effective consolidate therapy exists. Arguably, some subgroups of patients may benefit from secondary cytoreductive surgery at the time of second-look laparotomy. However, these patients likely have indolent growing tumors, amenable to cytoreductive efforts, and therefore may be the ones who do reasonably well with or without this operation.

The precise clinical role of intraperitoneal chemotherapy in the treatment of ovarian cancer is still evolving. As mentioned earlier, recent results from a prospective randomized trial have clearly demonstrated its effectiveness in the treatment of optimally cytoreduced stage III patients over conventional systemic therapy. Unfortunately, this represents only a small subset of ovarian cancer patients. However, this positive result has led to the consideration of the potential usefulness of this approach for other clinical settings such as consolidative therapy after minimal disease is found after a second-look laparotomy.

Future Directions

The future directions of clinical research related to ovarian cancer will focus on three issues: prevention, early detection, and treatment. All three areas will be aided by ongoing efforts in understanding the molecular basis of the development of ovarian cancer. Identification of genes such as *BRCA*-1, which are important for the initial events in ovarian epithelium, will be critical for the development of the genetic screening assays to identify high-risk patients. Characterization of the role of dominant and negative oncogenes active during the development of ovarian cancer will serve to identify important prognostic and possible "early detection" markers for these tumors. Finally, these genes and their products, in conjunction with growth factor and their receptors, will be important targets for future drug development. Agents that can replenish a missing critical function (tumor suppressor gene) or suppress activated biochemical pathways (growth factors, or dominant oncogenes) will represent a new class of agents that may play an important role in the treatment and prevention of ovarian cancer.

Vulvar Neoplasms

Jonathan A. Cosin, MD

Linda F. Carson, MD

Tumors of the vulva represent about 1% of all malignancies in women and about 5% of genital tract malignancies. In contrast to cancer of the cervix, whose incidence declines after the eighth decade, the incidence of vulvar carcinoma increases consistently with age. At least one third of women with vulvar cancer present at age 70 or older and the disease is rare before the age of 30. An exception to this is the occurrence of vulvar carcinoma in young, immunosuppressed women. Histologically, 85% to 90% of vulvar neoplasms are squamous cell carcinoma, 5% are malignant melanoma, and 4% are adenocarcinoma of the Bartholin gland. Sarcomas, invasive Paget's disease, and basal cell carcinoma compose most of the remainder. Vulvar intraepithelial neoplasia (VIN) and noninvasive Paget's disease represent the two types of intraepithelial disease found on the vulva. Most vulvar carcinomas do not appear to arise from intraepithelial lesions and instead arise in the background of either vulvar dystrophy or "normal" vulvar skin, the exception again being in young immunosuppressed women. Treatment is becoming more individualized, with greater emphasis now being placed on the patient's quality of life and psychosexual function, both during and after treatment.

Squamous Vulvar Intraepithelial Neoplasia

The incidence of VIN has been increasing over time, nearly doubling between the years 1973 to 1976 and 1985 to 1987. During this same time period there was a threefold increase in the incidence of VIN in women under the age of 35 years, while the rate of invasive squamous cell cancer of the vulva remained relatively stable. This trend has led to the recognition of VIN as a heterogeneous condition, with differing etiologies and different implications for the patient. Patients may present with vulvar pruritus, but many are asymptomatic. Lesions vary greatly in appearance. They may be flat, raised, pigmented, or white, and occasionally have a very irregular contour. Although some areas may be visible only after the application of 5% acetic acid, many are grossly apparent. All lesions should be evaluated

colposcopically to document the extent of disease.

Multifocal VIN is more common in younger patients, generally in their third and fourth decades of life. Risk factors include a history of genital warts or other sexually transmitted disease, smoking, and altered immune status. VIN is frequently associated with preinvasive or invasive lesions of the lower anogenital tract, especially as seen in transplant recipients and HIV-infected patients. Unifocal VIN is more prevalent in women in their sixth decade and beyond. Viral studies show lower rates of human papillomavirus infection than are seen in patients with multifocal disease. VIN is found to be associated with 20% to 30% of cases of vulvar carcinoma, but the exact proportion of these cases that will progress to invasive cancer is unknown. Progression rates are often quoted as low as 2% to 4%; however, these data are observed in previously treated patients. In contrast, progression of VIN to invasive cancer has been noted in series of untreated patients to be as high as 100%. This risk is higher in older patients (sixth decade) and in immunocompromised patients. Progression times are also reported to be relatively short, typically less than 10 years. Spontaneous regression is also noted to occur and is more common in younger patients, particularly when diagnosed during or shortly after pregnancy. For this reason, in the absence of cytologic atypia or evidence of invasion, lesions associated with pregnancy can be followed conservatively and need to be treated only if they persist for more than 6 months postpartum.

Colposcopy is critical to appropriate and successful diagnosis, treatment, and follow-up of these lesions. Multiple biopsies may be required to rule out invasion, particularly in the area of the posterior perineum, were microinvasion may be present in up to 10% of cases. Once invasion is ruled out, CO_2 laser vaporization is the treatment of choice for small to medium-size lesions. The vulva, unlike the cervix, has no glands, and treatment therefore is necessary to a depth of only 1 to 2 mm in non–hair-bearing areas, which corresponds to the second surgical plane or the base of the basement membrane. In hair-bearing areas, treatment should extend to 2 to 3 mm to include deeper structures such as skin appendages. A CO_2 laser, set at 20 to 25 watts with superpulse (25 to 40 watts without the superpulse feature) with a minimum 2-mm spot size will provide sufficient power to vaporize the tissue to the appropriate depth while minimizing damage to the surrounding normal tissues. Treatment should extend beyond the involved area to treat 3 to 5 mm of bordering normal skin. Most patients with limited disease can be treated under local anesthesia. Patients with more extensive disease and involvement of the anus or perianal tissues will require regional or general anesthesia. Postoperative pain control is best achieved with a combination of oral analgesics and sitz baths. Larger lesions or multiple lesions involving large areas are best treated by simple excision or skinning vulvectomy with split-thickness skin grafting. For older patients with vulvar atrophy, a simple vulvectomy with primary closure is often the best treatment.

Recurrences will occur in about 10% to 20% of patients—most in untreated areas—and can be treated with repeat vaporization or excision once invasive disease is ruled out.

Paget's Disease

Extramammary Paget's disease can occur anywhere in the body outside of the breasts but is most commonly found on the vulva. It is now believed to represent a group of neoplasms with multiple histogenetic origins. It may arise directly from pluripotent stem cells within the epidermis or by direct extension from an adenocarcinoma in the apocrine or eccrine glands, or it may metastasize from a remote malignancy, most commonly of gastrointestinal, breast, or genitourinary origin. Risk factors include being Caucasian and postmenopausal. As with VIN, patients commonly present with vulvar pruritus, which in the case of Paget's disease may precede the diagnosis by years. The characteristic lesion is grossly well demarcated with a velvety red appearance and scattered white patches representing areas of hyperkeratosis, although the appearance of lesions can be highly variable. Women with Paget's disease should also undergo evaluation to look for occult malignancies of the cervix, colon, bladder, gallbladder, and breast, which may occur in 30% of patients. An underlying adenocarcinoma has been reported in up to 100% of patients with perianal Paget's disease.

The treatment for Paget's disease is radical vulvectomy, including the epidermis and the dermis extending down to Colles' fascia. Paget's disease should not be treated with skinning vulvectomy, as there are frequently underlying apocrine adenocarcinomas. The lesion can grow horizontally and frequently is more extensive than is apparent grossly. Local recurrences are common; however, the prognosis for intraepithelial extramammary Paget's disease is excellent. It is bene-

ficial to have confirmed microscopically negative surgical margins via intraoperative frozen sections, as recurrences are three times more likely when the surgical margins are histologically positive. Recurrences can be managed by re-excision. For invasive Paget's disease, an inguinal-femoral lymphadenectomy should be performed in addition to a radical vulvectomy. Much like squamous carcinoma, the prognosis for invasive disease confined to the vulva appears good. However, for the one half of patients with invasive disease who present with regional node metastases, the prognosis is quite poor. For all patients, continued careful surveillance for adenocarcinomas involving the breasts or the gastrointestinal or genitourinary tracts must be practiced.

Squamous Cell Carcinoma

The lifetime risks for acquiring and dying from carcinoma of the vulva have been calculated to be 0.3 and 0.1, respectively. In contrast, the lifetime risk of dying from breast cancer is 32 times higher. Size and depth of invasion of the primary tumor, presence of lymph vascular space invasion, and regional lymph node metastases are the histopathologic features significantly correlated with survival. Unfortunately, delay in diagnosis is a common occurrence. Patients delay because of fear of cancer and minimization of symptoms, which are present for more than 6 months in two thirds of patients and longer than a year in a third. Physician delay occurs because of the similarity of the symptoms and the lesions to benign conditions such as lichen sclerosus as well as a reluctance to perform biopsies. Before treating any lesion on the vulva, a punch biopsy should be obtained from the center of the lesion, and extensive and multifocal lesions deserve multiple biopsies.

Treatment of Invasive Squamous Cell Carcinoma

The International Federation of Gynecology and Obstetrics issued new guidelines for the staging of vulvar cancer (Table 1), which recognizes that "microinvasion" can be defined for the vulva and allows for a modification of surgical resection. Patients with stage Ia lesions have a negligible incidence of lymph node metastasis and may, in the absence of lymph vascular invasion and clinically suspicious lymph nodes, be treated with radical local excision only. A radical excision of

TABLE 1. FIGO Staging of Invasive Cancer of the Vulva

T, N, M*	Stage		Description
Tis	0		Carcinoma in situ
T1 N0 M0	I		Lesions 2 cm or less in size confined to the vulva or perineum. No nodal metastasis
		Ia	Stromal invasion no greater than 1 mm†
		Ib	Stromal invasion greater than 1 mm
T2 N0 M0	II		Lesions greater than 2 cm, confined to the vulva or perineum. No nodal metastasis.
T3 N0 M0	III		Lesions of any size with
T1 N1 M0			Extension to the lower vagina and/or urethra
T2 N1 M0			and/or anus
T3 N1 M0			*and/or*
			Unilateral regional lymph node metastasis
	IV		
T4 N any M0		IVa	Tumor invades any of the following:
T1 N2 M0			Upper urethra, bladder mucosa, rectal
T2 N2 M0			mucosa, or pelvic bone
T3 N2 M0			*and/or*
			Bilateral regional lymph node metastasis
T any N any M1		IVb	Any distant metastases, including pelvic lymph nodes

°N—Regional (inguinal-femoral) lymph nodes
    N0 No regional lymph node metastasis
    N1 Unilateral regional lymph node metastasis
    N2 Bilateral regional lymph node metastasis
M—Distant metastasis
    M0 No clinical metastasis
    M1 Distant metastasis (including pelvic lymph nodes)
    †The depth of invasion is defined as the measurement from the epithelial-stromal junction of the adjacent most superficial dermal papilla to the deepest point of invasion.

some or all of the vulva is defined as one that extends to the periosteum of the pubic bone or the inferior fascia of the urogenital diaphragm. The specimen should include a 2-cm margin beyond the edge of the lesion.

The treatment of more advanced lesions is best individualized to the patient. For smaller lesions (T1 or T2), the vulvar excision can spare the clitoris if the lesion is more than 2 cm away. For larger lesions, treatment considerations include radical total or hemivulvectomy, neoadjuvant chemotherapy or radiation, or both, followed by radical surgery or, in some cases, pelvic exenteration. When choosing the most appropriate therapy for each patient, consideration must be given to her overall health status, the nature and location of the primary lesion, and presence or absence of metastatic disease.

Like the vulvar lesion, treatment of the regional lymph nodes must also be individualized. For T1 lesions with less than 1 mm of invasion (Stage Ia, microinvasive), the groin dissection may be omitted in the absence of clinically palpable lymph nodes. Ipsilateral inguinofemoral lymphadenectomy is appropriate with a 2-cm or smaller vulvar lesion that is located laterally and more than 2 cm from the clitoris or anus.

The risk of pelvic node metastases is insignificant if the inguinofemoral nodes are uninvolved. However, pelvic nodal metastases are present in up to one third of cases when three or more inguinofemoral nodes are microscopically involved, the groin nodes are clinically positive, or there is bilateral regional lymph node involvement. In these cases, adjuvant radiation therapy given to the groin and pelvis has demonstrated improved survival.

Early surgical complications associated with radical vulvectomy and bilateral inguinofemoral lymphadenectomy include wound infection, lymphedema, and thromboembolic disease. Potential late effects of treatment include urinary incontinence, vaginal stenosis, lymphedema, and impaired sexual function.

As with primary disease, the treatment for recurrent vulvar cancer must be individualized and based on disease site and type of prior therapy. Options for salvage therapy include surgery, radiation, and chemotherapy, used either alone or in combination.

Malignant Melanoma

Vulvar melanomas account for 1.3% of all melanomas in women. The median age at diagnosis is 66 years. Caucasian women experience a 2.6 relative risk for the development of malignant melanoma when compared with black women. While most lesions are pigmented, amelanotic melanoma can occur on the vulva and may be confused with squamous carcinoma or Paget's disease. Histologic differentiation is based on immunohistochemical markers including carcinoembryonic antigen (CEA) and S-100. According to data from the Gynecologic Oncology Group, capillary lymphatic invasion and central tumor location were the only factors significantly associated with lymph node metastases. The only independent prognostic factors for disease-free survival are tumor depth and lymph node status, and these factors are incorporated into the American Joint Committee on Cancer (AJCC) stage for malignant melanoma of the skin (Table 2). When the lymph node status is unknown, Breslow's depth of invasion (see Table 2) becomes the most significant predictor of survival.

Based on these data, treatment recommendations are wide local excision with at least a 1- to 2-cm margin for lesions less than 0.75 mm thick (approximately Clark's level III) that demonstrate no evidence of capillary lymphatic invasion. Larger lesions require at least a 2-cm margin and often necessitate at least a hemivulvectomy. In addition, a bilateral regional lymph node dissection is recommended, although its role is unproven. Although adjuvant therapy for advanced or recurrent disease has been disappointing, immunotherapy using interferon or interleukin-2 has shown promise in recent trials.

Bartholin's Gland Carcinoma

While the majority of the tumors arising in the Bartholin gland are squamous or adenoid cystic, adenocarcinoma and transitional cell types may occur. The lesions are often advanced at diagnosis because of their origin beneath the skin and because of delay in treatment due to misdiagnosis as simple inflammatory processes. Since Bartholin's gland abscesses are uncommon in older women, it is recommended that tissue diagnosis be obtained by excisional biopsy or office fine needle aspiration of any abscess occurring after the fourth decade. Treatment is guided by the same principles as that for squamous cell carcinoma and has excellent survival for early stage disease.

Basal Cell Carcinoma

Basal cell carcinoma accounts for about 2% of all vulvar cancers and is generally considered to follow an indolent course characterized by local invasion and infrequent metastases. The recommended treatment is wide local excision with the addition of regional lymph node dissections for lesions greater than 4 cm as all of the reported cases of lymph node metastases are in patients with these larger lesions. Keratinization is commonly found and differentiation must be made between keratinized basal cell carcinoma and basosquamous carcinoma, which has a much poorer prognosis.

Verrucous Carcinoma

A variant of squamous cell carcinoma, verrucous carcinoma is characterized by nests of well-

TABLE 2. Regional and Microstaging Systems for Melanoma

AJCC Stage*	Description	Level	Clark's Level of Deepest Invasion	Breslow's Thickness (mm)
Ia	Localized, <0.76 mm or Clark's II	I	Intraepithelial	<0.76
Ib	Localized, 0.76–1.5 mm or Clark's III	II	Papillary dermis	0.76–1.50
IIa	Localized, 1.51–4.0 mm or Clark's IV	III	Junction of reticular and papillary dermis	1.51–2.25
IIb	Localized, >4.0 mm or Clark's V	IV	Reticular dermis	2.26–3.0
III	Limited regional nodal metastases (only 1 regional lymph node basin)	V	Subcutaneous fat	>3.0
IV	Advanced regional metastases or any distant metastases			

*From Beahrs OH, Henson DE, Hutter RVP, and Kennedy BJ, eds: Philadelphia: JB Lippincott, 1992. American Joint Committee on Cancer Manual for Staging of Cancer, 4th ed.

differentiated squamous cells without invasion. It should be suspected when a condylomatous lesion is encountered in a postmenopausal woman. Regional and distant metastases are rare. Surgical excision is the treatment of choice, as these tumors are resistant to radiotherapy and may instead respond with more aggressive growth and metastasis.

Vulvar Sarcomas

Vulvar sarcomas constitute less than 2% of all vulvar malignancies. The most common histologic type is leiomyosarcoma. Presenting symptoms include a vulvar mass, pain, and bleeding. Metastatic disease at presentation is rare. Treatment is primarily by radical local excision. Local recurrences are common. Risk factors for recurrence include size of tumor, high mitotic count, and infiltrative versus pushing margins. Adjuvant chemotherapy and radiation have been useful for only certain histologic subtypes.

Metastatic Tumors

Most metastatic tumors to the vulva arise in the lower genital tract, with the cervix being the most common site of origin. Carcinomas of the breast, lung, and gastrointestinal tract have also been reported to metastasize to the vulva.

Conclusions

Tumors of the vulva are an uncommon but challenging disease for the clinician. With proper evaluation, treatment, and follow-up, the cure rate is high, especially for preinvasive and early-stage disease. As younger women are becoming increasingly afflicted with vulvar disease, treatment plans must become more flexible to maximize quality of life and psychosexual well-being without sacrificing cure rates.

Obstetrics

Amniocentesis for Antenatal Diagnosis of Genetic Disorders

Mark I. Evans, MD

Mark P. Johnson, MD

Arie Drugan, MD

In the 1970s, prenatal diagnosis emerged as a medical possibility. In the 1980s, the expansion of available technology made the offering of prenatal diagnosis the standard of care for patients with defined indications such as advanced maternal age. As the number of physicians and facilities who could deal with such patients rapidly increased, the specifics of the indications were liberalized. For example, the "magic number" for offering genetic amniocentesis fell from age 40, to age 38, and now to 35 or even lower. The development of other technologies such as alpha-fetoprotein and multiple marker screening has added more flexibility to the indications for offering prenatal diagnosis.

Indications for Offering Prenatal Diagnosis

Advanced Maternal Age

At a bare minimum, patients who will be 35 years of age at delivery must be offered the opportunity of having genetic amniocentesis or chorionic villus sampling (CVS). While most patients presenting for prenatal diagnosis are concerned about Down syndrome, in reality Down syndrome—while the most common diagnosis made—represents only about 50% of the abnormalities that are detected. Thus, counseling should be directed at the total risk of chromosome abnormalities for the maternal age (Table 1).

Previous Child with Chromosome Abnormalities

Several studies have looked at the risk of having a second baby with a chromosome abnormality.

While there are certain subsets of populations in which one of the parents has a balanced translocation that can raise the risk in subsequent pregnancies to the 10% to 15% range, in instances where both parents are found to have normal chromosomes, the risk for abnormalities in a subsequent pregnancy is approximately 1%, which is equivalent to the risk of a 38-year-old woman. Therefore, all patients who have had a previous child with Down syndrome, or any other chromosome abnormality, should be offered prenatal diagnosis regardless of their age.

History of Multiple Miscarriages

Several studies have addressed the issue of increased risk of a liveborn, aneuploid child follow-

TABLE 1. Chromosome Risks by Maternal Age at Midtrimester and at Term Delivery

Maternal Age	Trisomy 21		All Aneuploidy	
	Midtrimester	Term	Midtrimester	Term
20–21	1/1167	1/1167	1/368	1/526
22–23	1/1000	1/1429	1/350	1/500
24–25	1/875	1/1250	1/333	1/476
26	1/823	1/1176	1/333	1/476
27	1/778	1/1111	1/319	1/455
28	1/737	1/1053	1/304	1/435
29	1/700	1/1000	1/292	1/417
30	1/666	1/952	1/269	1/385
31	1/636	1/909	1/269	1/385
32	1/538	1/769	1/225	1/322
33	1/437	1/602	1/222	1/286
34	1/350	1/485	1/182	1/238
35	1/270	1/378	1/143	1/192
36	1/206	1/289	1/115	1/156
37	1/160	1/224	1/91	1/127
38	1/123	1/173	1/72	1/102
39	1/96	1/136	1/57	1/83
40	1/74	1/106	1/46	1/66
41		1/82		1/53
42		1/63		1/42
43		1/49		1/33
44		1/38		1/26
45		1/30		1/21
46		1/23		1/16
47		1/18		1/13
48		1/14		1/10
49		1/11		1/8

ing multiple miscarriages. From our own data and others, it would appear that women who have had two or more spontaneous losses, not attributable to other factors such as inadequate luteal phase, are at a somewhat increased risk of having abnormalities in a third or subsequent pregnancy. Therefore, we believe (although this is not a universally held opinion) that women with two or more miscarriages should be offered amniocentesis or CVS. Our own experience has suggested approximately a 1% detection rate of abnormalities, consistent with a risk rate for a 38-year-old patient.

Mendelian Disorders

Fluid obtained at amniocentesis can be used for the diagnosis of inborn errors of metabolism. However, such testing is laborious and expensive, so it is only recommended when the couple is identified to be at significant risk, such as having a previously affected child, or when carrier testing shows both parents to carry an abnormal trait. Carrier testing should be performed for patients of specific ethnic groups, for such disorders as sickle cell anemia in African Americans, Tay-Sachs in Jews, β-thalassemia in Mediterranean populations, and α-thalassemia in Southeast Asian populations, for whom the frequency of the abnormal gene is much higher than in the general population. (It should be noted that the list of diagnosable disorders is constantly expanding, and when the situation arises, contact with the appropriate authorities in a particular field is recommended.)

Increasing availability of molecular diagnosis of single-gene disorders, through the use of restriction fragment length polymorphism and gene probes, suggests that this method will be the future mainstay of prenatal diagnosis. Unlike enzymatic or biochemical assays, DNA material is similar in all cells, without tissue specificity. The use of molecular diagnosis would avoid confusion created by changes in the level of expression of specific enzymes as a result of hormonal changes in pregnancy. Molecular methods will also, among other factors, enhance the shift toward earlier diagnosis by CVS, as 1 mg of placental tissue contains many times more cells (and DNA) to analyze than the number of cells obtained from 40 mL of amniotic fluid, thus shortening the procedure-to-diagnosis interval.

History of Neural Tube Defects

Neural tube defects (NTD) such as spina bifida and anencephaly, occur in about 1 in 700 white

and 1 in 1000 African-American pregnancies. Amniocentesis to measure alpha-fetoprotein and sometimes acetylcholin-esterase is used for a definitive diagnosis in patients at high risk. However, the vast majority (about 95%) of all babies born with neural tube defects are born to couples who have no reason to suspect they are at any increased risk. Thus, inherent in a program to detect the vast majority of neural tube defects is the necessity to test all pregnancies. Clearly it is impossible to offer amniocentesis to all patients. Thus, the concept of maternal serum alpha-fetoprotein (MSAFP) screening was developed in the mid-1970s. For neural tube defects, approximately 3% of patients will either have one very significantly elevated MSAFP value (greater than 4 MOM [multiple of the median]) or two values, both of which are greater than 2.5 MOM. Of these 3% of patients, ultrasonography will find an obvious explanation for the elevations in approximately one half of the cases: twins, anencephaly, severe NTD, or most commonly, incorrect dates. The remaining 1.5% of patients are offered a genetic amniocentesis. In most large programs, including our own at Hutzel Hospital/Wayne State University, the pick-up rate for abnormalities is approximately 5% of patients who have the amniocentesis. It should be noted that even in a top-quality ultrasonography unit, approximately 10% to 15% of all defects may not be detected by the screening ultrasonograms. These data support the contention that amniocentesis is appropriate even if the ultrasonogram appears normal, although it would be appropriate to alter the odds when a good, thorough ultrasonogram is normal. Amniotic fluid alpha-fetoprotein and acetylcholinesterase remain the most sensitive tests available for detection of defects in these patients.

Amniotic Fluid Alpha-Fetoprotein

The association between elevated levels of alpha-fetoprotein (AFP) in amniotic fluid and open neural tube defects was first noted by Brock and Sutcliffe in 1972. Other abnormalities such as fetal teratomas, Meckel's syndrome, exstrophy of the cloaca, esophageal atresia, ventral wall defects, congenital skin defects, and fetal demise are also associated (at least in part) with elevated amniotic fluid AFP levels. The accuracy of prenatal diagnosis of NTD is improved by testing for acetylcholinesterase (AChE), a relatively specific neural tissue enzyme. The combination of amniotic fluid AFP and AChE has a false-positive rate of 1 in several hundred to 1000, as compared with a 5% to 7% false-positive AFP in clear amniotic fluid, and 16% false-positive AFP in bloody amniotic fluid.

Traditionally, amniotic fluid AChE was considered a bimodal test, positive results being frequently associated with fetal anomalies and negative results excluding such problems. With increasingly sophisticated laboratory techniques, a faint but true band can sometimes be detected in the specific AChE position on gel electrophoresis. This result is inconclusive, since in early pregnancy (less than 15 weeks' gestation), this result is commonly seen (approximately 10%), but less frequently associated with fetal anomalies (20%). Later in pregnancy, an increased AChE is rarely seen (2%), but an anomaly is detected in more than half these cases.

Multiple Marker Screening for Chromosomal Risk

The chance association in the mid 1980s that babies born with chromosome abnormalities such as Down syndrome tended to have lower than normal MSAFP values led to a complete re-evaluation of our assessment of genetic risk. Only 20% of babies with Down syndrome are born to women 35 years of age and older. Thus, despite the fact that for any given younger woman the risk of having a baby with a chromosome abnormality is lower than for an older woman, in total numbers, the vast majority of babies with chromosome abnormalities are born to women who have no presumed risk. The advent of the use of low maternal serum AFP allowed for the identification of approximately one third of the 80% of women under the age of 35 carrying fetuses with Down syndrome to be identified. In total, including the 20% of women over age 35, about 45% of such pregnancies could be identified. While clearly this was a vast improvement over age risk alone, there was much more that could be done. In the late 1980s, the concept of using additional markers, particularly human chorionic gonadotropin (hCG) and unconjugated estriol (E3), were introduced, and although there is considerable controversy in the literature as to whether double screening (AFP + hCG) is better or worse than triple screening (AFP, hCG, + E3), most studies suggest that about 60% of the total of Down syndrome cases can be identified through the use of multiple marker screening—that is, 20% of women over age 35, plus about 40% of the 80% under age 35. Throughout the 1990s, numerous papers have touted one screening methodology over an-

other. It is very clear, however, and all physicians must understand, that there are some cases of Down syndrome that will be picked up by either double or triple screening, some that will be missed by both, some that will be detectable by double and missed by triple, and some that will be detectable by triple and missed by double. There is no one uniformly agreed upon protocol. Just because a particular case was not detected does not mean the screening was done wrong, nor would it be appropriate to infer that another method of screening should have been done. From a population point of view, the answer lies in what percentage sensitivity there is for what percentage of patients told to be at risk, and judgments cannot be made on an individual case basis.

Many investigators are attempting to further improve screening. At the millennium there will be several new markers, which will undoubtedly come and go. We believe that as new markers come on board, estriol will quietly fade to the background, and there will be combinations of anywhere between two and five markers being used. Promising parameters currently include the following:

- Pregnancy-associated placental proteins, which seem to be very effective in the first trimester but not beyond
- Free beta, which is the associated form of hCG, which in the second trimester is probably equivalent to the total intact beta, but seems to be better in the late first and early second trimester
- Neutrophil alkaline phosphatase, which in earlier published data has the highest detection sensitivity (80%)
- Inhibin, and the α subunit of hCG

We predict that ultimately clinicians will order aneuploidy screening without specific tests being ordered, and that the laboratory will run an appropriate panel of tests as a function of the gestational age at which the test is being ordered, and perhaps the maternal age of the patient. Another dramatic change will be the concept of using ultrasonographic data in affect as a laboratory test. It has been clearly shown that there are certain markers, such as nuchal membranes in the first trimester, which convey significant risk of aneuploidy, and that such risk can be calculated into an overall algorithm of risks for patients.

Some investigators, and in fact some jurisdictions, have proposed that rather than allow patients to go primarily to amniocentesis or CVS, that biochemical screening should be done first to determine risk. From a public health point of view, it has been shown that if maternal age 35 were eliminated as a criteria for invasive testing and replaced with screening, overall the detection frequency would go up for the same number of invasive procedures performed in the population. However, in American society, we believe that patients now over 35 who have a "right" to such services would not take kindly to having that "right" removed. A further elaborate discussion is beyond the scope of this chapter.

Technical Aspects of Amniocentesis

Amniocentesis was traditionally performed at or beyond 16 weeks' gestation, when the uterine fundus is well above the pelvic brim, and the amount of fluid around the fetus is about 200 mL. However, with advances in technology, all dogmas are being called into question, with a shift toward earlier procedures.

The amniocentesis procedure should be preceded by a genetic counseling session that includes evaluation of family pedigree and genetic risks, and explanation of advantages and risks of the procedure. Amniocentesis should be performed by an obstetrician trained and experienced in the procedure. A detailed level II ultrasonographic examination should assess gestational age, fetal and placental location, and the volume and location of pockets of amniotic fluid. The preferred site of needle insertion is then chosen. After sterile preparation of the lower abdominal skin, a 20- or 22-gauge, 3.5-inch spinal needle with stylet is commonly used to penetrate the abdominal layers to the amniotic cavity. The needle should be inserted quickly, directly, and to the depth needed. The experienced operator should be able to feel the needle passing through different tissue layers until the amniotic membranes are penetrated. Injection of a local anesthetic into the needle path is, in our opinion, not necessary, as it may be more uncomfortable for the patient than the actual amniocentesis. Stopping every centimeter to assess location on the ultrasonographic screen only adds to the discomfort and may raise the risks. If possible, the selected needle path should avoid the placenta and stay away from the fetus, although a significant difference in pregnancy outcome has not been noted between transplacental and nontransplacental amniocentesis. Transplacental amniocentesis should be avoided, if reasonably possible, in Rh-negative women even though the

risk of Rh isosensitization is probably only slightly increased by transplacental passage of the needle with disruption of fetomaternal circulation. Pooled data from several studies estimate the risk of Rh isosensitization associated with amniocentesis in Rh-negative women with Rh-positive fetuses to be 1% to 2.5% above the background risk for these patients. Blood type and Rh status should be known prior to amniocentesis, and women with Rh-negative antibody screening should receive 300 μg of Rh immunoglobulin following the procedure.

When the needle tip is satisfactorily placed into a pocket of amniotic fluid, freely flowing fluid will be obtained when the stylet is removed. The first milliliters of amniotic fluid are aspirated in a syringe and discarded, to minimize the risk of contamination by maternal cells in the needle pathway. If blood is present in the first drops and subsequently clears, the bloody aliquots are also discarded. Twenty to 30 mL of amniotic fluid are then gently aspirated into a different syringe, transferred into sterile tubes or maintained in the original syringes, and transported at room temperature to the laboratory.

Although there are a few highly skilled operators who were trained in amniocentesis before ultrasonography was routinely used, real-time ultrasonography should be used to guide needle penetration during the amniocentesis procedure. A decrease in the frequency of bloody taps, multiple needle insertions, and failure to obtain amniotic fluid have been noted with ultrasonographic guidance. Continuous ultrasonographic guidance may be especially helpful for the relatively inexperienced operator, may decrease the incidence of fetal trauma and fetal loss from the procedure, and may help identify potential technical problems such as membrane tenting during the procedure. (In the last case, rotating the needle while inserting it may help.)

The ultrasound transducer should be directed so that the beam is parallel to the needle track. The beveled end of the needle is usually identified as a bright spot. Aseptic conditions may be maintained by using sterile coupling gel and placing the transducer into a sterile plastic bag or glove.

Patients are released after a brief period of observation and ultrasonographic documentation of fetal viability. Although patients are allowed to return to normal activity following amniocentesis, strenuous exercise and sexual activity should probably be deferred for 2 to 3 days. Patients are instructed to report signs of amniorrhexis, vaginal bleeding, regular uterine activity, or infection.

Safety and Complications of Amniocentesis

Clinical

Amniocentesis is a relatively safe procedure with severe maternal complications almost non-existent. The frequency of procedure-related amnionitis is quoted to be 0.1%. Vaginal leakage of amniotic fluid is experienced in 1% to 2% of women but usually resolves within 48 to 72 hours. Persistent and significant amniotic fluid leakage is rare but may lead to oligohydramnios and, as a result, fetal deformities and pulmonary hypoplasia. Pregnancy loss related to the procedure in experienced hands is 0.2% to 0.5% over and above the spontaneous pregnancy loss rate at 16 weeks' gestation (estimated to be 3%). When comparing amniocentesis groups to control subjects, a US collaborative study did not find an association between pregnancy loss and amount of fluid removed or number of procedures performed (on same individual on different days). The only significant associations were found with frequency of vaginal bleeding following the procedure and number of needle insertions.

Difficulties in Cytogenetic Interpretation

Cytogenetic analysis of amniotic fluid cells accurately reflects the fetal status in over 99% of cases. However, the clinical interpretation of cytogenetic results may not always be conclusive. While in most cases concrete information can be given to the prospective parents, when inversions, translocations, or mosaic karyotypes are involved, the expected phenotype may be unclear. Comparison with parental karyotypes is frequently needed to clarify the clinical picture. If one of the parents is the carrier of the same inversion or balanced translocation, the parents may be reassured that the phenotype most probably will be normal. If, however, the abnormality occurred in the product of conception de novo, the situation is of great anxiety for both patients and physicians, as the exact risk is not known.

Differentiation between cytogenetic abnormalities that truly reflect fetal chromosome aberrations from those that are the result of laboratory artifacts may be difficult. Two to 3% of all amniotic fluid cell cultures show at least one hypermodal cell (more than 46 chromosomes). Chromosome number 20 is one of the five chromosomes most frequently involved in pseudo mosaicism in cultured amniotic fluid cells. Fortunately, the majority of cases (85%) were associated with grossly normal phenotypes. There is evidence that an extraembryonic origin (trophoblastic nondisjunction) is the acting mechanism in most of these cases, and the mosaicism is not represented in fetal tissue.

To identify true mosaicism, finding hypermodal cells in different culture flasks, or in at least two colonies, is necessary. Multiple cells with the same abnormality in a single flask or colony are seen in about 0.7% of cases. Multiple abnormal cells in multiple flasks or colonies have frequencies of 0.2%. However, even in these cases, the mosaicism will not always be reflected in fetal blood chromosomes. Gosden et al. investigated chromosomal mosaicism in amniotic fluid cell cultures using simultaneous lymphocyte cultures from fetal blood sampling. Fetal blood chromosomes were normal in 15 of 16 autosomal trisomy mosaicisms and in all eight sex chromosome trisomy mosaicisms. When mosaicism for structural chromosomal rearrangements and for marker chromosomes was investigated, amniotic cell culture results were correct in 5 of 11 cases of translocation or inversion, and in 4 of 6 cases with de novo supernumerary marker chromosomal mosaicism. Although these results do not exclude a chromosomal mosaicism confined to a specific fetal tissue, the follow-up of mosaicism in cultured amniotic cells by fetal blood sampling helps to avoid termination of pregnancy of some normal fetuses. Fetal blood karyotypes obtained via cordocentesis may increase insight into the phenotype of chromosome rearrangement that can potentially cause mental retardation and multiple structural anomalies even in the mosaic form.

Multiple Gestation

Monozygotic twinning (MZ) is a relatively constant phenomenon across races, ages, and parities. Dizygotic twinning (DZ) shows ethnic and familial influences and increases in frequency with maternal age and parity. Among white North American women, the frequency of twin birth was 1 in every 87 in the 1980s, with about 70% of these twins being dizygotic. However, with the explosion of fertility drug use, some estimates suggest 1 in 45 pregnancies are multiples. It would be expected, therefore, that 1.2% to 2% of patients presenting for prenatal diagnosis have multiple gestations.

Monozygotic twins will virtually always be concordant to chromosome abnormalities, while DZ twins will almost always be discordant. As every twin has its own risk for chromosomal problems, the risk that at least one twin is abnormal should be quoted as approximately twice the age-related risk. Separate amniocentesis of each sac is necessary to assess the chromosomal status of each fetus.

The amniocenteses are performed after ultrasonographic identification of the membrane separating the two sacs. Using continuous ultrasonographic guidance, it is generally easy to sample the two sacs separately. If continuous ultrasonography is not used, injection of a dye like indigo carmine or Congo red into the first sac, after aspiration of amniotic fluid, is a helpful marker. Aspiration of clear fluid from the second sac, following insertion of dye into the first, indicates that the operator did not sample the same sac twice. Using this method, successful amniocentesis can be achieved in virtually all cases, and the amniotic fluid obtained can be analyzed for chromosomes and for AFP. Although data are still lacking on the interpretation of amniotic fluid AFP in twin gestation, a study of 73 twin pairs demonstrated that discordance (defined as an AFP difference of ≥0.2) (MOM) in amniotic fluid AFP results is more common in DZ than MZ twins. In same-sex twins, discordance between sacs is less common, but should be regarded with high suspicion for an abnormality in the high-AFP twin. AChE readily diffuses between sacs and cannot be used to determine which twin has an abnormality.

Discolored Amniotic Fluid

Brown- or green-tinged amniotic fluid is found in 1% to 6% of midtrimester amniocenteses. Karp and Schiller first reported this phenomenon and concluded that it has no clinical significance. Others, however, have reported high perinatal mortality associated with discolored amniotic fluid. Allen observed an incidence of discolored amniotic fluid in 4709 consecutive amniocenteses of 1.7%, and fetal mortality of 5%. An incidence of 3.5% for discolored amniotic fluid, and a 9% frequency of miscarriages in this group (compared to 1.6% frequency of miscarriages with normal-colored amniotic fluid) was noted by Zorn et al. Analysis by spectrophotometry, chromatography, and electrophoresis of discolored fluid samples indicates that in most cases the discoloring pigment is blood rather than fetal bowel contents. This seems to confirm a previous study by Hankins et al. in which the only statistically significant difference between control and test patients for presence of discolored fluid was bleeding prior to amniocentesis.

Early Amniocentesis

Increasing technical capabilities and patient preference for earlier and more private genetic diagnosis have motivated a shift from traditional amniocentesis, performed around 16 weeks' gestation, to earlier procedures: CVS and early amniocentesis. CVS is still not accessible to many patients who would use such services. An alternative approach for patients opting for early diagnosis is to perform an amniocentesis before the traditional gestational age. Advantages of early amniocentesis over CVS would include the ability to measure AFP and AChE. The biggest problem is defining what is "early" amniocentesis, as there are vast differences in techniques, background risks, and procedural risks in patients between 10 and 14 weeks. Earlier procedures require a sharp thrust into the cavity to avoid tenting membranes. The Canadian early amniocentesis trial has shown a 1% risk of talipes equinovarus, which is predominantly associated with fluid leakage. Other studies have confirmed these risks, and therefore amniocentesis should not be performed before 13 weeks. It is suggested that in the first trimester, chorionic villus sampling is safer and the procedure of choice. Also because of slower growth in culture of these earlier cells, disadvantages include a slower result time, particularly in biochemical or molecular disorders.

Alpha-fetoprotein measured in amniotic fluid samples from early gestation peaks at 12 to 13 weeks and then gradually declines, following the trend in fetal blood. High amniotic AFP values have been found with fetal structural anomalies but amniotic fluid AFP and AChE in early amniocentesis should be interpreted with caution.

We believe that the trend toward increasing public and professional demand for earlier prenatal diagnosis will continue and that, in the new millennium, first-trimester procedures by CVS will become the mainstay of prenatal diagnosis.

Management

Ninety-eight percent of all patients who present for prenatal diagnosis have normal test results. However, the reason for doing such testing is that the tragedy of the birth of a severely impaired child can sometimes be avoided. It should be made clear to all couples who present for prenatal diagnosis that no test can guarantee the birth of a healthy child; in addition, they should understand that they may be faced with a very difficult decision following the detection of an abnormality.

When prenatal diagnostic services were developed in the early 1970s, and the number of physicians who could perform the testing and the number of laboratories who could process specimens were few and far between, those services had to be prioritized to those patients who were at the greatest risk. There were also often added requirements, that is, that the patients would agree to have an abortion if an abnormality were detected. While there may have been some logic to such a requirement when services were extremely scarce, it is generally believed today that such a requirement is inappropriate both from medical and ethical standpoints. It is a generally held concept that the decision to seek information should have no bearing what the couple decides to do with the information once it has been obtained.

When an abnormality is discovered by the laboratory, this information should be relayed to the couple as soon as possible, preferably by meeting the patient in person rather than by telephone contact. Only in the rarest of circumstances should devastating information be given by telephone. Patients should be seen within a matter of hours as it is less than ideal to relay the potential of bad news on a Friday and schedule a meeting for the following Wednesday. When relaying bad news, the first step is to remind couples that the reason they sought prenatal diagnosis was to have this information as soon as possible and to allow them the legal option of termination of pregnancy, if they so choose. It is then imperative that the diagnosis and its ramifications be explained in as thorough and nonjudgemental a fashion as possible. The couple can then be told what options are available to them including continuation of pregnancy, termination of pregnancy, or obtaining more information as appropriate.

Gestational age time factors are, of course, a critical element, particularly for traditional midtrimester amniocentesis in which the procedure has been performed between 16 and 17 weeks' gestation, with results taking approximately 3 weeks. Thus, at 20 weeks, the legal limitations of abortion need to be considered as these may vary from jurisdiction to jurisdiction. Furthermore, by 20 weeks, the patient is visibly pregnant and has usually felt the baby moving, and the bonding process has accelerated. At that point the termi-

nation of pregnancy of an otherwise wanted conception can be extremely emotional and traumatic, and it is incumbent upon the counseling team to provide emotional support as best as possible, and to make the patient and couple aware of more complete services if they are available.

In our experience, approximately 50% of patients who are confronted with the diagnosis of a serious abnormality will elect to terminate a pregnancy. There is a correlation between the severity of the anomaly and the likelihood of patients choosing to terminate. A 100% rate or a 0% rate in any one center would suggest inappropriate counseling with biases toward one option. It is extremely important that the commonly asked question. "What would you (the professional) do in this situation?" not be answered and that the health care providers make a great effort not to expose their own biases. Couples should be told that they will be emotionally supported no matter what their decision, and that they will receive further appropriate medical care. In our opinion, a center that does prenatal diagnosis must have either a personal commitment to perform such terminations of pregnancies or a solid relationship with another physician who will. There is no situation more terrifying to couples than to discover a fetal abnormality and be told by the physician who performed the amniocentesis that he or she does not do abortions, or does not believe in abortions, and will not help them to arrange for such.

Amniotic Fluid Embolism

Steven L. Clark, MD

Amniotic fluid embolism (AFE) is an uncommon obstetric disorder with a mortality rate of 60% to 70% and is a leading cause of maternal death. AFE is classically characterized by hypoxia, hypotension, or hemodynamic collapse and coagulopathy. Despite numerous attempts to develop an animal model, AFE remains incompletely understood. Nevertheless, the past decade has seen several significant advances in our understanding of this enigmatic condition.

Hemodynamic Alterations

In humans, an initial, transient phase of hemodynamic change involving both systemic and pulmonary vasospasm leads to a more often recognized secondary phase involving principally hypotension and depressed ventricular function. The mechanism of left ventricular failure is uncertain. Work in the rat model suggests the presence of possible coronary artery spasm and myocardial ischemia in animal AFE. On the other hand, the global hypoxia commonly seen in patients with AFE could account for left ventricular dysfunction. The in vitro observation of decreased myometrial contractility in the presence of amniotic fluid also suggests the possibility of a similar effect of amniotic fluid on myocardium.

Pulmonary Manifestations

Patients suffering AFE typically develop rapid and often profound hypoxia, which may result in permanent neurologic impairment in survivors of this condition. This hypoxia is likely due to a combination of initial pulmonary vasospasm and ventricular dysfunction. In both animal models and human experience, however, this initial hypoxia is often transient. Initial profound shunting as well as rapid recovery is often seen. In survivors, primary lung injury often leads to the adult respiratory distress syndrome and secondary oxygenation defects.

Coagulopathy

Patients surviving the initial hemodynamic insult may succumb to a secondary coagulopathy. The exact incidence of the coagulopathy is unknown. Coagulopathy was an entry criterion for inclusion in the initial analysis of the National AFE Registry, but several patients were submitted to the registry who clearly had AFE but did not have clinical evidence of coagulopathy. In a similar manner, a number of patients have been observed who developed an acute obstetric coagulopathy alone in the absence of placental abruptio and suffered fatal exsanguination without any evidence of primary hemodynamic or pulmonary insult.

The coagulopathy associated with severe placental abruption and that seen with AFE are probably similar in origin and represent an activation of the coagulation cascade following exposure of the maternal circulation to a variety of fetal antigens with varying thromboplastin-like effects.

Pathophysiology

In a recent analysis of the National AFE Registry, a marked similarity was noted between the clinical, hemodynamic, and hematologic manifestations of AFE and both septic and anaphylactic shock. Clearly the clinical manifestations of this condition are not identical; fever is unique to septic shock and cutaneous manifestations are more common in anaphylaxis. Nevertheless, the marked similarities of these conditions suggest similar pathophysiologic mechanisms. Both of these conditions involve the entrance into the circulation of a foreign substance (bacterial endotoxin or specific antigens), which then results in the release of various primary and secondary endogenous mediators (Fig. 1). Similar pathophysiology has also been recently proposed in nonpregnant patients with pulmonary fat embolism. It is the release of these mediators that results in the principal physiologic derangements characterizing these syndromes. These include profound myocardial depression and decreased cardiac output described in both animals and humans; pulmonary hypertension, demonstrated in lower primate models of anaphylaxis; and disseminated intravascular coagulation, described in both human anaphylactic reactions and septic shock. Further, the temporal sequence of hemodynamic decompensation and recovery seen in experimental AFE is virtually identical to that described in canine anaphylaxis. An *anaphylactoid* response is also well described in humans and involves the nonimmunologic release of similar mediators. It is also intriguing that 41% of patients in the AFE registry gave a history on admission to the hospital of either drug allergy or atopy.

Arachidonic acid metabolites are known to cause the same physiologic and hemodynamic changes observed in human AFE. Further, in the rabbit model of AFE, pretreatment with an inhibitor of leukotriene synthesis has been shown

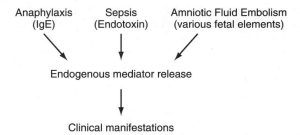

Figure 1. Proposed pathophysiologic relation between amniotic fluid embolism, septic shock, and anaphylactic shock. Each syndrome may also have specific direct physiologic effects. (From Clark SL, Harkins GD, Dudley DA, et al: Amniotic fluid embolism: Analysis of the national registry. Am J Obstet Gynecol 1995;172:1158–1167.)

to prevent death. These experimental observations further support the clinical conclusions of the National AFE Registry analysis that this condition involves the anaphylactoid release of endogenous mediators, including arachidonic acid metabolites, which result in the devastating pathophysiologic sequence seen in clinical AFE.

Earlier anecdotal reports suggested a possible causal relationship between hypertonic uterine contractions or oxytocin use and AFE. Although disputed on statistical grounds by Morgan in 1979, this misconception persisted in some writings until recently. The historical anecdotal association between hypertonic uterine contractions and the onset of symptoms in AFE was made clear by the analysis of the National Registry. These data demonstrated that the hypertonic contractions commonly seen in association with AFE appear to be a result of the release of catecholamines into the circulation as part of the initial human hemodynamic response to any massive physiologic insult. Under these circumstances, norepinephrine, in particular, acts as a potent uterotonic agent. Thus, while the association of hypertonic contractions and AFE appears to be valid, it is the physiologic response to AFE that causes the hypertonic uterine activity rather than the converse. Indeed, there is a complete cessation of uterine blood flow in the presence of even moderate uterine contractions; thus a tetanic contraction is the least likely time during an entire labor process for any exchange between maternal and fetal compartments. Oxytocin is not used with increased frequency in patients suffering AFE compared with the general population, nor does oxytocin-induced hyperstimulation commonly precede this condition. Thus, authorities today, including the American College of Obstetricians and Gynecologists, have concluded that oxytocin use has no relation to the occurrence of AFE.

The syndrome of AFE appears to be initiated after maternal intravascular exposure to various types of fetal tissue. Such exposure may occur during the course of normal labor and delivery, after potentially minor traumatic events such as intrauterine pressure catheter placement, or during cesarean section. Because fetal-to-maternal tissue transfer is virtually universal during the labor and delivery process, actions by health care providers, such as intrauterine manipulation or cesarean delivery, may affect the timing of the exposure, but no evidence exists to suggest that exposure itself can be avoided by altering clinical management. Simple exposure of the maternal circulatory system to even small amounts of amniotic fluid or other fetal tissue may, under the

right circumstances, initiate the syndrome of AFE. This understanding explains the well-documented occurrence of fatal AFE during second trimester pregnancy termination at a time when neither the volume of fluid nor positive intrauterine pressure could be contributing factors.

Clinical Presentation

Clinical signs and symptoms noted in patients with AFE are described in Table 1. In a typical case, a patient laboring, having just undergone cesarean delivery, or immediately following vaginal delivery or pregnancy termination suffers the acute onset of profound hypoxia and hypotension followed by cardiopulmonary arrest. The initial episode is often complicated by the development of a consumptive coagulopathy, which may lead to exsanguination even if attempts to restore hemodynamic and respiratory function are successful. It must be emphasized, however, that in any individual patient, any of the three principal phases (hypoxia, hypotension, or coagulopathy)

TABLE 1. Signs and Symptoms Noted in Patients with Amniotic Fluid Embolism

Sign or Symptom	No. of Patients	Percent of Patients
Hypotension	43	100
Fetal distress°	30	100
Pulmonary edema or adult respiratory distress syndrome†	28	93
Cardiopulmonary arrest	40	87
Cyanosis	38	83
Coagulopathy‡	38	83
Dyspnea§	22	49
Seizure	22	48
Atony	11	23
Bronchospasm‖	7	15
Transient hypertension	5	11
Cough	3	7
Headache	3	7
Chest pain	1	2

°n = 30. Includes all live fetuses in utero at time of event.

  †n = 30. Eighteen patients did not survive long enough for these diagnoses to be confirmed.

  ‡n = 38. Eight patients did not survive long enough for this diagnosis to be confirmed.

  §n = 45. One patient was intubated at the time of the event and could not be assessed.

  ‖Difficult ventilation was noted during cardiac arrest in 6 patients, and wheezes were auscultated in 1 patient.

  From Clark SL, Harkins GD, Dudley DA, et al: Amniotic fluid embolism: Analysis of the national registry. Am J Obstet Gynecol 1995;172:1158–1167.

TABLE 2. Cardiac Arrest-to-Delivery Interval and Neonatal Outcome

Interval (min)	Survival (*n/n*)	Intact Survival (*n/n*[%])
<5	3/3	2/3 (67)
5–15	3/3	2/3 (67)
16–25	2/5	2/5 (40)
26–35	3/4	1/4 (25)
36–54	0/1	0/1 (0)

From Clark SL, Harkins GD, Dudley DA, et al: Amniotic fluid embolism: Analysis of the national registry. Am J Obstet Gynecol 1995;172:1158–1167.

may either dominate or be entirely absent. Clinical variations in this syndrome appear to be related to variations in both antigenic exposure and maternal response.

Maternal outcome is dismal in patients with AFE syndrome. The overall maternal mortality rate appears to be 60% to 80%. However, only 15% of patients survive neurologically intact. In patients progressing to cardiac arrest, only 8% survive neurologically intact. In the National Registry, no form of therapy appeared to be consistently associated with improved outcome.

Neonatal outcome is similarly poor. Among fetuses in utero at the time of onset of maternal symptoms, survival rate is approximately 80%. However, only half of these fetuses survive neurologically intact. There is a clear relationship between neonatal outcome and event-to-delivery interval in those women suffering cardiac arrest (Table 2).

Diagnosis

In the past, histologic confirmation of the clinical syndrome of AFE was often sought by the detection of cellular debris of presumed fetal origin either in the distal port of a pulmonary artery catheterization or at autopsy. However, several studies in the past decade suggest that such findings are commonly encountered even in normal pregnant women. In the analysis of the National AFE Registry, fetal elements were found in roughly 50% of cases in which pulmonary artery catheter aspirate was analyzed and in roughly 75% of patients who went to autopsy. The frequency with which such findings are encountered varies with the number of histologic sections obtained. In addition, multiple special stains are often required to document such debris. Thus the diagnosis of AFE remains today a clinical

one; histologic findings are neither sensitive nor specific. It is interesting to note that similar conclusions have recently been drawn regarding the diagnostic significance of histologic findings in patients with pulmonary fat embolism.

Treatment

Treatment remains disappointing, with an overall mortality rate of 60% to 80%. In the National Registry, we found no difference in survival among patients suffering initial cardiac arrest in small rural hospitals attended by family practitioners as compared with those suffering identical clinical signs and symptoms in tertiary level centers and attended by board-certified anesthesiologists, cardiologists, and maternal-fetal medicine specialists. Nevertheless, several generalizations can be drawn:

1. The initial treatment for AFE is supportive. Cardiopulmonary resuscitation is performed if the patient is suffering from a lethal dysrhythmia. Oxygen should be provided at high concentrations.

2. In the patient who survives the initial cardiopulmonary insult, it should be remembered that left ventricular failure is commonly seen. Thus, volume expansion to optimize ventricular preload and, if the patient remains significantly hypotensive, the addition of an inotropic agent such as dopamine seem most appropriate. In patients who remain unstable following the initial resuscitative efforts, pulmonary artery catheterization may be of benefit, to guide hemodynamic manipulation.

3. In patients suffering AFE with the fetus still in utero, careful attention must be paid to the fetal condition. In a mother who is hemodynamically unstable but has not yet undergone cardiorespiratory arrest, maternal considerations must be carefully weighed against those of the fetus. It is axiomatic in these situations, however, that where a choice must be made, maternal well-being must take precedence over that of the fetus.

4. In mothers who have progressed to frank cardiac arrest, the situation is different. Under these circumstances, maternal survival is extremely unlikely, regardless of the therapy rendered. In such women, it is highly unlikely that the imposition of cesarean section would significantly alter the maternal outcome. Even properly performed cardiopulmonary resuscitation

(CPR) (difficult at best in a pregnant woman) provides only a maximum of 30% of normal cardiac output. Under these circumstances, it is fair to assume that the proportion of blood shunted to the uterus and other areas in the splanchnic bed approaches zero. Thus the fetus will be for practical purposes anoxic at all times following maternal cardiac arrest, even during ideal performance of CPR. Because the interval from maternal arrest to delivery is directly correlated with newborn outcome, perimortum cesarean section should be initiated immediately on the diagnosis of maternal cardiac arrest in patients with AFE, assuming sufficient personnel are available to continue to provide care to the mother and deliver the baby. For the pregnant patient, the standard ABCs of CPR should be modified to include a fourth category: D, delivery.

Anesthesia for Obstetrics

Kathryn Zuspan, MD

An understanding of obstetric anesthesia and analgesia is critical to providing good obstetric care. No one form is ideal for all obstetric patients. In most cases a number of options may be appropriate.

Communication and teamwork between the obstetrician, anesthesiologist, and obstetric nurse are essential. An anesthesiologist who is aware of the obstetrician's concerns and plans for a patient is better able to tailor the patient's anesthesia and analgesia to appropriately meet these concerns as well as the patient's needs.

Obstetric anesthesia coverage should be provided by well-trained and experienced individuals, preferably anesthesiologists. *Anyone administering anesthesia or supervising a nurse-anesthetist must be able to recognize and manage all possible complications and must have up-to-date skills in intubation and resuscitation techniques.*

Maternal Physiology

Maternal physiology is altered early in pregnancy and returns to prepregnant baseline only about 6 weeks postpartum. These changes affect the pregnant patient's response to anesthesia and must be taken into consideration when choosing anesthesia or analgesia in this population. For example, the increased cardiac output inherent in pregnancy results in a more rapid induction of and emergence from general anesthesia.

Pregnancy significantly increases the patient's risks from anesthesia in several ways. For example, respiratory changes in pregnancy increase the patient's risk of hypoxia. Gastrointestinal tract changes increase the risk of vomiting and aspiration. Furthermore, the increasing size and weight of the gravid uterus heighten the risk of aortocaval compression and maternal hypotension in the supine position.

Labor Pain Relief

Labor is painful. Pain causes a maternal "stress" response, with an increase in autonomic activity, release of catecholamines, and a decrease in placental perfusion, resulting in fetal acidosis. This stress may also cause maternal hyperventilation, which leads to respiratory alkalosis, a compensatory metabolic acidosis, and thus fetal acidosis. In short, labor pain is not good for mother or neonate and expecting a woman to "tolerate" labor pain when there are so many good pain control options is barbaric.

There are a variety of techniques to relieve labor pain. No one form of analgesia is best for all patients. The more common techniques are discussed here briefly.

Lamaze

Lamaze, a relaxation technique, is a form of psychoprophylaxis. The patient is taught to concentrate on breathing techniques during the various stages of labor, which will distract and thus relieve discomfort. The husband or support person is taught to assist and encourage the patient through labor. Most patients find that this technique alone provides inadequate analgesia. Lamaze is often most effective in combination with other forms of analgesia.

Systemic Opioids

The use of systemic opioids is still the most common means of labor analgesia in the United States. Used in small doses to limit fetal exposure, these drugs often provide incomplete pain relief. The most popular agent is meperidine (Demerol) in a dose of 25 to 50 mg given intravenously every 1 to 2 hours or 50 to 100 mg intramuscularly given every 2–4 hours. This has a 5- to 10-minute onset of action when given intravenously, versus 30 to 45 minutes with an intramuscular dose. Maternal side effects include sedation, postural hypotension, pruritus, nausea and vomiting, obtundation of reflexes, and respiratory depression. Neonatal side effects include decreased fetal heart rate variability, impaired early breast feeding, neurobehavioral changes, and respiratory depression. The latter risk is greatest about 2 to 3 hours after drug administration.

Naloxone (Narcan) is the opioid antagonist of choice in obstetrics. The dose is 0.04 to 0.40 mg IV for adults and 0.1 mg/kg IV for neonates. The onset is in minutes, and the duration of action is 1 to 2 hours. The recommendation for naloxone is that it be used readily in depressed neonates who might be narcotized, but not routinely in all neonates. Naloxone should also be avoided in mothers who are opioid addicts and in neonates in whom its administration could induce acute withdrawal symptoms.

Other opioids commonly used are butorphanol (Stadol), nalbuphine (Nubain), fentanyl (Sublimaze), and morphine. Butorphanol and nalbuphine are synthetic opioid agonist-antagonist analgesics. The labor analgesic dose for butorphanol (1–2 mg), and nalbuphine (10 mg) is given intravenously. Both drugs provide analgesia and sedation. They differ from meperidine because of a reported "ceiling effect" on respiratory depression, that is, larger doses of these drugs cause less increase in maternal respiratory depression than are seen with increasing doses of other opioids.

Fentanyl is gaining popularity for labor pain control. It is a potent drug and thus used in small doses. A dose of 100 μg (0.1 mg) of fentanyl is approximately equivalent to 10 mg morphine or 75 mg meperidine. Fentanyl's advantage is its rapid onset and short duration of action when used in small doses. For active labor pain relief, the usual fentanyl dose is 50 to 100 μg IV repeated every hour as needed. One word of caution: fentanyl, sufentanil, and alfentanil are not the same drug. Sufentanil is five to 10 times more potent than fentanyl. Alfentanil is one third to one fifth as potent as fentanyl and has a faster onset and a shorter duration of action.

Morphine is seldom used in obstetrics because of its delayed onset and prolonged duration of action. An intravenous dose peaks in 20 minutes, and an intramuscular dose peaks in 1 to 2 hours. The duration of action for both is 4 to 6 hours. The fetus is more likely to have respiratory depression with morphine than with comparable doses of meperidine. Morphine is appropriate for a patient in early labor with intact membranes, making little progress and in pain. Given 10 to 15 mg of morphine, this patient will sleep and often awaken 3 to 4 hours later in good labor.

Sedatives and tranquilizers are often used to potentiate narcotics, allay anxiety, and promote sleep. The usual choice is hydroxyzine (Vistaril) 25 to 50 mg IM, which also has antiemetic qualities in the mother. The fetal effects include a decrease in beat-to-beat variability on the fetal heart rate pattern but no evidence of neonatal depression.

Paracervical Block

The paracervical block, another technique once used to provide analgesia in the first stage of labor, involves injecting local anesthetic into the vaginal mucosa at various sites on the cervix. Though maternal side effects are rare, neonatal side effects include a very high incidence of severe and prolonged fetal bradycardia. For this reason, paracervical blocks are seldom used for analgesia during labor.

Regional Analgesia

Lumbar Epidural Analgesia

According to the *Guidelines for Perinatal Care* (1997) by the American College of OB/GYN (ACOG) and the American Academy of Pediatrics, "of the various pharmacologic methods used for pain relief during labor and delivery, lumbar epidural block is the most flexible, effective, and least depressing to the central nervous system, allowing for an alert, participating mother."

There are many accepted benefits of epidural analgesia. Epidurals reduce labor pain and maternal stress, thus helping to maintain the fetal acid-base status. There is little direct effect on uteroplacental blood flow and tone as long as the maternal blood pressure is maintained. Epidurals may actually accelerate the first stage of labor in patients with dysfunctional labor. Patients are in better control during the second stage of labor. Finally, there is an anesthetic method in place in case a semi-emergent cesarean section is needed. Epidural anesthesia is known to be safer than general anesthesia for the mother and the neonate. In fact, in obese patients in whom intubation may be difficult, some authors suggest that an epidural should be placed early in labor so it will be available in the event that an emergency cesarean section is required.

There are controversies. Epidural analgesia is often blamed for prolonging the second stage of labor by taking away the urge and ability to push. This problem is averted by good coaching and by dosing the epidural with a dilute concentration of local anesthetics with or without opioids. Many articles in the literature also accuse epidural analgesia of increasing the incidence of dystocia and instrumented deliveries. Close scrutiny of these studies reveals major methodologic problems. Most of these studies are retrospective and not randomized. They compare women who received epidurals, often because of slower more dysfunctional labors, with women who received no epidurals, often due to rapid or uncomplicated labors. Other inherent biases include the increased likelihood of an elective forceps delivery (especially in teaching institutions) in patients with the effective perineal anesthesia provided by an epidural. Furthermore, intervention in the second stage usually occurred after 1 and 2 hours for multiparas and primiparas respectively. This is now known to be an inadequate trial period for spontaneous delivery. ACOG has revised the definition of "prolonged second stage" to 3 hours for primiparas and 2 hours for multiparas in patients with an epidural and a stable fetus.

A better approach to addressing this controversy is to examine the studies that compare statistics in obstetrics units before and after an active labor epidural service was established. A number of such studies demonstrate no increase in dystocia or instrumented deliveries. Some units documented a drop in the cesarean section rate since fewer patients (who were attempting vaginal birth after a prior cesarean section) were requesting surgical intervention due to discomfort.

The epidural can be initiated when the patient is in labor and notes discomfort and the obstetrician is committed to delivery. There is no need to wait for a particular cervical dilatation, although some physicians feel that the epidural should not be dosed during latent phase. The catheter for the epidural anesthetic is placed after the patient receives a bolus of 500 to 1000 mL of lactated Ringer's fluid. Aspiration of the catheter followed by a test dose of local anesthetic is used to check catheter placement. This practice helps rule out possible intravascular or subarachnoid placement of the catheter. Next, the full epidural dose is given in a fractionated manner: 5 mL boluses with at least 30 seconds between doses. The usual dose regimen involves

bupivacaine (0.05–0.25%) given in an initial bolus dose. Fentanyl (50 μg) or sufentanil 10 μg may be added to improve analgesia and decrease the concentration of local anesthetic needed. This reduces the amount of motor block. The epidural can be redosed at intervals or maintained with a constant infusion. The continuous infusion is typically with bupivacaine (0.05–0.125%), possibly supplemented with fentanyl (1–2 μg/mL) or sufentanil (0.2–0.4 μg/mL). After administration of the dose, the patient's blood pressure is monitored every few minutes for 20 minutes. With the sympathectomy that occurs as the epidural block sets up, hypotension is possible and can be avoided by increasing the intravenous fluid rate or by repositioning the patient. When this fails, ephedrine is used in 5 mg increments intravenously. The epidural anesthetic should be maintained throughout the second stage of labor and delivery. Possible side effects include failure to relieve pain, spotty or one-sided block, maternal hypotension, intravascular placement with possible local anesthetic toxicity, subarachnoid placement with related postdural puncture headache or high spinal headache, and epidural hematoma. Absolute contraindications to epidural anesthesia include patient's refusal or inability to cooperate, increased intracranial pressure due to a mass lesion, infection at the insertion site, clinical coagulopathy, uncorrected maternal hypovolemia, or unavailability of qualified medical personnel to perform the technique.

Spinal Analgesia

Spinal anesthesia for labor pain relief is gaining popularity. It has a variety of names, including intrathecal narcotics, intrathecal opioids, and subarachnoid analgesia. This procedure is performed either as a single shot technique or as a combined technique in which an epidural catheter is also inserted.

The *single shot technique* is especially useful for parturients in active labor, where spontaneous delivery is anticipated within 2–3 hours. A spinal needle is advanced into the subarachnoid space at the L3-4 or L2-3 level and drugs injected.

The typical dose possibilities are fentanyl 25 μg or sufentanil 10 μg with either bupivacaine 2.5 mg or morphine 0.25 mg. Morphine is becoming less popular for two reasons. Morphine provides little or no relief during second stage labor. It also does not prolong overall pain relief, yet it requires prolonged postpartum monitoring. Bupivacaine in this low dose usually does not preclude ambulation. Unlike morphine, bupivacaine also helps relieve some of the pain of second stage. Onset of relief is rapid. Redoses are rarely done. When necessary, however, the procedure can be repeated at intervals dependent on the drugs used.

In an effort to provide continuous pain relief, 27 gauge and smaller spinal catheters were developed. These were placed in the subarachnoid space via a spinal needle. A *continuous subarachnoid infusion* could then be maintained through delivery. Unfortunately, the Food and Drug Administration (FDA) reported eleven cases of neurologic injury associated with this continuous infusion technique. Five of these cases (using 5% lidocaine in 7.5% dextrose) resulted in cauda equina syndrome. One theory is that the microcatheter caused a slower injection rate, thus mixing less of the local anesthetic with cerebrospinal fluid. This resulted in higher sacral concentrations of local anesthetic, which could cause permanent neurologic damage. In May 1992, the FDA recalled all spinal microcatheters (27 gauge or smaller). These catheters will be reintroduced only after FDA-sponsored studies can demonstrate their safety.

The *combined spinal–epidural technique* offers the advantages of both spinal and epidural blocks. A small gauge pencil point needle is passed through an epidural needle placed in the epidural space. The spinal needle punctures the dura and deposits a small subarachnoid dose of, typically, fentanyl 25 μg or sufentanil 10 μg. The spinal needle is withdrawn and an epidural catheter is passed into the epidural space. This procedure can be done very early in labor. The patient gets pain relief as early as the latent phase but can still usually ambulate. The epidural catheter is then available for use for pain relief after the intrathecal dose wears off or in the event that an instrumented delivery is needed.

The side effects from spinal analgesia for labor are similar to those seen with epidural analgesia. These include pruritus, nausea and vomiting, urinary retention, drowsiness, postdural puncture headache, maternal respiratory depression, fetal heart rate changes (bradycardia), and maternal hypotension. As a result, patients receiving spinal analgesia should be monitored similarly to those receiving epidurals. These patients require intravenous access, a preload of non–glucose-containing Ringer's lactate solution, fetal heart rate monitoring, and maternal respiratory and blood pressure monitoring. There is also the possibility of some motor function weakness, so patients must be checked prior to any attempts at ambulation.

An intense postural headache, the *postdural puncture headache or spinal headache*, occurs at a higher rate (estimated at 13% to 50%) in the pregnant population. Use of smaller gauge (e.g., 24 to 27) spinal needles have been reported to decrease the headache rate. Recent development of the pencil point (versus the cutting edge) spinal needle has further improved the statistics. Three such commercially available needles, the 24 gauge Sprotte, the 24 or 25 gauge Whitacre, and the Gertie Marx needle all have decreased the risk to less than 2%. Occurring after dural puncture, the etiology of the headache is unknown. Bedrest following spinal anesthesia does not decrease the incidence of headache. It merely delays onset of the headache for the length of time the patient was flat. Therefore, it is no longer necessary to keep patients flat after spinal anesthesia. Treatment once the headache occurs includes (1) bedrest, analgesics, and fluids, (2) intravenous or oral caffeine, (3) epidural saline injection, or (4) an epidural blood patch. The blood patch involves performing an epidural on the patient at the level of the previous dural puncture. Blood from the patient is drawn and immediately injected through the needle into the epidural space. This is thought to create a clot "patch" over the dural puncture site until the dura seals over the puncture site. Relief is typically immediate in about 97% of cases.

Anesthesia for Spontaneous or Instrumental Vaginal Delivery

A few patients, especially multiparas who do not require an episiotomy, are quite happy without anesthesia for spontaneous vaginal delivery. Most patients, however, need some form of anesthesia. A variety of techniques are available.

Local Infiltration

For a spontaneous delivery local infiltration is useful prior to cutting and repairing an episiotomy. It involves injecting local anesthetic intradermally in the perineum at the episiotomy site. Lidocaine 1% is the usual drug choice. Other local anesthetics may be substituted.

The maximum safe dose of plain lidocaine is 4.5 mg/kg. A 1% lidocaine solution is 10 mg/mL. Thus the maximum volume of 1% lidocaine for a 70 kg patient, for example, is about 30 mL.

Pudendal Block

Pudendal block is useful for spontaneous or low forceps or outlet forceps vaginal deliveries. It is designed to anesthetize the internal pudendal and perineal nerves bilaterally in an effort to relax the perineal muscles and anesthetize the perineal skin. Lidocaine 1% is the most commonly used agent. Local infiltration, described earlier, may additionally be used to improve pain relief in the perineum.

Epidural Anesthesia

Epidural anesthesia is useful for spontaneous or instrumented vaginal deliveries. An epidural dose of local anesthetic, called a "perineal," "sit-up," or "top-up" dose, is used to attain motor block, perineal relaxation, and anesthesia. It is given late in the second stage of labor, with the patient in the sitting position. The epidural dose involves a larger volume (10–15 mL) and stronger concentration of local anesthetic than that used earlier in labor. Lidocaine 2% or 2-chloroprocaine 3% are typically used.

Spinal or Saddle Block

Spinal or saddle block anesthesia is useful for instrumented vaginal delivery. This form of spinal anesthesia is called "saddle block" because anesthesia is maximized in the anatomic areas that would touch a saddle if the patient were riding a horse. The traditional spinal technique is used, but a smaller dose of hyperbaric local anesthetic is given with the patient in the sitting position. The result is sacral anesthesia. Local anesthetics commonly used are lidocaine or bupivacaine. Precautions and contraindications are similar to those for epidural anesthetics.

Inhalational Analgesia

Inhalational analgesia is rarely used for spontaneous or instrumented deliveries. Oxygen and nitrous oxide with or without enflurane or methoxyflurane are inhaled continuously in low concentrations or intermittently in higher concentrations. This technique provides maternal pain relief; however, there is also a significant risk of maternal aspiration, respiratory depression, loss of consciousness, and neonatal depression.

Anesthesia for Cesarean Section

No matter what form of anesthesia is chosen, four main points are important. First, all obstetric patients are at significant risk of aspiration and thus aspiration pneumonitis. For prophylaxis, all patients should receive a preoperative oral dose of nonparticulate (clear) antacid; 30 mL of sodium citrate (Scholl's solution) or Bicitra is commonly used. Patients at greater risk may receive an H_2 antagonist, such as cimetidine 300 mg IM, or ranitidine 50 mg IV one hour preoperatively, and metoclopramide, 10 mg IV one-half hour prior to administering anesthesia.

Second, a left lateral wedge should be placed under the patient's right hip while she is supine on the operating room table. This practice produces left lateral uterine displacement and decreases the risk of aortocaval compression.

Third, patients must be well oxygenated. For cases involving local, spinal, or epidural anesthesia, the patient receives supplemental oxygen by face mask versus nasal cannula. For cases involving general anesthesia, the patient receives 100% oxygen by face mask for 3 minutes or four deep breaths before induction and intubation.

Finally, the choice of anesthesia for cesarean section depends on several variables. The medical status of the parturient and fetus should be considered, as well as the skills of the obstetrician and anesthesiologist. The emergent nature of the procedure is another variable. In cases of dire fetal distress, general anesthesia is often the best choice for rapidly initiating anesthesia. However, in cases of severe or chronic fetal distress, if an epidural catheter is already in place and time permits, then a short-onset local anesthetic, such as chlorprocaine or lidocaine, may be used to attain the epidural block, or a quick spinal anesthetic can be done.

The surgical time factor is another consideration. For regional anesthesia (spinal and epidural), the time period of concern is the uterine-incision-to-delivery (U-D) time. With U-D time of less than 3 minutes, there is a decreased incidence of low Apgar scores and fetal acidosis. For general anesthesia, the U-D time also needs to be less than 3 minutes. In addition, with general anesthesia, a second surgical time period is important. This is the abdominal-incision-to-delivery (A-D) time, which should be less than 8 minutes to avoid fetal acidosis and low Apgar scores.

The anesthetic techniques used for cesarean section include spinal, epidural, general anesthesia, and local infiltration of the anterior abdominal wall. The majority of cesarean sections in the United States are done with spinal or epidural anesthesia. Regional anesthesia tends to be a better choice because there are fewer risks related to aspiration or difficult intubation. There is less risk of neonatal depression due to drug exposure and there tends to be less maternal blood loss.

Epidural Anesthesia

The technique, precautions, and contraindications involved in epidural anesthesia for cesarean section are the same as those for labor, with a few key differences. Unlike with labor, the epidural anesthetic for cesarean section requires a greater preload of intravenous lactated Ringer's solution. An amount of 1500 to 2000 mL is appropriate. A stronger concentration and larger volume of local anesthetic are used, and the level of the block is extended to T4-6. Lidocaine 2% with epinephrine and bicarbonate is commonly used. The epidural catheter may be redosed at appropriate intervals during the cesarean section to maintain the surgical level of anesthesia.

A small amount of sodium bicarbonate is often added to the epidural local anesthetic to increase its pH. This increases the local anesthetic's speed of onset and duration of action. The potential hazard is the higher incidence of hypotension related to this faster onset. Epinephrine, which has some local anesthetic properties, may also be added to the epidural dose. It serves to enhance the block. Studies suggest that local anesthetics containing epinephrine 1:200,000 cause a decrease in uterine activity. Thus, for labor epidurals, epinephrine should only be used in the test dose.

Spinal Anesthesia

The technique, precautions, and contraindications involved in spinal anesthesia are similar for vaginal delivery and cesarean section. A preload of 1500 to 2000 mL of lactated Ringer's solution is needed. A larger dose of hyperbaric local anesthetic produces a level of anesthesia to T4-6.

General Anesthesia

All pregnant patients undergoing general anesthesia require intubation using a "rapid sequence induction." This involves using cricoid pressure and avoiding positive-pressure ventilation prior to intubation. The patient is extubated when she is awake and in control of her gag reflexes. These measures are used to avoid maternal aspiration.

Difficult intubation and aspiration remain the leading causes of death due to obstetric anesthesia. Obstetric patients are about eight times more likely to be difficult to intubate. Obese obstetric patients are at even greater risk of requiring an emergency cesarean section and being difficult to intubate.

A variety of drugs and techniques are used in general anesthesia. Some of the typical agents are discussed here.

Prior to induction, the patient receives 100% oxygen by face mask for 3 minutes or four deep breaths. Induction of anesthesia and intubation are done using thiopental and succinylcholine. Thiopental (Pentothal), a barbiturate, has a short-acting depressant effect on the central nervous system. Succinylcholine (Anectine), an ultra-short-acting skeletal muscle relaxant, facilitates endotracheal intubation.

Following intubation, anesthesia is maintained using oxygen, an inhalational agent and a muscle relaxant. Oxygen is given in a 50% to 100% concentration. Nitrous oxide, often withheld until after delivery, is added to reduce the chance of maternal recall and lower the inhalational anesthetic requirements. Low concentrations of enflurane (Ethrane) or isoflurane (Forane) serve to increase uterine blood flow and decrease the risk of maternal recall. In low concentrations, these agents do not cause neonatal depression or uterine bleeding. Different muscle relaxants are used, depending on the surgeon's speed. Succinylcholine (Anectine) is short acting, atracurium (Tracrium) and vecuronium (Norcuron) have intermediate duration, and pancuronium (Pavulon) has a long duration of action. Incidentally, these muscle relaxants cross the placenta but have no effect on neonatal respiration or Apgar scores. After delivery, narcotics and tranquilizers are used to deepen the level of anesthesia. The shorter-acting drugs, such as fentanyl (Sublimaze) and midazolam (Versed) are often chosen so that the mother will be alert postoperatively for bonding with the neonate. At the end of the cesarean section, the muscle relaxants (with the exception of succinylcholine) are reversed. This is done with one of the cholinesterase inhibitors. These anticholinergic drugs include pyridostigmine (Regonol), neostigmine (Prostigmin), or edrophonium (Tensilon). Glycopyrrolate or atropine is also given to block the bradycardia and excessive secretions often seen with the anticholinergic drugs.

Local Infiltration of the Anterior Abdominal Wall

Finally, local infiltration of the anterior abdominal wall is rarely used for cesarean section. This technique is appropriate for an emergency cesarean section when no one trained in anesthesia administration is available or when intravenous access is impossible. Gentle handling of the patient and the instruments is critical. A number of local anesthetics may be used as long as the maximum safe dose is known and observed. It usually takes 150 to 200 mL of drug to attain satisfactory anesthesia. Large volumes of any local anesthetic can lead to toxic reactions such as seizures and cardiac arrest and should be used cautiously. For example, 0.5% lidocaine with 1:200,000 epinephrine (100 mL) plus normal saline (100 mL) is commonly used. Note: When epinephrine is added to lidocaine, the maximum safe dose increases to 7 mg/kg.

Conclusion

In summary, obstetric anesthesia and analgesia involve a wide variety of drugs and techniques. New agents and procedures are constantly evolving. No one technique is best for all patients. Familiarity with all the options is key to good patient care. Teamwork between the obstetrician and anesthesiologist then assures delivery of the optimum in pain relief for each individual patient.

Asthma Management During Pregnancy

Jordan H. Perlow, MD

Epidemiology

Asthma is the most common pulmonary disease complicating pregnancy and may affect up to 5% of all pregnant women. The need for an understanding of the pathophysiology and management of asthma is emphasized by the presence of more than 10 million asthmatic people in the United States and several disturbing epidemiologic trends. The Centers for Disease Control and Prevention (CDC) recently reported a 40% increase in asthma-related death over the years 1980 to 1992. Interestingly, and importantly, female deaths increased more than the average, with female asthma-related mortality increasing 59%. During the same time interval, the CDC also reported that the prevalence of asthma has increased by 42% overall, and 82% for women.

Pathophysiology

Asthma is a lung disease with the following characteristics: airway obstruction that is at least partially reversible with or without treatment, airway inflammation, and airway hyper-responsiveness to a variety of intrinsic and environmental stimuli. These stimuli are varied and include environmental allergens (pollens, dust, mites, air pollutants), viral respiratory infections, irritants such as perfumes and paint vapors, food additives, exercise, and cold air. At the cellular level, these stimuli activate mast cells, epithelial cells, macrophages, eosinophils, and lymphocytes resulting in the release of inflammatory mediators (eg, leukotrienes, cytokines, platelet-activating factor), the activation of the autonomic nervous system, and smooth muscle contraction. These events lead to airway edema and narrowing, cellular infiltration, increased mucous secretion, airway plugging, and markedly increased mucosal and vascular permeability. The common clinical manifestations of asthma, including airway obstruction, dyspnea, cough, and wheezing are therefore a result of these complex events at the cellular and subcellular levels. In practice, the diagnosis of asthma is often made based on these clinical and historical factors.

Maternal-Fetal Outcome

With respect to the effects of pregnancy on asthma, it has been traditionally taught that asthma in pregnancy follows the "rule of thirds," with one third of patients each improving, demonstrating no change in disease acuity, or worsening. This is misleading, however, as the course of asthma in pregnancy is more accurately related to the pre-existing state of disease, with nearly 75% of patients with mild asthma having no change in their disease state in pregnancy, contrasted to a greater than 80% chance of exacerbation in pregnancy for severe asthmatics. Fortunately, labor and delivery do not appear to be a particularly vulnerable time for asthma exacerbation, as a study of nearly 400 asthmatic women found the risk to be 10%, with less than 50% of these patients requiring pharmacologic intervention.

Asthma has a significant impact on perinatal outcome. Retrospective descriptive and case-controlled studies indicate a wide variety of threats to the asthmatic pregnancy, including significantly increased risks for hyperemesis, preterm delivery, low birth weight, intrauterine growth restriction (IUGR), pre-eclampsia, and perinatal mortality. In severe asthma, maternal mortality has also been shown to be markedly increased. Perinatal outcome in pregnancies complicated by asthma may be linked to medication needs during pregnancy. A recent study investigating this concept found that among medication-dependent asthmatic pregnant women, increased risks for diabetes, preterm delivery, premature ruptured membranes, low birth weight, fetal distress, cesarean section, and neonatal admissions to the intensive care unit were noted when compared with control subjects. Patients chronically dependent on corticosteroids for asthma management had nearly a 75% chance of requiring antepartum hospitalization and were significantly more likely to incur these complications compared with patients not dependent on non-steroid medication. Recent encouraging information, however, indicates that patients who are actively managed during pregnancy may have a comparable perinatal prognosis to that of the nonasthmatic population.

Management Approach (Fig. 1)

The evolving understanding of the pathophysiology of asthma is shaping trends and recommendations in management. Asthma management has traditionally been based on the acute management of airway obstruction. New understandings with respect to the chronic nature of airway inflammation has led to a more prominent pharmacologic role for the anti-inflammatory drugs, including corticosteroids (both systemic and aerosolized) and cromolyn sodium. Based on the changing understanding of the pathophysiology of asthma and disturbing national epidemiologic trends with respect to asthma-related morbidity and mortality, the National Institutes of Health convened a working group (National Asthma Education Program) to provide guidelines to assist the clinician and patient in providing appropriate asthma care during pregnancy.

Asthma management in pregnancy should set out to accomplish the following goals: maintenance of normal or near normal pulmonary function, control of asthma symptoms (including nocturnal symptoms), maintenance of normal activity and exercise levels, prevention of acute exacerbations, avoidance of adverse medication effects, and the delivery of a healthy infant.

These goals are best achieved through the implementation of four components of manage-

ment: (1) patient education, (2) avoidance and control of asthma triggers, (3) pharmacologic therapy, and (4) objective measures for patient and fetal assessment and monitoring. The importance of patient education cannot be overemphasized. Besides providing critical information education provides the opportunity to build rapport, which enhances open communication and builds confidence within the patient, who should be encouraged to take an active role in her disease management. Education with respect to the relative safety of asthma medications is essential, and it should be emphasized that it is much safer for both the mother and her fetus to control asthma with appropriate medications than to avoid fetal exposure and risk disease exacerbation during pregnancy. Preconception counseling is encouraged. It is reasonable to acknowledge that no medication can be considered safe in absolute terms, while explaining that relatively few medications have been proven harmful during pregnancy. It would also be important to include a brief discussion of the background risk of congenital malformations overall. Other aspects of patient education include a review of proper medication dosing, use of a peak expiratory flow meter and metered-dose inhalers, and environmental control measures where appropriate. These aspects of patient education and informed consent to the treatment plan should be documented in the patient chart.

Objective measures of maternal and fetal status are essential for appropriate monitoring and assessment of asthma severity and are critical in determining the need for therapeutic interventions. While the measurement of the volume of air expired in 1 second from maximum inspiration (FEV_1) is the best measure of pulmonary function for making the assessment of severity of asthma, it is often difficult to measure in the outpatient (home) setting. The peak expiratory flow rate (PEFR) is the greatest flow velocity that can be obtained during a forced expiration starting with fully inflated lungs and correlates well with the FEV_1. Also, it is easily measured with an inexpensive portable meter and is valuable in providing insight into the course of asthma throughout the day, to discern circadian variations, detect deterioration, and allow for appropriate and timely therapeutic recommendations based on objective measures of severity. Regular use of a peak flow meter allows for the determination of the "personal best" peak flow rate over a period of time when disease status is optimally controlled. This allows important comparisons to be made in an objective manner when the patient's condition changes. The deter-

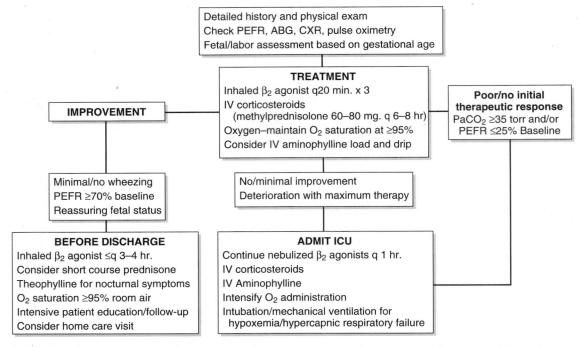

Figure 1. Asthma management during pregnancy. (Adapted from *Management of Asthma During Pregnancy*, National Asthma Education Program, National Institutes of Health. NIH Publication No. 93-3279A, March 1993.)

mination of the personal best PEFR is preferred to utilizing the normal PEFR range for women of 380 to 550 L per minute (unchanged in pregnancy); however, for patients presenting acutely, this normal range may be useful in determining severity of disease and effects of treatment. Patients with moderate to severe disease (defined subsequently) should self-monitor their PEFR twice daily to determine treatment efficacy and establish their "personal best." Fetal status is assessed periodically in the stable patient and acutely in the patient with an asthma exacerbation, especially in the late second and the third trimesters. Early ultrasonography is useful for accurate pregnancy dating. The importance of establishing early gestational age is emphasized by the frequent need to compare fetal ultrasonographic biometric data obtained serially in the second and third trimesters for the patient with moderate to severe disease or when IUGR is suspected. Asthma has been cited as an indication for antepartum fetal heart rate or biophysical testing. For the patient with mild disease (defined subsequently) whose course has been stable, with normal fetal growth and activity, this may not be necessary. Those patients with moderate to severe disease, evidence of IUGR, asthma exacerbation, or decreased fetal movement requires antepartum fetal heart rate or bio-

physical testing. Daily maternal assessment of fetal activity using an accepted protocol should be encouraged for all asthma patients.

Pharmacologic therapy for asthma during pregnancy is based on the principle of using the safest drug in the lowest dose via the most effective and least toxic route to effect an optimal therapeutic response. Pharmacologic management of asthma uses a "step-care" approach, in which the number and frequency of medications used are increased with increasing asthma severity. Once control is established and sustained, a reduction in therapy is considered. Drugs recommended to treat asthma in pregnancy include both steroid (oral prednisone, inhaled beclomethasone, intravenous prednisolone/hydrocortisone) and nonsteroidal (inhaled cromolyn sodium) anti-inflammatory drugs; bronchodilators, including inhaled β-agonists (albuterol, metaproterenol) and theophylline; the antihistamines chlorpheniramine and tripelennamine; decongestants including pseudoephedrine; cough suppressants with guaifenesin and dextromethorphan; and antibiotics, particularly ampicillin and amoxicillin. Cromolyn sodium is believed to exert its anti-inflammatory effect by preventing degranulation of pulmonary mast cells, thus inhibiting the local release of histamine, and other inflammatory stimuli of airway obstruction.

With respect to the effects of asthma medications during pregnancy on the fetus and perinatal outcome in general, a large experience with corticosteroids in humans has failed to suggest any increase in facial clefts or other congenital malformations. Chronic oral and parenteral use has been associated with decreased birth weight and a slight increase in premature delivery. It is always difficult, however, to determine whether these are medication-associated risks or risks associated with the disease itself. An extensive human experience with the inhaled corticosteroid beclomethasone has been reassuring, as it has been for cromolyn sodium. No fetal harm has been suggested with extensive human experience with β-adrenergic agonists in pregnancy. Similarly, human experience with theophylline has been extensive and has not demonstrated teratogenic effects.

One of the most important, yet often neglected, components of asthma management is the institution of efforts to control or avoid the patient's exposure to asthma triggers. Instituting this component is assisted by detailed history taking and pre-pregnancy allergen testing. Clearly, in all situations the elimination of tobacco smoke from the patient's environment is essential. Patients receiving immunotherapy ("allergy shots") may continue, but because of concerns for anaphylaxis, this therapy is not routinely initiated in pregnancy. Patients may need to develop strategies to avoid animal dander, house dust mites, cockroach antigens, pollens, and molds. Removal of pets, the encasing of pillows and mattresses in airtight covers, the weekly washing of bedding in extremely hot water, use of air conditioning and avoidance of air pollution are additional important measures. Furthermore, the influenza vaccine is recommended annually for all patients with moderate and severe asthma after the first trimester. Patients with asthma triggered by exercise should not be discouraged from regular exercise but rather should have therapy maximized with particular attention to pretreatment with cromolyn sodium or a β$_2$-agonist up to 1 hour prior to activity. With proper management, most patients should be able to participate in any activities they choose without experiencing asthma symptoms.

Treatment Strategies

Chronic mild asthma (Fig. 2) is defined as the occurrence of asthma symptoms (wheezing, coughing, and dyspnea) no more than twice per week with otherwise symptom-free intervals.

Treatment consists of inhaled β$_2$-agonists (two puffs every 4 hours as needed). Increased need for this therapy indicates a need for reassessing disease severity and treatment plan. *Chronic moderate asthma* patients are those individuals who have symptoms poorly controlled by periodic inhaled β$_2$-agonists, with symptoms often occurring more than twice per week. The PEFR may be diminished at 60% to 80% of personal best. These patients require a daily inhaled anti-inflammatory medication to suppress and prevent airway inflammation and airway responsiveness with either inhaled corticosteroids (beclomethasone two to five puffs twice to four times daily) or cromolyn sodium (two puffs four times daily or two sprays in each nostril twice to four times daily). A spacer should be used with the corticosteroid inhaler to increase medication deposition in the respiratory tract and reduce the risk of systemic side effects and oropharyngeal candidiasis. The patient should also be instructed to rinse her mouth after use. Several weeks of anti-inflammatory inhalational therapy may be needed before maximal effect is noted. A short tapering course of oral corticosteroids is indicated when asthma is not controllable by any combination of bronchodilators, cromolyn sodium, or inhaled corticosteroids, often characterized clinically by reductions in the PEFR, greater intolerance of exercise, and the development of nocturnal symptoms. Prednisone, 40 mg per day in single or divided dose for 1 week, followed by a period of tapering is suggested. The occurrence of nocturnal symptoms may be an indication for the addition of sustained-release theophylline (100–300 mg at bedtime) or oral terbutaline to the pharmacologic regimen. *Chronic severe asthma* is characterized by the patient who without adequate treatment has continuous symptoms, limited activity tolerance, frequent nocturnal symptoms, and frequent severe exacerbations. Consultation with a pulmonologist, allergist, or other physician with expertise in asthma care is recommended. These patients are managed with multiple medications at maximal doses. In addition to the pharmacologic recommendations for moderate asthma, cromolyn sodium may be used concurrently with inhaled corticosteroids. Oral prednisone is often required on a chronic basis and therefore these patients need increased surveillance for systemic effects as well as gestational diabetes and IUGR. Perinatology consultation may be desirable to assist in the management of these high-risk patients. Oral corticosteroids may be tapered following persistent high-dose inhaled corticosteroid therapy (800 μg or more per day). Theophylline (daily

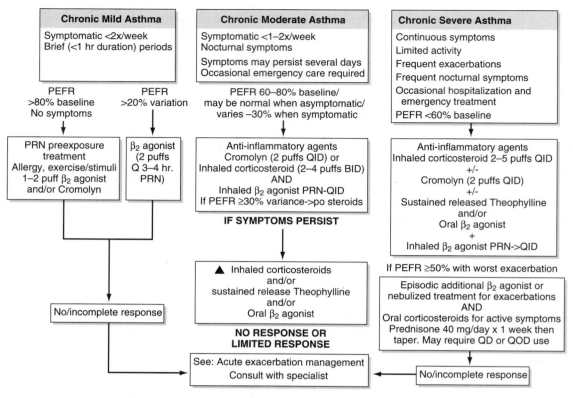

Figure 2. Outpatient management of chronic asthma during pregnancy.

dose to maintain therapeutic level of 8 to 12 μg/mL), a long-acting β_2-agonist (terbutaline 2.5–5.0 mg two to three times daily), or both may be helpful for these severe asthma patients. Caution is required when using theophylline concurrently with erythromycin, as this antibiotic decreases theophylline clearance, thereby increasing the risk of toxicity (nausea, vomiting, tachydysrythmia).

Acute Exacerbation

Unfortunately, despite optimal therapy and appropriate care, some women will experience acute asthma exacerbations during pregnancy. Urgent attention and treatment are imperative to prevent maternal and fetal hypoxia. The setting for this care is variable, depending on the severity of exacerbation and the gestational age. Home management should be limited to those women with normal fetal activity and for whom increasing the use of inhaled β_2-agonists to two to four puffs every 20 minutes brings about a relatively quick resolution of symptoms and a self-monitored PEFR greater than 70% of baseline personal best. Close follow-up is important,

as an increase or change in medication requirements is often necessary. If improvement is not complete or sustained, there is decreased fetal activity, or if the PEFR is less than 70% of the baseline personal best, in-patient evaluation is required. This may occur in the emergency department, labor and delivery department, obstetric intensive care unit (ICU), or medical ICU setting depending on hospital resources and clinical circumstances. A history is taken and physical examination is performed, assessing for cyanosis, the use of accessory muscles to breathe, and the patient's ability to converse or walk without significant dyspnea. Oxygen is administered and monitored with continuous pulse oximetry, with a goal of maintaining maternal oxygen saturation at greater than 95% (partial pressure of arterial oxygen [PaO_2] >60–70 torr), thus maintaining normal fetal oxygenation. Beware the arterial blood gas result demonstrating a "normal" partial pressure of arterial carbon dioxide ($PaCO_2$). Typically, you should expect a respiratory alkalosis and hypocarbia ($PaCO_2$ 27–32 torr) in the early stages of asthma exacerbation. Therefore, a $PaCO_2$ in the "normal range" indicates CO_2 retention and may be a prelude to impending respiratory failure. Continuous electronic fetal heart rate monitoring is applied, depending on the gestational age, or fetal viability is assessed with ultrasonography. The PEFR is determined and arterial blood gases are obtained. Intravenous hydration is begun. Pharmacologic interventions include inhaled β-agonist nebulization treatments (albuterol 0.5 mL of 0.5% inhalant solution mixed with 3 mL of sterile saline) repeated every 20 minutes or until the PEFR (checked after each treatment) is at 80% to 90% of baseline. Alternatively, 0.25 mg terbutaline may be administered subcutaneously every 20 to 30 minutes for up to three doses. Early initiation of intravenous corticosteroids (methylprednisolone 80 mg every 6 hours or hydrocortisone 100 mg every 6 hours) should be considered for patients who present on oral corticosteroids or those who do not demonstrate an immediate response to bronchodilator therapy. Patients who demonstrate a good response to this therapy as demonstrated by significant symptomatic improvement and a PEFR that returns to greater than 70% baseline may be considered for discharge with close outpatient follow-up and often a short course of oral corticosteroid. Those patients with a PEFR at 40% to 70% are considered for admission to the hospital and begun on intravenous corticosteroids while β₂-agonist therapy is continued hourly (in the absence of heart disease). Antibiotics should be administered at this point if there is suspicion of an infectious trigger of bacterial origin. Erythromycin is utilized to treat community-acquired pneumonia, while amoxicillin or ampicillin may be used to treat sinusitis or bronchitis. Patients with a PEFR of less than 40% baseline after treatment are admitted to the hospital, where β₂-agonist therapy is intensified and an aminophylline drip is begun (in years past, aminophylline was "first-line" therapy). Patients with severe respiratory distress, fatigue, and lack of any response to these therapies should be placed in an ICU setting and consideration given to early intubation. Continuous positive airway pressure may be beneficial, improving ventilation and clearing airway and interstitial edema through continuous positive pressure. Women with deteriorating mental status, paradoxical respiratory motion of the chest and abdominal muscles, or hypercarbia may be nearing respiratory failure, requiring endotracheal intubation and mechanical ventilation. While clinical judgment is best individualized, specific indications for intubation of the asthmatic gravida include inability to maintain PaO_2 greater than 60 torr despite supplemental oxygen, inability to maintain $PaCO_2$ below 40 torr, or evidence of maternal exhaustion. The pulmonologist, intensivist, and perinatologist may be indispensable consultants in managing these critical cases.

Labor and Delivery Management

Approximately 10% of asthmatic patients will have an asthma exacerbation during their labor and delivery. Anesthesiology consultation is suggested when the patient is admitted. Patients in labor should be kept well hydrated and continued on their previously scheduled regimen of asthma medications. Oral theophylline may be given intravenously and oral β₂-agonists may be given subcutaneously. Pulse oximetry may be considered to determine oxygen requirements. The patient who has been on oral corticosteroids should be treated with stress-dose parenteral corticosteroids (hydrocortisone, 100 mg every 6–8 hours) for labor or for cesarean section until 24 hours postpartum. The well-controlled stable asthmatic patient may be monitored for fetal well-being in the manner customary for the institution in which care is rendered. Patients with any degree of compromise should be managed with continuous electronic fetal heart rate monitoring. Induction of labor may be accomplished with oxytocin or prostaglandin E_2 products, as these have not been associated with bronchospasm. The management of postpartum hemorrhage is modified for the patient with asthma. Prostaglandin $F_{2\alpha}$ and methylergonovine are contraindicated, as they may precipitate bronchospasm. The use of oxytocin and rectal prostaglandin E_2 suppositories to control bleeding due to uterine atony is advocated.

Conclusion

While severe asthma exacerbations pose a serious threat to both maternal and fetal health, the preconceptional and perinatal management of the woman with asthma offers the opportunity to put into place therapeutic and educational interventions aimed at significantly improving the health of mother, fetus, and, ultimately, baby. A multidisciplinary approach to the provision of care incorporating obstetric care providers, maternal-fetal medicine specialists, pulmonologists, allergists, pharmacists, and nurse educators is encouraged. Further research is clearly needed to ultimately validate therapeutic regimens and determine whether other approaches or interventions are both safe and effective (eg, anticholinergics). Intensive educational efforts directed at nonobstetric health care providers are needed if we are to reverse the worrisome trends of increasing asthma prevalence and mortality and achieve optimal asthma treatment preconceptionally.

Breech Delivery

Tamerou Asrat, MD

Edward J. Quilligan, MD

Incidence

Overall, the incidence of breech presentation is said to be about 4% of the term deliveries and 15% to 20% of the preterm deliveries. Frank breech lies are most common in the term fetus whereas footling breech presentations represent the majority in preterm gestations. Footling breech has the highest rate of cord prolapse (15–18%), as compared to less than 0.5% in the frank breech.

Scope of the Problem

It has been clearly established that breech presentation in both term and preterm gestations is a bad prognostic variable in itself. There is a well-described association of breech presentation with fetal abnormalities (5–18%), aneuploidy, intrauterine growth restriction, and abnormal placentation (primary placenta previa). Estimates of the risk of perinatal mortality vary from 0 to 35 per 1000 births. Several authors have reported higher antepartum stillbirth and neonatal death rates with breech presentations regardless of the mode of delivery, even when corrected for the abnormality that may have caused the breech presentation.

In the United States, therefore, most clinicians are reluctant to consider a vaginal delivery of the breech fetus even in the absence of serious congenital anomalies or prematurity. This reluctance to deliver vaginally has resulted in significantly decreased experience in training programs, rendering "obstetric inexperience" yet another indication for cesarean sections.

Management Options

In most centers, breech presentation contributes about 10% to the overall cesarean delivery rate. A coordinated and concerted effort of identification of term breech presentations and implementation of external cephalic versions will convert nearly 50% of these breech presentations to vertex, and about 25% of the remainder can deliver vaginally, safely, without an increased risk to the fetus or mother.

External cephalic version (EVC) remains contentious, primarily owing to concerns raised by older studies that seemed to indicate an increased risk of fetal morbidity and mortality. However, the more recent literature indicates that ECV is a "safe" alternative in the management of term breech presentations, resulting in a marked reduction of cesarean sections without any statistically significant increase in short-term or long-term fetal morbidity. The most commonly reported risk to the fetus is a transient bradycardia, which leads to a cesarean delivery in less than 1% of cases.

In most centers, an ECV is attempted at 37 to 39 weeks with a success rate of 60% to 70%. Absolute contraindications to ECV include multiple gestation, antepartum hemorrhage, placenta previa, ruptured membranes, and "serious" fetal abnormalities. Relative contraindications include oligohydramnios, intrauterine growth restriction, previous cesarean section, macrosomia, and maternal obesity.

Prerequisites for ECV include a recent detailed ultrasonogram to confirm an intact fetus and adequate fluid volume; a reactive fetal heart rate tracing without decelerations; and informed consent, with the mother advised of the risks of rupture of membranes, cord and placental accidents, and, rarely, an emergency cesarean section. The mother should be on nothing-by-mouth status and have an intravenous line in place, and an anesthesiologist and facilities for a rapid cesarean section should be available nearby.

We recommend that all ECV be done in the hospital, in close proximity to the operating room. We usually use 0.25 mg of terbutaline given subcutaneously immediately prior to the ECV. The ECV should be done in one sitting by one operator and should not take more than 5 minutes. The longer the attempt, the higher the incidence of fetal bradycardia. Continuous or frequent (every 2 minutes) assessment of the fetal heart rate by ultrasonography is necessary. Acoustic stimulation with an artificial larynx may be used at the beginning or during the procedure to facilitate the version. We strongly discourage vaginal disengagement of the breech. Anesthesia, epidural or spinal, and intravenous sedation are not recommended, since the level of maternal discomfort is often used as a gauge of the amount of uterine manipulation. If the mother is Rh negative, full-dose RhoGAM is given, since feto-maternal hemorrhage has been reported in association with ECV. After ECV, whether successful or not, the fetus is monitored for 1 or 2 hours prior to discharge. Some authors have advocated continued antepartum testing, until delivery, despite the lack of data to support this degree of fetal surveillance. If the ECV was unsuccessful and the mother is to be delivered by cesarean section, the presentation should be rechecked immediately prior to the operation.

Vaginal Delivery of the Breech Fetus

While this chapter is not intended to be a step-by-step protocol for vaginal breech deliveries, there are certain prerequisites that must be adhered to in order to assure successful delivery and mitigate the risk of maternal and neonatal complications.

Vaginal delivery of breech presentation should be considered when the fetus is presenting as either frank or complete breech, is of an appropriate weight (2000–3900 g), does not have a hyperextended head, and makes normal progress through labor.

Although radiography or computed tomographic pelvimetry is seldom needed, clinical evaluation of the pelvis must be done and adequacy of the pelvis documented.

Most authors do not favor the use of oxytocin to initiate or augment labor, although this point is rather controversial among various clinicians.

Vaginal delivery should only be contemplated if immediate anesthesia and prompt cesarean section are available. Continuous fetal monitoring should be used in all cases and the delivery should be attended by a pediatrician and two experienced obstetricians.

The safe breech delivery of a term infant depends primarily on maternal expulsion efforts. Operator intervention should be minimal and limited. Injudicious traction will cause displacement of fetal limbs from their normal flexed position across the fetal body, promote hyperextension of the fetal head, and result in injury of soft tissue and body parts.

Total labor duration for the breech presentation should be similar to that in cephalic presentation.

We recommend liberal use of epidural anesthesia, since it will make manipulations in the second stage more comfortable and reduce the urge to push prior to full dilatation.

Finally, prior to undertaking a vaginal breech delivery, the clinician should discuss at great lengths with the mother and partner the risks and benefits of vaginal delivery versus elective cesarean section.

Chorioamnionitis

John W. Riggs, MD
Jorge D. Blanco, MD

Clinical Intraamniotic Infection

It is possible to be greatly confused by the many names for clinical, intrapartum, intrauterine infection that have arisen in recent years: chorioamnionitis, amnionitis, and intra-amniotic infection. Similar terms are used to describe the histologic findings of infection in the placenta and membranes. Most women with intra-amniotic infection (IAI) have histologic evidence of chorioamnionitis, but not all placentas with this finding come from women with IAI. The clinical diagnosis of IAI is made in only 0.5% to 10.5% of pregnancies, whereas histologic inflammation of the chorion and amnion is found in 20% of term and 60% of preterm pregnancies. The term "microbial invasion of the amniotic fluid" is also used to describe a preclinical phase of amniotic fluid infection. Although numerous studies are being done to discover the relationship between preterm labor and subclinical infection in the uterus, that discussion is beyond the scope of this chapter. The term intra-amniotic infection (IAI) will be used in this chapter to refer to the clinically diagnosed intrapartum infection. This clinical entity (IAI) is highly associated with maternal and neonatal morbidity, which can frequently be improved by timely diagnosis and treatment.

Defense Mechanisms

Natural defense mechanisms prevent the development of IAI in all but a few women and can be categorized as either natural barriers (cervical mucus and amniotic membranes) or natural amniotic fluid inhibitory properties. The thick, tenacious cervical mucus acts as a plug in the cervix and the amniotic membranes form an additional seal to the fetal cavity. Amniotic fluid has been shown to inhibit bacterial growth and to have antimicrobial properties. This property may vary depending on the ethnic population studied. Sixty-seven percent of sterilely obtained fluids from white patients were inhibitory, while only 33% of those from patients of African decent were. The inhibitory mechanisms of amniotic fluid also seem to work less well in infected than noninfected fluid. The relationship between amniotic fluid inhibitory activity and IAI was studied by Blanco and colleagues, who found that *Escherichia coli* was much less likely to be inhibited by the amniotic fluid from patients with IAI than from matched control subjects. This could be due to inhibitory factors that are deficient, impaired, or overwhelmed by the bacterial inoculum. For example, meconium impairs the infection-inhibiting properties of amniotic fluid, probably through diminished neutrophil phagocytic function.

Risk Factors

As mentioned, the amniotic membranes are a natural barrier to the ascent of pathogenic organisms, so most IAI is found after the membranes have ruptured. While hematogenous spread is possible, pathogenic organisms can more easily reach the amniotic cavity once this barrier is gone. However, access to the amniotic cavity is not sufficient to produce an infectious process.

Other factors predisposing to IAI have been identified, including duration of ruptured membranes, transcervical instrumentation, vaginal examinations, parity, and cerclage placement. How many cervical examinations, if any at all, can be performed safely remains unknown and controversial at this time. Newton and colleagues found nuliparity, duration of internal monitoring, and duration of ruptured membranes to be significant risk factors for IAI. About 20% of women with 28- to 32-week pregnancies with preterm premature rupture of the membranes develop IAI; however, in this population, factors other than the duration of ruptured membranes may have a stronger influence on the incidence of IAI. Women found to have group B streptococcal vaginal colonization within the 3 weeks preceding delivery have an increased risk of clinical IAI (odds ratio, 3.6; 95% CI, 2.1–6.2). This risk seems to rise with more pronounced colonization.

With intact membranes, it is possible that cervical manipulation with cerclage placement or membrane stripping may increase the risk of intra-amniotic infection. Charles and Edwards found a 2.6-fold increase in IAI if the cerclage placement was delayed until the late second tri-

mester. Treadwell studied 482 patients undergoing cerclage placement and found a 6% infection rate when the cervix was less than 2 cm but 41.7% when greater than 2 cm. In another case series of 33 women at 14 to 24 weeks' gestation with cervical dilation greater than 2 cm, 17 (51%) had positive amniotic fluid cultures. All patients with negative Gram stains received cerclage placement. IAI developed in 30% of patients whose amniotic fluid cultures were later positive. In a randomized controlled trial, stripping of the fetal membranes was associated with clinical IAI in 4 of 10 women, compared with 1 in 10 who did not receive such treatment. However, this result has not been found by other authors. Whether membrane stripping actually increases the risk of IAI has yet to be established, but these studies suggest an additive effect of cervical manipulation and exposure of the chorioamniotic membranes to the vaginal flora, possibly allowing bacterial invasion.

As mentioned earlier, the development of IAI in women via hematogenous route has been reported. Nine infants with evidence of early-onset listeriosis have been described, many of whom were born to clinically ill mothers. One patient with IAI, intact membranes, and transabdominal cultures growing *Listeria monocytogenes* has been described by Petrilli. Other organisms in which this route has been implicated are fusobacterium and group A streptococcus.

Iatrogenic IAI has been presumed to follow amniocentesis. A review of the available literature in 1968 describing the complications from 45 studies including 8300 amniocenteses found only three cases of amnionitis. This complication occurred at a rate of 0.6% and 1% in the two studies reporting amnionitis. Intra-amniotic infection following percutaneous umbilical blood sampling is likewise a rare occurrence complicating 0.7% of procedures.

Microbiology

As in most severe upper reproductive tract infections, IAI is a polymicrobial infection. A quantitative bacteriologic comparison of the amniotic fluid collected by intrauterine catheterization from 52 laboring women with clinical IAI and 52 matched control subjects was presented by Gibbs and colleagues. The infected patients' fluid grew an average of 2.2 isolates, and the organisms isolated from the infected group were more likely to be "highly virulent." The rates of isolation for this study are shown in Table 1. The most common high virulence isolates in the in-

TABLE 1. Amniotic Fluid Isolates in Patients with
Intra-amniotic Infection°

Microorganism	Incidence (%)
High virulence	
Bacteroides spp	33
Group B *Streptococcus*	15
Escherichia coli	13
Clostridium spp	12
Alpha streptococci	12
Peptococcus spp	10
Klebsiella spp	8
Fusobacterium spp	8
Low virulence	
Lactobacillus	38
Diphtheroids	19
Eubacterium lentum	12
Staphylococcus epidermidis	8

°$n = 52$.

fected group were *Bacteroides* species, group B streptococcus, and *E. coli*. Both aerobic and anaerobic organisms were isolated from half of the cases, only aerobes in 38%, and only anaerobes in 8%. Blood cultures were positive in 10.3% of infected women who were sampled and 4% of sampled neonates with strong similarities between blood and amniotic fluid cultures. So, patients with IAI are usually suffering from a bacterial infection with a bacterial spectrum that is similar to that of other genital tract infections.

At least two distinct bacterial spectra are prominent in IAI, one group consisting of predominantly enteric flora (as mentioned earlier) and one related to *Mycoplasma hominis*. Genital tract mycoplasmas are found more often in patients with IAI than uninfected control subjects (35% of infected and 8% of control cases grew *M. hominis*) and are associated with high-virulence anaerobic organisms and *Gardnerella vaginalis*. *M. hominis* is strongly associated with bacterial vaginosis. A study of 408 patients with IAI identified an association with bacterial vaginosis in some patients. The study found that bacterial vaginosis organisms (*M. hominis*, *G. vaginalis*, and anaerobes) were highly associated with each other. Also, women with premature ruptured membranes and bacterial vaginosis developed IAI significantly more frequently. The authors also observed an association between *E. coli*, other aerobic gram-negative rods, and enterococci and postulated that these represented two distinct sources of infection, vaginal or intestinal.

Other organisms have been reported in association with IAI, including *Ureaplasma urealyti-*

cum, *Candida* sp, and *Haemophilus influenzae*. Martin and colleagues described an association between chlamydial cervicitis and subsequent perinatal demise. Oshiro and colleagues infected murine cervices with *Chlamydia trachomatis* and found a 35% incidence of histologic chorioamnionitis and 19% incidence of intrapartum fetal demise. Chlamydial cervicitis, which is one of the most prevalent cervical infections, has an unknown effect on the incidence of IAI in humans.

Diagnosis

The accurate and timely diagnosis of intra-amniotic infection is important to avoid failing to treat infected mothers and fetuses but also to prevent the overuse of antibiotics in noninfected patients. Unfortunately, early diagnosis is difficult because clinical signs and symptoms of IAI occur late and are neither sensitive nor specific. To avoid a delay in diagnosis, a high index of suspicion should be maintained. Fever and maternal or fetal tachycardia, especially in the presence of ruptured membranes, suggest the diagnosis of IAI. The diagnostic criteria most commonly used for IAI are listed in Table 2. Table 3 lists the frequency of specific findings.

Laboratory evaluation of maternal blood or amniotic fluid can be helpful in diagnosing IAI, but no single test is diagnostic. Maternal leukocytosis, although found frequently, must be interpreted cautiously if the patient is in labor, and bacteremia is found in only 10% of patients with IAI. Amniotic fluid can be obtained from an intrauterine pressure catheter if the membranes are ruptured or via amniocentesis. When using fluid from an intrauterine pressure catheter, the first 7 to 10 mL should be discarded. Gram stain, culture, and cell count are the most commonly

TABLE 2. Clinical Diagnosis of Intra-amniotic
Infection

One of these:
  Fever (>37.8°C)
  Rupture of the membranes
and two or more of the following:
  Peripheral leukocytosis (white blood cell count
    >15000)
  Fetal tachycardia (fetal heart rate >160)
  Maternal tachycardia (pulse >100)
  Malodorous amniotic fluid
  Uterine tenderness
and no other apparent site of infection.

TABLE 3. Clinical Findings in Patients with Intra-amniotic Infection°

Finding	Incidence (%)
Rupture of membranes	98.2
Peripheral leukocytosis	86.1
Maternal fever	85.3
Fetal tachycardia	36.8
Maternal tachycardia	32.9
Foul-smelling amniotic fluid	21.6
Uterine tenderness	12.9
Foul-smelling neonate	9.4

°$n = 171$.

used tests, yet the diagnostic properties of these tests are not ideal. Women with the diagnosis of IAI have a higher frequency of bacteria and white blood cells in the amniotic fluid. The Gram stain is positive in 67.4% ($p < 0.001$) and leukocytes are present in 80.8% ($p < 0.001$) compared with 11.6% and 28%, respectively, in the uninfected laboring patient. While reasonably specific, a negative Gram stain does not rule out IAI, since it is negative in approximately 50% of infected patients. Because leukocytosis and bacteria on the Gram stain are common in the uninfected patient and can have a low sensitivity, these findings must be interpreted with care and when taken alone are insufficient to make the diagnosis of IAI.

To enhance the diagnostic utility of amniotic fluid sampling, many other diagnostic tests have been studied: leukocyte esterase, glucose *Limulus* amebocyte assay, gas-liquid chromatography, and interleukins. These tests involve amniocentesis and are most often indicated in diagnosing subclinical infection, such as might be associated with preterm labor. Leukocyte esterase is released in response to bacteria and can be measured in amniotic fluid by reagent strips. Glucose levels in amniotic fluid have been found to be decreased in patients with microbial invasion of the amniotic cavity. Interleukin-6 has received the most attention recently. It is one of many inflammatory cytokines that mediate the host's response to infection and is highly predictive of microbial invasion of the amniotic fluid and neonatal morbidity. Nevertheless, these tests may not be readily available and their role in assisting with the diagnosis or reducing maternal or neonatal morbidity is not yet clear.

Management and Outcome

Antibiotic treatment for IAI should be initiated once the diagnosis is made. Delivery is usually indicated. Maternal therapy is also therapy for the fetus and has been clearly shown to lower neonatal morbidity. Neonatal sepsis and pneumonia were found in 0% of infants whose mothers were treated for IAI intrapartum compared with 32% in infants of mothers whose treatment was delayed until postpartum. Delaying treatment was a more common management plan in the past because of the desire to optimize neonatal culturing. Although awaiting delivery to start antibiotics may provide a greater likelihood of isolating an organism in the neonate, there is a clear advantage to mother and baby from intrapartum treatment when it can be given.

Due to the variety of microbes found in this infection, broad-spectrum antibiotic coverage is desirable. The most established treatment regimen is ampicillin, 2 g IV every 6 hours and gentamicin 1.5 mg/kg IV every 8 hours. Penicillin G levels are one third the maternal level 120 minutes after administration. In contrast, ampicillin's concentration in the fetal compartment is comparable to that of the mother after the same time interval and therefore may be preferable. Delivery is usually indicated if labor has not begun spontaneously and if cesarean section is necessary; clindamycin 900 mg IV every 8 hours should be added after cord clamping to prevent puerperal infection. Cesarean section should be reserved for the usual obstetric indications. These antibiotics should be continued until the mother is afebrile for 24 to 48 hours. The use of single-agent, broad-spectrum antibiotics has not been studied in large, comparative trials. Given the spectrum of activity of newer generation cephalosporins and penicillins, it is possible that they may provide equally effective regimens.

Neonatal Outcome

While neonatal morbidity may be reduced by the antepartum initiation of antibiotics, it is not eliminated and is greatest in the preterm neonate. The incidence of respiratory distress is doubled and the mortality increased fourfold among infants born at 28 to 32 weeks who had preterm, premature ruptured membranes and developed IAI. The respiratory distress incidence was felt to be elevated because of the difficulty in distinguishing it from early-onset pneumonia. Other studies have found a higher rate of neonatal sepsis, mortality, intraventricular hemorrhage, and respiratory distress syndrome among appropriately treated preterm neonates with IAI. However, IAI in preterm neonates was not associated with developmental delays at 1 year of life.

At term, perinatal morbidity from IAI defined as pneumonia or sepsis may occur in up to 27% of infants born to mothers treated for IAI, depending on the definition of morbidity used. Although umbilical cord blood gas pH may be lower in neonates of mothers diagnosed with IAI, this decrease is not found when other variables such as induction of labor, length of labor, or mode of delivery are statistically excluded. Also, immediate operative delivery does not seem to improve neonatal morbidity when IAI is present. In contrast, perinatal mortality in full-term pregnancies treated for IAI is rare. For example, only two neonatal deaths were reported in a series of 131 term cases of IAI, both of which had noninfectious causes of death (meconium aspiration and transposition of the great vessels).

Maternal Outcome

Pre-existing intrauterine infection is a major risk factor for the development of postpartum infection in patients requiring cesarean section. To enhance the anaerobic coverage in such patients, clindamycin should be added after cord clamping. A prospective randomized study of patients with IAI found no difference in the endometritis rate between the group of patients whose treatment was augmented by clindamycin after delivery. However, clindamycin may prevent abscesses or septic pelvic thrombophlebitis in these same patients.

The progress in labor of women suffering with IAI has been studied. If treated promptly and aggressively, the maternal and neonatal outcomes are not altered by the interval from diagnosis to delivery; however, there are very few data on labor intervals greater than 12 hours. The majority of the cesarean sections in patients with IAI are indicated for dysfunctional labor. The presence of IAI is not an indication for cesarean section, although cesarean section occurs in up to 40% of affected patients. Whether IAI causes dysfunctional labor or dysfunctional labor predisposes to IAI is not clear. IAI is associated with labor that lasts an average of 5 hours longer and with a 40% cesarean section rate when diagnosed in women who already require oxytocin augmentation. In contrast, the cesarean section rate is not significantly higher when the diagnosis of IAI is made before oxytocin is needed. Patients who have a subclinical bacterial colonization of the amniotic fluid have a higher cesarean section rate if their cultures grow high-virulence organisms, as compared with those growing low-virulence organisms (57.9% vs. 25%, $p = 0.05$). IAI may

be a sequelae of dystocia, or dystocia may result from bacterial invasion of the amniotic cavity.

If cesarean section is necessary, the technique used is not altered by the presence of infection. With the development of modern aseptic technique and the availability of antibiotics, the use of the extraperitoneal cesarean section, cesarean hysterectomy, or the Portes procedure to limit intraperitoneal spread have been largely been replaced by the transperitoneal, transverse lower segment incision. This operation is less technically difficult and has a lower morbidity rate.

Conclusion

Numerous natural barriers protect women from intra-amniotic infection. Still, infection occurs in a substantial number of women each year. Many risk factors, such as the duration of ruptured membranes and transcervical instrumentation, have been identified. Early diagnosis is still difficult because clinical signs and symptoms occur late and are not highly specific nor sensitive. Nevertheless, timely diagnosis is crucial to avoid the adverse outcome of infection. As soon as the diagnosis is made, treatment should be initiated with antibiotics that will cross the placenta quickly. Delivery is usually indicated. Timely treatment will reduce but not eliminate neonatal morbidity, especially in the preterm neonate. The rate of cesarean section and maternal postpartum infectious morbidity are both increased, even when the condition is optimally treated. The current management of labor in these women does not differ from that of noninfected women, except for the addition of antibiotics.

Chorionic Villus Sampling for Prenatal Diagnosis

Marie H. Beall, MD

Chorionic villus sampling (CVS) is a procedure that has been proposed as an alternative to amniocentesis for prenatal diagnosis of chromosomal and some genetic disorders. CVS has the advantage that it is performed in the first trimester of pregnancy. In the late 1980s, CVS was being advocated as an alternative to amniocentesis, and the only issue commonly addressed was the difference in fetal loss rates between the two procedures. At the same time, access to the catheters used to perform CVS was strictly regulated, and CVS was more widely available in some areas than in others. Since that time, new information about possible sublethal fetal harm with CVS has become available, and maternal serum screening has moved much prenatal diagnosis into the second trimester. CVS has become much less common in all areas, especially in those where it was never popular.

Indications

Chorionic villus sampling may be performed for the determination of fetal karyotype in pregnancies complicated by (1) advanced maternal age, (2) a prior child with a chromosomal anomaly, (3) a known chromosomal abnormality (such as a translocation) in one of the parents, or (4) other complications known to increase the risk for fetal chromosomal anomalies. Karyotypic analysis also allows prediction of fetal sex in cases in which a sex-linked disorder is involved. CVS also provides a relatively large amount of viable fetal tissue suitable for DNA studies for the detection of genetic disorders. In addition to genetic "disorders," CVS has been used to predict the Rh status of the fetus in mothers with a history of severe isoimmunization. In a few cases, CVS diagnoses of fetal metabolic diseases have been used to plan fetal treatment, such as fetal bone marrow transplantation, although these treatments remain experimental at this time.

Chorionic villus sampling is not able to detect fetal neural tube defects or other abnormalities detected by the analysis of the amniotic fluid. In addition, CVS is performed at a gestational age that makes ultrasonographic examination for fetal anomalies problematic. Most CVS centers request that patients undergo an ultrasonographic examination in the second trimester of pregnancy, and many also recommend serum screening for neural tube defects.

Technique

Chorionic villus sampling may be performed by either the transcervical or the transabdominal route. Comparison of the two methods has shown little difference in outcome, although many centers report lower fetal loss rates when both procedures are available. The procedure is now performed at 10 to 12 weeks' gestation. No CVS procedure should be performed without an extensive genetic counseling session in which the

risks and benefits of the procedure are examined with the patient.

Transcervical CVS is performed by inserting a plastic catheter containing a wire obturator into the uterus through the uterine cervix under ultrasonographic guidance. In our center, patients are asked to undergo cervical cultures for gonorrhea and chlamydia, and vaginal cultures for group B Streptococcus. If at all possible, patients have an ultrasound scan before the day of the procedure, to establish the dates with certainty and to rule out a missed abortion. After receiving counseling and signing informed consent, the patient is asked to fill her bladder. In most cases, a full bladder is of benefit in performing transcervical CVS, as it straightens the angle between uterus and cervix. When the bladder is sufficiently full, the patient is placed in lithotomy position, a sterile speculum is placed, and a sterile vaginal prep is performed. The CVS catheter is then inserted under direct ultrasonographic guidance.

CVS catheters are produced commercially, but owing to the difficulty in obtaining the catheters, many centers make their own. In general, the catheter is smaller than an endometrial biopsy catheter and is not felt by the patient as it is inserted. It is imperative that the ultrasonography equipment be able to visualize the cervical canal, so that the catheter may be shaped to the correct curve, and so that the catheter may be visualized as it enters the uterine cavity. When the catheter has been maneuvered into the chorion frondosum, the obturator is removed, and a syringe containing a few milliliters of culture medium is attached. Gentle suction is then applied to the catheter as it is removed. The resulting tissue specimen is examined in the procedure room, and an additional pass is taken with a fresh catheter if insufficient tissue was obtained with the first pass. No more than two passes are performed at one time on any patient. Centers doing many CVS procedures report success rates over 97% in obtaining tissue with this technique.

After the CVS procedure, a brief ultrasound scan is performed to document fetal heart motion. The patient is informed that a small amount of vaginal spotting is common after this procedure. She is asked to immediately report any cramping, heavy bleeding, fever, or malaise. She is also asked to refrain from putting anything in the vagina for a period of 1 to 2 weeks. She is reminded of the need for second trimester evaluation for fetal neural tube defects. Finally, RhoGAM is administered if the patient is Rh negative.

Transabdominal CVS is performed with the

patient supine. After informed consent and abdominal prep, a spinal needle is inserted into the chorion. A minimum needle size of 20 gauge appears to be necessary to obtain sufficient tissue. When the needle is in position, the stylet is removed, and a syringe with a small amount of tissue culture medium is attached. With gentle suction and some working of the needle back and forth, a specimen is withdrawn. Again, the specimen is evaluated in the procedure room, and another pass is performed if necessary. The transabdominal CVS technique can be used in a wide variety of gestational ages; many centers use this technique for placental biopsy near term. The discussion of fetal risk may not necessarily apply to such late procedures.

After the procedure, the fetal heart motion is documented. The patient is informed that a limited amount of uterine cramping is expected after this procedure. She is asked to rest for 24 hours, and to refrain from intercourse for 3 days. She is asked to promptly report any prolonged cramping, heavy bleeding, fever, or malaise. She is reminded of the need for second trimester neural tube evaluation and given RhoGAM.

Other CVS procedures have been proposed. These have included the use of a needle endoscope to obtain tissue and transvaginal CVS through the posterior fornix of the vagina. None of these procedures is now in common use.

Risks and Benefits of CVS

Chorionic villus sampling originally became popular because it allowed much earlier prenatal diagnosis than was otherwise available. The original CVS protocols included "direct" karyotypes on the rapidly dividing fetal tissue, with results available in 2 to 3 days. Direct karyotypes are very expensive to perform, owing to the amount of work required in the laboratory, and they may be less accurate owing to the fact that they reflect the placental karyotype. For these reasons, fetal diagnosis based on direct karyptyping alone is no longer done in the first trimester, and the wait between procedure and results is similar for CVS and amniocentesis. Amniocentesis practitioners have also begun to offer this procedure earlier in gestation, meeting some of the need for earlier procedures. Finally, the need for first-trimester procedures has become less with the shift to maternal serum screening for Down's syndrome, which must (currently) take place in the second trimester.

An earlier diagnosis by CVS is of real benefit in some patients: Some centers have reported

fetal treatment with bone marrow transplantation. This technique requires first-trimester diagnosis of the affected fetus. In other cases, parents with a relatively high (25–50%) risk of recurrence of a genetic defect request CVS to avoid multiple second-trimester pregnancy termination procedures. Finally, some patients request CVS because their social situation prevents them from choosing pregnancy termination after the pregnancy becomes apparent. At present, no other technique can provide as early a diagnosis as CVS.

Karyotypes performed on CVS specimens are performed either on the cytotrophoblast, which reflects the karyotype of the placenta, or on the mesenchymal core of the villus. The mesenchymal core tissue is more directly derived from the fetus. CVS specimens have rarely yielded karyotypes that do not reflect the true fetal karyotype. These "false" karyotypes often result from cytotrophoblast (direct) preparations, but they may occur in any CVS preparation. These false results are often obvious, as they reflect chromosomal trisomies that are not compatible with a live fetus. The fact remains, however, that the need for follow-up after ambiguous karyotypic results is higher for CVS than for amniocentesis.

Chorionic villus sampling is an expensive procedure. Due to the dependence on maternal bladder filling, CVS procedures take several times longer than amniocenteses. In addition, laboratory technician time is required to dissect the fresh specimen, to prevent maternal tissue from being included in culture. This makes CVS more labor-intensive in the laboratory even if direct preparations of the chromosomes are not being performed. In our center, CVS cannot compete in a price sense with amniocentesis, with the result that insurers are reluctant to approve the procedure without special indications.

As with any invasive procedure, there are risks to the fetus from CVS. The risk of fetal death due to the procedure is generally believed to be 0.5% to 1%. There does appear to be a decreased risk of fetal loss in centers that perform many procedures, as compared with centers performing fewer. In addition, fetal loss is increased in pregnancies with vaginal bleeding in the week prior to the procedure, procedures requiring multiple sampling attempts, and procedures felt by the practitioner to be "difficult." Most centers do not report a difference in fetal loss rates between transcervical and transabdominal CVS, but many have reported an overall decrease in fetal loss when both modalities were available.

In 1991, the first report was published of

possible long-term fetal harm from CVS. Since then, there have been multiple reports of the association of CVS and transverse limb defects, including, in severe cases, the syndrome of oromandibular-limb hypogenesis, which includes limb and facial abnormalities. No prospective studies are available regarding this issue. Retrospective studies indicate that CVS is associated with this kind of limb defect. When CVS is performed prior to 10 weeks, the risk of limb defects is increased from about 0.03% to 0.2%, and whole limbs as well as facial defects may be involved. When CVS is performed after 10 weeks, the risk decreases to 0.07% (which may not be different than control), and the defects tend to be more distal, involving only the digits. For these reasons, CVS has been confined to pregnancies of greater than 10 weeks' gestational age. Information about the association of CVS with limb defects is part of any patient counseling session.

There are few known serious maternal risks associated with CVS. A few severe maternal infections following transcervical CVS were reported early in the development of the procedure; one was reported to require hysterectomy for treatment. At that time, the recommendation was made to use a new sterile catheter for each "pass." No further reports of maternal infections have been made, and this risk appears to be exceedingly low with current techniques. Less serious maternal side effects, such as uterine cramping, spotting, or discomfort with the procedure, may be quite common, depending on the technique used.

Conclusion

Chorionic villus sampling is a technique for first-trimester prenatal diagnosis that may be of significant benefit to selected patients. CVS has marked advantages for certain prenatal diagnostic patients, as it can be performed in the first trimester of pregnancy. An earlier procedure may increase the maternal sense of privacy and the safety of pregnancy termination while allowing additional time for the performance of complex laboratory procedures. At one time, CVS was very popular in some parts of the country for the performance of routine cytogenetic procedures. Increased understanding of the risks and shortcomings of the procedure have dampened this enthusiasm.

Chronic Hypertension in Pregnancy

Baha M. Sibai, MD

Definition and Classification

The prevalence of chronic hypertension in women of reproductive age is not known, and it likely varies according to the population race, maternal age, and leading mass indices. However, the incidence is particularly increased in obese women and in those older than 40 years of age. Chronic hypertension in pregnancy is defined as (1) hypertension that precedes pregnancy, (2) hypertension that occurs in pregnancy prior to 20 weeks' gestation, or (3) hypertension that persists beyond the sixth postpartum week.

The presentation of chronic hypertension implies either primary (essential) hypertension or secondary hypertension. Essential hypertension, which is not linked to a single etiology, accounts for 90% of the chronic hypertension seen during pregnancy. Secondary hypertension is due to an underlying abnormality, including renal disease, certain endocrine disorders, collagen vascular disease, pheochromocytoma, renal artery stenosis, or aortic coarctation.

In nonpregnancy, chronic hypertension is classified as mild (stage 1), moderate (stage 2), severe (stage 3), or very severe (stage 4). In contrast, during pregnancy, hypertension is usually classified as either mild or severe according to either systolic blood pressure (140–159 mm Hg versus ≥160 mm Hg) or diastolic blood pressure (90–109 mm Hg versus ≥110 mm Hg).

Management

The pregnancy outcome in patients with chronic hypertension receiving antihypertensive therapy depends on the severity of the hypertension. Antihypertensive treatment is necessary for the mother with severe hypertension to reduce the acute risk of cerebral hemorrhage or hypertensive encephalopathy. In addition, these patients are at increased risk for superimposed pre-eclampsia and require frequent antepartum assessment as well as antihypertensive therapy for blood pressure control.

The role of therapy in patients with mild uncomplicated chronic hypertension is uncertain, however. There are many prospective studies that have examined the pregnancy outcome in the treatment of mild chronic hypertension (Table 1). Although maximal blood pressure in pregnancy was lowered in mild chronic hypertensive patients on therapy, neither the controlled nor the uncontrolled studies have shown a reduction in the incidence of superimposed pre-eclampsia or abruptio placentae with the use of antihypertensive medications.

Therefore, to further delineate an approach to therapeutic management in pregnant patients with chronic hypertension, these patients can be divided into low-risk and high -risk groups (Table 2). This classification is based on patient history and clinical presentation.

Low-Risk Chronic Hypertension in Pregnancy

Chronically hypertensive patients who are considered at low risk (mild hypertension without target organ involvement or damage), have a

TABLE 2. Chronic Hypertension in Pregnancy: High-Risk Characteristics

Blood pressure >160 mm Hg systolic/110 mm Hg diastolic at <20 weeks' gestation
Maternal age >40 years
Duration of hypertension >15 years
Diabetes (class B to F)
Renal disease (all causes)
Cardiomyopathy
Collagen vascular disease
Coarctation of the aorta
History of stroke
History of congestive heart failure

favorable maternal and perinatal prognosis without the use of antihypertensive therapy. This observation was made in a prospective trial by Sibai and colleagues. Three hundred women with mild chronic hypertension were randomly assigned at 6 to 13 weeks' gestation to receive no medication or methyldopa or labetalol. There were no differ-

TABLE 1. Pregnancy Outcome in Randomized Controlled Trials of Chronic Hypertension

Study	Gestation at Entry (wks)	Gestation at Delivery (wks)	Birth Weight (g)	IUGR (%)	Pre-eclampsia (%)	Perinatal Death (%)
Leather et al.						
Control ($n=24$)	<20	36.5	2520	N/A	N/A	8.3°
Treated ($n=23$)		38.0	2840			0
Redman et al.						
Control ($n=107$)	20.6 ± 0.5	38.1 ± 0.2	3130 ± 49	N/A	4.7	1.9°
Treated ($n=101$)	21.9 ± 0.5	38.1 ± 0.2	3090 ± 60		6.7	1.0
Arias et al.						
Control ($n=29$)	16.4 ± 1.1	38.3 ± 0.4	3011 ± 103	14.2	10.3	3.4
Treated ($n=29$)	14.7 ± 1.0	38.1 ± 0.5	2926 ± 131	14.2	3.4	0
Weitz et al.						
Control ($n=12$)	<34	37.6 ± 0.5	2820	25	33.3	0
Treated ($n=13$)		39.0 ± 0.4	3140	0	38.4	0
Sibai et al.						
Control ($n=90$)	11.3 ± 0.2	39.0 ± 0.2	3123 ± 69	8.9	15.6	1.1
Treated ($n=173$)	11.2 ± 0.2	38.7 ± 0.2	3060 ± 72	7.5	17.3	1.2
Butters et al.						
Control ($n=14$)	15.9	39.5	3530	0	N/A	0
Treated ($n=15$)	15.8	38.5	2620	66		6
Gallery et al.						
Methyldopa ($n=27$)	32 ± 4.2	37.5 ± 3.1	2654 ± 821	N/A	7.4	7.4
Oxprenolol ($n=26$)	31 ± 9.1	38.0 ± 2.0	3051 ± 663		7.6	0
Fidler et al.						
Methyldopa ($n=22$)	23.9 ± 6.7	37.7 ± 2.3	2992 ± 732	N/A	9.1	4.5
Oxprenolol ($n=24$)	22.5 ± 7.2	37.1 ± 3.4	2715 ± 919		8.3	4.2

°Excludes second trimester loss.
  IUGR, intrauterine growth retardation; pre-eclampsia = blood pressure plus proteinuria; N/A = not available.
  Data are presented as mean ± SEM where available.

ences among the three groups in the incidence of superimposed pre-eclampsia, abruptio placentae, preterm delivery, and perinatal outcome. As a result, antihypertensive therapy in this low-risk group (95% of all pregnant women with chronic hypertension) may not be of added benefit in pregnancy. In fact, the potential association between low birth weight infants and the long-term use of β-blockers in pregnancy further discourages the use of these agents in treating patients with mild chronic hypertension. Because the trials performed to date do not establish a justification for treating low-risk chronic hypertension in pregnancy, antihyhypertensive therapy should be reserved for those patients who have chronic hypertension classified as high risk.

Although patients with low-risk hypertension do not require drug therapy, careful antepartum management and antenatal evaluation are still essential. About 50% of these women demonstrate significant reduction in blood pressure to normotensive levels during the second trimester. A further one third of the women will have no change in blood pressure in the second trimester, and the remaining 17% will demonstrate an increase in blood pressure (Fig. 1). At the initial prenatal visit, the importance and implications of hypertension in pregnancy should be discussed with the patient. The patient should be encouraged to avoid smoking and excessive caffeine consumption and should be advised about the benefits of proper nutritional intake.

During the course of pregnancy, the patient with low-risk hypertension should have outpatient assessment every 2 weeks in the second trimester and then weekly in the third trimester. However, the frequency of visits can be adjusted based on clinical findings. Maternal laboratory evaluation should include a 24-hour urine collection for protein and creatinine clearance in the first trimester. Further laboratory testing can follow in the subsequent trimesters depending on the patient's clinical course. For example, further laboratory testing may not be necessary in those patients whose blood pressure and clinical condition remain stable and in whom fetal growth continues to be reassuring. However, with the advent of clinical symptoms and signs of possible pre-eclampsia, immediate laboratory re-evaluation should be undertaken, and further management affected accordingly. A protocol for fetal evaluation in low-risk chronic hypertension is summarized in Table 3. Timing for delivery should be individualized to each particular clinical situation. However, patients with uncomplicated low-risk hypertension can usually continue the pregnancy until cervical ripening or until 41 weeks' gestation. Obvious indications for hospitalization include superimposed pre-eclampsia or a deterioration in fetal growth prior to 37 weeks, or both. If the clinical or laboratory status of the patient continues to worsen preterm delivery must be considered. Patients with a pregnancy of more than 37 weeks' gestation who develop

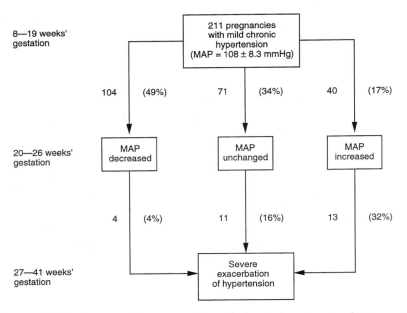

Figure 1. Serial changes in blood pressure in women with mild chronic hypertension during pregnancy. The flow chart represents the natural course in the absence of antihypertensive therapy.

TABLE 3. Antenatal Fetal Evaluation in Low-Risk Chronic Hypertension

Ultrasonogram (USG)	Nonstress Test (NST)/ Biophysical Profile (BPP)
Initial USG to confirm dates and/or anomalies	Initial NST/BPP at 34 weeks, then weekly
USG every 3–4 weeks starting third trimester for fetal growth	NST/BPP immediately with onset of pre-eclampsia
	NST/BPP before 34 weeks if history of prior fetal demise

superimposed pre-eclampsia or abnormal fetal testing or growth should also be considered for delivery.

High-Risk Chronic Hypertension in Pregnancy

Patients with chronic hypertension should be considered high-risk if they have severe hypertension or mild hypertension complicated by target organ involvement or damage. The specific characteristics that are considered as high-risk include blood pressure greater than 160 mm Hg systolic or 110 mm Hg diastolic prior to 20 weeks' gestation, or the presence of other clinical and laboratory abnormalities that reflect target organ involvement (see Table 2). It is important to note that a patient initially classified as low-risk early in pregnancy may eventually evolve into high-risk. Pregnancies in women considered high-risk are associated with increased maternal and perinatal complications (including superimposed pre-eclampsia, abruptio placentae, and prematurity.

Management of patients with chronic hypertension should ideally begin prior to pregnancy, whereby extensive evaluation and complete work-up is undertaken to assess the etiology and the severity as well as the presence of other medical illnesses (Table 4) and to rule out the presence of target organ damage of long-standing hypertension.

An in-depth history should delineate in particular the duration of hypertension and the use of antihypertensive medications, their type, and the response to these medications. As some medications that have potentially harmful effects on both the fetus and the mother are frequently used in the nonpregnant state (diuretics, angiotensin-converting enzyme inhibitors, atenolol), it is prudent to change these drugs to others with well-documented safety and to monitor the response of the patients to these medications. Also, attention should be given to the presence of cardiac or renal disease, diabetes, thyroid disease, and a history of cerebrovascular accident or congestive heart failure. A detailed obstetric history should include maternal as well as neonatal outcome of previous pregnancies with stresses on history of development of abruptio placentae, superimposed pre-eclampsia, preterm delivery, small-for-gestation infants, intrauterine fetal death, neonatal morbidity, and mortality. A detailed physical examination should include the following:

- General physical examination
- Funduscopic examination
- Measurement of blood pressure in the four extremities
- Measurement of blood pressure with changes in posture and after rest
- Detailed auscultation of chest and flanks
- Checking of pulses in the four extremities

Laboratory evaluation is obtained to assess the function of different organ systems that are likely to be affected by chronic hypertension, and as a baseline for future assessments. For all patients,

TABLE 4. Causes of Chronic Hypertension in Pregnancy

Primary essential hypertension, 90%
Secondary Hypertension, 10%
   Renal etiology
      Glomerulonephritis
      Interstitial nephritis
      Nephropathy
      Polycystic renal disease
      Renal transplant
      Renovascular disease
   Collagen vascular disease
      Lupus erythematosus
      Periarteritis nodosa
      Scleroderma
   Endocrine etiology
      Diabetes (with vascular involvement)
      Thyrotoxicosis
      Hyperaldosteronism
      Cushing's disease
      Pheochromocytoma
   Vascular diseases
      Coarctation of the aorta
      Vasculitis

these should include the following: urine analysis, urine culture and sensitivity, 24-hour urine evaluation for protein, and creatinine clearance, SMAC-20, complete blood count, and glucose tolerance test.

Selectively, the following assessments should be made:

1. If hyperglycemia or wide blood pressure swings are evident, a 24-hour urine evaluation for vanillylmandelic acid and metanephrines is recommended to rule out pheochromocytoma.
2. For patients with severe hypertension or significant proteinuria, chest radiograph, electrocardiogram, and antinuclear antibody and serum complement studies are indicated.
3. For patients with severe long-standing hypertension, or if there is a suspicion of heart disease, an echocardiogram is recommended.
4. Women with a history of poor pregnancy outcome (repetitive midpregnancy losses) and those with recent thromboembolic disease should be evaluated for the presence lupus anticoagulants and anticardiolipin antibodies.

Pregnancies in women with chronic hypertension and renal insufficiency are associated with increased perinatal loss and higher incidence of superimposed pre-eclampsia, preterm delivery, and fetal growth retardation. These risks rise in proportion to the severity of the renal insufficiency; women with severe renal insufficiency, particularly primary glomerular disease, risk rapid progression to end-stage renal disease during pregnancy or post partum. Thus, women with renal disease desiring pregnancy should be counseled to conceive before renal insufficiency becomes severe. For women with hypertension and severe renal insufficiency in the first trimester, the decision to continue pregnancy should not be made without extensive counseling regarding the potential maternal and fetal risks, particularly the potential need for dialysis during pregnancy or post partum. Women who elect to continue their pregnancies must be observed and managed at a tertiary care center with adequate maternal-neonatal care facilities.

Initial and Subsequent Prenatal Visits

Early prenatal care will ensure accurate determination of gestational age and the severity of hypertension in the first trimester, which have prognostic values for the outcome of such pregnancies. Furthermore, patients who are seen for the first time during pregnancy should be evaluated as discussed previously. At the time of initial and subsequent visits, the patient should be counseled regarding the following aspects as they pertain to her pregnancy:

- Instructed by a nutritionist regarding nutritional requirements, weight gain, and sodium intake.
- Instructed regarding the negative impact of maternal anxiety, smoking, and caffeine intake as well as drugs on maternal blood pressure and perinatal outcome.
- Counseled regarding the possible adverse effects and complications of hypertension during pregnancy.
- Counseled regarding the importance of frequent prenatal visits and their impact on preventing or minimizing the above adverse effects.

The management of antihypertensive therapy in these patients involves consideration of a therapeutic goal as well as patient understanding and compliance. Antihypertensive medications should be adjusted to keep the systolic blood pressure below 140 mm Hg and the diastolic blood pressure below 90 mm Hg. In those patients with mild hypertension and target organ damage, antihypertensive therapy is recommended for long-term maternal benefit.

The preferred approach for starting medical treatment in high-risk chronic hypertension is to initiate monotherapy whenever feasible. Methyldopa remains the drug of choice because it is the most extensively studied antihypertensive agent in pregnancy thus far. The dose of methyldopa ranges from 750 mg to 4000 mg/day, as titrated to blood pressure response. If this dose is ineffective or insufficient, then polytherapy can be instituted. Additional medications that we currently consider for use in patients with high-risk chronic hypertension are nifedipine (40–120 mg/day), followed by labetalol (300–2400 mg/day). Although the risk for low birth weight infants has been associated with the long-term use of β-blockers, we believe that the benefit of blood pressure control probably supersedes the risk of a low birth weight infant in this clinical situation. Diuretics may be used in a select group of patients who are known to be salt sensitive and in those with left ventricular diastolic dysfunction. However, diuretics should be discontinued if there is evidence of abnormal fetal growth or superimposed pre-eclampsia. Nevertheless, the associated risk of low birth weight infants in all pregnancies complicated by severe hypertension should not be overlooked. Therefore, close antenatal surveillance is recommended after 32 weeks' gestation in all patients with high-risk chronic hypertension.

Control of Postpartum Pain

Kathryn Zuspan, MD

Postpartum pain control has changed dramatically in the past 10 years. Patients now have a variety of options for pain relief after cesarean section. These include intravascular and intramuscular opioids, nonsteroidal anti-inflammatory drugs (NSAIDs), patient-controlled analgesia, and epidural or subarachnoid opioids.

Post-cesarean section patients differ from typical postoperative patients in three very important ways. First, they typically are anxious to be alert, oriented, and functional as soon as possible, to care for their newborns. Second, if breast-feeding, these patients are concerned about the type and quantity of analgesics they receive and potentially pass on in their breast milk. Third, compared with other postoperative patients, obstetrics patients tend to desire and demand more input and control of their care.

Post-cesarean section orders used to be somewhat standard. Patients received intramuscular injections of an opioid, typically demerol 50 to 75 mg IM every 3 to 4 hours as needed. Vistaril 50 mg IM was often added to improve pain relief and decrease the incidence of nausea and vomiting. This regimen is adequate but has a few key limitations. Patients are dependent on nursing personnel for injections, so relief may be delayed. Intramuscular injections may be uncomfortable. Furthermore, opioids typically cause drowsiness, which interferes with the new mother's ability to interact with her family and care for her baby. Patients also often experience some nausea or vomiting with these drug doses. Finally, these drugs may be transmitted via breast milk to the newborn.

Considering all these drawbacks, is there a place for intramuscular opioids in postpartum pain control? Absolutely. This technique is good for patients who noted satisfaction with intramuscular opioids after a previous cesarean section. In addition, there are a few patients who like the associated drowsiness and prefer to "sleep" through the first postoperative day. This technique is also useful for patients who do not qualify for other options.

Other options include NSAIDs, which have analgesic, anti-inflammatory, and antipyretic properties. They function by inhibiting prostaglandin synthesis. As a result, NSAIDs are particularly effective for uterine cramping. These "after-pains" can be especially painful for multiparous patients in the first 12 hours postpartum.

Since NSAIDs are weak acids, there is little concentration in breast milk. Ibuprofen is the best choice among this group because it also has a short half-life and breaks down into inactive metabolites. As a result, it has little effect on the breast-fed baby. Its use is supported by the American Academy of Pediatrics guidelines on drugs and breast feeding (1983).

The usual dose of Ibuprofen is 400 mg PO every 6 hours. Larger doses should be avoided. Adverse effects include gastrointestinal irritation, which can be avoided through the use of enteric-coated tablets. Because the drug may inhibit platelet aggregation, contraindications include bleeding disorders and vitamin K deficiency.

In short, ibuprofen is a mild analgesic, non-opioid option that is effective on uterine cramping, considered acceptable in breast-feeding mothers, and is one of the least expensive of the NSAIDs. Although good for "after-pains," ibuprofen alone is inadequate for post-cesarean section pain.

Ketorolac tromethamine (Toradol) is a new, more potent NSAID. It is equipotent to morphine and meperidine yet lasts longer and has no associated respiratory depression and no potential for abuse. It is the first parenteral NSAID for postoperative pain relief.

Like ibuprofen, ketorolac inhibits platelet aggregation and should be avoided in patients with bleeding disorders or vitamin K deficiency. It is contraindicated in asthmatics and in patients with a history of bronchospasm, nasal polyps, or renal failure. It should be used cautiously in patients with liver disease, since it may elevate liver functions. As with all NSAIDS, long-term use of large doses may cause renal dysfunction. Ketorolac is excellent for control of cramping pain. It can be used alone or in combination with an opioid. It is particularly helpful for managing postoperative pain in chemically dependent patients.

Because ketorolac is new, the American Academy of Pediatrics Committee on Drugs and Breast-Feeding did not evaluate it when it made its recommendations in 1983. Although it has a long half-life, it is broken down into inactive metabolites. Very small quantities of ketorolac are known to be excreted in breast milk. Nevertheless, the Food and Drug Administration recommended that the manufacturer add breast-feeding and labor and delivery patients to the list of contraindications for use of this drug.

In summary, ketorolac is a noncontrolled, potent, injectable NSAID. It is effective for immediate short-term postoperative analgesia, either alone or combined with an opioid. At this time, its use in breast-feeding mothers or in labor or delivery is controversial. The drug costs about 10 times more than an equivalent dose of morphine; however, its benefits outweigh some of this cost.

Patient-controlled analgesia (PCA) is another option for postoperative pain control. With this technique, a small PCA pump is connected to the patient's intravenous line. The PCA pump dispenses a small, preprogrammed dose of systemic drug, usually morphine or meperidine, when the patient pushes a button. The pump is programmed to dispense the analgesic up to a predetermined maximum dose per unit of time. After this amount, no drug is given until a preset period of time elapses. This eliminates the risk of overdose. A small continuous infusion can be added to the demand doses or demand dosing can be used alone.

The PCA technique has several benefits. It provides very good analgesia without dependence on nursing staff. No intramuscular injections are required. Although opioids are used, the doses are small and given frequently, thus there is less sedation, pruritus, and nausea. The greatest benefit is that patients like having control over their analgesia. Patients no longer need to request regular intramuscular injections in anticipation of possible future pain. With PCA, patients have immediate intravascular pain relief available when they decide they need it.

Meperidine and morphine are the typical agents used in PCA. Meperidine provides excellent analgesia and has a lower incidence of sedation, pruritus, and nausea and vomiting. A preliminary study by Wittels (1990) comparing both PCA drugs showed that the neonates from meperidine-treated mothers had lower neurobehavioral scores than those from morphine-treated mothers. Furthermore, normeperidine, an active metabolite of meperidine, was found in significant quantities in the breast milk of the meperidine mothers. Since post-cesarean section pain relief with morphine and meperidine are roughly equivalent, morphine appears to be the better choice for PCA in breast-feeding patients. The usual morphine dose is 1 mg bolus on demand with a 10-minute delay between boluses. If a basal rate is desired, the rate is 1 mg/hour. Thus the total morphine dose per hour is 6 to 7 mg.

Patient-controlled analgesia works well and is an appropriate technique for most patients. This includes women who are breast-feeding and women who had general or regional anesthesia. Although the PCA pump is a cost, there is a savings on nursing services.

The final options to consider are spinal and epidural narcotics. These popular techniques are possible only if the patient received a regional anesthetic for the cesarean section. Spinal opioids are injected at the time of the original subarachnoid injection prior to the cesarean section. Preservative-free morphine (0.15–0.25 mg) is added to the local anesthetic subarachnoid dose. Pain relief begins in about 1 hour and lasts 12 to 24 hours. Patients commonly complain of pruritus or nausea and vomiting. The rare complication is respiratory depression, which requires extra monitoring for about 24 hours.

Epidural opioids include fentanyl and morphine. These drugs are injected via the epidural catheter following delivery of the neonate. Fentanyl (50–100 μg) has an onset in 2 to 5 minutes and a duration of 4 to 6 hours. Preservative-free morphine (3 to 5 mg) has an onset in 1 hour and a duration of 8 to 24 hours. As with spinal opioids, patients may commonly experience pruritus, nausea, and vomiting. The incidence of itching is reported as 84%, with about half of these patients requiring antipruritic treatment with naloxone (Narcan) (0.2 mg IV) or nalbupine (Nubain) (10 mg IM). Both immediate and delayed respiratory depression, while rare, are possible, so these patients need additional monitoring.

Regional opioids provide a very effective analgesia; however, there are some drawbacks. First, if the patient's spinal or epidural anesthetic required supplementation for adequate surgical pain relief, then there is a good chance that a regional opioid will be less than adequate for postoperative pain control. Second, when spinal opioids are used, these are injected prior to delivery. Although studies suggest that this small dose has little or no effect on the neonate, the potential for neonatal exposure is present. Third, the side effects from this technique can be particularly annoying. Some patients will refuse future regional opioids because they found the itching so unpleasant. Finally, the extra surveillance to watch for respiratory depression may tax the nursing service.

Postoperative pain control with spinal and epidural opioids is ideal for many new mothers, including those who are obese or chemically dependent. Obese patients often require larger drug doses owing to their size. With regional opioids, a standard dose is all that is needed.

Furthermore, studies show that with epidural opioids, obese patients ambulate sooner, have less incidence of thrombophlebitis, and are discharged home an average of 1 day sooner. Chemically dependent patients typically have much larger opioid requirements to achieve pain relief. This technique provides pain control with just the standard dose. Although the opioid dose is small, these patients do need to be monitored for withdrawal and treated if these signs appear.

In summary, regional opioids provide a consistent and effective analgesia; however, they are limited by higher morbidity. The cost, including the use of nursing services, is comparable to that of the other options.

With all these pain control options, physicians should make their choice based on three factors. First, the patient should be evaluated and the appropriate technique selected. All options should be discussed with the patient, and she should have input as well as the final choice. Second, the physician should realize that no option will work well unless it has total nursing support. He or she should ensure that the labor and delivery and postpartum nurses are informed and feel comfortable and supportive of all the techniques. Third, physicians should realize that a combination of techniques may be the best choice for some patients. For example, the use of ketorolac may significantly decrease a patient's PCA requirements. Another example is the use of ibuprofen to control "after-pains" in patients receiving epidural or spinal opioids. A third example is combining ketorolac with an opioid to further improve patient satisfaction.

The best option for postoperative pain control really is the one that works well for the physician, in his or her practice setting, and with each individual patient. Postpartum pain control has improved significantly in the last decade. The ideal method has yet to evolve, but a number of options are now available. Patients and physicians should work together to decide on the optimal pain control technique for each individual case.

Diabetes Mellitus in Pregnancy

Steven G. Gabbe, MD

Mark B. Landon, MD

The overall incidence of insulin-dependent diabetes mellitus (IDDM) complicating pregnancy is approximately 0.1% to 0.5%. Gestational diabetes mellitus (GDM), which accounts for 90% of all cases of diabetes in pregnancy, occurs in 3% to 5% of the obstetric population.

Controversy still exists regarding the management of pregnancy complicated by diabetes mellitus. Careful regulation of maternal glycemia is generally well accepted. However, questions remain regarding the relationship between maternal glucose control and perinatal morbidity such as macrosomia in infants of diabetic mothers, as well as which techniques best predict antepartum fetal condition and maturity.

Risk Assessment

We formulate our program of patient care by first considering the potential risks to the patient and her infant. The most important consideration in assessing perinatal risk is the quality of maternal glucose control.

In addition, we utilize the White classification, focusing on the duration of diabetes and the presence and severity of vasculopathy (Table 1). Pregnancies complicated by diabetes mellitus may then be divided into three groups: (1) women with the recent onset of pregestational diabetes (White classes B and C); (2) patients with pregestational diabetes who have vascular complications (White classes D, F, R, and H); and (3) women with gestational diabetes who are treated with diet alone (class A_1) or who require both insulin and diet (class A_2). Nephropathy, particularly if associated with hypertension, is a significant risk factor, increasing the likelihood of superimposed pregnancy-induced hypertension and fetal growth retardation.

During the pregnancy, we also apply Pedersen's Prognostically Bad Signs of Pregnancy, remembering that ketoacidosis, pyelonephritis, pregnancy-induced hypertension, and poor clinic attendance or neglect on the part of the patient are more often associated with poor perinatal outcomes.

TABLE 1. White's Classification of Diabetes in Pregnancy

Class	Age at Onset (yr)		Duration (yr)	Vascular Disease	Insulin
A_1	Any		Any	None	Diet only
A_2	Any		Any	None	+
B	>20		<10	None	+
C	10–19		10–19	None	+
D	<10	or	>20	Benign retinopathy	+
F	Any	or	Any	Nephropathy	+
R	Any		Any	Proliferative retinopathy	+
H	Any		Any	Heart disease	+

+, insulin required.

Insulin-Dependent Diabetes Mellitus

Maternal Assessment

Ideally, we would like to see the woman with IDDM *prior to gestation* so that we may thoroughly assess her glucose control and determine whether significant vasculopathy exists (Tables 2 and 3). The patient considering a pregnancy should undergo an opthalmologic evaluation, have an electrocardiogram, and perform a 24-hour urine collection for creatinine clearance and protein excretion.

Poor metabolic control at conception and during embryogenesis is clearly related to the three-fold to fourfold increase in the number of major congenital malformations seen in pregnancies complicated by IDDM. In addition, maternal hyperglycemia may lead to a greater likelihood of spontaneous abortion. It is essential, therefore, that preconception counseling focus on establishing optimal glucose control and achieving a near normal glycosylated hemoglobin level. The obstetrician can explain to the nonpregnant patient techniques for self-blood glucose monitoring (SBGM), as well as the need for proper dietary management. Questions may also be answered for the patient and her partner regarding risk factors for complications and the plan for the general management of diabetes in pregnancy.

TABLE 2. Prepregnancy Care

1. Discuss contraceptive program
2. Assess patient's vascular status
3. Obtain optimal glucose control
4. Determine immune status against rubella
5. Check thyroid function
6. Evaluate psychosocial well-being

Detection of Fetal Malformations

Although poor glycemic control during embryogenesis, as reflected by an elevated glycosylated hemoglobin level in the first trimester, may increase the likelihood of a major fetal anomaly, it is our practice to evaluate *all* patients with IDDM in the following manner: a maternal serum alpha-fetoprotein level at 16 weeks, a detailed or targeted ultrasonographic examination of the fetus at 18 weeks, and an assessment of fetal cardiac structure by echocardiography at 20 weeks. We do not recommend that termination of pregnancy be advised on the basis of an elevated glycosylated hemoglobin value.

Strategies to Achieve Normoglycemia

During a normal pregnancy, maternal plasma glucose levels rarely exceed 100 mg/dL, ranging between fasting levels of 60 mg/dL and postprandial levels of 120 mg/dL. These values are our therapeutic objective in pregnancy complicated by IDDM (Table 4).

TABLE 3. Management of Insulin-Dependent Diabetes Mellitus in Pregnancy

Prepregnancy	Counseling
	Contraception
	Evaluate maternal vasculopathy
	Glucose control
First trimester	Screen for fetal anomalies
Second trimester	Assess fetal growth
Third trimester	Monitor fetal condition, maturation
	Timed delivery

TABLE 4. Target Glucose Levels in Pregnancy*

Before breakfast	60–90 mg/dL
Before lunch, supper, bedtime snack	60–105 mg/dL
Two hours after meals	≤120 mg/dL
2 AM to 6 AM	>60 mg/dL

*Mean capillary glucose levels should be maintained at 110 mg/dL or less.
  Glycosylated hemoglobin levels should be within the normal range for the individual laboratory.

The pregnant diabetic must utilize SBGM to achieve normoglycemia. We believe patients should monitor their glucose levels using both glucose-oxidase impregnated reagent strips *and* a glucose reflectance meter. Glucose determinations are made in the fasting state and before lunch, dinner, and bedtime. At least once each week, patients are asked to obtain a panel of postprandial values as well. Glycosylated hemoglobin measurements are performed in each trimester. The patient should also check her first voided morning urine for acetone to ensure adequate caloric intake.

We manage most patients with two insulin injections. A combination of intermediate-acting (neutral protamine Hagedorn [NPH], lente) and regular insulin before breakfast and at dinner time is the most commonly employed regimen. As a general rule, the amount of intermediate-acting insulin taken in the morning will exceed that of regular insulin by a 2:1 ratio. Patients usually receive two thirds of their total insulin dose at breakfast and the remaining third at dinner time. In an alternative regimen, the patient may take separate injections of regular insulin at dinner time and intermediate-acting insulin at bedtime to reduce the risk of nocturnal hypoglycemia. The latter may occur when the mother is in a relative fasting state while placental and fetal glucose consumption continues. As the third trimester approaches, maternal insulin requirements may increase 30% to 100%. Ketoacidosis is most common at this time. For this reason, patients with evidence of a respiratory or urinary tract infection should be promptly evaluated.

The effectiveness and safety of the continuous subcutaneous insulin infusion pump have been demonstrated for selected pregnant patients. This therapy should be reserved for highly motivated women whose diabetes cannot be controlled despite a program of multiple insulin injections. Because ketoacidosis and fetal death have occurred in association with pump failure,

we ask patients using a pump to check their glucose level at 2 to 3 AM.

In the average diet for a pregnant patient with IDDM, 20% of the calories are derived from protein, 35% from fat, and 45% from carbohydrate. In terms of caloric distribution, 25% of the calories are provided with breakfast, 30% with lunch, 30% with dinner, and 15% with a bedtime snack. Some patients may require snacks in the midmorning or midafternoon, or both, to prevent hypoglycemia. In such cases, we subtract 5% of the calories from breakfast and lunch, respectively. The average daily caloric intake for the pregnant diabetic woman will range from 2200 to 2400 calories, or approximately 35 kcal/kg ideal body weight. Patients who are restricted in activity or who demonstrate early excessive weight gain may require a lower caloric prescription. We advise our obese patients to avoid weight loss during pregnancy.

Program of Care

Most pregnant women with IDDM can be managed successfully as out-patients. In selected cases, we utilize hospitalization early in gestation to ensure optimal control through intensive education of the patient. Visits are usually scheduled at 2-week intervals in the first and second trimesters and weekly in the third trimester. At each visit, we carefully review the patient's glucose log book, assess her pattern of weight gain, and evaluate the blood pressure and urine protein. We usually increase or decrease the appropriate insulin dose by approximately 20%. For example, if the predinner glucose level is elevated, the morning intermediate insulin dose is increased by 20%. An elevation in the prelunch glucose level will require an increase in the morning regular dose. Should the patient have an elevated fasting glucose level, we ask her to check her glucose level at 2 to 3 AM. If that glucose level is high, more intermediate-acting insulin at dinnertime is usually needed. However, if the patient is found to be hypoglycemic during the night, her elevated fasting glucose level may reflect rebound hyperglycemia, and we will reduce the dinner-time dose of intermediate-acting insulin. We also instruct our patients to telephone us immediately if they experience episodes of hyperglycemia (higher than 200 mg/dL) or hypoglycemia (less than 50 mg/dL), or if they develop a febrile illness.

In patients found to have benign retinopathy during the first trimester, we schedule follow-up ophthalmologic examinations in the second and third trimesters. Proliferative retinopathy may require monthly examinations. We repeat the renal function studies at least once during each trimester.

Fetal Assessment

Biophysical techniques have proved most valuable in assessing fetal well-being. Ultrasonography is an extremely important tool that may be used to evaluate fetal growth, detect anomalies, and diagnose hydramnios. Ultrasonographic studies are repeated at 4- to 6-week intervals to assess fetal growth.

We initiate our program of antepartum fetal surveillance during the third trimester, when the risk of sudden intrauterine death is increased. Normal tests are rarely associated with intrauterine demise; that is, there are few false-negative results. Therefore, we find that this surveillance allows us to delay delivery and await fetal maturation (see Table 3). Of course, excellent control of maternal diabetes will also reduce the risk of fetal death and the frequency of abnormal test results.

We now use the non–stress test (NST) to follow our patients. NSTs are performed twice weekly, starting at 32 weeks of gestation in patients without vasculopathy. In women with nephropathy, testing may be initiated at 28 weeks of gestation or earlier, should compromised fetal growth become evident. Some clinicians now use the biophysical profile (BPP) as a primary screening technique. We prefer the NST but utilize the BPP or contraction stress test (CST) after a nonreactive NST. Such sequential fetal evaluation is necessary in fewer than 5% of our patients.

We believe maternal assessment of fetal activity is an easy and practical screen for fetal compromise and utilize this approach in all pregnancies complicated by diabetes. Beginning at 28 weeks of gestation, patients are asked to record fetal activity over a 12-hour period, usually from 9 AM until 9 PM. Ten movements should be noted during this period. If the length of time is found to increase before this number of movements is appreciated, or if fewer than 10 movements are recorded, heart rate testing is performed as soon as possible. Patients may also count fetal movement at several designated periods each day.

Timing of Delivery

We now feel comfortable following a select group of pregnant diabetics as out-patients until term.

Continued assessment of maternal glycemia using SBGM as well as out-patient heart rate testing has made this possible. Perinatal outcome has not been compromised by this approach, and the likelihood for the spontaneous onset of labor and vaginal delivery is increased. We want to emphasize, however, that in-patient care is still advisable for those patients with poor glycemic control, those with severe vascular complications, or those women requiring more intensive fetal surveillance.

If the patient's diabetes is well controlled and the findings on antepartum surveillance remain normal, we delay delivery until fetal pulmonary maturation has been completed, as documented by a mature lecithin to sphingomyelin (L:S) ratio and the presence of phosphatidylglycerol (PG). We perform an amniocentesis to document fetal pulmonary maturity when a patient has poor glucose control or questionable dates or before an elective delivery at less than 39 weeks' gestation. Each clinician must be familiar with the laboratory analysis of amniotic fluid in his or her institution and the neonatal outcome at various L:S ratios in the presence or absence of PG. Should amniotic fluid analysis fail to reveal fetal pulmonary maturity, and if antepartum fetal assessment remains reassuring, we postpone an elective delivery and repeat the amniocentesis in approximately 1 week.

We carefully consider the optimal route and timing of delivery for each patient. With excellent control, no evidence of hypertension or vasculopathy, reassuring fetal testing, and normal fetal growth, we will await the onset of spontaneous labor until 40 weeks of gestation. With any adverse factors, including maternal hypertension, a prior stillbirth, or poor control, elective induction or cesarean section is planned after pulmonary maturity has been documented.

When antepartum fetal testing suggests fetal compromise (nonreactive NST, row BPP score, or positive CST), immediate delivery must be considered. An amniocentesis should be performed, and in the presence of a mature L:S ratio, delivery should be accomplished. If the L:S ratio is immature, clinical management must be individualized. We also consider preterm delivery if the patient develops pregnancy-induced hypertension, rapidly worsening retinopathy, or renal failure.

Management of Labor and Delivery

A skilled neonatal team should be present at delivery. If adequate neonatal care cannot be provided, the patient should be transferred to a hospital with an appropriately equipped nursery.

During labor, continuous fetal heart rate monitoring is mandatory. Labor is allowed to progress as long as normal rates of cervical dilatation and descent are documented. To avoid shoulder dystocia, we consider an elective cesarean section when fetal weight is estimated to be 4250 g or more by ultrasonography. We also avoid midpelvic forceps or vacuum delivery after a prolonged second stage because of the high likelihood of shoulder dystocia in this setting.

To reduce the incidence of neonatal hypoglycemia, we maintain maternal capillary glucose levels below 120 mg/dL during labor and delivery. This objective requires careful attention to maternal glucose values, the glucose infusion rate, and insulin dosage. In general, glucose determinations are made every 1 to 2 hours at the bedside with SBGM techniques. A flow sheet to summarize these data is essential. We use a continuous infusion of insulin and glucose, mixing 10 units of regular insulin with 1000 mL of a 5% dextrose solution. An infusion rate of 100

to 125 mL/hr usually results in good glucose control.

In patients who undergo elective cesarean section, we schedule the procedure in the early morning. The patient is given nothing by mouth, and her usual morning insulin dose is withheld. Epidural anesthesia is preferred because it enables the anesthesiologist to evaluate the patient's mental status and detect potential hypoglycemia. In the postoperative period, an intravenous solution of 5% dextrose is administered, and glucose levels are monitored every 2 hours.

After delivery, when insulin requirements are usually reduced, we must avoid maternal hypoglycemia. Therefore, the objective of strict control used in the antepartum period is relaxed. Patients who deliver vaginally and who are able to eat a regular diet are given one half of their prepregnancy dose of NPH insulin on the morning of the first postpartum day. Frequent capillary glucose determinations indicate the need for coverage with regular insulin. If a patient has been given supplemental regular insulin in addition to the morning NPH dose, the amount of

---

TABLE 5. Management of Gestational Diabetes Mellitus

Screening for Gestational Diabetes Mellitus°

A 50 g oral glucose load is administered between week 24 and week 28, without regard to time of day or time of last meal, to all pregnant women who have not been determined to have glucose intolerance before week 24, except for those women with *all* of the following low risk characteristics: member of an ethnic group with a low prevalence of type 2 diabetes mellitus, age less than 25 years, normal weight, no known first-degree relatives with diabetes.

Venous plasma glucose is measured 1 hour later.

A value of 140 mg/dL or above in venous plasma indicates the need for a full diagnostic glucose tolerance test.

Diagnosis of Gestational Diabetes Mellitus°

A 100 g oral glucose load is administered in the morning after an overnight fast for at least 8 hr, but not more than 14 hr, and following at least 3 days of unrestricted diet (≥150 g carbohydrate) and physical activity.

Venous plasma glucose is measured at fasting and at 1, 2, and 3 hr. Subject should remain seated and not smoke throughout the test.

Two or more of the following venous plasma concentrations must be met or exceeded for positive diagnosis:

Fasting, 95 mg/dL
1 hr, 180 mg/dL
2 hr, 155 mg/dL
3 hr, 140 mg/dL

Postpartum Evaluation of Patients with Gestational Diabetes Mellitus†

A 75 g oral glucose load is administered under conditions described for a 100 g oral test.

Venous plasma glucose is measured at fasting and at 30-min intervals for 2 hr.

Normal	Impaired Glucose Tolerance	Diabetes Mellitus
Fasting <110 mg/dL	≥100–<126 mg/dL	≥126 mg/dL
and	*and*	*or*
2 hr <140 mg/dL	2 hr ≥140–<200 mg/dL	2 hr ≥200 mg/dL

°From Proceedings of the Fourth International Workshop-Conference on Gestational Diabetes Mellitus. Diabetes Care 1998;21 [Suppl 2]:B161.

NPH insulin given on the following morning is increased by an amount equal to two thirds of the additional regular insulin. With this method, most patients are stabilized within a few days of delivery.

Patients delivered by cesarean section receive regular insulin during the first 24 to 48 hours postoperatively to maintain glucose values below 200 mg/dL. As their diet is advanced, NPH insulin is administered based on the regular insulin requirement of the preceding day.

All patients are encouraged to breast-feed. Insulin requirements may be somewhat lower in lactating women.

Gestational Diabetes Mellitus

Gestational diabetes mellitus has been characterized as a state restricted to pregnant women in whom the onset or recognition of diabetes or impaired glucose tolerance occurs during pregnancy.

More than half of all patients who develop GDM lack the classic historical or clinical risk factors associated with this disorder. Therefore, we screen *all* pregnant women at 24 to 28 weeks of gestation by administering a 50 g oral glucose load followed by a glucose determination 1 hour later (Table 5). Patients need not be fasting for this test. An abnormal screening test must be followed by a 3-hour oral glucose tolerance test (GTT), the "gold standard" for the diagnosis of GDM (Table 5). We repeat the oral GTT at 32 to 34 weeks of gestation in women with a positive 50-g screen who initially exhibit a normal GTT but who have significant risk factors, including a previous history of GDM, obesity, or advanced maternal age. In addition, we repeat the GTT in those women who have one abnormal value on the first GTT.

Once the diagnosis of GDM is established, we start patients on a diet of 2000 to 2200 calories daily. Complex carbohydrates from foods high in soluble fiber provide 50% to 60% of total calories; protein, 10% to 20%; and fat, 25% to 30%. Simple sugars as found in concentrated sweets are eliminated from the diet. Fasting and 2-hour postprandial glucose levels are monitored at each weekly office visit. Patients are also asked to check their first voided morning urine for acetone. Most recently, we have used SBGM in patients with GDM as well. Patients are asked to check their fasting glucose level and several postprandial levels each day. If fasting capillary glucose levels exceed 95 mg/dL and/or capillary postprandial values are greater than 120 mg/dL,

treatment with human insulin is begun. Most patients can be treated with a single morning injection of approximately 20 U of NPH and 6 to 10 U of regular insulin. We do not recommend prophylactic insulin therapy in all cases of GDM.

We follow patients with GDM until 40 weeks of gestation, as long as fasting and postprandial glucose levels remain normal. If labor cannot be safely induced at 40 weeks, we initiate fetal surveillance with twice-weekly NSTs. In general, patients with GDM should be delivered by 42 weeks. The risk of intrauterine deaths and perinatal morbidity is greater in those with GDM who have had a prior stillbirth, who develop pregnancy-induced hypertension, whose diagnosis is delayed until late in pregnancy, or who have required insulin therapy in a prior gestation. In these patients, we initiate a program of fetal surveillance in GDM at 34 weeks of gestation similar to that employed in IDDM. As for women with IDDM, clinical assessment of fetal size and ultrasonography should be used to select those patients best delivered by cesarean section.

It has been recommended that all women with a history of GDM undergo a 75-g oral GTT several months after delivery to determine whether they still demonstrate carbohydrate intolerance (see Table 5). We have found a check of fasting and postprandial plasma glucose levels to be more practical, using cut-off values of 110 mg/dL and 140 mg/dL, respectively.

Postpartum Care

Contraceptive counseling is an important part of the care of the young diabetic woman. We recommend low-dose combined contraceptive pills or the progestin-only pill in young women who have no evidence of hypertension or vasculopathy. However, we do not prescribe these medications in women with vascular disease. In addition, we assess the patient's lipid levels prior to instituting oral contraceptive therapy. Women with a history of GDM may use certain triphasic oral contraceptives without developing carbohydrate intolerance or abnormal lipid profiles. The diaphragm and other barrier methods pose the least risk to the diabetic patient. Surgical sterilization may be appropriate after the couple has completed their family or in the patient with significant vasculopathy.

Drug Abuse in Pregnancy

Cynthia Shellhaas, MD

The true prevalence of substance abuse in pregnancy is difficult to assess because it varies with the population studied, but estimates have ranged from 7.5% to 20%. Polypharmacy is the rule rather than the exception; the concomitant abuses of alcohol and nicotine are especially common. Pregnancy-related problems include increased rates of poor fetal growth, developmental delay, neonatal withdrawal, and increased exposure to sexually transmitted diseases, especially human immunodeficiency virus (HIV) and syphilis. Fetal risks are compounded by the propensity of addicted patients to obtain little or no prenatal care.

Substance-abusing women who are pregnant and parenting have unique treatment needs. These women have experienced higher rates of sexual and physical abuse as children and are also more likely to abuse their own children. They are likely to be the children of substance-abusing parents and to have been introduced to drugs by a male partner. These women are at high risk to be involved with the legal system; they may be under scrutiny by child protective services or, in some states, even be subject to incarceration for delivering drugs to their fetus.

Such patients need to be identified before treatment can offered. At the time of the initial prenatal visit, each patient should be questioned in a nonjudgmental way about legal and illicit drug use, including tobacco and alcohol. The use of a screening questionnaire can be both helpful and nonthreatening to the patient. However, denial is an intrinsic component of addicted patients' behavior.

The following sections describe several of the most common drugs, with a focus on maternal-fetal effects. There are many confounders in assessing drug effects. They include the presence of polysubstance abuse, the effects of poor nutrition, having little or no prenatal care, the possibility of fetal infections especially from HIV or syphilis, a chaotic social environment, and exposure to trauma. Therefore, the long-term effects of many of these drugs are the subject of more speculation than scientific fact.

Alcohol

The fetal alcohol syndrome (FAS) was first identified and reported in 1973. It is the most common environmental cause of mental retardation. In the United States, approximately 12,000 children per year are born with FAS, with a fourfold increase in such cases from 1979 to 1992. There is no amount of alcohol consumption known to be safe in pregnancy, but the actual syndrome is seen in women with heavy alcohol consumption (ingestion of at least six 3-ounces drinks per day). Although the effects among light or moderate drinkers are less clear, intrauterine growth retardation (IUGR) and spontaneous abortion rates do appear to be increased among moderate drinkers.

The FAS has specific criteria that requires at least one feature from each of the following three categories in order to make the diagnosis:

1. Growth retardation before or after birth
2. A pattern of abnormal facial features or microcephaly, including shortening of the midfacial area (the nose and/or philtrum)
3. Central nervous system abnormality—mental retardation, developmental delay, or abnormal neonatal development.

Alcohol-related birth defects (ARBDs) include such structural abnormalities as ophthalmologic or otic anomalies, cardiac septal defects, hemangiomas, undescended testes, and hernias. There are also increased rates of spontaneous abortions, decreased immune function, hearing impairment, and developmental delay. FAS and ARBDs are especially harmful in relation to the central nervous system. Neuronal differentiation may be delayed or inhibited by ethanol. The specific effects of alcohol are dependent on the timing of alcohol exposure during pregnancy and the alcohol dose. Since there is no treatment for FAS, the goal for practitioners is prevention. The first step is identification of mothers at risk. Self-reporting of alcohol consumption is almost always underestimated on direct questioning. It may be helpful to proceed more indirectly by obtaining a family history of alcohol usage and then assessing the individual for signs of increased tolerance to alcohol effects. One of the simplest ways to do the latter is to use the T-ACE questionnaire:

- T   How many drinks does it take to make you feel high? (*Tolerance*)
- A   Have people *annoyed* you by criticizing your drinking?
- C   Have you felt you ought to *cut down* on your drinking?
- E   Have you ever had to drink first thing in the morning to steady you nerves or to get rid of a hangover (*eye-opener*)?

Two or more positive answers are highly suggestive of alcoholism. Use of disulfiram as an intervention is contraindicated in pregnancy owing to possible association with teratogenic effects, specifically limb defects. Referral should be to an alcohol rehabilitation program, especially one with both in-patient and out-patient treatment capabilities, or to Alcoholics Anonymous.

Cocaine

Cocaine is derived from the *Erythroxylon coca* plant of South America. Although it has a medical use as a topical anesthetic, cocaine is a stimulant and is more widely used illicitly, especially in its free base form, as "crack cocaine." Its subjective effects include intense euphoria and alertness, increased confidence, heightened sexual feelings, and indifference to previously noted anxieties. These feelings rapidly change to despondency and despair. Euphoria is restored by the next dose of the drug. The euphoria or "rush" is due to cocaine's ability to increase the actions of dopamine in the limbic system and cortex. Cocaine, especially crack, is extremely addictive, and its usage has virtually become an epidemic among pregnant women. Cocaine is able to block reuptake of catecholamines by the neuronal end plate, thus lengthening their effects. The adrenergic stimulation and subsequent vasoconstriction may cause tachycardia and hypertension. Its use is associated with poor prenatal care and increased risks of abruption, prematurity, growth retardation, and, secondarily, fetal death and distress.

Cocaine has a short half-life of 60 to 120 minutes, depending on route of administration. Metabolites of cocaine can be found in the maternal urine for 24 to 72 hours after use. Cocaine rapidly crosses the placenta by simple diffusion, where it then affects the fetus. Fetal blood pressure and heart rate are increased by cocaine, and there is an increase in fetal cerebral blood flow that seems to be related to direct effects of cocaine on fetal cerebral vessels. Fetal intestinal blood flow is also adversely affected by cocaine administration. Evidence concerning cocaine-associated malformations is contradictory. At least in mice and rats, there would appear to be a dose-related increase in central nervous system, cardiac, genitourinary, and limb abnormalities. In humans the strongest association is with genitourinary malformations. The proposed mechanism relates vasoconstriction and hypoperfusion with subsequent hypoxia and vascular disruption. The most common central nervous system sign is decreased intrauterine brain growth manifesting as microcephaly, giving cocaine an association with a form of asymmetric IUGR. There may also be an association with disorders of midline neuronal migration leading to an increase in agenesis of the corpus callosum. The long-term fetal neurologic and cognitive sequelae of cocaine use are unknown, and speculation is confounded by many other variables.

Nicotine

Approximately 22 million American women were noted to be smokers in 1993. The vast majority began smoking before the age of 18 years. Most women continue smoking during pregnancy, although most decrease the amount. Smoking is the single most common cause of impaired fetal growth. The effects are dose-dependent, with an average decrease in birth weight of approximately 200 g. Fifteen to 25% of fetuses of smokers have IUGR. The effects may be ameliorated or even reversed in the index pregnancy if the patients stops smoking. Tobacco contains over 1500 compounds; of these, nicotine and carbon monoxide are considered to be responsible for most adverse pregnancy outcomes. Carbon monoxide forms carboxyhemoglobin, which inhibits the release of oxygen into fetal tissues. Nicotine-induced release of catecholamines leads to repetitive episodes of transient vasocontriction of the uterine and potentially the umbilical arteries. Cyanide decreases intracellular oxygen utilization, and compounds such as the aromatic hydrocarbons and cadmium may impede placental function. The decrease in appetite experienced by many smokers may also contribute to poor maternal weight gain with subsequent low birth weight. The poor pregnancy outcomes associated with nicotine include, but are not limited to, low birth weight—related either to prematurity or to intrauterine growth restriction, premature rupture of the membranes, preterm labor, placental abruption, spontaneous abortions, and placenta previa. Post-delivery complications include persistent failure to thrive secondary to poor breast feeding, increased risk of sudden infant death syndrome, asthma, frequent respiratory infections requiring hospitalization, and attention deficit disorder.

Many communities have smoking cessation programs, either hospital-based in respiratory therapy departments or sponsored by organizations such as the American Heart Association and the American Lung Association. Smoking patients should be counseled as to their risks and encouraged to participate in such programs.

Opiates

The opium alkaloids have been in use for many hundreds of years. The development of the hypodermic syringe led to their illicit intravenous use, with subsequent rise in infections such as HIV, hepatitis, and endocarditis. There are approximately 9,000 to 10,000 births in the United States per year to narcotic-addicted women. In addition to perinatal morbidities such as low birth weight, pregnancy-induced hypertension, and third-trimester bleeding, the neonatal complications include withdrawal syndrome, postnatal growth deficiency, microcephaly, neurobehavioral problems, and an increased risk for sudden infant death syndrome. Replacement of the illicit drug with methadone maintenance therapy is the only legal alternative to continued perinatal narcotic abuse. Withdrawal or detoxification is not recommended in pregnancy because of the risk of concomitant fetal withdrawal and possible fetal death. A delayed and prolonged neonatal withdrawal syndrome is seen in most cases of maternal methadone usage. A gradual taper (2 to 5 mg/week) to a goal of 20 mg/day may be attempted in the second trimester, but the women should be maintained using the lowest possible dose that still maintains the women in a comfortable state.

Summary

In conclusion, addiction is a chronic disease with a high rate of recidivism. Although it affects all sectors of the population, pregnant and parenting women comprise a special group with unique needs. Each woman requires an individualized treatment plan, but comprehensive services should include high-risk prenatal care with additional treatment modalities such as individual, group, and family therapy. These women also need strong social service support with encouragement toward education and job training. Residential treatment for the women and their children should also be available to alleviate the social problems faced by these patients.

Dysfunctional Labor

William D. Fraser, MD, MSC, FRCSC
Michel Boulvain, MD, PhD

Dysfunctional labor, also known as dystocia, is one of the most frequent and most challenging problems faced by the obstetrician. Care that is provided to women in normal labor can have an important impact on peripartum outcomes, especially on labor duration, progress of cervical dilatation and descent, requirement for operative delivery, and women's satisfaction regarding the birth experience.

Dysfunctional labor can result from (1) abnormal fetal size, presentation, or position; (2) abnormal pelvic size and shape, including pelvic tumors; (3) abnormal uterine activity; or (4) increased soft tissue resistance. Certain of these conditions are potentially preventible or amenable to medical intervention. Others can be the consequence of inappropriate interventions (eg, inappropriate induction of labor). Accurate diagnosis and the careful planning of subsequent management is important to avoid unfavorable outcomes.

Assessment in Early Labor

Women who present to the labor ward in early labor usually do so because of a perceived need for support and care. It is important for labor wards to develop clearly defined strategies regarding the diagnosis of labor, criteria for admission, the type and timing of medical procedures that are performed in early labor, and the support that is provided to women. Admission assessment and triage should be carried out by experienced personnel so that women are oriented to the level of obstetric care that is most appropriate to their needs. Women who are not yet in active labor may be better cared for in a "pre-labor" area that is less intensive than the labor ward and where there is ready access to simple comfort measures and nutrition. Specific criteria for the diagnosis of labor such as the duration and frequency of contractions, the presence of show, membrane status and cervical dilatation (ie, 3 cm) have been recommended. Although there have be no published trials to compare differing admission criteria, the flexible application of such criteria is likely to facilitate the process of providing care.

Assessing Progress in the First Stage

The rate of labor progress should be assessed within the context of a woman's total well-being. Among women who experience spontaneous vaginal delivery, there is wide variation in the normal rate of labor progress, both in the first and second stages. The latent phase of labor is particularly subject to normal variation in its duration. There is no evidence that a prolonged latent phase is detrimental to the mother or her baby. Because latent phase disorders are most often not associated with problems in the active phase or second stage of labor, clinicians should avoid performing cesarean for dystocia during the latent phase. Factors influencing labor duration, such as cervical status at labor onset, whether labor is spontaneous or induced, and the presence and type of epidural analgesia, should be taken into consideration when evaluating progress.

The partogram, a method of documenting vaginal examinations that are performed at predetermined intervals, has been recommended as a tool for screening and diagnosis of dystocia. It is not clear whether screening for dystocia by regular vaginal examinations performed at predetermined intervals and early medical intervention based on the results of these assessments result in an improvement in obstetric outcomes. However, the partogram may be useful as a guideline in clinical decision making and as a document that facilitates the peer review process.

Criteria for the Diagnosis of Dystocia

While there are no universally accepted criteria for the diagnosis of dystocia, the recommendations of the Canadian Consensus Panel on Aspects of Cesarean Birth would appear to be the most appropriate guidelines currently available. These guidelines suggest that for a patient to be considered to have dystocia, cervical dilatation of 3 cm must have been achieved, and, following this, there should be a period of at least 4 hours during which cervical dilatation is less than 0.5 cm per hour. This definition, although relatively conservative, will result in as many as one third of nulliparous women being labelled as having dystocia. This definition of dystocia is very similar to that proposed in the partogram, which has been recommended by a consensus committee of the Division of Family Health of the World Health Organization. Certain studies indicate that a significant proportion of women who experience spontaneous vaginal delivery do not enter the active phase of labor until 5 cm dilatation is achieved. Thus, not all women who go beyond the limits of normality established by this definition require medical intervention.

Active Labor: The Active Management of Labor

The Active Management of Labor has been advocated as a means of preventing dystocia and reducing cesarean section. This approach to care involves several components, including selective admission to the labor ward, support from caregivers, early amniotomy, and early oxytocin. Randomized controlled trials of early amniotomy and early administration of oxytocin have shown a modest reduction in the duration of labor; however, they did not show improvements in maternal or fetal morbidities. In contrast, psychosocial support during labor has been shown to be associated with a reduction in cesarean section and operative vaginal delivery along with improved fetal outcomes. Thus, expectant management of slow labor progress in the latent phase with an emphasis on psychological support, physical comfort measures, and ambulation is an acceptable approach to care. We prefer to avoid artificial rupture of the membranes as long as labor is progressing normally. Routine early amniotomy may be associated with an increase in variable decelerations, leading to obstetric interventions.

Medical Intervention for the Treatment of Dystocia

Despite the absence of evidence from clinical trials, amniotomy is likely to be proven an effective method for the treatment of mild forms of dysfunctional labor due to uterine hypotonia. While oxytocin has been a mainstay in the medical treatment of dystocia, there are few controlled trials demonstrating its benefit. There is no evidence that the early use of oxytocin for minor delays in labor progress confers advantages over a selective approach to oxytocin use. Neither is there evidence that high-dose oxytocin protocols are better than low-dose protocols. Further studies are required. However, given the frequency of uterine dysfunction in association with delayed progress in labor, an adequate trial of augmentation with oxytocin should be implemented prior to any consideration of cesarean section for dystocia. Intrauterine pressure catheter monitoring should be reserved for women for whom the evaluation of contraction frequency is difficult because of obesity, or in cases in which progress remains abnormally slow despite an adequate trial of the conventional oxytocin augmentation regimen.

Once the decision has been made to intervene medically for delay in labor progress, whether by amniotomy, oxytocin augmentation, or both, adequate time must be allowed to observe for a clinical response to treatment. Depending on the starting dose and rate of increase of oxytocin, 2 to 3 hours may be required to achieve therapeutic concentrations in maternal serum. In the majority of cases, a therapeutic level is achieved at doses of 10 mU/min or less. Once a therapeutic level has been achieved, a further period of observation is required to assess for a clinical response. Particularly when oxytocin is commenced at cervical dilatations of less than 5 cm, the time interval from initiation of treatment to achieving a clinical response (ie, an increase in cervical dilatation) may be considerable.

Several regimens of oxytocin infusion have been proposed, including "rapid methods" (doubling the dose or increasing it by 2 to 4 mU/min every 15 minutes) and "slow methods" (increasing the dose by 1 mU/min every 30 minutes). While neither scheme has been shown to be clearly superior to the other, higher dose regimens are associated with an increased risk of uterine hyperstimulation.

Second Stage

Traditionally, 2 hours have been considered to be the upper limit of normal for the duration of the second stage of labor in nulliparous women. Recent information indicates that the mean duration of the second stage is prolonged in association with epidural analgesia use. In the presence of epidural, there does not appear to be an association between the duration of the second stage and the risk of adverse neonatal outcome. Clinicians should avoid placing artificial limits on the duration of the second stage when epidural analgesia is present. As long as there is progress, as measured by descent of the fetal head, and fetal and maternal status remain satisfactory, expectant management of the second stage is the preferred approach to care.

For women with continuous epidural analgesia, a strategy of delaying the time of commencing pushing until the fetal head is visible at the perineum is an effective approach to reduce the frequency of operative intervention. This approach has recently been evaluated in a multicenter randomized clinical trial.

In the presence of abnormal progress in the second stage, careful assessment of the fetopelvic relationship may help in deciding on subsequent management. Uterine activity augmentation by oxytocin may correct dystocia due to uterine hypotonia, which is frequent in the presence of epidural anesthesia. Excessive soft tissue resistance or fetal malposition may be amenable to vacuum extraction or forceps delivery. The treatment of absolute fetopelvic disproportion will be cesarean section. The correct diagnosis of these conditions is essential to avoid maternal and fetal injury.

Strategies to Reduce Cesarean Section for Dystocia

Dystocia remains the most frequent indication for primary cesarean section. Rates of cesarean section for dystocia are more than two times higher in North America than in many Western European countries, even after adjusting for factors such as baby's birth weight and the use of epidural anesthesia. Among hospitals providing the same level of obstetric services, wide variations in cesarean section rates are observed. There is no evidence that higher rates of cesarean section confer benefits to the newborn. These observations clearly suggest that cesarean section rates in many centers require critical scrutiny with a view to safely reducing rates.

Physician practice patterns have been shown to be among the strongest risk factors for cesarean section for dystocia. Attempts to modify practice patterns have included initiating peer review and providing public access to hospital cesarean rates. Requesting a second opinion has been suggested as a strategy to reduce cesarean rates. This approach is currently being tested in the context of a clinical trial.

Ectopic Pregnancy

Gary H. Lipscomb, MD
Frank W. Ling, MD

Since 1970, the incidence of ectopic pregnancy in the United States has steadily increased from a rate of 4.5 per 1000 pregnancies to 19.7 per 1000 pregnancies. In 1992, the last year for which statistics are available from the Centers for Disease Control and Prevention, there were an estimated 108,800 cases of ectopic pregnancy. During this time period, the death rate declined almost tenfold, most likely as a result of earlier detection. Nevertheless, ectopic pregnancy still accounts for 9% of all pregnancy-related deaths. Considering the increasing incidence, the continued decrease in the death rate is certainly a result of earlier detection. Earlier detection has been made possible by more sensitive and specific radioimmunoassays for the beta subunit of human chorionic gonadotropin (hCG), serum progesterone screening, high-resolution transvaginal sonography, and the widespread availability of laparoscopy.

Probably the most important factor responsible for the dramatic rise in ectopic pregnancy has been the increase in pelvic inflammatory disease (PID). Therefore, patients being treated for an acute episode of PID should be informed of this increased risk and should be screened for ectopic gestation in any subsequent pregnancy.

Applying the diagnostic and treatment algorithm developed at the University of Tennessee, Memphis (Fig. 1), the use of laparoscopy for the diagnosis of ectopic pregnancy is virtually eliminated. With the advent of methotrexate as an effective medical treatment, surgical treatment with its attendant anesthetic and operative risk is minimized. Each of the components of the algorithm and the manner in which they are used are discussed in detail here.

Serum Progesterone

Serum progesterone can be used as a screening test for abnormal pregnancy because progesterone concentrations associated with ectopic pregnancy are lower than those associated with intrauterine pregnancies (IUP). Despite findings in earlier studies, there is no clear-cut level of serum progesterone that identifies a normal IUP from an ectopic pregnancy. Considerable overlap exists in progesterone values for normal and abnormal pregnancies. One to 2% of abnormal pregnancies (abortions or ectopic pregnancies) are associated with a progesterone level of 25 ng/mL or greater, while viable IUPs have been noted with levels as low as 3.9 ng/mL.

In early versions of the nonlaparoscopic protocols, serum progesterone was utilized extensively to screen for ectopic pregnancy, and to identify candidates for dilatation and curettage (D&C). Serum progesterone is helpful, but not diagnostic, in identifying a nonviable pregnancy. Thus, a low progesterone level alone is not diagnostic of ectopic pregnancy, but levels below 5.0 ng/mL

are highly suspicious of an abnormal pregnancy, be it intra- or extrauterine. As a result, serum progesterone has a more limited role in the diagnosis of ectopic pregnancy than previously thought.

Human Chorionic Gonadatropin

Using currently available quantitative assays, hCG can be detected in maternal serum 8 days after the luteinizing hormone (LH) surge. Using qualitative enzyme-linked immunosorbent assays (ELISA), hCG can be detected by urine pregnancy tests in first-voided maternal urine by day 21 of the menstrual cycle. The mean doubling time for serum hCG in a normal IUP has been shown to be 1.4 to 1.98 days. However, in patients with an ectopic pregnancy, the hCG will typically rise at a much slower rate.

Based on studies of doubling times, serum level hCG will rise by at least 66% in 48 hours in 85% of normal pregnancies (one standard deviation from the mean). Thus, 15% of normal IUPs will rise less than this in 48 hours. However, a rise of less than 50% is more than 3 standard deviations from the mean and would be associated with an abnormal pregnancy 99.87% of the time. Since the interassay variability of hCG is 10% to 15%, a change of less than this amount is considered to be a plateau. Plateaued levels are the most predictive of ectopic pregnancy.

Levels of hCG play a pivotal role in determining interpretation of other the other diagnostic modalities. Levels of 50,000 or greater are rarely (<0.1%) associated with an ectopic pregnancy. At hCG levels of 2000 mIU/mL or greater First International Preparation (1st IRP), transvaginal ultrasonography can visualize an intrauterine sac in all normal IUPs. Patients with an abnormal rise in hCG (<50% in 48 hours) or plateaued levels (±15%) may undergo D&C without fear of interrupting an ongoing intrauterine pregnancy. A fall in hCG level following D&C or a plateaued or rising level after D&C indicates the presence of persistent trophoblastic tissue.

Vaginal Ultrasonography

Vaginal ultrasonography permits visualization of a gestational sac at much lower hCG titers than with transabdominal scanning. The minimal hCG titer at which a sac should always be seen is not known, but an experienced transvaginal sonographer should always visualize a viable IUP at an hCG titer of 2000 mIU/mL. Vaginal ultrasonog-

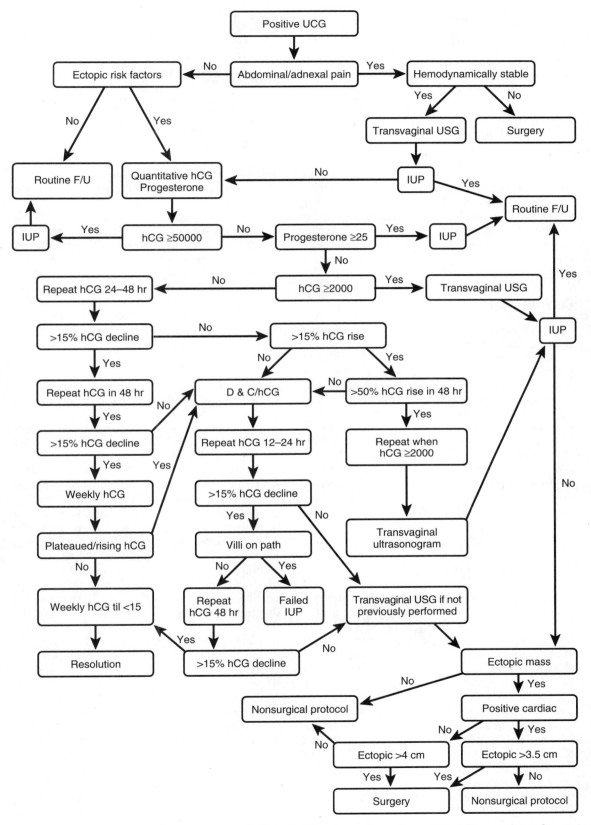

Figure 1. Ectopic pregnancy diagnostic protocol. D & C, dilatation and curettage; F/U, follow-up; hCG, human chorionic gonadotropin; IUP, intrauterine pregnancy; UCG, urinary chorionic gonadotropin. (Developed by the University of Tennessee, Memphis, 1996.)

raphy can also accurately image oviducts and ovaries such that ectopic pregnancies and their dimensions can be defined. The addition of color Doppler transvaginal sonography aids in earlier detection of an intrauterine gestation and allows better visualization of an ectopic gestation. Color Doppler scanning can help differentiate among a completed abortion, incomplete abortion, and an early IUP before visualization of a gestational sac.

The ultrasonographic identification of an intrauterine gestational sac essentially excludes an ectopic pregnancy. Transvaginal ultrasonography can also identify an ectopic pregnancy greater than 4 cm in greatest dimension, or the presence of adnexal cardiac activity in ectopic pregnancies larger than 3.5 cm, both relative contraindications to methotrexate therapy.

Culdocentesis

Culdocentesis offers no clinical utility when considering diagnostic and therapeutic options for ectopic pregnancy, as 45% to 60% of unruptured ectopic pregnancies have a positive culdocentesis, while also being associated with a 15% false-positive rate. Culdocentesis is useful in the diagnosis of hemoperitoneum but not ectopic pregnancy. Historically, culdocentesis was used to decide whether to perform a laparotomy, such as if blood was found, or to proceed with diagnostic laparoscopy. With new instrumentation, laparoscopy is now a viable treatment option even in the presence of hematoperitoneum. As a result, the utility of culdocentesis has been eliminated.

Dilation and Curettage

Dilatation and curettage allows identification of chorionic villi and thereby essentially eliminates the diagnosis of ectopic pregnancy, except in the rare case of heterotopic pregnancy (<1 in 15,000). By identifying villi, D&C also eliminates giving methotrexate to a patient with a failed IUP. D&C was originally used extensively in our ectopic protocol, but to reduce the cost and potential surgical morbidity of D&C, we have eliminated D&C in patients with appropriately falling hCG level. If a D&C is performed, the diagnosis of an ectopic pregnancy can be delayed by several days unless a frozen section on the uterine contents is obtained. A serum hCG drawn at the time of D&C followed by a repeat level in 12 to 24 hours, as indicated in the algorithm shown in

Figure 1, can substantially reduce this time factor.

Methotrexate

Methotrexate has been used extensively for the treatment of trophoblastic disease, and placental tissue left in situ after an abdominal pregnancy. The first reported use of methotrexate for ectopic pregnancy was in 1982. Since that time, multiple reports describing the use of methotrexate for treatment of ectopic pregnancy have been published.

The initial series using methotrexate for the medical treatment of ectopic pregnancy used multiple doses of methotrexate alternating with citrovorium rescue factor during a prolonged hospital stay. Subsequently, experience at the University of Tennessee and other sites has demonstrated that medical management of ectopic pregnancies can be performed on an out-patient basis. Using a multidose regime, a success rate of 96% with 100 patients was reported from our institution.

Single-Dose Methotrexate Protocol

A subsequent protocol using single-dose methotrexate has been developed. Currently almost 300 patients have been treated with this protocol with a success rate of 93%. This success rate is particularly noteworthy since the previous limit on the size of an ectopic gestation that could be treated has been relaxed despite liberalization in the size of ectopic pregnancies treated. This success rate is similar to that obtained when a multidose protocol was followed.

Before treatment with methotrexate, patients must be counseled extensively about the risk and benefits of treatment, the expected course and duration of treatment, as well as the importance of follow-up. All patients are screened with a baseline hCG, Rh factor, complete blood count, serum glutamic-oxaloacetic transaminase, and creatinine and blood urea nitrogen levels. White blood cell counts of less than 1500 or elevation in the renal or liver function values more than twice the upper limit of normal are contraindications to treatment with methotrexate. Methotrexate is given in a dose of 50 mg/m² based on actual body weight. The day methotrexate is given is considered day 1. A repeat hCG is performed on days 4 and 7. If the hCG level declines less than 15% between days 4 and 7, a second dose of methotrexate is given and the protocol restarted at a new day 1. A repeat blood count and serum glutamic-oxaloacetic transaminase are obtained before redosing. If the hCG level declines 15% or greater, hCG titers are followed weekly until the level is less than 15 mIU/mL. If the hCG level declines less than 15% in any week, repeat methotrexate dosing is performed.

During treatment, patients are required to avoid intercourse, alcohol, folate-containing vitamins, and pelvic examinations. Approximately 75% of patients will experience an episode of increased pain during treatment, most likely due to tubal abortion. Patients are advised to take ibuprofen 800 mg and lie down. If significant relief does not occur in 1 hour, patients are asked to return for re-evaluation. Hemodynamically stable patients with severe pain are admitted and observed with serial hematocrits. As noted previously, 45% to 60% of patients with unruptured ectopic pregnancy will have blood in the pelvis; this is not a reason for surgical intervention.

The natural history of ectopic pregnancy is high variable. At one extreme there is acute pain, hemorrhage, shock, and even death. At the other, in an asymptomatic patient, the implantation may undergo resorption or tubal abortion. When hCG titers are falling and there is no evidence of tubal rupture, nonintervention offers freedom from chemotherapy toxicity, or surgical morbidity. Success rates have been reported to be from 70% to 100%. At our institution, all patients with tubal ectopic pregnancies without cardiac activity have at least two hCG level measurements before treatment. Patients with falling levels are followed conservatively as long as hCG levels fall appropriately.

Fetal Fibronectin: Its Role in Obstetrics

Thomas J. Garite, MD

Premature delivery remains the leading cause of perinatal mortality and major morbidity. Despite the availability of tocolytic drugs, aggressive surveillance techniques, and other treatment and prevention strategies, no change has been observed in the premature delivery rate since we began keeping records on this issue. Obstetric clinicians face many problems in dealing with this critical problem. Correct methods of identifying patients at risk, such as previous history, demographic factors, and detection of early signs and symptoms are generally neither sensitive nor specific. Once premature labor is actually diagnosed, current treatment regimens are hampered by several difficulties. Some leading causes of premature delivery, such as PROM, are at present unresponsive to treatment. Many patients with premature labor, who might otherwise be good candidates for tocolytic treatment, present in advanced labor, too late for effective intervention. Those who do present early enough are often clinically indistinguishable from patients with irrelevant contractions that are not destined to lead to true premature labor and delivery.

It is apparent that a noninvasive clinical tool that assists the clinician in the early and accurate identification of premature labor would be immensely valuable to the clinician and have the potential to lead to substantial improvement in our success in dealing with this most challenging and frustrating problem.

Over the last 5 years, a new test, fetal fibronectin (fFN) identified in vaginal secretions, which promises to more accurately identify and actually predict premature labor, has been described and tested and has been approved by the Food and Drug Administration (FDA) and is now available for clinical use. Fibronectins are a family of abundant, multifunctional, and ubiquitous proteins. Plasma fibronectin, produced in the liver, has oncotic, coagulation, and opsonic and other immune-related functions. Cellular fibronectin is an insoluble extracellular matrix protein. Many other antigenically distinct forms of fibronectin have been identified. In 1985, a new isoform of fibronectin was identified and described as *oncofetal fibronectin,* which was found exclusively in certain malignant tumors and in fetal tissues, including placenta and amniotic fluid.

This protein is present in fetal tissue throughout pregnancy. Immunohistochemical studies of placenta and membranes localize this protein to the extracellular matrix of the extravillous trophoblast and decidua basalis adjacent to the intervillous space. In membranes, such studies reveal a somewhat more diffuse distribution of fFN, however, as with the placenta most fFN is concentrated at the junction of the decidua and the chorion. It appears that fetal fibronectin plays a role in the establishment of the extracellular interface between the mother and fetus and perhaps is important in placental cleavage following delivery.

Most of the clinical applications of this test stem from the physiologic knowledge that antigenically recognizable portions of this protein leak through the cervix into the vagina, usually 2 to 3 weeks before the onset of labor. At first it was thought that this might be a "microleak" of amniotic fluid, as amniotic fluid concentrations of fFN are particularly high. Immunohistochemical tests revealed the decidual/trophoblastic matrix junction fFN to have disappeared in these patients, apparently as the result of proteolysis occurring in the natural course of the process of labor.

This test has been approved by the FDA for use in assisting the clinician with improved accuracy of the diagnosis of impending premature delivery in both symptomatic and asymptomatic patients.

Symptomatic Patients

Patients who present in premature labor often pose both a diagnostic and a management dilemma. The diagnosis of premature labor in patients with regular contractions and advanced cervical dilation is not a difficult diagnostic problem, but therapy is usually unsuccessful because labor has progressed too far. For those with irregular contractions or nonspecific symptoms and lesser degrees of cervical dilation, especially 2 cm or less, the accuracy of the diagnosis of preterm labor is often in question. Even when the entire clinical picture is known, including past history, coexisting risk factors such as twins, associated findings such as vaginal bleeding, and the physician's best clinical judgment is used, often as many as 50% of patients in placebo-controlled studies go onto term. Conversely, when in the physician's best judgment the patient is thought not to be in premature labor and she is sent home, as many as 20% of these patients will subsequently deliver prematurely. Thus the need for a more accurate diagnostic addition to our clinical acumen is needed in this group of patients.

This test has now been studied by numerous authors for testing patients with symptoms of possible premature labor and minimal cervical dilatation. The test, done on vaginal and cervical secretions during speculum examination and prior to the first digital examination is highly accurate in predicting premature delivery within 1 to 2 weeks with sensitivities of over 85% and negative predictive values of 99.5% (a 1 in 200 chance of delivering within a week in a patient with a negative test).

Thus, symptomatic patients who are found to be positive for fFN might be more likely to

benefit from more aggressive therapy, more careful and close surveillance, corticosteroid administration to reduce neonatal complications of prematurity, and triage to a hospital capable of caring for a baby of the gestational age being evaluated. The patient with a negative test result might be observed longer before implementing any therapy; pharmacologic intervention might be avoided completely and imposing interventions such as bedrest, oral tocolytics, discontinuing work, and daily nurse contact with or without home contraction monitoring might be avoided.

Screening for Asymptomatic Patients

Over the past decade, perhaps the most promising approach to changing the prematurity rate has been the development of risk assessment techniques identifying patients at high risk for prematurity. Once the high-risk patient has been identified, using various strategies of more intense surveillance may allow earlier identification and intervention for premature labor once it does occur. Most risk identification techniques rely on demographic variables, previous history, and various findings during prenatal care, such as twins or polyhydramnios. As discussed previously, the success of such risk identification varies among populations.

Since fFN was shown to be an accurate predictor in symptomatic patients, it was only logical for investigators to ask the question as to whether this test might be useful in predicting premature delivery in asymptomatic patients. Numerous studies have now been performed and patients, both high-risk and low-risk, who are subjected to fFN testing every 1 to 2 weeks have been shown to have improved prediction of premature delivery. Generally speaking, patients with one or more positive tests before 34 weeks' gestation have a many-fold increase in the rate of premature delivery. As many as 50% of patients delivering prematurely will have at least one positive test. And most importantly, in the majority of patients who never have a positive test, the prematurity is at or below the rate of prematurity in the general population.

These data do appear to be similar in low-risk and in high-risk patients, but because of the low prevalence of prematurity in low-risk patients and the absence of intervention trials, routine screening in low-risk patients cannot be advocated. Although there are no intervention trials, it is clear that the presence of a positive test, in already high-risk patients, will enhance the clinician's ability to more appropriately assess these patients for risk. Then in the high-risk patients, with any positive test, increased and more aggressive surveillance should have the potential for improving outcome. Whether we can actually accomplish this awaits clinical intervention trials; however, at this time, it is clear that continued negative testing allows the clinician to avoid unnecessary interventions, such as discontinuing work, complete bedrest, oral or continuous subcutaneous pump tocolytic therapy, and even hospitalization.

In reality, many patients with premature delivery will fall somewhere in between symptomatic and asymptomatic. They may experience subtle symptoms such as pelvic pressure, or examination reveals cervical shortening. The management of these most difficult patients can be greatly enhanced by fFN testing.

Predicting Labor at Term

The appearance of fFN in the cervicovaginal secretions occurs before the onset of labor by about 2 weeks, and this is true whether labor ensues prior to term or at term. This is apparently the reason that in the initial study of fFN we found that most patients normally have fFN present near term. Thus, one exciting application of the fFN study in patients near term has been studied. Since post-date pregnancy is one of the most vexing clinical problems in the otherwise normal obstetric patient, and management and surveillance strategies are often contemplated well before the 42nd week, a test that could predict whether patients will deliver at term or later might be quite useful clinically. In patients studied during the 39th week of gestation, those with positive tests virtually all delivered before 41 weeks and over half of those with negative tests went beyond 41 weeks. Perhaps inteventions in those with negative tests, such as aggressive cervical ripening, might even decrease the incidence of prolonged pregnancy and thus prevent its complications.

Prediction of Successful Induction of Labor

Another vexing problem for the everyday practicing clinician is predicting the successful induction of labor. Other than historical factors such as parity, the only currently applicable clinical tool to determine which patients can have labor successfully induced is the status of the cervix or Bishop score. It is clear that the patient with a well-dilated and effaced cervix will generally be easily induced and that her risk for cesarean section for dystocia is not increased over that for spontaneous or noninduced labor. Unfortunately the predictability of successful labor induction with lower Bishop scores is poor, especially in nulliparous patients; and patients who have labor induced with low Bishop scores, especially of 5 or less, have longer labors and a higher likelihood of operative deliveries. Furthermore, many patients in nonurgent or semielective situations, in which induction would be the better choice if a safe, easy, and effective induction could be assured, have unfavorable cervices. Several recent studies suggest that testing for vaginal or cervical fFN may add to our ability to determine which patients will have labor most successfully induced. In general, patients with a positive fFN have shorter labors, less need for multiday inductions, and lower cesarean section rates with induced labor than those with negative tests. Therefore it would appear that fFN also has a very promising application in determining which patients who might benefit from labor induction will have shorter and more successful labor and deliveries.

Summary

Initially this test was manufactured as an ELISA and is done in regional clinical laboratories with turnaround times of around 24 hours. A rapid test has been approved by the Federal Drug Administration that will significantly enhance our ability to use this test in patient care, especially in symptomatic patients. Thus it appears that we now have a powerful new tool added to our clinical armamentarium for dealing with the problem of prematurity; and perhaps to deal with other clinical problems such as post-date pregnancy and induction of labor. Much further study is needed to discover exactly how specific interventions performed in the setting of a positive or a negative fFN will affect outcome. Nevertheless, management can only be improved by more precise and accurate diagnosis and it is clear that fFN can improve our diagnostic accuracy.

Gastrointestinal Disorders of Pregnancy

Daniel Hollander, MD

Approximately one half of the population of the United States suffers from one or more gastrointestinal problems. Therefore, it is not surprising that pregnant women often experience some gastrointestinal symptoms. These complaints may have preceded pregnancy, may be exacerbated by pregnancy, or may have arisen as a complication of pregnancy.

Both diagnostic and therapeutic approaches are somewhat limited in a pregnant woman because they pose risks to the fetus and its development. The diagnosis of gastrointestinal dysfunction often involves radiologic studies but since these studies should be avoided during pregnancy, ultrasonographic studies or endoscopy must be used as alternative diagnostic approaches.

In this discussion, I deal with the most common gastrointestinal problems seen in pregnancy. I do not cover the pathophysiology of gastrointestinal disorders but concentrate instead on the unique clinical presentation, diagnostic alternatives, and therapeutic options of the more common gastrointestinal problems during pregnancy.

Esophagitis

Approximately one third of the adult population suffers from some degree of esophagitis, with heartburn as its most common symptom. Heartburn is caused by the reflux of gastric contents into the esophagus and oropharynx. Why gastric contents reflux into the esophagus in patients with esophagitis is not clear, but it is often attributed to esophageal sphincter dysfunction, disordered motility of the body of the esophagus, and perhaps an intrinsic defect in the ability of the esophageal mucosa to resist injury. Hormonal changes during pregnancy are thought to exacerbate esophageal reflux. Other factors that exacerbate esophagitis include the ingestion of aspirin or other nonsteroidal anti-inflammatory drugs (NSAIDs) or irritants such as alcohol and caffeine. At times, tablet medications of any kind may lodge in the esophagus and cause esophagitis.

The diagnosis of esophagitis in a pregnant woman relies heavily on a thorough medical history. Heartburn, the typical symptom, is usually worse after meals, or with the ingestion of fruit juices, or when the patient is reclining. If the history is very clear and typical of heartburn, there is no reason to perform additional diagnostic studies.

In the pregnant woman, the presentation of esophagitis may consist of anorexia, nausea, and vomiting. In some cases, "finer points" in the history may help; for example, retrosternal pain or discomfort that occurs when solid foods or very hot or very cold liquids are being swallowed or after fruit juices have been ingested may be an indication of esophagitis. However, if the history is not clear, the preferred diagnostic study is endoscopy. In addition, one must rule out the presence of cholelithiasis and other biliary problems that could cause nausea or vomiting by ultrasonographic diagnostic modalities.

The aim of therapy for mild to moderate esophagitis is to decrease acid reflux and to diminish gastric acidity. The patient should ingest antacids after meals, at bedtime, and as needed; avoid common mucosal irritants (alcohol and caffeine); limit the size and volume of meals; raise the head of the bed by 3 to 4 inches; and avoid eating before bedtime. These measures are effective for more than two thirds of pregnant women with mild, uncomplicated esophagitis. However, if the extent of esophageal inflammation is more severe or if there are complications such as esophageal ulcerations, these simple therapeutic measures may be insufficient.

Histamine receptor antagonists (eg, cimetidine, ranitidine, or famotidine) and the pump inhibitors omeprazole or lansoprazol are frequently prescribed for patients with complicated, severe esophageal reflux; however, the safety of these agents in pregnancy is not absolutely established and they should be used in pregnant women after a trial of antacids. Another drug that could be tried in pregnant women with esophagitis is sucralfate.

Sucralfate is a drug that increases esophageal mucosal resistance to injury and stimulates mucosal restitution and renewal. Sucralfate can be administered 1 hour before meals and at bedtime in conjunction with postprandial antacids and the other measures outlined earlier. It can be swallowed whole, chewed, or dissolved in water and mixed into a slurry.

Other drugs that are used in the therapy for esophagitis in patients who are not pregnant include metoclopramide and other prokinetic agents. These drugs act by stimulating esophageal contractions and peristalsis and by increasing the pressure of the gastroesophageal sphincter. Their safety in pregnancy is not established, and therefore they should not be used.

If the patient does not respond to these measures the diagnosis should be questioned and consultation with a gastroenterologist should be obtained to rule out the possibility of esophageal ulcerations or other intestinal problems that may mimic esophageal symptoms in a pregnant woman.

Nausea and Vomiting

Nausea and vomiting occur commonly in pregnancy, particularly during the first trimester, but can persist or appear at any stage of pregnancy. The pathogenesis of these complaints is not clearly understood, but hormonal changes in pregnancy may be an important initiating factor. Hormonal factors may cause abnormal motility of the stomach and proximal small intestine, which, in turn, is perceived by the patient as nausea and may result in vomiting. Not infrequently, nausea and vomiting are caused by esophagitis or gastritis. Less commonly, nausea and vomiting are symptoms of cholecystitis or even inflammatory bowel diseases, such as Crohn's disease. One should also include intestinal obstruction, intra-abdominal sepsis, and central nervous system lesions in the differential diagnosis of persistent nausea and vomiting.

The treatment of mild, first trimester nausea consists of several nonspecific measures that often result in significant but incomplete resolution of the symptoms. These include taking antacids before meals, eating small-volume meals, and avoiding mucosal irritants, such as alcohol and caffeine. Elevation of the head of the bed to prevent nocturnal reflux from the stomach into the esophagus may also help. If these measures do not relieve the problem, 1 g of sucralfate before meals and at bedtime should also be tried.

If the patient's condition does not improve with these relatively safe measures, ultrasonography of the abdomen should be performed to rule out gallstones, partial intestinal obstruction, and Crohn's disease. If the ultrasonographic examination is not helpful, upper endoscopy should be performed to look for esophagitis, gastritis, or duodenitis.

If a specific cause for the nausea cannot be found and the symptoms are not controllable with these measures, antiemetic medications may have to be used, especially if the patient is losing weight or becoming dehydrated. Generally, the safety of systemic antiemetics in pregnancy is not absolutely established. However, meclizine and promethazine (Phenergan) are drugs with proven efficacy and probable safety. They should be used cautiously, at the lowest effective dose, and in conjunction with the general therapeutic measures outlined earlier. As soon as the patient is feeling better, the systemic antiemetic drugs should be tapered off.

In patients with severe vomiting, dehydration, and weight loss (hyperemesis gravidarum), intravenous hyperalimentation should be used to provide fluid and nutrients. In patients in the second or third trimester with severe nausea and vomiting, prokinetic agents such as metoclopramide can be used. Since the safety of these agents in pregnancy is not clearly established, their use should be reserved for severe vomiting in the second or third trimester that does not respond to other measures.

Peptic Ulcer Disease

Peptic ulceration of the stomach or the duodenum occurs in approximately 10% of the population and is therefore a relatively common disorder. There is no evidence that peptic ulcers occur more frequently in pregnant women. Similarly, there is no evidence that pregnancy adversely affects the course of peptic ulcer disease. In fact, there is some evidence that estrogens have a protective effect against the formation of peptic ulceration and may accelerate the healing of peptic disease.

Ordinarily, the diagnosis of peptic disease hinges on the typical history of upper abdominal discomfort made worse by fasting and relieved completely or partially by eating. Similarly, the patient with peptic diseases typically obtains at least temporary relief by using over-the-counter medication such as antacids. Peptic ulcer disease also has a genetic component, and thus individuals with peptic discomfort may have other family members with documented peptic ulceration. The two diagnostic methods to substantiate and document the existence of the disease are radiographic studies of endoscopy. Upper gastrointestinal barium meal studies are relatively accurate in detecting the presence of gastric ulcerations but are quite inaccurate and insensitive to the presence of duodenal ulceration. Therefore, many physicians rely on the upper endoscopy. In the pregnant woman, upper gastrointestinal barium radiographic studies are contraindicated and should not be used. Upper gastrointestinal endoscopy, however, can be performed with very little risk to the pregnant woman. Most of the time, if a clear history is obtained that the patient's abdominal discomfort is relieved by eating and exacerbated by fasting, it can be reasonably concluded that the patient has a peptic ulcer. The physician might treat such a patient for 8 to 12 weeks without resorting to diagnostic studies. If the pain persists beyond 8 to 12 weeks or the pain is atypical, the physician should seek endoscopic or other diagnostic studies.

In the nonpregnant individual, the most commonly used drugs for peptic ulcer therapy are the histamine receptor antagonists, such as cimetidine, ranitidine, or famotidine, or the hydrogen potassium pump inhibitors omeprazole or lansoprazole. Histamine receptor antagonists should not be used as the first drug in the pregnant woman because the histamine receptor antagonists have receptors in many organs besides the stomach or duodenum, and they pass across the placenta into the fetus. Instead, antacids and sucralfate should be used first. Antacids containing aluminum, magnesium, or calcium carbonate are safe both for the pregnant woman and for the fetus. In controlled studies, antacids have been shown to be as effective as the histamine receptor antagonists in the treatment of acute peptic ulceration. Magnesium-containing antacids tend to cause laxation, while predominantly aluminum-containing antacids tend to cause constipation. Which type of antacid is used depends on the bowel habits of the pregnant woman. Calcium carbonate–containing antacids are equally as effective as aluminum or magnesium antacids and have the advantage of supplying extra calcium to the mother and fetus.

Sucralfate is also nonsystemic and can be used safely in the pregnant woman. This drug is not an antacid, does not cross the intestinal barrier, and is not likely to affect the fetus. It can be used four times daily both for the acute treatment of peptic ulcer disease and for the prevention of peptic ulcer recurrence. It does not influence bowel habits and is somewhat more convenient to use than antacids.

The newest type of medication used for the therapy of peptic ulceration as well as esophagitis is the hydrogen-potassium pump antagonists omeprazole and lansoprazole. These drugs are potent inhibitors of acid secretion. The safety of the pump inhibitors in pregnancy is not completely established and they should be used only after other drugs have failed.

Recently, an infectious etiology of peptic ulcer disease was described. The infective organism is *Helicobacter pylori*. Its eradication with antibiotics speeds the healing of peptic ulcerations and decreases the likelihood of ulcer recurrence.

It is difficult to eradicate *H. pylori* with antibi-

otics. To achieve eradication of the bacteria one must use two or three antibiotics at high dosages. Therefore, in the pregnant woman with peptic ulceration, one should reserve *H. pylori* eradication for patients not responding to the other modalities of therapy mentioned earlier. After delivery, one could electively use antibiotics to eradicate *H. pylori*.

Constipation

Constipation occurs frequently during the latter stages of pregnancy. The pathogenesis of this problem in pregnancy is not understood. Hormonal changes may contribute to abnormal motility of the colon and rectosigmoid, and the expanding uterus may form a mechanical obstacle to normal bowel evacuation. In addition, many women develop hemorrhoids or anal cryptitis as pregnancy progresses, resulting in pain on defecation and constipation.

The treatment of simple constipation without rectal abnormalities is to have the patient ingest bulk containing cellulose and other nondigestible residues (eg, Metamucil) and increase dietary intake of fiber by eating more fresh fruits and vegetables. These simple measures alleviate mild constipation in many pregnant women. In the past, stool-softening detergents, such as docusate calcium (Surfak) and docusate sodium (Colace), were used extensively to treat constipation. In controlled trials, these agents have not been shown to be better than placebos and therefore their use is not advocated.

In patients with hard stools and without rectal abnormalities, a plain tap-water enema can be helpful in addition to these measures. Lubricating rectal suppositories can also be very helpful in initiating defecation. If at all possible, irritant enemas (eg, Fleet enema) should be avoided since their use will abolish spontaneous defecation. Another approach to severe persistent constipation is to use hypersomatic solutions such as magnesium citrate or sodium phosphate to start evacuation. This approach should be used to supplement, not replace, the other measures mentioned. An alternative to the hyperosmotic cathartics is lactulose syrup, which works by the osmotic effects of its bacterial metabolites in the large bowel.

In patients whose constipation does not respond to these measures, the rectal area should be inspected, a digital examination should be performed, and anoscopy or sigmoidoscopy should be done.

Anal pain on defecation due to hemorrhoids,

fissures, or cryptitis may cause constipation. If abnormalities are found, the patient should use lubricating rectal suppositories twice daily after a 20-minute sitz bath. If the hemorrhoids do not respond to these measures, the patient should be referred to a gastroenterologist or a proctologist.

The gastrointestinal disorders discussed here are the most common ones seen during pregnancy. Less common problems, which I have not discussed, require more specialized diagnostic approaches and therapeutic measures. A gastroenterologist should assist the obstetrician in the management of these patients.

Genital Tract Trauma

Edward Newton, MD

Epidemiology

Genital tract trauma is one of the most common obstetric morbidities after vaginal delivery. The morbidities include acute injury (laceration, bleeding, hematomas, and infection), dyspareunia, pelvic floor relaxation, and urinary stress incontinence. In prospective studies, acute trauma occurs with sulcus tears or posterior lacerations (including episiotomy) in approximately one of two women. Labial tears occur in one of four. Injury of the rectal sphincter or rectal mucosa or cervical lacerations occur in 0.5% to 5% of deliveries. Maternal death from genital tract trauma is uncommon unless uterine rupture is involved. However, a life-threatening hemorrhage occurs. In most cases, this is a complication heralded by external blood loss in the face of a contracted uterus, or an atonic uterus with rapid response to oxytoxic drugs, but rapid relapse into hemorrhage. Occasionally, interfascial blood loss is occult from a paravaginal, ischiorectal, or parauterine hematoma. Perineal pain and rectal pressure may be the only symptoms prior to shock associated with perigenital hematoma.

Other risks associated with genital tract trauma are perineal infections, dyspareunia, urinary stress incontinence, and fistula formation. Episiotomy infection occurs in about 5% of cases. Although 90% of patients will return to sexual relationships within 3 months postpartum, 20% of women will complain of discomfort with sexual activity. Twenty percent of women will have involuntary loss of urine at 3 months postpartum. However, long-term prospective studies of stress incontinence after genital tract trauma have not been performed.

Fistulae of the urinary tract or bowel are a rare complication of delivery. They are related to pressure necrosis or trauma. Prolonged obstructed labor causes pressure necrosis 7 to 10 days after delivery. Anteriorly, the fetal head compresses the trigone, bladder neck, and upper urethra against the symphysis, and a fistula forms as the necrotic tissue sloughs. Less frequently, a similar complication occurs posteriorly; the rectum is compressed against the sacral promontory and a high rectal vaginal fistula occurs.

The incidence of obstetrically related fistulae has dropped with the advent of safer cesarean section. Destructive manipulation of a dead fetus and complicated forceps operations have been largely eliminated, and rarely is obstructed labor neglected for days in Western countries. In Third World countries, fistula formation from pressure necrosis remains a problem in rural obstetrics.

Genital tract trauma, perigenital hematomas and lacerations, is classified into four types based on location: vulvar, perivaginal, vulvovaginal, and supravaginal. Extension of the episiotomy, vaginal sulci lacerations, and cervical trauma are most common. A variety of conditions predispose to development of genital tract injury: young primipara, fetal macrosomia, abnormal presentation (occiput posterior, breech), precipitous labor, abnormal pelvic structure (narrow subpubic angle, straight sacrum), abnormal soft tissue (scar), obstetric manipulation, and uncontrolled delivery.

Management

After every vaginal delivery, especially operative deliveries of a large fetus, a systematic examination of the perineum, sulci, and cervix should be undertaken after the placenta is delivered. First, the vulva and labia should be examined. Common locations for injury are in the periclitoral area and labia minora. Second, the lateral sulci, upper vagina, and cervix are examined for lacerations or hematoma. This is accomplished by depressing the perineum with two or three fingers, inspecting the upper vagina, and examining the cervix for integrity. The cervical examination is best accomplished by progressive clamping with ring forceps through its entirety. Vaginal injury usually occurs at 4 and 8 o'clock in sulci, over the ischial spines, and 3 and 9 o'clock on the cervix. Third, the injuries to the posterior perineum and anal mechanisms are examined. These may be an extension of the episiotomy. At this point, an evaluation of sphincter integrity and rectal mucosal integrity should be established by a double-gloved finger in the rectum. During this examination, the ischiorectal fossae can be examined for hematoma formation. Fourth, after the examination is complete, all lacerations should be carefully recorded in the progress notes, including the location and need for suture.

Anterior lacerations of the perineum usually involve stretch tears of the labia. The urethral meatus and clitoris may be involved. Individual vessels are clamped and ligated with small polyglycolic suture. A general ooze may be treated with ice and pressure after the skin repair. When bleeding occurs close to the clitoris, it is important not to place a suture into the body of the clitoris, as a hematoma and subsequent dyspareunia may result. The skin and mucosa are reapproximated to restore normal anatomic relationships.

Posterior lacerations of the fourchette and vagina are classified by degree of injury. A first-degree laceration involves only the vaginal mucosa. Second-degree lacerations involve the bulbocavernosus, superficial, and deep transverse perineal muscles. Third-degree lacerations (partial or complete) involve the rectal sphincter, and fourth-degree lacerations involve the rectal mucosa. European literature includes the rectal mucosa injury into third-degree lacerations.

Posterior perineal trauma is the most common type of genital tract injury. Episiotomy with or without extension constitutes the major portion of the injuries. Episiotomy has been performed in the past to reduce the incidence of genital tract trauma. As a consequence, it is the most common operation in women. Between 1.5 and 2.5 million episiotomies are performed each year in the United States. About 70% of primiparous and 30% of multiparous women undergo episiotomies. In the United States, a midline episiotomy is preferred because of easier repair, better healing, less postpartum pain, less dyspareunia, and reduced blood loss; however, a mediolateral incision has the benefit of a lower rate of extension into the rectum.

Recent literature has brought the benefits of episiotomy into serious question. Rather than reducing genital tract trauma, midline episiotomies have been associated with increased rates of third- and fourth-degree lacerations and subsequent rectovaginal fistulae and rectal incontinence.

The prevention of pelvic relaxation is a second reason given for routine episiotomy. This reasoning has been based on older, poorly controlled retrospective reviews of pelvic relaxation. Adequate study of this subject would need to control for parity, age, medical conditions, fetal position, presentation, birth weight, mode of delivery (forceps), and anesthesia. In a randomized study by Sleep and coworkers (1984) that compared restricted versus a liberal policy toward episiotomy, the incidence of episiotomy was 10% in restricted use, and 51% in liberal use of episiotomy. Nineteen percent of patients in the restricted policy group and 19% in the liberal policy group had involuntary loss of urine after 3 months; 6% had to wear vulvar pads. This study and others suggest that there is no relationship between episiotomy and the prevention of stress incontinence.

In summary, scientific reasoning does not support the routine use of episiotomy. The selective indication for the use of this operation includes fetal distress, instrumental deliveries, macrosomic infants, and abnormal presentation or position. Midline episiotomies are associated with less discomfort and improved healing, but with a higher incidence of fourth-degree extension than are mediolateral episiotomies.

The repair of posterior lacerations is directed toward restoration of normal anatomy and function. The key points are the identification and repair of rectal mucosal injury, restoration of the anal sphincter, and prevention of hematoma formation. Insertion of a double-gloved finger into the rectum is essential to rule out mucosal injury and aid in repair of mucosal injury.

Longitudinal lacerations of the vaginal sulci are common (10–15%). Individual bleeding vessels are isolated and ligated. The mucosa is reapproximated with a 2-0 or 3-0 running, locking suture (polyglycolic or chromic). The line of suture should always be in the longitudinal rather than transverse plane, so as to prevent scar constriction of the vaginal caliber. The anchoring suture of the laceration should be placed 0.5 cm above the apex to prevent hematoma formation. A rectal examination after the procedure will identify mucosal compromise or stitch incorporation.

The repair of a fourth degree extension starts with a closure of the rectal mucosa with interrupted, inverting 4-0 polyglycolic sutures. A second layer of closure reapproximates the levator ani muscles with interrupted or running 2-0 polyglycolic acid sutures. The ends of the anal sphincter muscle are grasped with Allis clamps and a figure-of-eight suture of 2-0 polyglycolic acid is used to reapproximate each quadrant of the capsule. The deep perineal muscles are reapproximated with interrupted 2-0 polyglycolic acid sutures. The vaginal mucosa, superficial perineal muscles, and skin are repaired in standard fashion.

The long-term prognosis for fourth degree laceration is usually good. Between 1% and 5% of these patients will have decreased sphincter tone, and 1 in 300 patients will develop a retrovaginal fistula. The retrovaginal fistula may develop as late as 8 months post partum. Recent data suggest that once the perineal wound is free of active infection and induration, that it can be repaired in a secondary fashion with a good expectation for success. In the past it was felt that the repair should be delayed until the defect is epithelialized and is free of infection (6–8 weeks).

Perineal infection (episiotomy wound infection) can be life-threatening. Although stitch abscesses and minor wound infections occur in 0.5% to 5% of procedures, maternal death has been associated with perineal infection. Fetal cases are associated with a history of a fourth-degree laceration and increasing perineal pain on the third to fourth day postpartum. On physical examination, there is perineal induration and asymmetric vulvar edema. Erythema of the lower abdomen, buttocks, and thigh implies a fascial extension. Signs of systemic disease may be late; the patient's temperature may be greater than 38°C and her white blood cell count may be greater than 25,000. The wound must be explored as soon as possible. Necrotic tissue must be excised until bleeding tissue is recognized. This may involve extensive surgery. High-dose antibiotics are given intravenously early in treatment, for example, penicillin 10 million units q6h, gentamicin 1.5 mg/kg q8h, and clindamycin 900 mg q8h.

Perigenital hematomas are an additional life-threatening complication. The vessels of the perineum are engorged during delivery and are only loosely attached to the underlying structures. When these vessels are lacerated, they retract well away from the wound edge or laceration. If they are not recognized, a hematoma can form. The loose areolar fat tissue offers little resistance to hematoma formation. Repair of perineal lacerations and hematomas must be directed to securing these vessels. For example, in the repair of a vaginal laceration or espisiotomy, the first stitch of the mucosal repair is placed well above the apex of the laceration.

The incidence of perigenital hematomas is difficult to determine. It varies a great deal with the care with which this complication is examined and reported. Older studies with a higher incidence of instrumental delivery showed a higher incidence. In the late 1950s, the rate was

as high as 1 in 300 deliveries. In a series of 47 perigenital hematomas, 45% were perineal or vulvovaginal, and 53% were perivaginal. Perineal hematomas often resulted from a bleeding vessel within the episiotomy site. Perivaginal hematomas tended to occur over the ischial spines and were related to instrumental delivery. Most commonly they occurred on the right side and were between 2 and 4 inches in diameter. The most common symptoms were rectal pain and pressure with radiation to the coccyx. Seventy-seven percent were diagnosed within 8 hours of delivery, although 9% were found 5 to 10 days post partum. Of these, 19% of the patients developed shock, and 43% required blood transfusion.

The management of perigenital hematoma depends on the timing, location, and severity of the symptoms. Hematoma of the episiotomy site developing within 4 to 6 hours should be opened, the vessel ligated, and the episiotomy resutured. A small (<5 cm) perivaginal hematoma should be watched carefully for enlargement. The patient should have serial hematocrit determination, rectovaginal examinations, and determination of vital signs. Enlargement or hemodynamic instability indicates a need for cervical exploration. With the patient under adequate anesthesia, a longitudinal mucosal incision is performed over the hematoma. Transverse incisions may lead to vaginal constriction from scar formation. Hematoma is evacuated and the individual vessels ligated. The dead space mucosa are closed with simple sutures of 3-0 polyglycolic acid. The vagina is tightly packed for 12 hours and a Foley catheter is placed to relieve urinary tract obstruction.

A supravaginal hematoma is an extension of a hematoma from a perivaginal area, or more commonly from the broad ligament trauma with uterine rupture or cesarean section. The management often requires exploratory laparotomy. The presence of a cervical or vaginal laceration extending beyond the fornix is an indication for immediate laparotomy. Occasionally, a nonexpanding broad ligament hematoma can be observed. Continued bleeding is treated with supportive transfusion and exploration. Arterial embolization using invasive radiology is a new and often successful alternative to immediate surgery.

Cervical lacerations are related to three factors: prior surgery, cervical manipulation during transition, and instrumental delivery. Cerclage and cone biopsy are the most common antecedent operations. Precipitous delivery in the presence of a cerclage can lead to annular amputation of the cervix. Often bleeding will be minimal, otherwise a running locking stitch of 3-0 polyglycolic acid will accomplish hemostasis. Cervical lacerations that occur during cervical manipulation or instrumental deliveries are linear and extend toward the vaginal reflection at 3 and 9 o'clock. After a vaginal delivery, the cervix should be assessed for laceration. When there is adequate anesthesia, the cervix is progressively visualized with ring forceps. In an unmedicated vaginal delivery, perineal discomfort may be limiting. Palpation of the cervical ring can be used to screen for lacerations. In cases of postpartum hemorrhage, the vagina and cervix should always be examined. Linear cervical lacerations are repaired only if they are bleeding or extend into the upper one third of the vaginal cervix. The cervix is stabilized with ring forceps and repaired with interrupted through-and-through sutures of 2-0 polyglycolic acid. If the laceration extends beyond the vaginal reflection, a full exploration is recommended.

Group B Streptococcus in Pregnancy

George D. Wendel, Jr, MD
F. Gary Cunningham, MD

Asymptomatic carriage of group B β-hemolytic streptococcus (GBS or *Streptococcus agalactiae*) is common in women, especially in the vagina and rectum. The Vaginal Infections and Prematurity Study Group reported that 15% to 20% of more than 8000 pregnant women from five clinical centers had a positive lower genital tract culture done between 23 and 26 weeks' gestation. GBS has been associated with a variety of maternal complications. Increased rates of GBS colonization have been observed in older, low parity, indigent, non-white women. Apparently, health behaviors and sexual activity do not fully explain differences in GBS carriage rates among pregnant women. GBS urinary infections occur, but mainly as asymptomatic bacteriuria, rather than as cystitis or pyelonephritis. In the setting of asymptomatic bacteriuria, women are presumed to be heavily colonized with GBS and may have higher rates of neonatal colonization and disease.

The organism has been implicated in several adverse pregnancy outcomes, including preterm labor, prematurely ruptured membranes, clinical and histologic chorioamnionitis, and puerperal sepsis. GBS also causes fetal and neonatal colonization and symptomatic infections. The role of GBS in overt maternal infection is less well-defined. Intrapartum colonization with GBS is an important independent risk factor for chorioamnionitis, but not endometritis. The risk of chorioamnionitis increases in a stepwise fashion from light to heavy GBS vaginal colonization. There have also been reports of wound infection, cellulitis, fasciitis, osteomyelitis, endocarditis, and mastitis caused by GBS.

Epidemiology

Half of newborns of carrier women become colonized almost immediately at birth. Serious neonatal infections with GBS are at least as prevalent as those from coliform organisms, and since the 1970s, neonatal GBS infections have increased remarkably. In Victoria, Australia, these infections caused one third of perinatal deaths due to infection.

It is clear that intrapartum fetal transmission from the colonized mother may lead to severe neonatal sepsis soon after birth. The overall attack rate of early-onset sepsis is about 1 to 2 per 1000 of all births. It is 10 per 1000 for babies born to colonized mothers, and approaches 40 per 1000 if there is preterm labor and delivery, prolonged membrane rupture, or intrapartum fever. Although preterm or low birth weight infants are at highest risk, more than half of the cases of neonatal sepsis are in term neonates.

Neonatal Sepsis

With septicemia from GBS that characterizes early-onset disease, signs of serious illness usually develop within 6 to 12 hours of birth. These include respiratory distress, apnea, and shock. At the outset, therefore, the illness must be differentiated from idiopathic respiratory distress syndrome. The mortality rate with early-onset disease is about 10% and preterm infants fare less well. Unfortunately, it is not uncommon for surviving infants to exhibit neurologic sequelae apparently sustained during hypotension from the sepsis syndrome. Late-onset *disease* usually manifests as meningitis a week or more after birth. These cases are most often caused by serotype III GBS organisms. The mortality rate, although appreciable, is less for late-onset meningitis than for early-onset sepsis. Here again, neurologic sequelae are common in survivors.

Screening

Until recently, there was no comprehensive agreement concerning universal screening or treatment for maternal GBS carriage. Targeted screening of "high-risk" women was not found effective by the Vaginal Infections and Prematurity Study Group. A major problem with universal screening and attempts to eradicate the GBS colonization is a high recurrence rate. Because of a high colonization rate combined with a relatively low attack rate, screening is not considered to be cost-effective by most. In lieu of universal screening, the American College of Obstetricians and Gynecologists (ACOG) recommends intrapartum administration of ampicillin or penicillin G (clindamycin or erythromycin for penicillin-allergic women) based on the presence of clinical risk factors to include (1) preterm labor, (2) preterm prematurely ruptured membranes, (3) prolonged membrane rupture for greater than 18 hours, (4) sibling affected by symptomatic GBS infection, or (5) intrapartum maternal fever.

In a comparative study of two different time periods, implementation of the American Academy of Pediatrics' guidelines for prevention of GBS infection was found to be not effective in decreasing early-onset newborn disease. Because of these problems, efforts have been directed at intrapartum rapid screening techniques and treatment schemes designed to prevent neonatal colonization, and thus sepsis. Most have concluded, however, that rapid GBS identification tests are ineffective.

Treatment and Prophylaxis

In an early study, absence of early-onset GBS sepsis was observed in 130,000 newborn infants given 50,000 units of aqueous penicillin G intramuscularly at birth as prophylaxis against gonococcal ophthalmia. A prospective study of nearly 19,000 infants was then carried out at Parkland Hospital. Half of these infants were randomly assigned to receive aqueous procaine penicillin G intramuscularly within 1 hour of birth as prophylaxis against ophthalmia neonatorum and also to evaluate its impact on GBS infections. The incidence of streptococcal disease was significantly lowered in those given penicillin. It was worrisome, however, that the incidence of infection and mortality caused by penicillin-resistant nonstreptococcal organisms marginally increased.

It was subsequently reported that such penicillin prophylaxis was of little benefit in preventing early-onset group B disease in low birth weight neonates. Many preterm infants who did poorly were subsequently found to have positive cord blood cultures for GBS. Thus, in these already covertly infected fetuses, single-dose prophylaxis failed to adequately treat ongoing neonatal infection. These findings also served to emphasize the important association of GBS with preterm delivery.

Emphasis was next placed on intrapartum treatment of mothers found to be colonized near the time of delivery. In a randomized clinical trial, intrapartum and neonatal ampicillin treatment of colonized mothers was associated with decreased neonatal colonization (9% versus 51%) and early-onset sepsis (0% versus 6%) in infants born to treated women compared with untreated control subjects. In another study, over 30,000 Australian clinic patients were screened at 32 weeks, and asymptomatic carriers were treated intrapartum with intravenous penicillin. Nearly 27,000 private patients were not screened. Although there were no GBS infections in neonates of clinical patients, by contrast, there were 27 infections and 8 deaths in the unscreened private control group.

In another two studies, screening cultures were performed at around 28 weeks' gestation. Culture-positive women were treated in labor only if they developed risk factors. Using this approach, one half to two thirds of cases of neonatal sepsis were prevented. Choice of antimicrobials may prove to be important. Penicillin and ampicillin-resistant Enterobacteriaceae infections have been observed. For these reasons, some recommend penicillin G intrapartum prophylaxis.

Recommendations for Prophylaxis

In 1996, the ACOG recommended that until there are further data to support a definitive strategy for prevention of GBS infection in the neonate, it would seem appropriate for clinicians to adopt one of two prophylactic strategies. The first approach utilizes intrapartum antibiotics based on clinical risk factors as ACOG originally described. The second strategy was proposed by the Centers for Disease Control and Prevention (CDC) in 1996. Group B streptococcal urogenital cultures are obtained in all women beginning at 35 to 37 weeks' gestation and those with a positive culture are treated with penicillin G intrapartum. If women deliver prior to this time, they should be given intrapartum penicillin if they have one of the previously mentioned clinical risk factors. The CDC also recommends that previous infants with GBS disease and maternal antepartum GBS bacteriuria both are indications for intrapartum prophylaxis.

Current Practices

Because of confusion, conflicting opinions, and lack of definitive data, there has been no universal approach to GBS screening and treatment. Various university hospitals surveyed indicated that strategies, including implementation of the guidelines of the ACOG were incorporated between late 1992 and 1995. At Parkland Hospital, we were concerned about antimicrobial resistance and maternal morbidity from universal treatment. In early 1995, we adopted a universal GBS prevention program. It followed ACOG guidelines for intrapartum ampicillin prophylaxis of high-risk pregnancies and added neonatal penicillin for infants delivered from high-risk mothers. Infants of any gestational age with signs at birth of neonatal sepsis are not given penicillin prophylaxis; instead antimicrobial treatment is begun after blood cultures are obtained. Asymptomatic infants of low-risk and high-risk mothers (who received intrapartum ampicillin) are administered aqueous penicillin G in the delivery room or within an hour of birth in the nursery. The dosage is 25,000 units for a birth weight of less than 2000 or 50,000 units for a birth weight over 2000 g. The injection is administered after drying the infants, removing any visible maternal blood, and thorough alcohol cleansing of the anterior thigh.

This approach was chosen after reviewing surveillance studies from Parkland Hospital and the Dallas area from 1972 through 1992. There were low early-onset GBS infection rates (0.63 per 1000 live births) from 1981 through 1986, when universal neonatal penicillin G prophylaxis was utilized. The incidence of late-onset GBS disease was unaffected by penicillin prophylaxis. Neonatal sepsis caused by penicillin-resistant organisms or mortality in the penicillin-treated infants was not increased. Importantly, nearly two thirds of cases of early-onset GBS sepsis were in term newborns.

Our GBS prevention program is aimed at universal prophylaxis of each delivery, either maternal ampicillin in GBS high-risk settings or neonatal penicillin G in low-risk situations. Thus, our practice is similar in principle to the 1996 CDC guidelines in recognizing the need for prevention of GBS disease both in high-risk situations and at the low-risk term delivery. Thus, intrapartum antimicrobials are given to women (and their fetuses) with high-risk factors. Rather than performing GBS cultures at 36 weeks to identify low-risk women who may be colonized at a term delivery, we administer prophylaxis to all low-risk term infants. The current hospital cost of a single dose of penicillin G in either dose is $0.14. Thus, the annual costs of the neonatal penicillin program are less than $2000, even if each of the 13,500 deliveries received penicillin prophylaxis. This program costs less than one hospitalization for uncomplicated neonatal GBS septicemia. In the first year of the prophylaxis program, early-onset GBS disease was decreased from 1.6 cases per 1000 live births the previous year to 0.4 per 1000 live births.

Prevention

Because some protection against serious neonatal infection is conferred by maternal antibody, it is logical that vaccination with capsular polysaccharide antigen may prove efficacious. From preliminary findings, maternal immunization to type III antigen produces antibody in about 60% of women. The Institute of Medicine has cited vaccine development as attainable and as a priority.

HELLP Syndrome

James N. Martin, Jr, MD
Everett F. Magann, MD

In the spectrum of patients with severe pre-eclampsia and eclampsia, there is a subset with laboratory evidence of hemolysis, hepatic dysfunction, and thrombocytopenia. Considered secondary to microangiopathic hemolytic anemia that is initiated by ill-defined stimuli, this occurs in approximately 10% of patients with severe pre-eclampsia and up to 50% of patients with eclampsia. This potentially lethal complication of pre-eclampsia was given the acronym of HELLP by Weinstein in 1982, primarily to assist clinicians in appreciating this insidious condition. It can present either as the primary expression of the pre-eclampsia process in pregnant patients or as a secondary phenomenon in others with complicated sepsis, adult respiratory distress syndrome, renal failure, and multiple organ disease with disseminated intravascular coagulation (DIC). Untreated disease will progressively worsen with liver damage, hemorrhage, or rupture, DIC, and multiple organ failure.

The natural history of this disorder is characterized by an initial phase of slow progression followed by an accelerative phase. A decreasing platelet count usually is the initial abnormality detected. Mild thrombocytopenia (platelets >100,000 ≤150,000/μL) can persist for a variable interval of time before an accelerative phase (average daily rate of fall 40,000/μL) is observed into the range of severe thrombocytopenia (midphase >50,000 ≤100,000/μL and late phase ≤50,000/μL). Modest elevations of lactate dehydrogenase (LDH), indirect bilirubin, and aspartate aminotransferase (AST) follow the initial appearance of thrombocytopenia. These worsen rapidly as the liver and vascular tree are progressively affected by microangiopathic hemolytic anemia. Because LDH reflects both the extent of hemolysis and hepatic dysfunction, this laboratory determination and the platelet count are the two most important laboratory tests for disease assessment and surveillance. Variable amounts of hypertension, proteinuria, and edema usually accompany the disease, but these are not in direct proportion to the underlying severity of the HELLP process. The most severe morbidity and mortality associated with HELLP syndrome is encountered when the platelet count falls below 50,000/μL. In the absence of corticosteroid therapy, the disease process usually reaches its nadir 24 to 48 hours after delivery of the placenta, at which time healing in the hepatic and hematologic systems begins the recovery process. Thus, the worst clinical expression of this disorder usually is manifested during the puerperium.

Based on the natural history of HELLP syndrome, for clinical purposes it is conveniently subdivided into an early mild phase when the platelet count is greater than 100,000/μL but less than or equal to 150,000/μL (Class 3), a middle accelerative phase when the platelet count is greater than 50,000/μL but less than or equal to 100,000/μL (Class 2), and a late severe phase when the platelet count is less than 50,000/μL (Class 1).

There are 12 steps to the effective management of patients with HELLP syndrome:

1 Make the Diagnosis

The typical gravida with HELLP syndrome presents with malaise, right upper quadrant/upper abdominal discomfort or pain, recent excessive weight gain, a wide pulse pressure often with systolic hypertension >140 mm Hg and a diastolic pressure less than 90 mm Hg, along with a variety of other nonspecific signs and symptoms including nausea/vomiting. Parameters of pre-eclampsia such as diastolic hypertension, proteinuria, and nondependent edema may not be present at diagnosis and may never be detected in a minority of patients. Some pre-eclamptic patients with HELLP syndrome therefore are erroneously diagnosed with other disease entities. Most patients are preterm, usually in the 26- to 34-week gestational range; they are multiparous or primigravidas with about equal frequency. Late in the course of disease the patient may present with eclampsia (one in six eclamptic patients have HELLP syndrome), hematuria, bleeding from the gums, or severe pain in the abdomen, flank, or shoulder. One in five patients with HELLP syndrome will be diagnosed for the first time during the puerperium.

2 Completely Evaluate the Mother

To make the diagnosis, the suspicious clinician should perform a complete blood count on any patient with possible pre-eclampsia or any other gravid patient with signs, symptoms, or a clinical situation possibly related to HELLP syndrome. Thrombocytopenia, if present, must be associated with other laboratory evidence of hemolysis and hepatic dysfunction to make the diagnosis. In the absence of liver dysfunction, the patient with thrombocytopenia could have gestational thrombocytopenia, immune thrombocytopenia, or another platelet disorder. With HELLP syndrome LDH is high normal or above normal in association with increased values for other tests of hepatic dysfunction such as AST and alanine aminotransferase (ALT). In general, these enzymes increase in amount as the parturient patient becomes more thrombocytopenic. When the platelet count is less than 100,000/μL (Class 1 and 2 HELLP), the LDH usually exceeds 600 IU/L and the AST to ALT ratio is often greater than 2:1 and variably elevated. Evidence of DIC with prolongation of prothrombin and partial thromboplastin times is usually not encountered until late in the disease process (Class 1 HELLP). Usually no renal impairment is present other than variable degrees of proteinuria and hyperuricemia. Hypoglycemia is rare and the total bilirubin rarely exceeds 3 mg%.

In addition to the basic laboratory screening for HELLP syndrome (complete blood count [CBC], urinalysis, LDH, AST, ALT, uric acid, serum creatinine, and indirect and total bilirubin), the managing physician might test for the presence of cocaine or amphetamines, since these can be associated with a pseudo-HELLP syndrome. Severe nutritional and folate deficiency can be causative. More extensive laboratory testing includes screening for lupus erythematosus, Coombs' positive hemolytic anemia, and pancreatitis. Baseline arterial blood gases, pulse oximetry, cultures of the urine and cervix, syphilis serology, hepatitis, and HIV testing may be performed for patients with advanced Class 1 and 2 HELLP syndrome. Serial surveillance of maternal disease status (CBC with platelets, LDH, AST) is repeated as often as every 8 to 12 hours during active disease.

Mothers at highest risk of developing significant maternal morbidity with HELLP syndrome are those who exhibit LDH >1400, uric acid >7.8, AST >150, and/or urine protein of 4+.

3 Evaluate Fetus and Delay or Facilitate Delivery

Because all patients with HELLP syndrome are considered to have severe pre-eclampsia, delivery of the placenta with elimination of the residual gestational decidua is the eventual goal of management. The timing of delivery is determined by the severity of the maternal and fetal condition, the clinical response to treatment, and fetal maturity. Hospitalization of the patient with HELLP syndrome is imperative, with maternal transfer to tertiary care recommended, particularly for very preterm gestations or advanced disease.

Within several hours of diagnosis, an assessment of fetal gestational age (usually by ultrasonography) and well-being (non-stress test, contraction stress test, and/or biophysical profile), as well as a determination of disease extent in the mother, is completed. Corticosteroids for fetal lung maturation and arrest of maternal disease progression are given in double-strength doses (dexamethasone 10 mg IV) soon after admission and repeated every 12 hours until delivery. Presently, we initiate delivery attempts (1) within 24 hours in all patients with Class 1 or 2 HELLP who show no response to dexamethasone therapy; (2) in any patient with a gestational age of 34 weeks or greater; and (3) when there is any evidence of significant maternal or fetal compromise (see Fig. 1). Patients with Class 2 or 3 HELLP syndrome at less than 34 weeks' gestation without obvious maternal-fetal compromise are observed closely for disease progression despite steroid therapy and delivered if the platelet count trends downward toward the Class 1 range of 50,000/μL or less or if the maternal or fetal condition worsens significantly.

4 Control Blood Pressure

Hydralazine is the drug of choice for blood pressure control when systolic pressure exceeds 160 mm Hg or diastolic pressure exceeds 100 mm Hg. The target pressure range is 130 to 160 over 80 to 100 mm Hg. An intermittent bolus intravenously in 5 mg increments works best in our hands.

5 Prevent Seizures with Magnesium Sulfate

Eclamptic convulsions frequently occur in patients with HELLP syndrome. Utilization of intravenously infused magnesium sulfate in the manner traditionally recommended for all patients with severe pre-eclampsia probably acts in multiple roles to prevent seizures, relax the peripheral vascular beds where microangiopathic hemolytic anemia is most active, and enhance renal blood flow.

6 Manage Fluid to Protect the Kidneys

The combination of vasospasm and the loss of endothelial vascular integrity with severe pre-eclampsia and HELLP syndrome narrows the margin of tolerable intravascular volume excess or deficiency, particularly in relation to the kidney. Careful attention is given to alternating liters of 5% dextrose/half-normal saline and 5% lactated Ringer's solution at approximately 100 mL/hr to maintain urine output at 20 mL/hr or greater (usually 30 to 40 mL/hr). Electrolytes are evaluated at least daily with adjustments in fluid made accordingly. Too little fluid intake may exacerbate a vasoconstricted, contracted intravascular volume and insult the kidneys; too much fluid intake may exceed the limits of vascular compensation and overflow into pulmonary and peritoneal low pressure spaces as pulmonary edema and ascites. Central lines are avoided in these patients unless renal output is unresponsive to conservative fluid management with one or two fluid boluses of 500 mL and vascular volume status remains uncertain.

7 Exercise Conservative Transfusion Therapy

Blood products are transfused very conservatively. Generally, packed red cells are administered only for hematocrit determinations of less

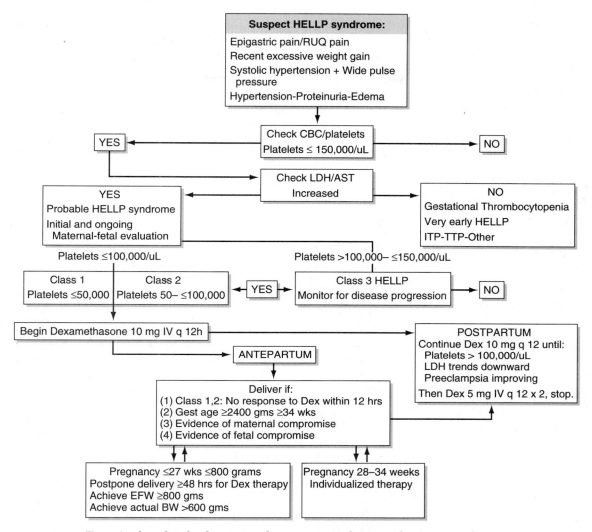

Figure 1. Algorithm for diagnosis and management of suspected HELLP syndrome.

than 22% with maternal hemodynamic instability. Blood replacement at surgery follows traditional guidelines, with transfusion during or soon after cesarean delivery more likely if the preoperative hematocrit is 25% or less and blood loss is above normal. A 6- or 10-unit platelet transfusion is administered immediately preoperatively if the platelet count is 40,000/μL or less (not the usual <50,000/μL recommendation) before cesarean delivery (≤20,000/μL vaginal delivery) or if there is evidence of deficient clotting, active bleeding, or bruising. Intermittent platelet transfusion of 6 to 10 units is utilized in the first 48 hours post-cesarean to maintain a platelet count of 20,000/μL or greater. Use of dexamethasone dramatically reduces the need for blood product transfusion.

Rarely, plasma exchange therapy utilizing a cell separator and 3 to 4 L of fresh frozen plasma is employed in the infrequent patient who fails to show evidence of spontaneous disease resolution within 3 to 5 days' postpartum or if atypical perinatal complications develop such as senso-rium changes, adult respiratory distress syn-drome, or severe multiple organ damage. The use of high-dose dexamethasone around the time of delivery until disease resolution is apparent has almost completely displaced the need for plasma exchange therapy.

8 Labor and Delivery

The utilization of effective cervical ripening agents in association with high-dose dexametha-sone to temporarily arrest the HELLP process can facilitate attempts to deliver the patient vaginally, a preferable mode of delivery since cesarean birth is a hazardous undertaking. If a patient with HELLP syndrome is ≥34 weeks' gestation, attempted delivery is undertaken very soon after the diagnosis is made; if at less than 34 weeks, postponement of delivery for 48 to 96 hours is undertaken if the mother and fetus remain stable so that fetal lung maturation can be achieved (see Fig. 1). Generally, laboring patients are not tocolyzed. All patients usually are treated with dexamethasone even if immediate delivery is contemplated so that morbidity and the possible need for transfusion can be minimized. Cesarean delivery is undertaken for obstetric indications such as fetal malpresentation if efforts at cervical ripening and labor induction fail and if the patient's severe pre-eclampsia or HELLP syndrome deteriorate rapidly into a Class 1 condition despite dexamethasone, and if vaginal delivery is not soon expected.

Use of conduction analgesia is relatively contraindicated if platelets are less than 100,000/μL or the bleeding time is prolonged, or both. During labor, maternal analgesia is provided by intermittently infused butorphanol or meperidine with promethazine. Vaginal delivery is undertaken with local infiltration analgesia but usually without pudendal block; cesarean delivery is performed under balanced general anesthesia. Intramuscular injections and central lines are minimized. Antibiotic coverage is provided for cesarean delivery, particularly if any form of transfusion therapy is utilized. Careful attention to hemostasis is given during abdominal delivery. Low vertical incisions are often used in preterm pregnancies with poorly developed lower uterine segments to minimize the risk of incision extension laterally and to provide adequate area for atraumatic delivery of the fragile fetus. The vesicouterine peritoneum is not closed, a Smead Jones fascial closure or mass closure is frequently utilized, and the skin and subcutaneous tissue are either left open or closed over a Jackson-Pratt drain perforating the skin separate from the incision. If ascites is encountered at surgery, central line placement is considered to help guide fluid management and plans are made to follow more intensively the patient's cardiorespiratory, renal, and fluid status during the ensuing 48 hours. Exploration of the upper abdomen is very gently undertaken in view of the increased risk of hepatic rupture in Class 1 patients and those with epigastric pain.

9 Fetal and Neonatal Care

HELLP syndrome is primarily a disease of prematurity. Owing to the relatively impaired fetoplacental circulation common to all mothers with severe pre-eclampsia, the fetus is in a precarious position that is best assessed by continuous electronic fetal monitoring once the diagnosis of HELLP is made. Maternal referral to an appropriate venue for optimal maternal and neonatal care is recommended prior to delivery, especially in the very preterm pregnancy and the patient with Class 1 HELLP syndrome (if stable). Once the mother's platelet count decreases to less than 50,000/μL, the incidence of fetal or neonatal intracranial hemorrhage increases considerably, particularly in the preterm gestation. Assessment of the neonatal platelet count is recommended.

10 Manage Postpartum Period

All patients with severe pre-eclampsia/eclampsia and HELLP syndrome are intensively monitored in an appropriate site for 24 to 48 hours or longer and until (1) the platelet count begins to trend upward and the LDH downward, (2) the patient begins to diurese greater than 100 mL/hr consistently, (3) hypertension is well controlled with orally administered hydralazine (25–75 mg q 6 hr) in the less than 150 mm Hg systolic and less than 100 mm Hg diastolic range, and (4) clinical improvement is obvious in the absence of any specific complication or concern. After delivery, attempts to keep diastolic blood pressure no higher than 100 and no lower than 80 are encouraged. Laboratory tests for disease surveillance (CBC with platelets, LDH) and general evaluation—electrolytes and renal and liver function testing—are repeated frequently until recovery is assured. Usually this trend begins within 48 hours or almost always within 72 hours postpartum. Intravenously infused magnesium sulfate is continued until the patient's microangiopathic hemolytic anemia shows evidence of recovery. Dexamethasone 10 mg IV q 12 hours is continued until recovery is apparent and then discontinued, with 5 mg IV q 12 hours × 2 over the last 24 hours of treatment. Coagulation testing of prothrombin, partial thromboplastin time and fibrinogen is rarely performed unless the platelet count decreases below 50,000/μL or there is active bleeding.

11 Be Watchful for Hepatic/Renal/ Respiratory Failure

Reflective of disease severity, patients with progressively fewer platelets in HELLP syndrome are increasingly at risk for maternal morbidity and mortality. The mother with severe or long-standing epigastric pain unresponsive to steroids is at high risk for hepatic hemorrhage and/or rupture; her management should be aggressive pregnancy termination with intensive surveillance for signs and symptoms of hypovolemic shock. If liver rupture occurs, appropriate therapy (surgical hemostasis or vascular occlusion therapy) must be instituted rapidly. The mother with significant blood loss due to hepatic hemorrhage, rupture, cesarean birth, or postpartum hemorrhage is at high risk for acute renal failure and acute respiratory failure. Rapid, timely normalization of blood volume with replacement fluids and blood products is necessary to avert insult to compromised endothelial, alveolar, and glomerular tissue. Intake and output are carefully monitored and manipulated. When tachypnea (>24 respirations/minute) develops, pulmonary consultation is requested and intensive pulmonary therapy including oxygen is undertaken. In the "neglected" patient with advanced disease who is received late in transfer, aggressive plasma exchange therapy may be necessary to "cleanse" the circulation of debris and facilitate rapid reduction of the disease process.

12 Counsel for Future Pregnancy

A recurrence rate of HELLP syndrome up to 25% has been observed. The risk of recurrence in a subsequent pregnancy is highest for patients who developed very preterm, Class 1 HELLP syndrome analogous to the situation with very preterm, severe pre-eclampsia. Low-dose aspirin (80 mg/day) can be used from 6 to 36 weeks in patients with previous Class 1 or 2 HELLP syndrome, particularly if it was virulent or complicated, for instance, by placental abruption or hepatic hemorrhage.

Summary

The management of HELLP syndrome in pregnancy is undergoing change and the proper place of high-dose corticosteroids such as dexamethasone in the overall scheme of care is under intense study. Early aggressive and sustained use of this agent until disease recovery is apparent as a cornerstone of therapy to minimize maternal and fetal risk. The three-class scheme of classification both emphasizes the natural history of the disorder and functions as a framework for the clinician. Transfer of the undelivered mother to tertiary care while she is still in the Class 3 range, especially with a preterm pregnancy, is advisable

not only for neonatal considerations but also for optimization of maternal care. The gravida who develops virulent, Class 1 HELLP syndrome with multiple organ dysfunction or failure can tax the resources and expertise of even the most high-powered perinatal centers.

Human Immunodeficiency Virus in Pregnancy

Patrick Duff, MD

Several conditions have traditionally caused great concern among obstetricians; their approximate prevalence is listed in Table 1. Many millions of dollars are spent annually in efforts to prevent these disorders. Unfortunately, the human immunodeficiency virus (HIV) epidemic has now increased to the point that HIV infection in pregnancy is more common than any of these conditions. The prevalence of HIV infection even in low-risk populations is close to 1 in 1000. In high-risk populations, the prevalence may approach 1% to 2%. Although HIV infection occurs primarily in large and medium-sized metropolitan areas, no geographic locale or selected patient population is exempt. Accordingly, all obstetricians must become familiar with the diagnosis and care of women with this devastating illness.

Antepartum Care

All patients should be offered voluntary serologic testing for HIV infection. Mandatory testing is virtually unenforceable and probably would serve to drive away from the health care system the very individuals who are most in need of prenatal assessment. Selective screening of only those pa-

TABLE 1. Prevalence of Selected Obstetric Complications

Condition	Approximate Prevalence (No. of Pregnancies)
Congenital rubella syndrome	1 in 300,000
Neonatal herpes infection	1 in 20,000 to 1 in 7,500
Abdominal wall defects	1 in 10,000 to 1 in 5000
Down syndrome	1 in 1000
Open neural tube defect	1 in 1000 to 1 in 500

tients who acknowledge high-risk behavior will fail to identify up to half of infected patients. Counseling should be provided prior to and after testing.

Patients who test seropositive require extensive additional counseling regarding the social, economic, and medical aspects of their disease. This counseling is best accomplished by a multidisciplinary team composed of social worker, nutritionist, obstetrician, and medical infectious disease specialist or immunologist. A referral for treatment of drug addiction should be made, if indicated. Patients who smoke should be urged to quit. The patient should be encouraged to inform other family members, particularly her sexual partner, of her condition. The latter individual should be offered serologic testing for infection. If he is seronegative, the couple should be advised to use protective condoms and spermicides when having intercourse so that the male partner does not subsequently become infected.

The patient should be advised that, in the absence of intervention, approximately 20% to 30% of infants born to seropositive mothers develop HIV infection. Risk of vertical transmission is increased if the mother is overtly ill or severely immunocompromised, if she has previously delivered an infected infant, or if her viral load is high.

The option of pregnancy termination should be discussed. Women should be informed that pregnancy per se does not appear to accelerate the progression of HIV infection, but that HIV infection is associated with an increased frequency of obstetric complications such as preterm delivery, preterm premature rupture of membranes, intrauterine growth restriction, and postpartum infection.

The patient should be tested for other sexually transmitted diseases such as gonorrhea, chlamydia, herpes, syphilis, and hepatitis B, C, and D. She also should have serologic testing for cytomegalovirus and toxoplasmosis. She should be offered vaccination for influenza, pneumococcal infection, hepatitis A, and hepatitis B and observed frequently for opportunistic infections such as candidiasis, *Mycobacterium avium* complex (MAC), and *Pneumocystis carinii* pneumonia. She also should have a tuberculin skin test with an appropriate intradermal control to be certain that she is not anergic. If the test is positive or anergy is present, a chest radiograph should be taken to rule out active tuberculosis. If the chest radiograph is negative, daily chemoprophylaxis with isoniazid (INH), 300 mg orally, and pyridoxine (vitamin B_6), 50 mg orally, should be administered. If the chest radiograph is positive, multidrug chemotherapy is indicated, and treatment should be supervised by a pulmonary medicine or infectious disease consultant.

At the time that HIV infection is first diagnosed, the patient should have a CD_4 count and determination of viral load (HIV-RNA-PCR). She then should be offered treatment with three antiviral agents. Although there is no definitive evidence yet that multidrug therapy reduces the rate of perinatal transmission of HIV more than that achieved by zidovudine monotherapy, recent studies clearly indicate that multidrug therapy is more effective than single-dose therapy in inhibiting viral replication and prolonging survival of the adult.

Table 2 lists the many drugs now available for treatment of HIV infection. Based on considerations of efficacy, cost, and maternal and fetal safety, a reasonable three-drug regimen in pregnancy would be zidovudine, lamivudine, and nelfinavir. The first two drugs can be administered together in a fixed dose combination as Combivir (zidovudine, 300 mg, plus lamivudine, 150 mg) twice daily.

HIV-infected patients also should receive prophylactic antibiotics to protect against certain opportunistic infections. Specific guidelines are summarized in Table 3.

Intrapartum Care

During labor, every effort should be made to avoid procedures that might result in breaks in the skin or mucous membranes of the infant. Therefore, amniotomy, attachment of the scalp electrode, and determination of scalp blood pH should not be performed unless absolutely necessary. The effect of cesarean delivery on risk of perinatal transmission has not been precisely delineated, particularly in patients receiving multiagent antiviral chemotherapy. Accordingly, cesarean should be performed only for accepted obstetric indications.

Precautions should be taken to protect health care workers from contact with potentially infectious body fluids. To accomplish this objective, obstetric attendants should observe universal precautions for all patients. Needles should not be recapped and should be deposited in puncture-proof containers. Caps, masks, eye shields, water-repellent gowns, and double or reinforced gloves should be worn for all surgical procedures. Mechanical suctioning devices should be used to remove secretions and meconium from the neonate's airway.

TABLE 2. Antiviral Agents for Treatment of HIV Infection

Agent	Usual Adult Dose	Remarks	Cost of 30 Day Treatment
Nucleotide Analog			
Adefovir dipivoxil	120 mg qd	Principal adverse effects are GI irritation, elevation in transaminase concentrations, and decrease in serum carnitine level	Not yet available
Nucleoside Analogs			
Abacavir	300 mg bid	Most serious adverse effect is a hypersensitivity reaction (2–5% of patients).	$350.00
Didanosine (DDI, Videx)	200 mg bid	Most serious adverse effects are pancreatitis and peripheral neuropathy.	$194.00
Lamivudine (3TC, Epivir)	150 mg bid	Adverse effects are similar to those of zidovudine but are less frequent. Drug is eliminated by renal excretion.	$230.00
Stavudine (d4T, Zerit)	40 mg bid	Main adverse effect is peripheral sensory neuropathy.	$254.00
Zalcitabine (ddC, HIVID)	0.75 mg q8h	Most serious adverse effect is peripheral neuropathy. Pancreatitis also can occur. Least potent of the nucleoside analogs.	$207.00
Zidovudine (Retrovir)	300 mg bid	Main adverse effect is marrow suppression.	$287.00
Non-nucleoside Reverse Transcriptase Inhibitors			
Delavirdine (Rescriptor)	400 mg tid	Most common side effect is rash; it usually is less severe than the one associated with nevirapine. Hepatitis also can occur.	$222.00
Nevirapine (Viramune)	200 mg bid	Most common adverse effect is rash. If the rash is extensive, the drug should be permanently discontinued. Hepatitis is a rare side effect.	$248.00
Efavirenz (Sustiva)	600 mg qd	Most common adverse effects are rash and CNS changes. The drug is teratogenic and should not be used during pregnancy.	$410.00
Protease Inhibitors			
Amprenavir	1200 mg bid	Most common adverse effects are rash and GI irritation.	To be released in 1999
Indinavir (Crixivan)	800 mg q8h	Well tolerated. Most serious adverse effect is nephrolithiasis. Most common side effect is GI upset. Less expensive than ritonavir.	$450.00
Nelfinavir (Viracept)	750 mg tid	Clinical efficacy data are limited. Most common adverse effects are diarrhea, fatigue, poor concentration.	$557.00
Ritonavir (Norvir)	600 mg q12h	Most likely drug in this class to cause adverse effects. Can be given in a convenient twice-daily dosing regimen. Major side effect is GI irritation. Should be taken with meals. It has major potential for interactions with other drugs.	$668.00
Saquinavir (Invirase and Fortovase)	600 mg tid	Least effective of the protease inhibitors. Should not be used as monotherapy. Drug has low oral bioavailability and must be taken with a high-fat meal.	$572.00

TABLE 3. Guidelines for Prophylaxis for Selected Opportunistic Infections

Condition	Indication for Prophylaxis	Antibiotic
Pneumocystis carinii pneumonia	Prior infection or CD_4 <200/mm³	Trimethoprim-sulfamethoxazole-DS, one PO qd indefinitely
Toxoplasmic encephalitis	Positive serology and CD_4 <100/mm³	Trimethoprim-sulfamethoxazole-DS, one PO qd indefinitely
Tuberculosis	Positive PPD (>5 mm reaction)	Isoniazid, 300 mg PO qd plus pyridoxine, 50 mg PO qd × 12 mo
Disseminated infection with *Mycobacterium avium* complex	CD_4 <50/mm³	Azithromycin, 1200 mg weekly
Cryptococcosis	CD_4 <50/mm³	Fluconazole, 200 mg PO qd indefinitely

Postpartum Care

During the postpartum period, patients in developed nations should be advised to bottle-feed their infants because of the risk of transmission of HIV infection by breast milk. They also should be cautioned to avoid contact between their body fluids and open lesions on the infant's skin or mucous membranes.

The most important aspect of postpartum care is counseling concerning responsible sexual and family planning practices. Since HIV infection is not curable, women should be offered secure contraception or sterilization. Anal intercourse and unprotected intercourse should be discouraged, and patients should be advised to avoid sex when they are having their menses or when they or their partner have vesicular lesions (e.g., herpes, syphilis, chancroid) on the genitalia. The patient's pivotal role in transmission of a life-threatening infection should be emphasized, and the dangers of sexual promiscuity should be highlighted. Finally, the obstetrician must be certain that comprehensive long-term care is coordinated for both the infected mother and her infant.

Hyperemesis Gravidarum

Janet D. Larson, MD
William F. Rayburn, MD

Vomiting during the first half of gestation accompanies approximately half of all pregnancies. Persistent vomiting is known as hyperemesis gravidarum if it causes weight loss and fluid, electrolyte, and acid-base imbalances. This condition is estimated to occur in 0.5 to 10 per 1000 gestations. The peak occurrence is between the 8th and 12th week of pregnancy. No known relation exists between the incidence of hyperemesis and race, socioeconomic status, or prenuptial conception.

Evaluation

Vomiting is under the control of two distinct medullary centers in the brain: the vomiting center and the nearby chemoreceptor trigger zone. Listed in Table 1 are pregnancy, gastrointestinal, genitourinary, and miscellaneous causes for vomiting. With each cause, any combination of three major factors may be involved: impulses arising from the gastrointestinal tract, central or cerebral impulses, and chemical materials transported in the blood.

The specific etiology of hyperemesis gravidarum is unknown. Proposed causes include disturbances of carbohydrate metabolism, vitamin B deficiencies, endocrine imbalances, and genetic incompatibility. Each has been studied clinically, but none has been proven definitively. Since hyperemesis is more common in multifetal gestations and molar pregnancies, a relationship with elevated maternal serum levels of human chorionic gonadotropin (hCG) has been proposed. Measurements of hCG levels in affected patients have yielded conflicting results with levels being higher, lower, or similar to those of uncomplicated pregnancies.

Along with weight loss, chronic hypovolemia and dehydration may lead to a rise in maternal pulse rate, fall in blood pressure, dryness of the tongue, loss of skin elasticity, and ketotic odor of

TABLE 1. Evaluation of Persistent Vomiting During Pregnancy

Cause	Test
Pregnancy	
Multifetal gestation	Ultrasonography
Hydatidiform mole	Serum quantitative beta human chorionic gonadotropin
Gastrointestinal	
Reflux disorder	Serum chemistry
Hepatitis	Profile
Biliary tract disease	Serum thyroid hepatitis panel
Pancreatitis	
Inflammatory or obstructive bowel disease	
Genitourinary	Urinalysis
Pyelonephritis	
Uremia	
Miscellaneous	
Drug toxicity	Urine drug screen
Diabetic ketosis	
Hyperthyroidism	Thyroid function tests
Vestibular disorders	
Central nervous system lesions	

the breath. Diplopia, disorientation, uncoordinated movements, and coma may be rarely found due to hepatorenal failure. Laboratory findings, as shown in Table 1, may reveal ketonuria, increased urine specific gravity, elevations in the hematocrit and blood urea nitrogen, hyponatremia, hypokalemia, hypochloremia, and metabolic alkalosis with paradoxical aciduria. Mild increases in bilirubin and other liver function tests may also be present.

Unquestionably, psychological factors contribute to this condition. Circumstances to consider would include an unsuitable diet, poor communication with the father-to-be and family, poor communication with the obstetrician, stress and doubts about continuing the pregnancy, and inadequate information about pregnancy. It is important to attempt to determine whether the patient is looking for a secondary gain similar to that seen in conversion reactions.

Therapeutic Considerations

Hyperemesis gravidarum is a diagnosis of exclusion and other causes of vomiting must be ruled out or, if found, treated. Therapy as early as possible seems warranted. The average weight of newborns is significantly lower in patients experiencing hyperemesis. A relation between nutrition and teratogenicity has been suggested, but congenital anomalies and hyperemesis are open to criticism.

The fetus can utilize ketones, which are readily transmitted across the placenta, as a source of energy. While there is considerable evidence that ketones can be readily utilized by the fetus, there are no direct experimental data showing that ketones are toxic. Regardless of whether they produce any adverse effect, ketones appear to be a clinical marker of an unfavorable environment for the fetus.

Nutrition Advice

Ideally, early treatment of nausea and vomiting during pregnancy will prevent progression to hyperemesis gravidarum. The obstetrician should give emotional support, since poor communication with the patient and inadequate information about pregnancy are correlated with nausea and vomiting. Initial intervention should include reassurance and the recommendation of multiple small meals, sufficient in fluid and calories to prevent dehydration and ketonuria. Although not proven to be effective, liquids are recommended between, rather than with, meals. Liquid meals and sports drinks are often tolerated. Recommendations to increase the amount of carbohydrates and to decrease the amount of fats, spicy foods, and caffeine in the diet have been published, as well as the advice to avoid bothersome odors. Simply fulfilling a food craving may help on the premise that the patient would not crave something that would make her more nauseated.

Vitamin supplementation, as a means of relieving hyperemesis, is not known to be beneficial. Prenatal vitamins contain 2.5 mg of vitamin B_6 or pyridoxine, which may be taken daily. A larger daily dose using a 50 mg or 100 mg pill has been found in one study to reduce the findings of nausea and vomiting. No association between vitamin B_6 and congenital anomalies has been reported.

Psychotherapy

Consideration should be given to evaluating the patient for psychosocial pathology. Early psychologic intervention could contribute greatly, as well as being cost-effective when compared with in-patient medical treatment. Psychotherapy is recommended if personality variables or if marital or family conflicts seem to play a major role. Social work assistance is often helpful in decreasing the stress from inadequate financial support, housing, and social support.

When pregnant women do not respond to the medical and supportive care by the obstetric and nursing staff, a psychiatric evaluation is advisable. Supportive psychotherapy entails establishing a positive relationship, frequent reassuring conversations, and encouraging the expression of thoughts and feelings. Hypnotherapy consists of a trance induction and suggestions for comfort in the gastrointestinal tract, the desirability of feeling substance in the stomach, and the ability to retain and digest food. Behavior modification provides positive reinforcement for retaining food and gaining weight through granting desirable considerations, such as visitors, radio and television, and ambulating in or outside the hospital room. Studies on psychotherapy as an adjunct to the treatment of hyperemesis gravidarum have been scarce, however, and when controlled, have examined series that are too small to provide valid comparisons of treatment differences.

Drug Treatment

The value of drug therapy, if any, is at the stage of intractable vomiting, when any of the present antiemetic agents may be used to counter the feeling of nausea. By beginning medication at the onset of intractable vomiting, progression to hyperemesis gravidarum may be prevented. Several medications have been prescribed, but none has been clearly shown to be most preferred. Listed on Table 2 are examples of such medications. Many of these drugs are hypnotics with antihistamine properties or are used for motion sickness. Serious cardiovascular, hematologic, or dermatologic side effects are rare. Extrapyramidal effects, such as spasms of the neck, observed with certain antiemetics (e.g., metoclopramide, prochlorperazine), may be reversed with diphenhydramine.

Adequate or well-controlled studies about antiemetics are lacking during pregnancy. Reproductive studies in rodents and rabbits, using high daily oral doses, reveal no evidence of impaired fertility or harm to the fetus. While no direct fetotoxic effects are observed in humans and animals, sporadic abortions occur among patients with significantly reduced food intake. Epidemiologic studies about diphenhydramine, promethazine, and meclizine during early gestation have failed to associate drug use with an increase in congenital anomalies. Case reports in humans have not reported adverse pregnancy outcomes for women who took either metoclopramide or histamine-receptor antagonists. We were unable to locate reports about serotonin 5-HT3 blockers during gestation.

A single medication should be prescribed initially, beginning with the lowest daily dose, which is increased until vomiting is reduced or has subsided. A combination of drugs is necessary when a maximal dose of a single agent is insufficient. The medication is routinely taken before meals and at bedtime.

TABLE 2. Examples of Antiemetic Agents and Common Administration

Agent	Administration
Phenothiazine	
Promethazine (Phenergan)	25 mg PO or IV q 4–6 h
Prochlorperazine (Compazine)	10 mg PO or IM tid, qid
Piperazine antihistamine	
Meclizine (Antivert)	25 to 50 mg PO bid, qid
Antihistamine	
Diphenhydramine HCl (Benadryl)	25 to 50 mg PO bid, qid
Histamine-receptor antagonist	
Famotidine (Pepcid)	10 to 20 mg PO or IM q 12 h
Ranitidine (Zantac)	75 mg PO bid 60 mg IV q 6–8 h
Dopamine antagonist	
Metoclopramide (Reglan)	10 to 15 mg PO bid to qid
Serotonin 5-HD blocker	
Ondansetron (Zofran)	32 mg IV q 4–8h 8 mg PO tid
Inhibitor of gastric secretion	
Omeprazole (Prilosec)	20 mg PO q d

Hospitalization and Home Therapy

If vomiting persists despite out-patient therapy, weight loss, ketonemia, dehydration, electrolyte imbalance, and possibly hepatic and renal damage may result. Hospitalization is indicated for parenteral fluid and electrolyte replacement and, in some cases, hyperalimentation. The differential diagnosis of intractable vomiting must be reconsidered to exclude any underlying disease. A low-dose infusion of promethazine may be helpful. The addition of an intravenous multivitamin supplement has been reported to cease hyperemesis within 24 hours. Putting the gut at rest is a staple of therapy, with a gradual reintroduction of the diet after vomiting has ceased. Psychosocial counseling must be reconsidered.

Parenteral hyperalimentation is indicated after symptoms of nausea and vomiting persist and the standard peripheral venous crystalloid solutions fail to maintain and restore an anabolic state. Favorable pregnancy outcomes have been reported using a combination of dextrose, fat, protein, vitamins, trace elements, and electrolytes. Except for the need of additional calories for pregnancy, the daily nutritional requirements for hyperalimentation would be the same as in a nongravid patient. Administration of a peripheral intravenous lipid system should precede the central intravenous route unless long-term administration (i.e., more than 14 days) is contemplated or renal impairment exists. Much expense and possible toxic, metabolic, and infectious complications require careful monitoring.

Hyperemesis usually resolves by 20 weeks' gestation. However, symptoms may rarely persist throughout pregnancy. Small-bore nasogastric feeding tubes, along with antiemetic medications, have been reported successful. If necessary, long-term hyperalimentation may be undertaken with central intravenous placement. Consideration may be given to sending a stable patient home with enteral or parenteral nutrition. Most communities have the capability of home health care with hyperalimentation and visiting nurse services.

Hypertensive Diseases of Pregnancy: Role of Calcium and Low-Dose Aspirin

Andrea G. Witlin, DO
Baha M. Sibai, MD

Definition and Classification

Pre-eclampsia is a form of hypertension that is unique to human pregnancy and is a major cause of maternal and perinatal morbidity and mortality worldwide. The incidence of pre-eclampsia ranges between 5% and 10% in primigravidas and between 3% and 5% in multiparas. The incidence is increased with multifetal gestation and in women with previous pre-eclampsia. Our comprehension of the etiology of pre-eclampsia remains elusive. This lack of understanding complicates our efforts to establish effective screening programs and thus to reduce the incidence of pre-eclampsia and its associated morbidity and mortality.

Screening for Pre-eclampsia

The ideal screening test should identify an important and prevalent disease. The disease should be able to be identified at an early and recognizable stage. Furthermore, an acceptable treatment should be available for the disease that is being screened for. The screening test should be safe, reliable, and acceptable to the population being screened and should be available at a reasonable cost. Pre-eclampsia certainly meets the first criterion as an important disease that many practitioners have spent lifetimes attempting to conquer. However, the ideal screening test for early detection of pre-eclampsia has eluded us.

Populations at greatest risk for the development of pre-eclampsia include young, nulliparous women from lower socioeconomic environments. Although this describes a subgroup of women at greatest risk, it excludes many women who will ultimately develop pre-eclampsia.

A review of the world literature reveals that more than 100 clinical, biophysical, and biochemical tests have been recommended to predict or identify women at risk for the development of pre-eclampsia. The results of the combined data and lack of agreement between serial tests suggest that none of these clinical tests is reliable for use as a screening test. Several prominent tests will be reviewed.

Since hypertension is the hallmark of pre-eclampsia, it was thought that elevations in blood pressure early in gestation may be helpful in predicting those women destined to develop pre-eclampsia. The value of mean arterial blood pressure determinations in the second trimester of pregnancy had been investigated for its role in predicting pre-eclampsia. Unfortunately, the sensitivity of mean arterial pressure readings ranged from 0% to 99% and the specificity ranged from 53% to 97% for development of pre-eclampsia. Likewise, the "rollover test" had been evaluated for its role in prediction of pre-eclampsia with sensitivities ranging from 0% to 93% and specificities ranging from 54% to 91%. The results from these various studies suggest that although both of these tests are inexpensive and simple to perform, neither is sufficiently reliable for use as a screening test in clinical practice. Moreover, even if the women at risk are identified, what can be done to prevent pre-eclampsia from occurring?

The angiotensin infusion test, as first described by Gant, utilizes an exogenous infusion of angiotensin II and identifies those women with an increase in diastolic blood pressure greater than 20 mm Hg as being at risk for development of pre-eclampsia. Vascular sensitivity to angiotensin II increases as early as 18 weeks' gestation in women who become pre-eclamptic. This gestational age is far earlier than when pre-eclampsia generally becomes clinically apparent. Although early reports of the angiotensin infusion test were encouraging, subsequent studies have failed to duplicate these results as being predictive for the development of pre-eclampsia. Moreover, the test is expensive, complex and invasive and therefore would not be acceptable for screening large numbers of women.

Plasma cellular fibronectin is an insoluble glycoprotein present in the extracellular matrix, produced by endothelial cells and fibroblasts, and released into the circulation after endothelial injury. It is elevated in women with pre-eclampsia, with the elevations being seen as early as the second trimester. Although there is a significant difference between women with pre-eclampsia and control subjects, there is a large overlap in the values between the two groups, thus limiting clinical application.

Urinary calcium excretion has been shown to be decreased at term in women with pre-eclampsia. Reduced urinary calcium excretion has also been noted several weeks prior to the development of pre-eclampsia. The mechanism for this is unclear. A positive predictive value of less than 50% limits the value of this test for early prediction of pre-eclampsia.

Uterine artery Doppler studies have identified a diastolic notch early in the second trimester in women destined to develop pre-eclampsia. Although this test is safe and acceptable for screening pregnant women, it is somewhat expensive and limited by the personnel required for performing it. Once again, positive predictive values are quite low—less than 30%.

A combination of epidemiologic factors and clinical and laboratory tests may predict some of the women destined to develop pre-eclampsia. As described, many of these tests do not meet the criteria for the ideal screening test. Once again, we are limited in our abilities to prevent pre-eclampsia even in those women whom we identify as being at high risk.

Prevention of Pre-eclampsia

A major impediment for development of effective prevention programs for pre-eclampsia is the incomplete understanding of the etiology and pathophysiology of the disease. Recent prevention strategies have focused on areas related to pathogenesis of the disease: affecting the heightened vascular sensitivity to pressor substances as described earlier and altering prostaglandin synthesis to limit endothelial injury.

Various drug and dietary manipulations have been recommended for prevention of pre-eclampsia. No efficacy has been found for salt restriction, diuretic therapy, or high protein diets. Moreover, dietary sodium restriction and diuretic therapy reduce blood volume without reducing the frequency of hypertension.

Zinc deficiency has been studied, since zinc is an essential element in oxidative metabolism, DNA/RNA synthesis, immunocompetence, and membrane stabilization. Zinc deficiency at the time of conception is associated with teratogenesis. Low levels of zinc have been associated with adverse pregnancy outcomes such as intrauterine growth restriction and pre-eclampsia. Conflicting reports exist regarding the benefits of zinc supplementation during pregnancy. Moreover, zinc deficiency is extremely rare in humans, so routine zinc supplementation cannot be recommended at this time.

Magnesium is essential in cyclic adenosine monophosphate–dependent membrane transport, glycolysis, and genetic transcription and translation. There is some suggestion that antepartum magnesium supplementation may improve perinatal outcome. Current data are conflicting. As magnesium deficiency is rare, routine supplementation is not recommended at this time.

Serum calcium homeostasis is under hormonal control. Enhanced calcium absorption from the gut and physiologic hypercalciuria occur during pregnancy. In conjunction with fetal calcium needs, this suggests a need for maintaining adequate dietary calcium intake during pregnancy (1200 mg elemental calcium per day). Several studies have suggested an increase in blood pressure in those patients with decreased dietary calcium. The mechanism for this calcium-related hypotensive effect is unclear. The effect may be mediated through altered levels of parathyroid hormone with resultant decrease in intracellular ionized calcium. This in turn may relax the myocyte and produce arteriolar relaxation and blood pressure reduction.

Epidemiologic studies suggest an inverse relationship between dietary calcium intake and maternal blood pressure and the incidence of pre-eclampsia and eclampsia. The blood pressure–lowering effect of calcium was thought to be mediated by alterations in plasma renin activity and parathyroid hormone. In addition to the arteriolar relaxation as described earlier, uterine smooth muscle relaxation may also occur. Calcium supplementation was also shown to reduce angiotensin II vascular sensitivities in such pregnancies.

Two recently published meta-analyses found calcium supplementation in pregnancy effective in reducing both systolic and diastolic blood pressure (odds ratio, 0.44; 95% CI, 0.33–0.59) with a trend toward reducing the incidence of pre-eclampsia (odds ratio, 0.34; 95% CI, 0.22–0.54). However, the beneficial effect of calcium on major maternal and fetal morbidity and mortality remains unsubstantiated. These studies vary according to population studied (low risk or high risk for hypertension), definition of hypertensive disorders of pregnancy, study design, gestational age at enrollment, sample size in each group (range, 22–588), and dose of elemental calcium used (156–2000 mg/d). No adverse effects of calcium supplementation have been identified (Table 1).

Recently, a large multicenter trial (sponsored by the National Institute of Child Health and Human Development) to assess the benefits of calcium supplementation in healthy nulliparous women has been completed. This study included about 4600 nulliparous women who were assigned to take either 2 g of elemental calcium or a matching placebo. The incidence of pre-eclampsia as well as hypertension was similar in both groups.

Enhanced platelet activation with imbalance of thromboxane and prostacyclin is associated with the vasospasm and activation of the coagulation-hemostasis systems seen in pre-eclampsia. Thromboxane is associated with platelet aggregation and vasoconstriction, whereas prostacyclin is associated with platelet aggregation and vasodilation. Aspirin inhibits the synthesis of prostaglandins by irreversibly acetylating and inactivating the enzyme cyclooxygenase. Platelets, unlike endothelial cells that have a nucleus, are incapable of resynthesizing the enzyme. In vitro studies suggest that platelet cyclooxygenase is more sensitive to inhibition by very low doses of aspirin (<80 mg) than vascular endothelial cyclooxygenase. Therefore, treatment with low doses of aspirin could alter the balance between prostacyclin and thromboxane. A review by Dekker and Sibai suggests a beneficial effect for prophylactic ingestion of low-dose aspirin (60–81 mg/d) for the reduction in incidence and severity of pre-eclampsia. The inference from these studies is that the enhanced vascular responsiveness to angiotensin II infusions may be mediated by an imbalance in thromboxane and prostaglandin I_2 production and may be corrected by ingestion of low-dose aspirin in women at high risk for pre-eclampsia.

Hauth and colleagues studied 604 healthy nulliparous women randomly assigned at 24 weeks' gestation to receive either 60 mg/d of aspirin or placebo. The incidence of pre-eclampsia was significantly lower in the aspirin-treated group; however, there were no differences regarding gestational age at delivery, neonatal birth weight, or frequency of fetal growth restriction or preterm delivery.

A subsequent multicenter study by Sibai and colleagues included 2985 healthy, nulliparous women, randomly assigned at 13 to 26 weeks' gestation to aspirin (60 mg daily) or placebo. This study showed a reduction in the incidence

TABLE 1. Effect of Calcium Supplementation on the Incidence of Pre-eclampsia

Study	Calcium (%)	Control (%)	Odds Ratio and 95% Confidence Interval		
			0.1	1	10
Villar	4	11			
López-Jaramillo	0	24			
Montanaro	2	10			
Villar	0	3			
López-Jaramillo	0	24			
Belizán	3	4			
Sanchez-Ramos	14	44			
Typical Odds Ratio	0.29	0.18–0.47			

of pre-eclampsia by 26% percent in the aspirin treated women. Again, there were no differences in mean gestational age at delivery, birth weight, frequency of fetal growth restriction, or frequency of preterm delivery. Moreover, a significantly higher incidence of abruptio placentae was identified in women receiving aspirin. Despite a reduction in the incidence of pre-eclampsia, perinatal outcome was not improved with such therapy.

The Collaborative Low-Dose Aspirin Study in Pregnancy (CLASP) trial is a multinational randomized trial involving 9364 women. Women selected for the study were deemed at sufficient risk of pre-eclampsia or intrauterine growth restriction for the use of low-dose aspirin to be contemplated, but without clear indications for or against its use. The women received either low-dose aspirin (60 mg/d) or placebo, with randomization occurring between 12 to 32 weeks' gestation. The two study groups failed to identify a difference regarding the incidence of pre-eclampsia, intrauterine growth retardation, abruptio placentae, or perinatal deaths. The aspirin-treated group did have a lower incidence of preterm delivery.

The ECCPA trial (Estudo Colaborativo para Prevencao da Pre-eclampsia com Aspirina) from Brazil randomized 970 women at significant risk for development of pre-eclampsia to low-dose aspirin (60 mg/d) or placebo. The women selected for this study were at significant risk for development of pre-eclampsia or its sequelae, but were without clear indications for or against the use of aspirin. Randomization occurred at 12 to 32 weeks' gestation. There was no significant reduction in the incidence of pre-eclampsia nor was an increased incidence of abruption identified (Fig. 1).

Recently, a multicenter trial, sponsored by the National Institute of Child Health and Human Development, has been completed evaluating the effect of low-dose aspirin in high risk women (previous pre-eclampsia/eclampsia, chronic hypertension, class B–F diabetes, multifetal gestation). Over 2500 women were randomly divided into two groups administered either 60 mg aspirin or a matching placebo. The women were enrolled between 13 and 28 weeks of gestation. Low-dose aspirin did not reduce the incidence of pre-eclampsia or improve perinatal outcome in this group of women at high risk for development of pre-eclampsia.

Collectively almost 12,000 pregnant women have been randomly assigned to receive aspirin therapy. No reduction has been found in this group in the incidence of pre-eclampsia. Nor has there been a reduction in intrauterine growth restriction, neonatal death, or preterm delivery, or an improvement in birth weight or gestational age at delivery.

Safety of Aspirin in Pregnancy

The major effects of aspirin are related to the inhibition of prostaglandin synthesis in various body tissues. Arachidonic acid is liberated from membrane phospholipids by the action of phospholipase A_2. Arachidonic acid is then converted by the cyclooxygenase pathway into prostaglandin (PG) G_2, which serves as the precursor to various biologically active prostaglandins. Aspirin inhibits the synthesis of the cyclic endoperoxide PGG_2 by irreversibly acetylating and inactivating the enzyme cyclooxygenase. These effects in turn will result in simultaneous inhibition of the synthesis of four active substances (PGG_2, $PGF_{2\alpha}$, prostacylin, and thromboxane) that have major actions during pregnancy. This nonselective inhibition is usually seen following the chronic use of pharmacologic doses of aspirin (>325 mg/d).

There are numerous reports describing an association between prenatal aspirin ingestion and several adverse effects in the mother, fetus, and the newborn. The maternal side effects include antepartum and postpartum hemorrhage, prolonged bleeding time, and prolonged gestation and labor. Reported fetal effects include oligohydramnios, fetal growth restriction, closure of the ductus arteriosus, and stillbirths. Neonatal complications include various bleeding disorders and persistent pulmonary hypertension.

In contrast, there are minimal to no side effects reported with the use of low-dose aspirin in pregnancy. The majority of randomized trials found no difference in the incidence of abruptio placentae between the aspirin treated and the placebo-treated women (Fig. 2). None of the studies reported an increased frequency of post-

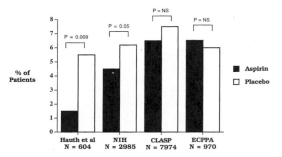

Figure 1. Incidence of pre-eclampsia.

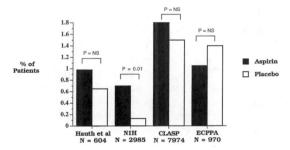

Figure 2. Incidence of placental abruption.

partum hemorrhage, prolonged gestation, or prolonged labor. The incidence of fetal growth restriction, oligohydramnios, and stillbirths were not increased with the use of low-dose aspirin in any of the reported trials. In addition, no instance of in utero closure of the fetal ductus was reported. Moreover, many women in these trials received epidural anesthesia without report of epidural hematoma. The incidence of neonatal bleeding complications was similar between the aspirin- and placebo-exposed neonates. The CLASP Collaborative study data of infants exposed to low-dose aspirin are reassuring about its safety when therapy was started after the first trimester. Although an adverse effect cannot be excluded, congenital malformations, major motor deficits, and severe neuromotor or developmental delay were not identified.

Summary and Recommendations

Calcium ingestion during pregnancy appears safe. Since it is a nutrient that many pregnant women fail to ingest in adequate amounts, calcium supplementation may be recommended to any pregnant women who does not appear to be ingesting the current recommended dietary allowance (RDA) for calcium of 1200 mg/day of elemental calcium. Further supplementation above the RDA to 2000 mg/day could be considered for selected high-risk women.

Some benefits from the use of low-dose aspirin during pregnancy are reported, although some of the findings have been contradictory. Currently, the routine use of low-dose aspirin in low-risk, nulliparous woman is not justified, since the beneficial effects are marginal. Women with chronic hypertension, multifetal gestation, and insulin-dependent diabetes may benefit from low-dose aspirin therapy during pregnancy. However, this remains unproved by current studies.

Certain women may be considered at increased risk for development of severe pre-eclampsia and its complications and may thus derive a potential benefit from low-dose aspirin or supplemental calcium therapy. These groups include women with previous severe pre-eclampsia resulting in fetal demise, previous pre-eclampsia occurring during the second trimester, severe chronic hypertension, renal disease, class F–R diabetes, or antiphospholipid antibody syndrome. The decision to utilize aspirin therapy may be considered for the woman requesting therapy following informed consent.

Hypothyroidism

Jorge H. Mestman, MD

Hypothyroidism may be defined as the constellation of symptoms and signs resulting from insufficient action of thyroid hormones at tissue levels. With rare exception, it is the result of decreased thyroid hormone synthesis. The clinical spectrum varies from an asymptomatic and mild form to the severe myxedema presentation.

Hypothyroidism may be caused by an intrinsic disease of the thyroid gland (primary hypothyroidism), by a hypothalamic or pituitary disease with impairment in the secretion of thyroid-stimulating hormone (TSH) (secondary hypothyroidism), or by peripheral resistance to thyroid hormone action. The most common etiologies of primary hypothyroidism include chronic or Hashimoto's thyroiditis; surgical ablation for Graves' disease, nodular goiter, or thyroid carcinoma; radiation therapy for Graves' disease; and primary or idiopathic myxedema (considered by some to be the endstage of Hashimoto's or Graves' disease). Congenital hypothyroidism is due to thyroid dysgenesis or dyshormonogenesis and occurs in about 1 in 4000 births.

Primary hypothyroidism occurs at all ages but peaks at 40 to 60 years. It is more common in women, with a ratio of men to women between 1:4 and 1:7.

Secondary hypothyroidism is rare and accounts for fewer than 5% of all cases of hypothyroidism. In most cases, other pituitary hormones are affected; postpartum pituitary necrosis, or Sheehan's syndrome, and destruction of the pituitary gland by tumor or radiation therapy are the most common causes.

Clinical Findings

Clinical symptoms vary from patient to patient. The presenting symptoms may be minimal or absent or, rarely, so severe that the patient presents with stupor or myxedema coma. Symptoms include fatigue, cold intolerance, mild weight gain, lethargy, lack of ambition, depression, arthralgias, muscle cramps, decrease in hearing, hoarse voice, and constipation. Abnormal menses with excessive bleeding is common; anovulation is not uncommon, although spontaneous pregnancies have been reported; on occasion, the patient may present with galactorrhea-amenorrhea syndrome. On clinical examination, findings may be minimal; periorbital edema is a frequent complaint, particularly on arising; the skin may be pale and of a yellowish color and is generally dry, rough, and sometimes scaly; the scalp hair becomes thin and may fall out; typically, there is a delay in the relaxation phase of tendon reflexes. Bradycardia is common, and blood pressure may be normal, although mild hypertension is not unusual. Examination of the neck may reveal a scar from a previous thyroidectomy, a goiter, diffuse or nodular; or no palpable thyroid tissue in patients with primary myxedema or previous ^{131}I treatment.

Diagnosis

The diagnosis of primary thyroid failure is confirmed by a low free thyroxine index (FT_4) in the presence of high serum levels of TSH. Positive antimicrosomal antibody titer is seen in patients with Hashimoto's thyroiditis, and lower titers are seen in those with primary myxedema. In patients with secondary hypothyroidism, serum TSH concentration is within normal limits; in such cases, other pituitary hormones are also deficient. Serum triiodothyronine determination is of no value in the diagnosis of hypothyroidism; the values may be within normal limits in almost 30% of cases.

Hypothyroid patients may present with other laboratory abnormalities. Anemia, macrocytic or normochromic, is not infrequent and responds to thyroid therapy. Liver enzymes may be slightly elevated. Serum creatine phosphokinase can reach five or six times the upper limit of normal. Electrocardiographic changes include low voltage ST segment depression, and occasionally T wave inversion.

Variants of Hypothyroidism

Subclinical Hypothyroidism

Subclinical hypothyroidism is defined as normal FT_4 in the presence of elevated serum TSH levels (usually not greater than 20 μU/dL). Most of these patients are asymptomatic, and this represents the first stage of thyroid failure. It is estimated that this condition occurs in 5% of the population, with a prevalence in women older than 60 years of age of close to 15%. There is a progression to overt hypothyroidism at a rate of 5% a year. This progression appears to be more likely to occur in those patients with positive thyroid antimicrosomal titers at the time of the diagnosis.

Transient Hypothyroidism

Although most hypothyroid patients require thyroid replacement therapy for life, transient hypothyroidism has been recognized following an episode of subacute thyroiditis, painless thyroiditis, postpartum thyroiditis, or ^{131}I therapy for Graves' disease. In most cases, the symptoms are not severe enough to require thyroid therapy. Thyroid tests return to normal spontaneously.

Treatment of Primary Hypothyroidism

One of the most gratifying experiences in medical practice for the physician as well as the patient is the diagnosis and treatment of thyroid failure. Thyroid hormone therapy will correct all the symptoms and signs caused by thyroid deficiency, with few or no side effects. The preparation of choice is L-thyroxine, since it produces constant serum concentrations of both thyroxine (T_4) and triiodothyronine (T_3), has to be taken only once a day, and is well tolerated. Several principles should be followed before therapy is started: (1) most patients will need lifelong replacement therapy; (2) therapy should be started with low dosage, especially in the elderly and in those with heart disease; and (3) the goal is to achieve euthyroidism with normalization of the thyroid tests.

The normal replacement dosage varies between 0.075 and 0.2 mg/day of L-thyroxine. It has been calculated to be about 1.7 μg/kg of body weight per day. The physician should be aware of the potential difference in L-thyroxine content between several generic preparations on the market; one study indicated that most, but not all, of the generic brands contain the stated amount of L-thyroxine.

In patients with newly diagnosed hypothyroidism and with significant symptoms, it is advisable to start with small dosages, 0.025 to 0.05 mg/day, increasing the dosage every 2 to 4 weeks. The goal is to normalize serum TSH levels and FT_4; it takes approximately 4 to 6 weeks for the serum TSH level to return to normal. Once the proper dosage is achieved, thyroid tests are repeated at regular intervals to assess the proper replacing dosage. Recent reports suggest the potential risk for bone demineralization in women taking excessive amounts of thyroid hormones.

During pregnancy, patients on thyroid replacement therapy may need an adjustment of the prepregnancy thyroid dosage. It is advisable to perform complete thyroid function tests in hypothyroid patients on replacement therapy. In about 50% of them, the dosage of L-thyroxine needs to be increased.

Treatment of Secondary Hypothyroidism

It is imperative to assess pituitary function completely before thyroid hormone is administered to patients with secondary thyroid failure. Isolated TSH deficiency is rare; the administration of thyroid medication to patients with adrenal insufficiency without replacement with cortisol may precipitate an adrenal crisis. The daily amount of L-thyroxine does not differ from that of patients with primary thyroid failure.

Idiopathic Thrombocytopenic Purpura

Robert F. Burrow, MD

Idiopathic thrombocytopenic purpura (ITP) is a common disorder of young women; consequently, physicians often manage pregnant patients with ITP. The disease is caused by autoantibodies directed to platelet-specific antigens. The immunoglobulin G (IgG)–coated platelets are cleared by the reticuloendothelial system, and if increased production by the bone marrow cannot compensate, thrombocytopenia results. Because the IgG autoantibody crosses the placenta, the fetus is also at risk for thrombocytopenia.

The diagnosis of ITP is one of exclusion. The ITP patient has isolated thrombocytopenia and unless concomitantly iron-deficient from blood loss, has normal red cell and white cell morphology. A bone marrow aspirate is normal with adequate or increased numbers of megakaryocytes. Coagulation studies are also normal, except those

affected by thrombocytopenia. No other cause for thrombocytopenia, such as drug ingestion or lupus erythematosus, is documented.

Clinical Presentation

Idiopathic thrombocytopenic purpura can present in one of three ways. A few patients have an abrupt onset of hemostatic impairment with petechiae, purpura, and nosebleeds. Questioning often reveals that the patient has had bruising for months before the episode, indicating the chronic nature of the disorder. The bleeding episodes sometimes are precipitated by the ingestion of an antiplatelet agent such as aspirin or alcohol. Not infrequently, the illness is preceded by several weeks by an upper respiratory tract infection. These patients require immediate treatment to raise the platelet count to safe levels.

The condition may also present with a long history of insidious and relatively mild hemostatic impairment. The patient often describes easy bruising for many years and prolonged bleeding from minor trauma. These patients may or may not require treatment.

Finally, ITP may present by the identification of asymptomatic thrombocytopenia during routine laboratory testing. This is an increasingly common way for ITP patients to be identified, especially in pregnancy, in which complete blood counts are routine. Most of these patients do not require treatment. It is nearly impossible to differentiate ITP patients from patients with incidental thrombocytopenia of pregnancy; however, maternal platelet counts consistently less than 70×10^9 per liter are compatible with the diagnosis of ITP. Patients with ITP are at risk for having thrombocytopenic infants, whereas those patients with incidental thrombocytopenia will in all likelihood deliver well infants. As we believe that maximum risk to the ITP-affected infant is as a neonate, cord sampling at birth is soon enough to identify at-risk infants.

Thrombocytopenia is conventionally defined as a platelet count less than 150×10^9 per liter; however, in pregnancy this level is best considered to be less than 100×10^9 per liter. This reasoning stems from several observations. First, in a 1-year study of consecutively defined normal patients, we found that the mean platelet count at delivery was 225×10^9 per liter with the 2.5th and 97.5th percentile being 109 and 341×10^9 per liter, respectively. Second, a continuation of this study, which now encompasses over 21,000 deliveries, has demonstrated that 5% of normal-term pregnant women (approximately

1000 patients) have a platelet count between 100 and 150×10^9 per liter at delivery. Only one of their infants had a cord platelet count at birth less than 50×10^9 per liter. This infant had Down syndrome and a congenital marrow problem and had no sequelae secondary to the thrombocytopenia. Finally, observations in the last 6 years have shown that of the ITP patients (71 patients) cared for in this institution, only 10 had platelet counts between 100 and 150×10^9 per liter at delivery. Thus there was a 1% chance that a maternal platelet count between 100 and 150×10^9 per liter was ITP with a fetus potentially at risk. To counter this slight chance, we recommend that infants produced by pregnancies identified with platelet counts of 100 to 150×10^9 per liter have a cord platelet count at birth to identify those at possible risk.

Of patients with thrombocytopenia of less than 100×10^9 per liter at delivery, we have recorded an equal prevalence of ITP and incidental thrombocytopenia; however, the majority of incidental patients had platelet counts greater than 70×10^9 per liter. Thus, with no prepregnancy history and without sign of hemostatic impairment, a maternal platelet count less than 70×10^9 per liter is most likely ITP.

Management

The management of incidental thrombocytopenia associated with pregnancy is not unlike that of the patient in the nonpregnant state. No treatment during pregnancy is required unless the thrombocytopenia is severe, for example a platelet count less than 50×10^9 per liter. Even at counts less than 50×10^9 per liter, if the counts have been stable and there is no immediate threat of hemostatic impairment (ie, delivery), often no treatment is indicated. Aspirin and nonsteroidal anti-inflammatory medications are best avoided.

Since almost all patients with ITP have chronic disease, the long-term impact of any proposed treatment should be considered. For this reason, corticosteroids represent a satisfactory short-term therapy, but are unacceptable as long-term support. The mainstay of treatment of ITP in nonpregnant patients is prednisone, 1 mg per kg as a starting dose, which is reduced with clinical response, which usually occurs within 1 to 2 weeks. In pregnant patients, corticosteroid therapy offers little risk to the fetus but there are potential side effects for the mother, including gestational diabetes, postpartum psychosis, hypertension, and osteoporosis. These side effects can be kept at a minimum by using the lowest possible dose.

During pregnancy, we prefer to use high-dose intravenous IgG. The majority (60–80%) of patients with ITP will have a rise in the platelet count following the administration of intravenous IgG. The usual dose is 1 g/kg administered over 8 hours on one day. This dose will raise the platelet count in about 50% of the patients. If the platelet count does not rise, an additional 1 g/kg can be given 2 to 3 days later. The rise in platelet count following intravenous IgG is more rapid than the rise following corticosteroids; consequently, it is the treatment of choice for patients with serious bleeding complications or if the maternal platelet count must be rapidly raised prior to surgery or delivery. The advantage of intravenous IgG is that it is a safe and benign treatment. Although minor side effects such as headache occur, serious complications such as viral infections are rare. However, intravenous IgG seldom produces a cure, and it is relatively expensive.

Splenectomy should be performed in the nonpregnant state. If absolutely indicated in pregnancy, splenectomy is best done in the second trimester, a time interval providing the best surgical exposure and least risk of obstetric complications. However, corticosteroids and intravenous IgG usually circumvent the need for splenectomy in pregnancy.

The prevalence of antepartum hemorrhage is not increased in ITP, but there is a slightly increased frequency of postpartum hemorrhagic complications. These are not due to uterine bleeding but are almost always secondary to lacerations, episiotomies, and bleeding from surgical sites. Surgical hemostasis must be meticulous and midline episiotomies are preferred for vaginal deliveries.

Platelet transfusions should be considered only to control life-threatening hemorrhage or if there is excessive blood loss not controlled by normal hemostatic maneuvers at cesarean section. In these circumstances, 6 to 12 units may be given, but the expected rise in platelet count of 10×10^9 per liter per unit is unusual because of the ongoing immune destruction.

Neonatal Risks

Because IgG is transported across the placenta, some infants of ITP mothers will be thrombocytopenic. Of those affected, the degree of thrombocytopenia varies dramatically. The risk for the infant has been exaggerated by small series bias and by the reporting of platelet nadirs, which occur 2 to 5 days into neonatal life. Decisions on delivery clearly should be determined by the fetal platelet count, which can only be determined by scalp sampling, cordocentesis, or cord sampling at delivery. We do not attempt to identify thrombocytopenic infants while in utero using cordocentesis or during labor with scalp sampling because we believe these maneuvers may actually increase the risk to mother and child. Instead, the infant's cord platelet count is obtained immediately at birth and treatment and follow-up are based on this level and the subsequent platelet counts.

Our experience supports the literature. Of 71 infants, 5 (7%) had cord platelet counts less than 50×10^9 per liter. Four were born vaginally and one by cesarean section for a primigravida breech. None of the 71 infants suffered morbidity or mortality.

Review of maternal factors used to predict the fetal platelet count shows that there was no correlation among maternal platelet count, the level of platelet-associated IgG (bound or unbound), maternal treatment with corticosteroids or intravenous IgG, and the fetal platelet count. Patients with prior splenectomies may be a special risk group, as identified by our literature review, but our clinical experience has not confirmed this relationship.

Our review of the literature failed to demonstrate one intrauterine event attributable to ITP, or to present a convincing argument supporting the use of routine cesarean section in ITP pregnancies. Thus, delivery should be conducted according to obstetric indications. Maternal platelet counts less than 70 to 100×10^9 per liter at term can be elevated by intravenous IgG, or a short course of corticosteroids, enabling the mother to have all analgesic options and ensuring adequate hemostasis. It is usually relatively easy to raise the platelet count to ensure hemostatic competency, but occasionally the cost (IV IgG) or the risk (corticosteroid) do not enable us to raise the count to a level at which anesthetists are content to place epidurals.

As the pregnancy and delivery are managed identically, it is not essential to differentiate antenatally between new-onset asymptomatic ITP (onset in the pregnancy without history) and incidental thrombocytopenia. The postpartum maternal platelet count will determine the etiology. If the maternal platelet count does not rise to normal levels postpartum or if the neonatal platelet count is low or falls neonatally, then the diagnosis of new-onset ITP is supported.

Intrauterine Growth Retardation

Nancy A. Callan, MD

Intrauterine growth retardation (IUGR) is an important cause of perinatal morbidity and mortality. To optimize outcome, it is essential for the clinician caring for the obstetric patient to understand the diagnosis and management of this complication. Intrauterine growth retardation is defined in the obstetric literature as birth weight less than the tenth percentile for gestational age. Since the weight of some normal individuals will be less than the tenth percentile, one of the keys to management is to recognize those whose small size is secondary to pathologic conditions and who will benefit from antenatal intervention and surveillance.

Risk Factors

Growth abnormalities in the fetus and newborn are the result of multiple etiologies. The exact cause in a particular individual may be difficult to determine, yet a knowledge of cause can improve one's ability to develop the proper management plan. The risk factors for IUGR can be divided into maternal, fetal, and placental conditions (Table 1). The clinician needs to be aware of these risk factors, their impact on fetal growth, and the appropriate prenatal evaluation to accurately diagnose IUGR and manage this potentially lethal complication.

In the antepartum period, an assessment of maternal risk factors such as previous history of an IUGR infant, maternal habits including smoking or use of illicit drugs, maternal weight gain, prepregnancy weight, or the existence or development of maternal medical conditions that may lead to impaired fetal growth should be undertaken. At every obstetric visit, an estimate of fetal size and the appropriateness of size should be made whether or not there are risk factors. This can be done with an assessment of fundal height or clinical estimate of fetal weight. If maternal, fetal, or placental risk factors are present or develop, then ultrasonography is used in addition to clinical assessment to make the diagnosis of IUGR.

Diagnosis by Ultrasonography

Obstetric ultrasonography has improved the ability to make the diagnosis and to manage the

TABLE 1. Conditions for Intrauterine Growth Retardation

Maternal	Fetal	Placental
Previous IUGR infant	Multiple gestation	Chronic abruptions
Low pre-pregnancy weight	Congenital abnormalities/	Premature aging/infarction
Poor weight gain	echogenic bowel	Placenta previa
Poor nutrition	Chromosomal abnormalities	Chorioangioma
Low socioeconomic status	Single gene disorders	Abnormality in cord insertion
Medical conditions	Congenital infections	
Pre-eclampsia		
Chronic hypertension		
Renal disease		
Diabetes with vascular involvement		
Collagen vascular disease		
Anemia/hemoglobinopathies		
Hyperthyroidism		
Cyanoic heart disease		
Infections		
Cytomegalovirus		
Toxoplasmosis		
Rubella		
Herpes		
Syphilis		
Habits		
Smoking		
Alcohol abuse		
Illegal drug use (cocaine, heroin)		
Obstetric		
Elevated serum alpha-fetoprotein with		
normal ultrasonogram		
Decreased growth by clinical estimate		
Chronic abruption		
Multiple gestations		
Uterine abnormalities (septations,		
bicornuate uterus)		

pregnancy at risk for or complicated by IUGR. If risk factors do exist in a pregnancy, a baseline ultrasonogram can be obtained at 18 to 20 weeks to establish gestational age. Obtaining an ultrasonographic study at this point in gestation yields not only an accurate assessment of gestational age but also an opportunity to carefully examine for fetal anomalies. Although ultrasonograms obtained in the first trimester may be slightly more accurate in dating the pregnancy, evaluation for anomalies at this early stage is more limited and requires considerable skill. In the presence of significant risk factors, serial ultrasonograms can be obtained if there is concern regarding clinical growth or at 28 to 32 weeks' gestation as the next baseline study with subsequent follow-up scans to determine fetal growth.

A knowledge of the characteristics of normal fetal growth is helpful in interpreting obstetric ultrasonographic findings. The maximum velocity of fetal skeletal growth occurs at approximately 22 weeks' gestation. Antenatally, skeletal growth parameters include the biparietal diameter, head circumference, and the femur length. The maximum velocity of soft tissue growth in the fetus occurs later, at approximately 33 weeks' gestation. The abdominal circumference is the most commonly used antenatal soft tissue parameter. Thus, an earlier insult would result in a fetus in which both skeletal and soft tissue growth are affected. With an insult occurring later in gestation, soft tissue growth is primarily affected, with skeletal growth relatively spared.

There have been attempts to classify IUGR as symmetric, if skeletal and soft tissue growth are proportionate, or as asymmetric, if soft tissue growth is more affected than skeletal growth. Symmetric IUGR has been related to an earlier insult and asymmetric to a later one. While there may be considerable overlap in these categories, they can be helpful in defining an etiology and establishing a management scheme. In evaluating fetal growth, it is important to look at the estimate of fetal weight and the pattern of growth, as opposed to depending only on the composite gestational age, which merely reflects an average of skeletal and soft tissue parameters. For example, if the abdominal circumference lags behind the biparietal diameter or femur length, this may be indicative of abnormal growth and warrants careful follow-up with serial growth studies.

A variety of ultrasonographic parameters are used in evaluating fetal growth. Biparietal diameter, head circumference, and femur length have been used to determine gestational age but are not adequate to diagnose IUGR. An estimate of fetal weight is superior and can be obtained using a variety of formulas that include evaluation of soft tissue and skeletal parameters. The most commonly used formulas include biparietal diameter, head circumference, abdominal circumference, and femur length. All formulas involve a similar range of error, in which the standard deviation ranges from 8% to 12%.

The ratios of head circumference to abdominal circumference, which varies with gestational age, and femur length to abdominal circumference, which remains constant after 22 weeks, are used to examine the pattern of growth and found to be elevated in fetuses with asymmetric IUGR or at risk for developing IUGR. Those fetuses with symmetric IUGR will have normal ratios. If, on obstetric ultrasonogram, a fetus is found to be of normal weight but has an elevated ratio, consideration should be given to a follow-up scan for growth in 2 to 4 weeks to evaluate the adequacy of growth.

Placental grading, a means of defining the maturity of the placenta, has been used to predict an increased antepartum risk and can be used in evaluating fetuses at risk for IUGR. The placental grades are 0 to 3 and include an assessment of the chorionic plate and the degree and pattern of echogenicity within the placenta. A grade 3 placenta, the most mature, may be found in up to 15% of normal pregnancies after 36 weeks. If found prior to 34 weeks or with an estimate of fetal weight less than 2700 g, it is abnormal and is in some cases predictive of IUGR or a fetus at risk of developing IUGR. By convention, if a placenta exhibits two grades, it is given the more mature grade.

In mild to moderate IUGR, the transcerebellar diameter (TCD) or the ratio of transcerebellar diameter to abdominal circumference (TCD/AC) have been used to diagnose IUGR. The use of these measures has been controversial, but in mild to moderate cases, the TCD is felt to reflect gestational age, and the TCD/AC ratio is ele-

vated. In severe cases, because of progressive involvement of the brain, the ratio may be normal. Delayed appearance of the distal femoral epiphyses on ultrasonogram has also been described with IUGR.

An assessment of amniotic fluid volume by ultrasonography is important in the diagnosis and management of IUGR. The amniotic fluid index, which is the sum of the largest fluid pockets without cord in the four quadrants of the uterus, is used. In IUGR, the amniotic fluid volume may be normal, decreased, or increased. Oligohydramnios in IUGR is an ominous sign, indicative of hypoxia and acidosis as the blood is shunted away from the fetal kidneys, with a decrease in fetal urine production resulting in decreased fluid.

In addition to measurements of growth, IUGR should lead to a careful ultrasonogram to look for fetal congenital anomalies and abnormalities of the placenta or uterus. Congenital anomalies, chromosomal abnormalities, and single gene disorders all may be associated with IUGR. In particular, the finding of a congenital anomaly, polyhydramnios, or the early onset of IUGR should lead to counseling the patient regarding the need for studies of karyotype. If an amniocentesis is performed for karyotype or other genetic studies, the clinician should consider sending the fluid for viral studies, especially cytomegalovirus.

The finding of isolated echogenic bowel in the second trimester has been associated with cystic fibrosis, aneuploidy, or IUGR developing in the third trimester. When the work-up excludes cystic fibrosis and aneuploidy, the patient should be followed to determine fetal growth through the use of serial obstetric scanning. This is also the case for the patient with an elevated maternal serum alpha-fetoprotein level and a normal second trimester ultrasonogram, in whom increased morbidity has been found, including IUGR.

Neonatal Outcome

Neonatal outcome varies according to the etiology of the IUGR, the gestational age at delivery, and the presence of antenatal or perinatal complications. Immediate morbidity includes perinatal asphyxia, meconium aspiration, hypoglycemia, hypothermia, hypocalcemia, and hyperviscosity. Long-term sequelae seem to depend on the severity of the growth abnormality, the time when growth restriction occurred, and whether the infant was preterm or full term. Those born preterm are more likely to have major disabilities; however, the majority of both preterm and term

IUGR infants are of normal intelligence. Learning deficits occur more frequently in the IUGR infant than in those whose weight is appropriate for gestational age. The risk of morbidity is increased in those that experience antepartum or peripartum complications; thus the antepartum and intrapartum management of these pregnancies is very important.

Antepartum and Intrapartum Management

The clinical suspicion of IUGR, whether it is based on the presence of risk factors or clinical findings, should be confirmed by ultrasonography. An attempt to determine etiology should be undertaken. This would include attention to the obstetric and maternal medical history, ultrasonogram to exclude congenital anomalies, karyotype or other genetic studies, and possibly viral studies. Baseline maternal studies include an evaluation for anemia, renal function, the presence of collagen vascular disease, antiphospholipid antibodies, toxicology screening, and, if clinically indicated, thyroid function studies.

Treatment involves correction of maternal factors such as poor nutrition, smoking cessation or drug abuse treatment, and treatment of medical conditions including hyperthyroidism, hypertension, and the antiphospholipid antibody syndrome. Bedrest has long been the mainstay of treatment, providing for increased blood flow to the uterus. Other modalities are controversial; these include low-dose aspirin therapy and high-calorie or high-protein diets.

The antepartum and intrapartum management of the IUGR fetus is critical for a successful outcome. Assessment of the adequacy of fetal growth is done through the use of obstetric ultrasonography. Because of the range of error of this technique, serial studies should be performed no more frequently than every 2 to 3 weeks. More frequent studies do not offer helpful information regarding the adequacy of growth. Evidence of poor head growth or minimal increase in fetal weight or the presence of oligohydramnios may, depending on gestational age, warrant delivery.

Because the fetus with IUGR is considered high risk, twice-weekly antepartum testing is recommended. This antepartum testing should include an assessment of amniotic fluid volume and a program of non-stress testing with amniotic fluid index, alternating with biophysical profile, has been useful. Biophysical testing should begin when the fetus is viable and the diagnosis of IUGR has been made. Serial scanning for growth is performed every 2 to 3 weeks to look for progressive growth.

The timing of delivery of the fetus depends on the gestational age and results of fetal testing. Fetuses with IUGR should be delivered prior to term, or if the fetus is viable, when fetal testing indicates fetal distress. Using these criteria, a premature delivery of a viable fetus may be warranted in the face of nonreassuring fetal testing. Care must be taken to ensure that the gestational age has been accurately determined. If delivery is to be induced prior to 39 weeks for reasons other than poor fetal testing, lung maturity studies should be performed on the fetus.

Current Doppler technology has allowed the study of a number of fetal vessels, both arterial and venous. Abnormalities of the umbilical artery waveform have been proposed as a predictor of poor outcome in high-risk pregnancies, especially IUGR. Various indices have been used in the evaluation, which include the systolic to diastolic ratio, the resistance index, and the pulsatility index. These are elevated in the face of low diastolic flows as found in certain types of fetal compromise. Especially important in predicting those with progressive compromise is the absence of end-diastolic flow or reverse end-diastolic flow. In the IUGR fetus, while umbilical artery waveforms may show increased resistance, decreases in cerebral vascular resistance have been found. The ideal use of Doppler in the management of high-risk pregnancies is controversial, and most authors recommend that a combination of ultrasonographic biometry, biophysical testing, and Doppler be used in the antepartum management of the IUGR fetus. Once the decision for delivery is made, intrapartum management requires careful fetal heart rate monitoring to avoid problems associated with the birth process.

The successful management of the pregnancy complicated by fetal growth restriction requires attention to early identification, antenatal surveillance, and careful intrapartum monitoring. The obstetrician needs to be aware of possible risk factors, diagnostic criteria, and the use of current technology to optimize outcomes.

Laboratory Diagnosis of Pregnancy

Donald E. Pittaway, MD, PhD

With the development of sensitive assays for human chorionic gonadotropin (hCG), specific laboratory tools for the diagnosis and management of early pregnancy are now available to clinicians. Although several hormones and other substances are produced in pregnancy, only the measurement of hCG has been used clinically to detect and monitor early pregnancy. In normal pregnancies, hCG becomes measurable approximately 7 to 10 days after ovulation and increases exponentially in a nonlinear fashion to peak levels that range between 80,000 and 100,000 mIU/mL at approximately 8 weeks after the last menstrual period. The levels then decline to about 20,000 mIU/mL by about 20 weeks and remain at this lower range of hCG concentration until term.

The most important function of the laboratory evaluation of hCG is to document a conception by establishing the presence or absence of trophoblastic activity. This function can now be achieved in 99% to 100% of pregnancies. The failure to detect a pregnancy may occur (1) because the hCG concentration is less than the sensitivity of the test, which is approximately 25 to 50 mIU/mL for rapid urine tests, 10 to 25 mIU/mL for qualitative blood tests, and 5 to 10 mIU/mL for the most sensitive quantitative blood tests; or (2) because of a laboratory malfunction or error. With assays now using antibodies that recognize the β-subunit of hCG, cross-reaction with other similar hormones like luteinizing hormone, follicle-stimulating hormone, and thyroid-stimulating hormone is generally less than 1%, which eliminates this source of false-positive tests. The detection of hCG (a positive test) in the absence of a pregnancy occurs with certain hCG-producing conditions such as a gestational trophoblastic neoplasm, certain nontrophoblastic carcinomas, and some benign gastrointestinal tract disorders such as ulcerative colitis, gastric or duodenal ulcer, and regional enteritis. Substances that interfere with assays occur rarely (1 in more than 13,000 tests), and when suspected, can be confirmed by using an alternative method (for example, a false-positive serum test often will be accompanied by a negative urine test) or by performing serial dilutions of the serum and demonstrating concentrations that do not correspond to the anticipated levels from the dilutions (nonlinearity).

TABLE 1. Human Chorionic Gonadotropin (hCG) Levels in Normal Pregnancy

Gestational Age	Mean hCG Concentration (mIU/mL)	Range (mIU/mL)
Anticipated day of menses	106	39–166
+2	221	55–408
+4	470	147–941
+7	2138	686–4708

To interpret a single quantitative hCG result, the clinician must know what form of hCG is being measured, that is, β-subunit or intact molecule, and whether the assay method is standardized against the Second International Standard (IS) or the Third IS (formerly the First International Reference Preparation, IRP). Most laboratories provide this information with reference values when reporting hCG results to assist the clinician. Yet considerable variation in hCG production from one normal pregnancy to another does occur, as seen in the values listed in Table 1 for a total β assay using the third IS.

When the last menstrual period is unknown or unreliable, however, estimates of the gestational age can be made within approximately 3 to 6 days for the first 49 days using the following formula:

$$\text{Gestational Age (day)} = 5.073 \ln (\text{hCG concentration}) - 0.1322$$

Serial hCG determinations may be helpful in determining whether the pregnancy is normal or abnormal (impending abortion or ectopic gestation). The rise of hCG concentrations occurs exponentially at a decreasing rate, with estimates of the mean doubling time (the time interval in days required for the value to double) for the postmenstrual days 23 through 35, 35 through 42, and 33 through 49 being 1.6, 2.0, and 2.5 days, respectively. Use of the 85% upper limits of the mean doubling time, which are 2.2, 2.6, and 3.5 days, respectively, results in a sensitivity (the probability that the doubling time will be abnormal in an abnormal pregnancy) of 75% and specificity (the probability that the doubling time will be normal in a normal pregnancy) of 93% in detecting abnormal pregnancies in asymptomatic women. One method to calculate the doubling time can be accomplished with a scientific calculator using a natural logarithm function:

$$\text{Doubling time (days)} = \frac{(\ln 2)}{(\text{Time interval in days})/\ln (hCG_2/hCG_1)}$$

Another method requires the use of a straight edge with the nomogram shown in Figure 1. When an abnormal doubling time is observed, an abnormal pregnancy is likely and further evaluation to determine the site of the pregnancy is required. When serum hCG concentrations are greater than 1500 to 2000 mIU/mL (Third IS or First IRP), transvaginal sonography (TVS) can detect an intrauterine gestational sac, which, when present, virtually excludes an ectopic pregnancy since a combined intrauterine and extrauterine pregnancy is very unlikely (fewer than 1 in 4000 pregnancies). One exception to this rare occurrence is a pregnancy resulting from an assisted reproductive technique, which has an approximately 1% chance of being heterotopic. In women in whom the hCG concentrations are greater than 2000 mIU/mL and no intrauterine sac can be seen on TVS, an ectopic pregnancy, a completed spontaneous abortion, trophoblastic disease, or a false-positive test result should be

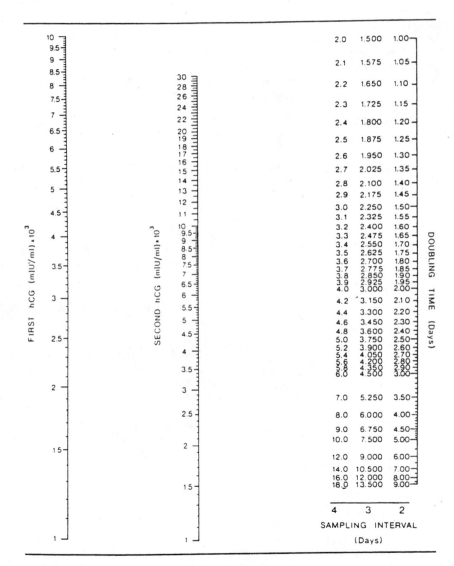

Figure 1. Nomogram for estimating doubling times of hCG in paired serum samples obtained between 2 and 4 days apart. (From Fritz MA, Guo S: Doubling time of human chorionic gonadotrophin (hCG) in early pregnancy: Relationship to hCG concentration and gestational age. Fertil Steril 1987; 47:584. Reproduced with permission from the American Society of Reproductive Medicine.)

considered. In addition, progesterone determinations (if excluding women receiving clomiphene citrate, human menopausal gonadotropins, or progesterone) may also be used to evaluate an early pregnancy since (1) a serum concentration greater than or equal to 25 ng/mL is seen in only 1% of abnormal pregnancies; (2) values less than 15 ng/mL suggest an abnormal pregnancy; and (3) concentrations less than 5 ng/mL are consistent with a nonviable pregnancy, either intrauterine or extrauterine.

The laboratory evaluation of an abnormal pregnancy by itself cannot identify the site of a pregnancy. In the woman at risk for or with symptoms suggesting an ectopic pregnancy, a high index of suspicion, the examination and sonographic findings, and in some patients in-office curettage or culdocentesis are necessary to support performing a laparoscopic evaluation. Nonetheless, in women with the following laboratory and clinical findings, a definitive diagnosis must be established:

1. A hemodynamically unstable patient or a falling hemoglobin
2. Abnormally rising or falling hCG concentration with signs and symptoms of an intra-abdominal process
3. Progesterone levels less than 5 ng/mL with an increasing hCG and either no chorionic villi on curettage or signs and symptoms of an intra-abdominal process
4. Sonographic identification of an extrauterine gestational sac or findings consistent with an ectopic pregnancy such as an adnexal mass separate from the ovary or increased cul-de-sac fluid
5. When no intrauterine sac can be detected by TVS when the hCG concentrations are greater than 2000 mIU/mL

Monitoring the decline of hCG levels may be helpful in the following situations: (1) when an ectopic pregnancy is suspected and histologic confirmation of an intrauterine pregnancy is lacking; (2) after conservative surgical treatment of a tubal pregnancy; and (3) after methotrexate therapy of a known tubal pregnancy. With the initial half-life of less than 1 day, hCG concentrations will be 20% or less of a preoperative or intraoperative value 48 to 72 hours later when removal of the trophoblastic tissue is fairly complete. If hCG concentrations are greater than 20%, persistent trophoblastic activity can be inferred and continued monitoring of the hCG levels and the patient's clinical status should be performed. Although persistent trophoblastic activity does not indicate that a resolving ectopic pregnancy will

become a problem or that a hemorrhage within a previously operated tube will occur, this finding nonetheless is associated with a higher frequency of complications and requires continued hCG monitoring and close observation of the patient and may require intervention such as reoperation or methotrexate therapy. With methotrexate as a primary treatment or as an adjunct, a 15% or greater decrease in 24 to 48 hours is considered a positive response, allowing continued out-patient monitoring and withholding of additional methotrexate. With a stable or rising hCG concentration, additional methotrexate injections may be required for successful treatment. A complete resolution of the ectopic pregnancy may be concluded when hCG concentrations are less than 15 mIU/mL, although rare tubal hemorrhages have been observed even at these very low levels.

In summary, in the patient at risk for or with symptoms suggesting an ectopic pregnancy, active management to determine whether the pregnancy is a normal, intrauterine pregnancy or an abnormal pregnancy that is intrauterine or extrauterine is foremost. The early detection of an ectopic pregnancy can reduce maternal mortality, excessive blood loss, the need to excise the involved fallopian tube, and even the need for surgical intervention with the alternative of medical therapy with methotrexate. Even though recent investigations have provided laboratory information to assist the clinician in the diagnosis and management of an ectopic pregnancy, the most effective use of the laboratory in the evaluation of a potentially abnormal pregnancy requires both the interpretation of the laboratory results within the clinical setting and the integration of the information with the historical, physical, and sonographic findings.

Pancreatitis in Pregnancy

W. Scott Melvin, MD

E. Christopher Ellison, MD

Pancreatitis is a common affliction resulting from inflammation of the pancreas, causing abdominal pain, nausea, retroperitoneal edema, and, rarely, extensive necrosis and death. Pancreatitis affects pregnant women at the same rate as their nonpregnant counterparts. It has been estimated to occur in about 1 in 1000 pregnancies and it is more common in the primigravid female than the multigravid. Pancreatitis is most often caused by biliary stone disease and recognition can be delayed secondary to the common and nonspecific symptoms of abdominal pain and nausea. Diagnosis is confirmed by serum enzyme determination, and ultrasonography can visualize the causative biliary disease. Symptomatic care and bowel rest result in prompt resolution in the vast majority of cases. Definitive surgical treatment for gallstones is performed electively during the second trimester or postpartum. The prognosis is favorable for both mother and baby, and recurrences are prevented by treating the cause of the pancreatitis.

Etiology

Early in this century, pancreatitis was commonly thought to be a result of idiopathic inflammation of the gland. Currently, alcohol abuse is recognized as the major cause of pancreatitis and its complications. Biliary stones that transiently obstruct the pancreatic duct are also a common cause of pancreatitis and represent the number one cause of pancreatitis in the gravid female. Together, alcohol abuse and gallstones account for over 90% of pancreatitis cases. Hyperlipidemia, sometimes exacerbated by the hormonal milieu of pregnancy, can cause pancreatitis, and should be evaluated in affected patients. A plethora of other etiologies exist for pancreatitis, including drug side effects, postoperative effects, and trauma.

Gallstones are common in Western cultures and occur in about 15% of the adult population. Gallstone formation, or cholelithiasis, is more common in females than in males. Changes in the maternal state predispose to developing cholelithiasis for several reasons. First, elevated serum estrogen levels cause elevations in the bile cholesterol level, resulting in a more lithogenic environment. Second, elevated levels of progesterone result in hypotonia of the gallbladder, allowing sluggish bile flow and resulting in stasis and subsequent stone formation. It is these stones that travel into the common bile duct and, in their passage through the ampulla of Vater, cause obstruction of the pancreatic duct. Resulting edema in this area can cause prolonged ductal dysfunction, or the stone can become impacted in the ampulla, causing persistent pancreatic duct obstruction and fulminant pancreatitis.

Hypertriglyceridemia is a recognized physiologic effect secondary to the hyperestrogenemia of pregnancy and also a recognized cause of pancreatitis. However, rarely do the physiologic changes associated with pregnancy alone cause pancreatitis. Most patients who develop severe hypertriglyceridemia during pregnancy are found to have pre-existing familial hyperlipidemia. This pre-existing condition, exacerbated by the physiologic effect of elevated serum estrogens, can result in extremely high levels of triglycerides and resultant severe, life-threatening pancreatitis. Patients with known familial hyperlipidemia should be carefully counseled, both prior to becoming pregnant and while pregnant, of the risk, albeit low, of developing pancreatitis. Strict diet control is effective in reducing elevated levels of serum triglycerides and preventing complications. Patients at risk should be screened during the first trimester, and elevated triglyceride levels should be treated if necessary. Triglyceride levels greater than 400 mg/dL should be considered elevated and carefully evaluated and followed for potential pancreatitis. Pancreatitis often appears as the triglyceride level approaches 2000, although it sometimes can be found with lower levels.

The other etiologic factors causing pancreatitis during pregnancy are numerous and rare but need to be investigated in patients who present with pancreatitis and no identifiable major risk factor. In patients who have no known identifiable cause, it is often reasonable to assume that biliary stone disease is not visualized.

Diagnosis

Presenting symptoms of pancreatitis are nonspecific and are common complaints of pregnancy. Abdominal pain, nausea, vomiting, and back pain are frequent. Persistence or unusual severity of these symptoms should lead the physician to further investigation. Prodromal symptoms in the patient's history may suggest alcohol use, symptomatic cholelithiasis, or a history of hyperlipidemia, which should place pancreatitis in the differential diagnosis. Physical examination in early pancreatitis is usually nonspecific and is associated with no changes in vital signs and only mild epigastric tenderness. Advanced cases can present after massive fluid sequestration, resulting in hypotension, tachycardia, fever, prostration, respiratory failure, jaundice, oliguria, and a distended tender abdomen. Diagnostic laboratory evaluation reveals hyperamylasemia.

Blood serum testing should be performed on obstetric patients who are at risk for developing pancreatitis or who present with persistent abdominal pain, nausea, and vomiting. Initial laboratory evaluations should include a complete blood count, serum electrolytes, calcium, phosphate, and especially glucose. Liver function tests, amylase, and lipase should be evaluated. Serum amylase and serum lipase levels are not altered physiologically during pregnancy. An elevated amylase level diagnoses pancreatitis; however, the increment of elevation does not predict the severity of the disease. In fact, mild pancreatitis secondary to gallstone disease results in amylase levels of over 1000 and can be quite self-limited. Amylase itself is not an organ-specific enzyme and can be elevated secondary to a multitude of conditions that should be included in the differential diagnosis of this population, including perforated peptic ulcer, acute appendicitis, ectopic and ruptured ectopic pregnancy, and salpingitis. Serum amylase can also be found to be elevated in nonabdominal processes such as parotitis, renal failure, diabetic ketoacidosis, or pneumonia.

Serum lipase may be a more sensitive and specific indicator of pancreatic inflammation. Serum lipase can become elevated prior to and remain elevated after amylase levels are normal. Other laboratory tests are helpful in limiting the diagnosis and directing therapy. Specifically, the physiologic leukocytosis of pregnancy may be further elevated by pancreatitis alone or represent an infective process. Anemia should be evaluated and carefully treated. Electrolyte disturbances secondary to dehydration are common. If pancreatitis is severe, marked deviations from the normal are seen in calcium, magnesium, and phosphate levels. Glucose homeostasis, already altered physiologically in pregnancy, can be severely disturbed by the addition of pancreatitis. Arterial blood gas determination should be obtained in severe cases. Noninvasive methods for obtaining arterial oxygen saturation can be used.

Liver function tests can provide information regarding biliary tract disease and provide a baseline for monitoring liver function. Mild elevation of the alkaline phosphatase and even of total bilirubin are common with choledocholithiasis and cholecystitis. Pronounced elevation of the bilirubin requires further evaluation to rule out persistent obstruction of the common bile duct. Serum triglyceride levels can be elevated secondary to pancreatitis or pregnancy; at higher levels they may represent the causative agent in pancreatitis. In addition, hyperlipidemia secondary to pancreatitis, left untreated, can lead to further pancreatic ischemic injury.

Ultrasonography plays an important role in the diagnosis and management of pancreatitis, particularly in the pregnant patient in whom the use of ionizing radiation for imaging would be discouraged. Ultrasonography of the biliary system provides a high resolution image and is highly sensitive in detecting gallstones. The presence of gallstones without other obvious causes completes the search for the cause of the pancreatitis. Gallstones can be seen by ultrasonography in the gallbladder proper, within the cystic duct or the common bile duct, or at the ampulla. The gallbladder wall can be evaluated for thickness or surrounding fluid suggestive of acute cholecystitis. The size of the common bile duct can be measured. An enlarged common bile duct indicates possible ductal obstruction. Evaluation of the pancreas may reveal peripancreatic edema, glandular enlargement, or, in some cases, calcification of the pancreas, indicating previous pancreatitis. Ultrasonographic evaluation of the gravid uterus, fetus, and placenta can easily be performed, ruling out ectopic pregnancy and monitoring the developing baby. Free fluid within the abdomen is abnormal and associated with severe cases of pancreatitis as well as other diagnoses such as late appendicitis and perforated ulcer.

Treatment

The management of pancreatitis in pregnancy is challenging because the physician must treat two patients. The physiology of normal pregnancy can complicate the observed compensatory mechanisms seen in nonpregnant patients. Initial treatment begins simultaneously with diagnostic testing. Bowel rest and intravenous hydration are the minimal initial steps in the management of patients with persistent abdominal complaints, beginning even while the diagnosis remains uncertain. Although most patients respond well to this therapy alone, some will need more intensive therapy. Surgical therapy is reserved for those few patients who develop pancreatic abscess or necrosis. Definitive therapy for the underlying cause is deferred until the appropriate time.

Pregnancy causes an increase in cardiac output, increase in heart rate, and increased resting minute ventilation. Hypervolemia near term increases circulating blood volume as much as 45% over the volume in nonpregnant control subjects. This hypervolemia is protective to maternal homeostasis and allows a blood loss of near 30% without reducing arterial blood pressure. However, with this amount of blood loss, placental blood flow may be decreased by 10% to 20%. The physician must keep this in mind and recognize that the normotensive mother may still have severely compromised fetal blood flow. Appropriate resuscitation may include a much larger fluid volume than would be appropriate for the nonpregnant female.

Intravenous hydration for pancreatitis initially replaces lost fluid, and then maintains adequate circulating volume as fluid loss continues. An isotonic fluid solution such as lactated Ringer's is the appropriate first choice. Electrolyte determination should help guide fluid replacement as electrolytes, especially potassium, can be severely deranged secondary to pancreatitis or when combined with persistent vomiting. Hyperglycemia can result or be exacerbated by pancreatitis. Intravenous insulin should be given and blood glucose carefully monitored to maintain blood glucose levels below 200 mg/dL. Dextrose-containing intravenous solutions should not be used early. Dextrose can be added as maintenance therapy when the initial resuscitation period is complete. Urine output is a reasonable indicator of adequate fluid replacement; however, this parameter can be in error when associated with osmotic polyuria secondary to hyperglycemia. Pregnancy alone can cause peripheral edema, a cardiac ejection murmur, and cardiomegaly. Therefore physical examination may be unreliable in evaluating an adequate fluid resuscitation. When pancreatitis is severe, the patient may present with hemodynamic compromise and severe dehydration. Invasive monitoring is indicated in these patients to help evaluate the adequacy of resuscitation. Placing invasive monitors (i.e., A-line, Swan-Ganz catheter) should not in any circumstances delay aggressive fluid replacement in the hypotensive patient. Pancreatitis causes pancreatic edema and retroperitoneal sequestration of fluid. As much as one third of the circulating blood volume can be sequestered in the retroperitoneal space in severe cases. Pancreatic necrosis and perhaps ongoing pancreatitis is propagated by ischemic injury, which needs to be prevented by improving blood flow by ensuring adequate circulating volume.

Nasogastric suction does not affect the outcome or clinical course of pancreatitis but is recommended for all patients who exhibit vomiting and is strongly recommended for pregnant patients, who are at higher risk for esophageal reflux and who may have compressed gastric reservoirs. Pain relief is necessary in pancreatitis and adequate relief is usually achieved with parenteral narcotics. Gastric hyperacidity is not a result of pancreatitis, but complications from gastritis and stress ulcerations need to be prevented with antacids. The use of prophylactic antibiotics during the course of acute pancreatitis is controversial. Most authors now recommend broad-spectrum coverage such as imipenem for cases

of significant pancreatitis. Therapeutic antibiotic usage is indicated in those patients who develop signs and symptoms of sepsis, pancreatic necrosis, or pancreatic abscess. The ability to control pancreatic secretions or alter the course of pancreatitis is limited. Use of H_2 blockers, somatostatin analogue, and apoprotinin have been advocated by some; however, no definitive benefit has yet been established and therefore these would not be recommended, especially when these agents have undetermined effects on the developing fetus.

Peritoneal lavage has been shown to alter the course of acute severe pancreatitis when established early in its course. However, because of the inability to identify the patient who could benefit from this, peritoneal lavage is not generally recommended, unless the patient develops multisystem organ failure from severe hemorrhagic pancreatitis. In pregnancy, peritoneal lavage has not been reported. Adequate caloric and protein intake need to be provided to replete depleted protein stores and maintain fetal growth. When enteral nutrition is reinstituted within 5 to 7 days of presentation the resultant malnutrition will be minimal. However, if symptoms or hyperamylasemia persist, then total parenteral nutrition should be started via a central venous catheter.

A typical clinical presentation of pancreatitis is abdominal pain, perhaps following biliary colic that is persistent and severe, prompting evaluation. Hyperamylasemia is noted and resolves with the abdominal pain in 3 to 5 days of bowel rest and intravenous hydration. Little other alteration in laboratory values or physical parameters are noted. Resumption of alimentary nutrition results in no further abdominal pain. However, 10% to 15% of patients who present with gallstone pancreatitis develop a worsening clinical picture that should be noted within the first 48 hours of diagnosis. Various formulas and parameters have been devised to predict patient outcome and mortality; however, these are not valid in the pregnant female. Different parameters used to evaluate and predict a worsening clinical picture include Ranson's criteria, which evaluate age, white blood count, blood glucose level, liver function, decreasing hematocrit, an elevated blood urea nitrogen, a decreasing calcium level, decreasing arterial oxygen saturation, or a large fluid requirement. Other studies indicate that hypotension, hyperpyrexia, hypoalbuminemia, and an elevated prothrombin time would predict a poor outcome. Patients who demonstrate a clinical course consistent with progressive pancreatitis need intensive monitoring, nursing, and continual fetal monitoring.

Respiratory failure is reported to be a complication in 15% to 55% of severe cases of pancreatitis. It is unclear what component of severe pancreatitis leads to this respiratory failure. The decreased lung capacity of pregnancy may exacerbate the poor gas exchange and relative hypoxia caused by pancreatic inflammation. Most patients' oxygen deficits can be corrected by simple supplemental oxygen. Careful monitoring can prevent maternal hypoxia with resulting fetal hypoxia. A few patients will have markedly decreased arterial oxygen tensions and some of these will need to have mechanical ventilation to cover this deficit.

Pancreatic necrosis secondary to severe inflammation and ischemia of the gland is associated with respiratory failure and a massive fluid requirement. In addition, necrotic tissue can secondarily become infected. Pancreatic abscess occurs in 5% to 10% of cases of severe pancreatitis. Abscess formation is suggested by fever, leukocytosis, and a hemodynamic profile consistent with sepsis. Repeat ultrasonographic examination can reveal areas of liquefied necrotic debris or abscess, identified by air bubbles. Surgical intervention is reserved for these few patients. The diagnosis of pancreatic abscess also requires surgical therapy. Criteria for surgical intervention are met when patients exhibit a persistent downward clinical course despite maximum medical support. Débridement and drainage of a grossly necrotic pancreas and retroperitoneum are performed. Wide drainage of all regions with placement of sump drains is recommended by some, while packing with planned re-exploration is advocated by others. Mortality for both mother and baby in this subset of patients is high.

The first episode of gallstone pancreatitis requires that cholecystectomy be performed to prevent recurrent disease. The definitive surgical treatment for gallstones is performed when acute pancreatitis has resolved. No benefit has been demonstrated in reduced morbidity, mortality, or duration of pancreatitis if cholecystectomy and common duct clearance are performed during the acute phase of the illness. Usually cholecystectomy should be performed within the same hospitalization for the first episode of biliary pancreatitis. This is modified during pregnancy. If biliary pancreatitis develops and resolves during the first trimester, definitive therapy should be delayed and electively performed during the second trimester. This approach, preventing surgery in the first trimester, presents less risk to the fetus and avoids a prolonged wait, reducing the risk of recurrence. Third-trimester biliary pancreatitis can be electively treated in the postpartum period. Obviously, emergent surgery should not be delayed if indicated during the first, second, or third trimester. Laparoscopic cholecystectomy and intraoperative cholangiogram can be safely performed in the gravid female. There has been no documented clinical adverse affects to the fetus caused by laparoscopy and it is widely practiced. However, there is no irrefutable proof that laparoscopy is safer for the fetus than open surgery.

Summary

Pregnancy does not cause pancreatitis. Some pregnant patients who develop severe or persistent abdominal pain, nausea, and vomiting are found to have pancreatitis. The diagnosis is suspected if patients have previous gallstone disease or hyperlipidemia and is confirmed by the finding of hypermylasemia. Several days of bowel rest with intravenous hydration results in resolution of the symptoms and normalization of the laboratory values in most cases. Some patients will have a fulminant course requiring intensive care, parenteral nutrition, and even operative intervention. Cholecystectomy is indicated for biliary pancreatitis but can be scheduled so that the risk to the pregnancy is minimal. A favorable prognosis is forecast for the majority of patients who respond to initial therapy.

Postpartum Hemorrhage

John C. Hauth, MD

Incidence and Significance

Normal maternal blood loss during the 24 hours following birth has been directly measured and indirectly estimated to range from 500 to 600 mL following a vaginal and 800 to 1000 mL after a cesarean delivery. Thus, the standard definition of a postpartum hemorrhage as greater than 500 mL is actually less than the average blood lost following most vaginal and all cesarean deliveries. Whereas only 5% of parturients have a measured blood loss of greater than 1000 mL following an uncomplicated vaginal delivery, the average blood loss following an elective repeat cesarean section is approximately 1000 mL. Elective cesarean sections comprise only 5% to 10% of all cesarean sections; other indicated cesarean sections are at increased risk of a postpartum hemorrhage. Thus, over 50% of the more than 1 million women who require a cesarean delivery each year will lose more than 1000 mL of blood following delivery. Normal maternal blood volume expansion is approximately 1500 mL. Thus, the first postpartum day's hematocrit, in more than 75% of women who have a vaginal delivery, will be higher than that obtained prior to delivery. In approximately 50% of women who require a cesarean delivery, the first postpartum day's hematocrit is similar to that prior to delivery. In practice, the amount of blood lost following delivery is imprecisely estimated. A postpartum hemorrhage is clinically suspected in circumstances of uterine, vaginal, or cervical lacerations and in all instances in which the uterus does not promptly and firmly contract following delivery of the placenta. Confirmation of a postpartum hemorrhage occurs with continued vaginal or uterine blood loss in combination with maternal hemodynamic changes (hypotension or tachycardia), oliguria, and with the requirement for maternal blood replacement or the occurrence of a significant postpartum anemia.

Obstetric hemorrhage accounted for 331 of 2067 (13%) reported maternal deaths in the United States from 1974 to 1978. Of these, 114 of the 331 were due to uterine atony. The frequency of maternal morbidity due to postpartum hemorrhage is less defined but is appreciable. Morbidity includes transfusion-related hepatitis, transient or permanent renal damage, acute respiratory dysfunction and capillary leak syndromes, and abscess formation secondary to infection of pelvic hematomas. Not infrequently, these women require additional surgical procedures, including repair of an abdominal wound dehiscence caused by subfascial bleeding, drainage of vulvar or vaginal hematomas, and hysterectomy to control the hemorrhage.

Diagnostic Considerations

Because of the frequency and severity of these complications, all obstetric training programs emphasize expertise in recognizing conditions that predispose to postpartum hemorrhage. This includes the accurate and prompt assessment of the differential causes and the prevention or minimization of the occurrence of postpartum hemorrhage.

Continued vaginal or uterine bleeding following delivery of the placenta mandates prompt palpation of the uterine fundus to assess atony

and inspection of the cervix, vagina, and perineum for lacerations or hematoma formation. Common causes of postpartum hemorrhage include uterine atony; uterine rupture; low-lying placenta; retained placenta; trauma to the cervix, vagina, or perineum; uterine inversion; and inadequate coagulation.

Predisposing Conditions

Many conditions increase the likelihood of a postpartum hemorrhage from uterine atony. These include prolonged labor with or without uterotonic agents, chorioamnionitis, low-lying placenta, uterine overdistension (multifetal pregnancy, hydramnios), large uterine leiomyomata, hypertensive disorders with or without $MgSO_4$ therapy, and uterine relaxant usage, such as halogenated inhalation agents.

Trauma of the uterus or vagina at the time of delivery may also predispose to postpartum hemorrhage. These conditions include the use of low or midforceps or the use of rotational forceps such as Kielland or modified Scanzoni. Precipitous vaginal delivery, vaginal rigidity, or situations with partial vaginal obstruction, such as marked vaginal condyloma acuminata, a transverse or midline vaginal septum, or prior vaginal repair with excessive scar formation may also predispose to hemorrhage. Finally, cesarean section following prolonged labor with marked thinning of the lower uterine segment and impaction of the fetal head, improper technique in cesarean delivery of the fetal vertex, and placenta previa increase the likelihood of postpartum hemorrhage.

Prevention

Atony

Postpartum hemorrhage due to uterine atony is more frequent in patients with the conditions listed; however, atony can also occur in otherwise low-risk women after an uneventful spontaneous vaginal delivery. Thus, it has become almost universally accepted to use a uterotonic agent, prophylactically, immediately following delivery of the placenta. Prendiville and colleagues, in a review of nine clinical trials, concluded that uterotonic drugs used routinely reduce the incidence of postpartum hemorrhage by 40%. They estimated that for every 22 women given a prophylactic uterotonic drug following delivery of the placenta, one postpartum hemorrhage could be prevented. *Williams Obstetrics,* 18th edition, notes that 20 U of oxytocin in 1000 mL of lactated Ringer's solution, at 200 mU of oxytocin per minute, usually proves effective. Our clinical experience has confirmed these recommendations. We have extended this policy to recommend the routine use of an even more concentrated oxytocin infusion for those women with the predisposing conditions for postpartum uterine atony; 60 U of oxytocin in 1000 mL of lactated Ringer's solution at 500 mU/min. We do not recommend the use of an undiluted intravenous bolus of 5 or 10 units of oxytocin following delivery of the placenta because of the potential for maternal hypotension.

Trauma

Postpartum hemorrhage can occur as a result of extension of the uterine incision during a cesarean delivery. These lacerations may result in appreciable blood loss and increased maternal morbidity that includes bladder and, infrequently, ureteral damage. All lacerations should be promptly sutured. Prevention of uterine trauma during cesarean delivery is dependent on the skill and experience of the operator. The uterine incision should be of sufficient size to preclude laceration of the uterine vessels with delivery of the fetus. Forcible delivery of the fetal head or shoulders through too small a uterine incision may result in extensive lacerations of the lower uterine segment. In addition, various techniques are available for elevation of a fetal head that is impacted in the vaginal inlet, so as to preclude uterine and vaginal lacerations. These include vaginal assistance with elevation of the presenting fetal part, cephalad traction on the anterior fetal shoulder, anterior vaginal pressure to dislodge and elevate the presenting fetal part prior to the operator's inserting his or her hand into the uterus, and the occasional use of a vacuum traction device to deliver the vertex in circumstances with limited abdominal or uterine exposure may also be of benefit. Lastly, the operator must elevate and flex the fetal head through the uterine incision without depressing the back of his or her hand against the inferior margin of the lower uterine segment.

Trauma to the cervix, vagina, and perineum during vaginal delivery can be minimized by careful attention to forceps application, use of adequate pelvic muscle relaxation prior to an operative delivery, and skillful delivery of the fetal head with extension and anterior traction once the vertex has passed under the symphysis.

Management of Postpartum Hemorrhage

If uterine hemorrhage continues without evidence of cervical, vaginal, or perineal causes, then a manual exploration of the uterine cavity should be performed to assess uterine contractibility and to exclude a uterine rupture or retained placental tissue. A uterine perforation or extensive laceration requires prompt laparotomy and repair. If exploration of the uterus is normal and the bleeding is due to uterine atony, as is most frequently the case, additional uterotonic agents are indicated.

Treatment
General

After a postpartum hemorrhage is diagnosed clinically due to uterine atony, supportive and general measures are begun. These include uterine massage, placement of two large-bore intravenous catheters, administration of either intravenous crystalloid or packed red cells as needed, placement of a Foley catheter to monitor hourly urine output, and testing to exclude coagulation abnormalities. This should include a maternal prothrombin time, partial thromboplastin time, platelet count, and fibrinogen level. Uterine packing and uterine lavage with warm saline have both been utilized with occasional success. If they are to be used, it should be briefly before curettage or laparotomy.

Pharmacologic

At our institution, in addition to the general measures outlined, postpartum hemorrhage due to uterine atony is initially treated by increasing the oxytocin concentration to 60 to 80 U/L at a rate of 1000 mL/hr. We then use 0.2 mg of an ergot alkaloid intramuscularly (ergonovine maleate [Ergotrate maleate] or methylergonovine maleate [Methergine]), except in women with hypertension. This dosage can be repeated once within 15 minutes. If uterine atony persists, we give a prostaglandin (PG), either as a 20-mg PGE_2 vaginal suppository or 0.25 mg of 15-methyl $PGF_{2\alpha}$ (Prostin/15M) intramuscularly. Injection of 15-methyl $PGF_{2\alpha}$ can be repeated every 15 to 60 minutes for up to three doses. Prior maternal asthma or cardiac dysfunction are relative contraindications to the use of prostaglandins. Also, PGE_2 is contraindicated in maternal hypotension and the 15-methyl $PGF_{2\alpha}$ is relatively contraindicated in hypertension.

Surgical

If bleeding persists from uterine atony despite these measures, most practitioners would perform an exploratory laparotomy with ligation of both hypogastric or ascending branches of the uterine arteries or would proceed to a hysterectomy. The choice of procedure will depend on the parity of the patient and her desire for childbearing, the extent of hemorrhage, and, most important, the experience and judgment of the surgeon. If life-threatening hemorrhage continues, hysterectomy frequently is the quickest and safest procedure for the patient. The main indication for hysterectomy in patients with postpartum hemorrhage is failure to respond to medical therapy. Emergency hysterectomy for obstetric hemorrhage was attributable to atony, accreta, uterine rupture, or extensive laceration in 96% of the cases in a series reported by Clark. A less invasive surgical alternative has been infrequently reported. By placing a catheter in the hypogastric and uterine vessels, a radiologist may be able to identify the bleeding site and inject either stabilized blood clots or gel foam to embolize the offending vessels. This is less likely to be successful with uterine atony than with continued bleeding following pelvic surgery.

Transfusion for Obstetric Hemorrhage

Every obstetric provider should be able to detail precisely his or her criteria for initiating red cell transfusions, for determining when transfusion has been sufficient, and for monitoring the continued adequacy of the maternal intravascular volume. All too frequently, phoned orders for repeated bolus crystalloid infusions have resulted in appreciable maternal morbidity and even death as a result of marked delays in the replacement of the maternal red blood cell volume.

Transfusion therapy is used to prevent or treat hemorrhagic shock and its consequences. Blood loss estimated to be greater than or equal to 1500 mL represents approximately 25% of a pregnant woman's total estimated blood volume (6000 mL). There are many clinical circumstances in which a pregnant patient might benefit from transfusion of red blood cells before the blood loss has reached such levels. In the pregnant patient, the circulating blood volume must be maintained and therapy should be directed at maintaining an adequate cardiac output and tissue perfusion.

Before delivery, red blood cell transfusion may be indicated in women with active or arrested hemorrhage and with consideration of her hemodynamic status and clinical conditions, such as the following:

- Appreciable bleeding continues
- Signs or symptoms of hypovolemia are present (e.g., shock)
- Oliguria and vasoconstriction persist

The endpoint of red cell transfusion therapy will vary with the clinical situation. Monitoring a hematocrit of greater than or equal to 30% and a urine output of 30 mL or more per hour generally has been recommended as a goal of therapy in a pregnant patient who is actively bleeding or who is at continued risk for significant obstetric hemorrhage, such as with a placenta previa. In a clinically stable patient who has responded appropriately to therapy, however, the decision to transfuse should be based on individual circumstances.

Following delivery, if active bleeding has ceased, transfusion can be withheld despite laboratory determinations of significant anemia, as in patients with normal tissue perfusion, including a normal urine output (>30 mL/hr) and no appreciable postural hypotension or tachycardia. The patient's compensatory mechanisms of increased erythropoiesis and plasma volume expansion will correct the red blood cell deficit.

The adequacy of transfusion therapy should be monitored by evaluation of the patient for signs and symptoms of shock to include maternal pulse and blood pressure. A further reassuring test (tilt-test) in women with a normal pulse in the recumbent position is to compare that pulse with one obtained sitting. If they are similar (less than a 20 beat-per-minute difference), in general, the intravascular volume is sufficient at that time. The hematocrit is measured sequentially, and urinary output is measured and recorded. A urinary output of greater than or equal to 30 mL/hour and a hematocrit of greater than or equal to 30% generally reflect adequate renal perfusion and circulating oxygen-carrying capacity, respectively. Both tissue perfusion and oxygen-carrying capacity can be adequate at lower levels in otherwise stable patients *without continuing blood loss.*

Post-Term Pregnancy

Tamerou Asrat, MD
Edward J. Quilligan, MD

Definition

Strictly defined, a pregnancy is considered post-term if it exceeds 294 days (42 weeks) because of the rapidly accelerating risk of fetal morbidity and mortality beyond 42 weeks.

Scope of the Problem

Prolonged pregnancy is a common obstetric problem. Four to 14% (average 10%) of women reach 42 weeks and 2% to 7% (average 4%) reach 43 weeks and beyond.

The rate of maternal, fetal, and neonatal complications increases exponentially with advancing gestational age, with perinatal mortality beginning to rise between 41 and 42 weeks, doubling at 43 weeks, and being four to six times higher at 44 weeks than at term.

The maternal complications include a more than twofold increase in the cesarean delivery rate and its attendant risk of hemorrhage, infections, and wound breakdowns.

Fetal and neonatal complications include a higher incidence of antenatal and intrapartum fetal distress, intolerance to labor, meconium aspiration syndrome, and birth trauma from macrosomia. Ten to 20% of post-term fetuses will demonstrate growth restriction from placental insufficiency. These neonates appear emaciated, with loss of subcutaneous fat and muscle mass along with epidermal desquamation and meconium-stained fingernails and membranes. On the other hand, 20% to 25% of post-term neonates weigh over 4000 g at birth and about 5% over 4500 g, resulting in a higher rate of birth injuries due to difficult instrumented deliveries and shoulder dystocia.

Management Strategies: Avoiding Common Pitfalls

Errors in dating pregnancies remain a common source of frustration because significant numbers of pregnant patients enroll in prenatal care clinics late in gestation. In situations in which the diagnosis of post-term pregnancy is equivocal, we recommend initiating fetal surveillance, primarily to assess the amniotic fluid volume. A normal or adequate amniotic fluid volume is a reassuring finding and allows expectant management with continued fetal surveillance.

As a rule, redating of pregnancies based on a late second or third trimester ultrasonographic evaluation should be avoided, since it may lead to iatrogenic prematurity or delayed intervention, leading to poor outcome.

Most clinicians initiate fetal testing between 41 and 42 weeks' gestation. The clinician may choose one of several modalities of antenatal fetal surveillance, including twice-weekly non-stress testing (NST), twice-weekly modified biophysical profiles (MBPP), weekly contraction stress tests, and twice-weekly biophysical profile.

Regardless of the method of fetal surveillance employed, it is critical to assess the amniotic fluid volume at a minimum of once a week, preferably twice weekly. At our institution we use the MBPP twice weekly. The MBPP consists of the NST (as a marker of acute hypoxia) and amniotic fluid index (AFI) (as a measure of chronic hypoxia). Oligohydramnios (AFI <5 cm) should prompt delivery of the post-term pregnancy.

It must be emphasized that weekly NST offers no benefit over no fetal surveillance. NST should be done twice weekly. When interpreting the NST, the clinician must pay close attention to spontaneous decelerations, since several studies have demonstrated that the majority of poor perinatal outcomes are found in this group of patients.

Several randomized trials of routine induction versus expectant management along with antepartum fetal surveillance have now shown that induction of labor between 41 and 42 weeks will reduce the risk of perinatal death significantly and slightly decrease the rate of cesarean births. Despite these encouraging results there remains a strong resistance against routine induction of labor at 41 to 42 weeks, particularly if the cervix is unfavorable.

Prostaglandin E_2 (PGE_2) cervical gel (Prepidil) is now approved by the Food and Drug Administration for preinduction cervical ripening. Prepidil contains 0.5 mg of PGE_2 and is administered intracervically every 6 hours for two to three doses. Various centers are experimenting with different dosages and modes of delivery of the medication to increase the rate of successful inductions.

Recently a few studies have demonstrated that the presence of fetal fibronectin (fFN) in the cervicovaginal secretions at 40 weeks and beyond is positively correlated with a higher rate of successful inductions. Indeed, a plausible scenario in the future might include routine testing for fFN at 41 to 42 weeks. In those patients found to be fFN-positive, labor will be induced, whereas those who are fFN-negative will be managed expectantly if the antepartum surveillance tests remain reassuring.

Prior to proceeding with induction of labor, the clinician must rule out the possibility of fetal macrosomia. Admittedly, ultrasonographic evaluation of the fetus, this late in pregnancy, is a highly insensitive tool for assessment of estimated fetal anatomy. These limitations notwithstanding, we recommend that the option of cesarean delivery be discussed if the estimated fetal weight, either by ultrasonography or by Leopold maneuvers, is thought to be over 4500 g.

In the intrapartum period, electronic fetal monitoring should be done routinely. Amniotomy should be done as soon as it is safely feasible. This allows for the early detection of meconium-stained fluid. We recommend that saline amnioinfusion be used liberally in cases of "thick" meconium or in the presence of variable decelerations, secondary to oligohydramnios and cord compression. Studies have shown that amnioinfusion in such settings reduces the rate of cesarean sections for fetal distress and meconium aspiration. Caution must be exercised in interpreting the fetal heart rate tracing during labor. While variable decelerations secondary to cord compression may respond to saline amnioinfusion, repetitive late decelerations are indicative of placental insufficiency and hypoxia and do not correct with amnioinfusion. The post-term, growth restricted fetus with oligohydramnios, meconium-stained fluid, and late decelerations is indeed at significant jeopardy and we recommend a liberal use of cesarean sections for delivery of this category of post-term fetuses.

Pre-eclampsia

Frederick P. Zuspan, MD

Pre-eclampsia/eclampsia is a disease of unknown etiology peculiar to human pregnancy, beginning after the 20th week of gestation and cured by delivery of the products of conception. The pathophysiology has been well established, but the etiology is unknown. Pre-eclampsia is divided into pre-eclampsia (mild), pre-eclampsia (severe), and eclampsia (i.e., a patient with pre-eclampsia who develops a generalized seizure within the first 7 days postpartum).

The Committee on Terminology of the American College of Obstetricians and Gynecologists lists the following classifications:

1. Pre-eclampsia—mild and severe
2. Chronic hypertension
3. Chronic hypertension with superimposed pre-eclampsia/eclampsia
4. Transient or gestational hypertension

Diagnosis

The International Society for the Study of Hypertension in Pregnancy and the World Health Organization have a more complicated classification of acute hypertension in pregnancy. Basically, the diagnosis of pre-eclampsia is made in a woman who, after 20 weeks of gestation, has a blood pressure that exceeds 140/90 mm Hg, with the presence of more than 0.3 g/L of urinary protein. If there is less protein or an absence of protein, the diagnosis of gestational hypertension is made. When the pre-eclamptic patient develops generalized convulsions, a diagnosis of eclampsia is then made.

Antecedent findings in pre-eclampsia often include a rapid weight gain of more than 5 or 6 pounds in 1 week, an increase in diastolic blood pressure of greater than 15 mm Hg, and an increase in systolic blood pressure of greater than 30 mm Hg. However, the diagnosis of pre-eclampsia cannot be made until objective findings of a blood pressure that exceeds 140/90 mm Hg and more than 0.3 g/L of protein is present in the urine.

Severe pre-eclampsia is diagnosed when one or more of the following situations exist:

1. Diastolic blood pressure that is persistent and exceeds 110 mm Hg and systolic pressure greater than 170 mm Hg
2. Protein excretion greater than 3 g/day
3. Clonus in reflexes
4. Oliguria of less than 400 mL/day associated with an increase in serum creatinine level
5. Platelet counts lower than 100,000
6. Abnormal liver enzymes
7. Cerebral or visual disturbances
8. Persistent, severe epigastric or right upper quadrant pain
9. Pulmonary edema or cyanosis

It should be noted that 20% of women have eclampsia with blood pressures of less than 140/90 mm Hg and no proteinuria. Not all women with mild pre-eclampsia develop severe pre-eclampsia/eclampsia.

Patients with severe pre-eclampsia/eclampsia must be considered to be in an acute emergency situation and are treated accordingly.

Pathophysiology

The major target organs are the cardiovascular system, demonstrating vasospasm and an increase in blood pressure; the kidneys, demonstrating a renal lesion known as glomeruloendotheliosis and manifested by significant proteinuria; and the uteroplacental bed, demonstrating failure of the spiral arteries to dilate, and a lack of adrenergic denervation. More likely than not, there is an inappropriate immune response between the trophoblastic tissue and the musculoelastic tissue of the spiral artery that does not permit appropriate invasion by the trophoblasts—hence, less dilatation of these vessels.

The organs secondarily shocked include the reticuloendothelial system, which demonstrates a decrease in platelets. The liver may manifest degenerative changes evidenced by an increase in the liver enzymes and, eventually, jaundice with a rise in the bilirubin level. The brain may manifest cerebral edema or hemorrhage. As a generalization, the organs secondarily shocked, when involved, indicate very serious disease for the mother, which may result in death.

Four to 6% of pregnant patients will develop pre-eclampsia, of which 85% are nulligravidas. There are certain observed associations in individuals who have a higher propensity for developing pre-eclampsia, including

1. Multiple gestation with hyperplacentosis, as also seen in diabetes and macrosomia, carries a twofold to threefold increase in the disease. Women who have chronic hypertension or chronic renal disease also have a twofold to threefold increase in the disease. The first term pregnancy, in contrast to the second pregnancy, has an incidence of some 4% to 6% worldwide.
2. It has been shown that a recessive gene can cause "recurrent pre-eclampsia"—hypertension in subsequent pregnancies in selected patients who have had eclampsia.
3. The working woman, who may lack sufficient bedrest, has a twofold increase in the development of pre-eclampsia.

Therapy
Gestational Hypertension

The patient who has less than 300 mg/L proteinuria but has a blood pressure of 140/90 mm Hg is diagnosed as having gestational hypertension. It is permissible for this patient to be treated at home with the use of bedrest and observation. The use of diuretics or a low-salt diet does not seem to improve the disease. If the patient is near term (i.e., 37 to 42 weeks) and the cervix is favorable, induction of labor may be appropriate.

Mild Pre-eclampsia

This diagnosis is made when the blood pressure is greater than 140/90 mm Hg and there is more than 0.3 g/L of protein in the urine. The patient should be hospitalized and removed from the environment in which she developed pre-eclampsia. She may or may not need to be delivered, depending on multiple factors, including gestational age, size of the baby, condition of the cervix, and her response to hospital therapy. At least two studies point out that the perinatal morbidity and mortality in gestational hypertension and mild pre-eclampsia are no different from those in normal pregnancy. Problems exist only when the fetus becomes compromised; the fetus may or may not be small for gestational age or may or may not show intrauterine growth retardation. Baseline laboratory studies include a complete blood count with platelet count, serum creatinine level, liver function profile, and serial urine protein determinations. The blood pressure is evaluated for change four times during the day. The blood pressure should be taken in the upper arm of the patient, who is sitting; the systolic, the muffled fourth Korotkoff's sound, and the disappearing fifth Korotkoff's sound are utilized, and all three are recorded.

The World Health Organization recommends using the fourth Korotkoff's sound, as do European clinics, but the fifth sound is routinely used in the United States. If all three are recorded, any confusion should be eliminated. If the patient's arm measures greater than 35 cm in circumference, a thigh cuff should be used. Otherwise, an erroneously high value will be obtained.

The patient should remain in the hospital if she tends to be agitated and noncompliant. The assumption should be made that the severe forms of the disease are preventable, since it is known that eclampsia carries with it a maternal mortality in the United States of 0.5% to 1% and a fetal mortality of 10% or less. The major problems for the fetus are prematurity and the need to deliver the patient early because of maternal indications or fetal distress.

Severe Pre-eclampsia/Eclampsia

It should be assumed that this is an emergency and requires the benefit of continuous health care in a closely observed situation. The principles of therapy include prevention of seizure once the patient is hospitalized; prevention of hazards for the mother, such as stroke; and prevention of hazards for the fetus (i.e., stillbirth or neonatal death). There is no therapy that is beneficial to both the mother and the fetus, but the one that affects the fetus least and gives the mother the greatest benefit is parenteral magnesium sulfate. This is the standard of care in the United States for preventing convulsions. Recently, a multicentered study of more than 1600 eclamptic patients confirmed the efficacy of magnesium sulfate and this has now become the worldwide recommendation.

Magnesium Sulfate

It must be assumed that magnesium sulfate is a potentially dangerous drug if given intravenously too fast. If the intravenous method of administration is chosen, which we prefer, it should take 3 to 5 minutes to give the intravenous loading dose of 4 to 6 g.

Magnesium sulfate is excreted principally by the kidneys; hence, urinary output must be observed carefully. It can be counteracted by intravenous calcium (1 g) if excessive magnesium is administered. It depresses activity at the myoneural junction and prevents convulsions, but it is not an antihypertensive drug. It will, however, help stabilize the blood pressure. Magnesium crosses the placenta and is usually in equilibrium with the fetus.

Magnesium has two benefits other than preventing convulsions. It has recently been found to decrease platelet aggregation, and it increases uterine blood flow and more likely than not is protective for the fetus.

Specific Information

A loading dose of magnesium sulfate, 4 to 6 g, should be administered intravenously, depending upon the size of the patient. The dose should take 3 to 5 minutes to give, and then the magnesium sulfate is given by a controlled infusion device, 1 to 2 g/hour intravenously. This regimen has been termed the Zuspan method of administering magnesium sulfate, and the following is known as the Pritchard method.

A loading dose of 20 mL of 20% magnesium sulfate (4 g) is administered intravenously over a 3-minute period. This dose is immediately followed by 20 mL of 50% magnesium sulfate, half (5 g or 10 mL) injected deeply in the upper outer quadrant of each buttock through a 3-inch 20-gauge needle. The maintenance dose is 10 mL of 50% magnesium sulfate (5 g) administered intramuscularly in alternating buttocks every 4 hours. Both of these methods were used in the large multicentered study.

Both regimens assume that the patient is literally a bioassay preparation, and their effectiveness is based on the following three conditions: (1) that the reflexes are present but hypoactive; (2) that respirations are not significantly depressed; and (3) that urine output is at least 100 mL in 4 hours.

This use of magnesium sulfate has been the standard of care in the United States for at least 40 years and has been adopted in other parts of the world. The reason for its value is that the patient is easy to manage and does not require other forms of therapy. There is little evidence of difficulty with airway problems, whereas with some forms of therapy, tracheostomy is needed. The fetus is less depressed, and it is a simplified method for the health care team.

The fetus may appear to be floppy on delivery, but the Apgar scores are usually good. The magnesium in the baby is excreted within 48 hours.

Control of Blood Pressure

Antihypertensive agents should be used if the diastolic blood pressure consistently exceeds 100 mm Hg. There are others who use a diastolic blood pressure of 110 mm Hg, but I have found that a more aggressive approach to the control of the blood pressure is beneficial.

The drug used is hydralazine, given in 5 mg bolus injections intravenously, and the blood pressure is then monitored by a Dynamap monitor at 3- to 5-minute intervals. If the blood pressure is not acceptably lower in 20 minutes, 100 mg of hydralazine is put in a plastic bag containing 200 mL of saline, and an infusion pump then administers the dose, with the blood pressure titrated to the point at which the diastolic pressure is in the vicinity of 80 to 90 mm Hg. Alternate drugs include labetalol (α, β blocker) intravenously in 20 mg increments or nifedipine, a calcium channel blocker, given orally in 10 mg increments. The drugs should be titrated to the blood pressure desired.

The fetal heart must be monitored at this time. If the blood pressure is lowered precipitously, fetal distress may occur.

Delivery

Once the patient who has severe pre-eclampsia/eclampsia is admitted to the hospital, baseline laboratory studies should be done and should include a complete blood count with platelet count, electrolyte values, a clotting profile, liver function studies, and a serum creatinine level. The results of these tests should be obtained within several hours, and a decision must then be made about whether or not the patient should be delivered and, if so, by what route. As a generalization, in someone who has severe pre-eclampsia/eclampsia, delivery is the treatment of choice. There are exceptional cases of patients remote from term (<30 weeks) who are not delivered, but in general, major problems for the fetus may result if delivery is not accomplished.

Evaluation should also include ultrasonography of the baby and a reaction of the baby's heartbeat to movement. The vaginal route of delivery is preferred, and the majority of patients whose babies weigh more than 1200 g should be delivered in that manner. If, after 8 to 12 hours of oxytocin administration, delivery has not been achieved, a cesarean section would be in order.

An amniocentesis is done on selected patients to determine pulmonary maturity if the baby has a gestational age of less than 34 weeks. Glucocorticoids to enhance pulmonary maturity may be given if delivery can wait for 48 hours.

Anesthesia

The simplest forms of anesthesia, such as local infiltration or pudendal block, are best. However, if a cesarean section is done, two options exist: (1) general endotracheal anesthesia using thiopental or succinylcholine or (2) epidural anesthesia. If an experienced obstetric anesthesiologist is available, epidural anesthesia is the route of choice. If extensive antihypertensive medication is given, the block may create a fall in blood pressure; an adequate fluid level prior to the epidural is desirable. Spinal anesthesia is definitely contraindicated.

Once the patient is taken to the operating or delivery room, the magnesium sulfate and hydralazine should accompany her there during the process of the delivery. Electronic fetal monitoring should also be done until the patient is delivered. Once delivery has been achieved, it is necessary to maintain the magnesium sulfate therapy for at least 24 hours postpartum, and then the dose should be gradually diminished.

Deaths in Pre-eclampsia/Eclampsia

Death for the fetus may occur because of prematurity. If hypoxia does not exist during labor and delivery, the fetus should do reasonably well if it has a gestational age of more than 30 weeks. The problems that befall the fetus are those of prematurity, not particularly those of the disease.

Maternal deaths in pre-eclampsia/eclampsia are due to an underestimation of the severity of the disease, an overconfidence in the use of polydrug regimens, and a reluctance to deliver the patient.

Prevention

Until a specific etiologic agent can be found, we must be content to implement measures to try to prevent severe disease from occurring. We understand the pathophysiology of the disease well, and therapy should be directed to correct this. These issues include the following:

1. Suggest that all pregnant patients spend at least 1.5 hours a day in the lateral recumbent position. This increases uterine and renal blood flow as well as decreases endogenous catecholamines.
2. Identify the potentially high-risk patient (first term pregnancy, family history of hypertension, chronic hypertension or renal disease, diabetes, and multiple gestation). Then institute a more intensive surveillance plan for prenatal care in these patients.
3. Utilize home blood pressure determinations. If a systolic blood pressure increase exceeds 30 mm Hg or a diastolic exceeds 15 mm Hg, assume that this patient may develop pre-eclampsia in the future and needs closer observation.
4. Decrease maternal anxiety by having a well-informed patient.
5. Insist on a protein intake that will at least achieve a zero nitrogen balance (1 g of protein per kilogram of body weight per day).
6. Hospitalize the patient if she has pre-eclampsia, then individualize her care.

The efficacy of using 2 g of calcium per day or low-dose aspirin (60 mg) has yet to be proved, but both agents look promising at this time in high risk and potentially at risk patients as preventive measures to decrease the incidence of severe disease in selected patients.

Premature Rupture of Membranes

Thomas Garite, MD

Premature rupture of membranes (PROM) is defined as rupture of the fetal membranes prior to the onset of labor, regardless of gestational age, and is one of the most common and most controversial problems facing the obstetric clinician today. This diagnosis complicates about 8% to 10% of all pregnancies. At term, PROM is probably a physiologic event associated with weakening of membranes that occurs as term nears. Complications associated with this problem in the term patient include maternal and fetal infections and the risk of umbilical cord compression, which may lead to fetal asphyxia and even fetal death. Preterm PROM accounts for about one third of the total cases of PROM and is etiologically responsible for 20% to 50% of preterm births, depending on the population. In addition to the complications seen at term, preterm PROM also results most often in preterm labor and delivery. In pre-viable gestational stages, an additional complication may occur, termed the *fetal deformation syndrome,* which includes pulmonary hypoplasia, intrauterine growth retardation, and facial and limb deformities, all due to prolonged oligohydramnios.

A history of a large gush of watery fluid from the vagina with continued leakage is consistent with PROM, and history alone is accurate for this diagnosis in over 90% of cases. Any patient, regardless of gestational age, with a history consistent with PROM, should be examined promptly to confirm the diagnosis. Confirmation of the diagnosis is made by speculum examination, which reveals pooling of fluid in the posterior fornix. A dark blue color change on a strip of Nitrazine paper is used to confirm the alkaline pH of the amniotic fluid. If there is any question of the diagnosis, a sample of the fluid is smeared on a slide, allowed to dry, and viewed under a microscope, which reveals a "ferning" pattern. Ultrasonography can also be used to confirm oligohydramnios. Unless the patient is clearly having active and painful contractions, every effort should be made to avoid digital endocervical examination, as the rate of infection is increased in both mother and newborn with digital examination. At the time of speculum examination, depending on the gestational age, additional tests may be done, including cultures for Group B streptococcus (GBS), chlamydia, and gonorrhea,

and amniotic fluid may be taken for fetal lung maturity testing.

Once the diagnosis is confirmed, the next step is to establish the gestational age, as this is generally the most critical first step in determining the appropriate management. History, prenatal records and previous ultrasonographic examinations should be reviewed. In preterm patients or in any patient whose gestational age is in question, an ultrasonographic examination is done following confirmation of the diagnosis, to confirm gestational age; determine fetal lie; evaluate amniotic fluid volume; rule out anomalies; and, when appropriate, perform fetal biophysical profile testing. Once gestational age is established, the remainder of management is based principally on which gestational age group the fetus falls into.

Management at Term

When PROM occurs at term, the onset of labor occurs within 24 hours in over 90% of patients. However, as membrane rupture becomes prolonged (>24–48 hours) the incidence of both chorioamnionitis and fetal sepsis increases. This increase in fetal sepsis results in a two- to three-fold increase in perinatal mortality; therefore, most management schemes have been developed to avoid prolonged rupture of membranes by inducing labor with oxytocin after allowing the patient some reasonable period of time to go into labor spontaneously. A recent trend advocating expectant management, avoiding digital examinations, has gained some favor, but generally outcomes are equal or better and patient satisfaction is greater when labor is induced within 12 to 24 hours of spontaneous PROM. Even more recently, studies have shown that inserting prostaglandin in the vagina following admission results in spontaneous labor more often or within a shorter time period and reduces the need for and increases the success of oxytocin induction.

Our protocol for patients whose history is consistent with possible PROM is as follows. The patient is asked to come into the hospital or office immediately and she is evaluated to confirm the diagnosis with speculum examination. Once the diagnosis is confirmed, she is evaluated for labor, fetal distress, or chorioamnionitis. These are evaluated clinically with history and physical examination and initially external electronic fetal heart rate monitoring. Fetal distress, in the setting of PROM, is usually due to umbilical cord compression due to oligohydramnios. Amnioinfusion is the ideal treatment for this constellation of PROM, oligohydramnios, and variable decelerations and once labor is established should be instituted early and liberally. Chorioamnionitis in the setting of PROM, more specifically addressed elsewhere in this textbook, is treated with antibiotics such as gentamicin and ampicillin and if the patient is not in labor, delivery should be expedited with oxytocin induction. However, the indications for or timing of cesarean section should not be altered by the presence of chorioamnionitis. Spontaneous labor is the desired outcome following PROM and therefore should be gratefully acknowledged.

In the case of a patient with PROM at term (≥36 weeks for the purpose of this diagnosis) who is not in labor and not clinically infected and in which the fetal heart rate is reassuring, our practice is to immediately insert prostaglandin, either using a 3 mg prostaglandin E_2 suppository prepared in our own pharmacy or using the continuous release pessary known as Cervidil. (The intracervical preparation is avoided because of the theoretical concern of introducing infection, although data to support or refute this concern are lacking.) If the suppository is used, it may be repeated in 6 hours if labor does not ensue. In either case, after 12 hours (for Cervidil, the string is removed), if the patient is not in labor, oxytocin induction is instituted. For all patients, it should be remembered that the latent phase is not associated with worse outcomes until it becomes prolonged at about 18 hours. Therefore the patient should be given that long to enter the active phase of labor before being subjected to cesarean section for failed induction. Once the active phase of labor is achieved, these patients are managed as any other laboring patients. The only exception is that antibiotics (eg, penicillin or ampicillin) should be used to prevent neonatal GBS sepsis in mothers with either unknown GBS culture status after 18 hours of membrane rupture or all patients with positive GBS cultures after 36 weeks.

Management at 32 to 35 Weeks

In patients with gestation of 32 to 35 weeks, survival exceeds 90% to 95% if delivery occurs, but complications of prematurity are common. However, should chorioamnionitis occur, not only does mortality increase by two- to threefold, but complications of prematurity and fetal sepsis increase similarly. Therefore the ideal aim is to deliver the fetuses destined to either do well in the nursery or to develop chorioamnionitis and to expectantly manage the rest to buy time for further maturity.

Again, the diagnosis is confirmed, cultures are taken, and an aliquot of amniotic fluid from the vagina is sent for laboratory determination of phosphatidylglycerol if delivery is not imminent. Patients in labor, those with chorioamnionitis, and those with fetal distress are delivered immediately and managed as described with term PROM. For those not in labor and with no infection or fetal distress, management depends on fetal lung maturity status. The phosphatidylglycerol can be measured with a slide agglutination test and results can be available in less than 1 hour. If the results are positive, labor should be induced unless vaginal delivery is otherwise contraindicated. If the results are negative, amniocentesis should be done for lecithin/sphingomyelin ratio or other tests of fetal lung maturity, as PG is often negative in the face of mature fetal lungs. At the time of amniocentesis, an aliquot of amniotic fluid is sent for Gram stain, culture, and glucose level. Patients with lecithin/sphingomyelin ratios or other test results indicating maturity are delivered by induction or cesarean section where indicated. Patients with occult intra-amniotic infection indicated by bacteria on Gram stain or glucose levels less than 15 mg/dL at these gestational ages are also probably best managed by delivery. Antibiotics should be started and induction initiated, reserving cesarean section for the usual obstetric indications. For those in whom amniocentesis is not done, another alternative for ruling out infection, particularly fetal sepsis, is the biophysical profile (BPP). However, if the fetal heart rate exhibits reactivity (accelerations of the FHR in response to fetal movement), there is no need to perform a complete BPP, as reactive fetuses will virtually always have otherwise reassuring BPPs. Patients with immature lung profiles and no indication of infection are managed expectantly in the hospital with daily evaluation for labor, infection, and fetal well-being. A prolonged daily non-stress test with particular attention to reactivity for absence of infection and the absence of variable decelerations due to oligohydramnios will provide good reassurance of fetal well-being. These patients are ultimately then delivered either for spontaneous labor, infection, or nonreassuring fetal status. Alternatively, fetal maturity tests may be repeated every 1 to 2 weeks and delivered when mature. Once these patients are in active labor they should be given antibiotics to prevent GBS transmission to the baby unless a recent positive culture is negative. As these patients are at high risk for umbilical cord compression in labor, amnioinfusion can be used either prophylactically or therapeutically with a very liberal threshold for starting promptly once variable decelerations do begin.

Management at 25 to 31 Weeks

For patients in the 25 to 31 weeks gestational age group, maternal risks are similar to those outlined in the previous section, but the major risk to the fetus is mortality and major morbidity from prematurity. Therefore the aim for these patients is to prolong pregnancy as long as it is safe to do so and to ameliorate complications of prematurity. Initial evaluation and management are similar to those used for patients at 32 to 35 weeks' gestation, except there is little point in doing amniocentesis in these patients as lung maturity is unlikely. While some clinicians use tocolytics, there is no evidence of benefit in PROM and we do not use them except to facilitate maternal transport. Recently the National Institutes of Health recommended corticosteroids in this group with PROM. Betamethasone 12 mg IM, two doses administered 24 hours apart or dexamethasone 6 mg IM or IV every 12 hours for four doses may be given and repeated every week until the end of the 31st week. Finally, there is now reasonably good evidence that antibiotics given prophylactically prolong gestation by an average of a week and may also decrease the likelihood of maternal and fetal or neonatal infection. Since there is some fear of increasing the chance of infection with resistant organisms with this approach, antibiotics should only be used when the likelihood of benefit clearly outweighs such risk. Thus the group of patients at these very early gestational ages, where a week is likely to make a substantial difference, is ideal for this therapy. The ideal antibiotic and length of therapy have not been determined. We currently use Unasyn 2 g every 8 hours for 2 days followed by Augmentin 500 mg four times a day for 5 additional days. The remainder of management is essentially the same as with the expectantly managed 32- to 35-week group.

Management at Less Than 25 Weeks

Patients with PROM at less than 25 weeks' gestation are very difficult to manage. The risk of complications due to PROM at this gestational age is substantial both to mother and fetus. The chance of ending up with a live baby who ultimately survives is about 30%, with the vast majority of mortality caused by prematurity, and many of the survivors will suffer neurologic damage from prematurity. About 15% to 30% of these babies will succumb to the fetal deformation syndrome. Maternal risks of chorioamnionitis exceed 40%, many will require dilatation and curettage and blood transfusion for retained placenta following delivery, and the risk of major complications of sepsis and even maternal death are substantial. Thus, after extensive counseling, the mother is faced with an extraordinarily difficult choice. She may elect to terminate the pregnancy, a reasonable option given the maternal risks and low likelihood of going home with a healthy baby. Alternatively, she may accept the risks and elect to be managed expectantly. If so, she may be managed at home since there is little to offer the fetus until after about 25 weeks. While there is some temptation to be selective in these patients based on attempts to delineate the degree of certain risks, efforts to date have not yielded satisfactory alternatives to do so. For example, many ultrasonographic formulas have been developed to predict pulmonary hypoplasia, but no single formula or combination of formulas has resulted in sufficient accuracy to be clinically useful. Similarly, while earlier gestational age at membrane rupture and more severe degrees of oligohydramnios are associated with worse outcome for both mother and fetus, there is great overlap and the difference is not great enough to be useful to the patient in making the decision to terminate or continue. If termination is chosen, the patient may be managed as with any second trimester induced abortion, the good news with PROM being that induction times are shorter and success rates are greater than with intact membranes. If the patient elects to continue the pregnancy, she should maintain bed rest, take her temperature frequently, and come in for fever, signs of labor, or decreased fetal movement. Once the fetus reaches a viable gestational age, the mother may be hospitalized and the patient can then be managed as outlined for patients at that gestational age.

Summary

Premature rupture of membranes is one of the most common and, from a management standpoint, one of the most controversial issues in obstetrics today. Once the diagnosis is made, the management generally depends on the gestational age of the patient at the time of rupture. In general, the treatment is aimed at avoiding the complications of infection or fetal distress and, in cases of the early gestation, at safely prolonging pregnancy in selected and appropriate patients. Prophylactic antibiotics have great potential to improve outcome in the very early gestation. Other management issues, such as the use of corticosteroids and tocolytics, remain controversial.

Preterm Birth

Jay D. Iams, MD

The Importance of Preterm Birth

Complications of preterm birth account for more than 70% of fetal and neonatal deaths annually in babies without anomalies. Prematurity is a major cause of developmental delay, visual and hearing impairment, chronic lung disease, and cerebral palsy. Babies born before 37 weeks' gestation (259 days from the first day of the mother's last menstrual period, or 245 days after conception) are *premature,* regardless of birth weight. An infant who weighs less than 2500 g at birth is said to be *low birth weight* (LBW), regardless of gestational age. Very low birth weight (VLBW) infants weigh less than 1500 g at birth. Rates of LBW and VLBW newborns in blacks are consistently about twice as high as corresponding rates in non-blacks, even when corrected for maternal age and income. The neonatal mortality rate is higher for male than for female VLBW infants. Morbidity in surviving premature infants may include respiratory distress syndrome, intraventricular hemorrhage, bronchopulmonary dysplasia, patent ductus arteriosus, necrotizing enterocolitis, sepsis, apnea, and retinopathy of prematurity. Long-term neurologic morbidity is a significant concern for VLBW infants who survive. Table 1 displays the frequency of major

morbidities for infants born weighing less than 1500 g in 1991 and 1992.

Epidemiology and Pathogenesis of Prematurity

Diagnoses that precede a preterm delivery include obstetric problems (e.g., preterm labor, preterm ruptured membranes, pre-eclampsia, abruptio placenta, multiple gestation, placenta previa, fetal growth retardation, excessive or inadequate amniotic fluid volume, fetal anomalies, amnionitis, incompetent cervix), and maternal medical problems such as diabetes, asthma, drug abuse, and pyelonephritis. Maternal characteristics associated with preterm delivery include maternal race (black more than non-black), poor nutrition, low prepregnancy weight, a history of previous preterm birth, inadequate prenatal care, strenuous work, high personal stress, anemia (hemoglobin < 10 g/dL), cigarette smoking, bacteriuria, genital colonization or infection (e.g., bacterial vaginosis, *Neisseria gonorrheae, Chlamydia trachomatis,* mycoplasma, and ureaplasma), cervical injury or abnormality (e.g., in utero exposure to diethylstilbestrol, a history of cervical trauma), uterine anomaly, fibroids, excessive uterine contractility, and premature cervical dilation of greater than 1 cm or effacement of 80% or greater.

Spontaneous versus Indicated Preterm Delivery

The clinical disorders listed have been usefully organized into two broad categories called *spontaneous* and *indicated* preterm births, based on the clinical presentation that led to premature delivery. Approximately 75% of preterm births occur "spontaneously" after preterm labor (PTL),

TABLE 1. Major Neonatal Morbidity in VLBW Infants According to Birth Weight

	501–750 g	751–1000 g	1001–1250 g	1251–1500 g
Number of infants	869	982	1153	1275
Respiratory distress (%)	89	83	58	39
Intraventricular hemorrhage (Grade III/IV) (%)	25	16	8	3
Necrotizing enterocolitis (%)	6	6	5	4
Hospital stay (average) for survivors (days)	123	89	64	44

Data from Fanaroff AA, et al: Am J Obstet Gynecol 1995;173:1423.

preterm premature rupture of membranes (preterm PROM), or related conditions. The spontaneous preterm delivery category also includes deliveries after amnionitis, with or without preterm PROM, and patients with reduced competence of the cervix. Indicated preterm births follow medical or obstetric disorders that place the fetus at risk, such as acute or chronic maternal hypertension, diabetes, placenta previa or abruption, and intrauterine growth restriction. Indicated preterm births account for 20% to 30% of births before 37 weeks' gestation. The distinction between indicated and spontaneous preterm births is useful because it has led to an understanding of spontaneous preterm birth as a syndrome that includes PTL, preterm PROM, amnionitis, and low or abnormal cervical competence. Spontaneous preterm births are more common among women who are indigent, poorly nourished, black, or who have a history of genital infection, in particular bacterial vaginosis. In parous women, the risk of spontaneous preterm birth is increased if there is a history of prior preterm delivery. The recurrence risk rises as the number of prior preterm births increase, and increases still further as the gestational age at delivery of the prior preterm birth decreases. Each factor considered by itself has a low predictive value for spontaneous preterm delivery. More than half of spontaneous preterm births occur in women who have no obvious risk factors. These diverse risk factors influence the rate of premature delivery by increasing the chance that an inflammatory "injury" will occur at the maternal-fetal interface. The fetal membranes and decidua, in response to an inflammatory insult (usually infectious or ischemic), produce cytokines that elicit production of prostaglandins E_2, $F_{2\alpha}$, and thromboxane A_2 that in turn stimulate uterine contractions, and may initiate release of proteases that can injure the membranes and underlying decidua, finally resulting in cervical ripening, dilation, or membrane rupture. The intensity and duration, gestational age, and host response to the injury all affect the likelihood of preterm birth. A single risk factor, such as triplets gestation, may be sufficient to initiate labor or rupture of membranes, but multiple factors are usually involved in singleton pregnancies. A good analogy may be made to atherosclerotic cardiovascular disease: In atherosclerotic vascular disease, the underlying pathology is complete or partial occlusion of a blood vessel caused by the combined influence of cholesterol, smoking, blood pressure, and so on. In spontaneous preterm birth, the pathologic event is an inflammatory injury to the decidua and membranes. Both

occur not as the consequence of a single risk factor but rather as the final product of multiple cumulative risk factors acting together.

Prevention and Treatment of Preterm Labor

Tertiary care of preterm labor includes prompt diagnosis and labor suppression to delay delivery long enough to allow (1) referral to an appropriate regional care site and (2) treatment with medication such as corticosteroids or antibiotics to reduce neonatal mortality and morbidity caused by respiratory distress syndrome and group B streptococcal infection, respectively. Secondary care, selection of patients with increased risk for surveillance or prophylactic treatment, has included risk scoring systems, early diagnosis programs, and prophylactic interventions such as tocolytic drugs, progesterone supplementation, antibiotics, and reduced physical activity. None of these have been found clearly effective when used prophylactically. Primary care, the elimination or reduction of risk in an entire population, is not yet possible for spontaneous preterm birth because effective interventions have not been demonstrated.

Initial Evaluation of Preterm Labor

Women with preterm labor may have diverse complaints, ranging from obvious labor to seemingly minor symptoms such as increased pelvic pressure or vaginal discharge, occasional spotting, or an awareness of painless contractions. Any complaint of persistent abdominal or pelvic symptoms between 18 and 35 weeks should be evaluated promptly. The first step is determining whether membrane rupture has occurred, because both maternal and fetal risks of continuing the pregnancy are heavily influenced by the status of the membranes. Evaluation of fetal maturity and gestational age is the next concern. Because pulmonary immaturity is the most frequent cause of serious newborn illness and death, an estimation of fetal pulmonary maturity is important. If the quality of obstetric dating is good and intrauterine fetal well-being is not compromised, the likelihood of neonatal respiratory distress syndrome can often be satisfactorily estimated from the gestational age alone. Amniocentesis to assess fetal pulmonary maturity is important when dates are uncertain or when fetal jeopardy may occur by continuing the pregnancy (e.g., when membranes have ruptured, fetal heart patterns are not reassuring, or growth restriction is suspected). Amniocentesis may also be indicated for fetal chromosome analysis if PTL is complicated by polyhydramnios or a suspected anomaly, or for culture, glucose, and Gram stain when amnionitis is suspected.

Diagnosis of Preterm Labor

The diagnosis of PTL is based on persistent uterine contractions and change in the dilation or effacement of the cervix by digital examination. However, the accuracy of these criteria is poor. Approximately 40% of women diagnosed by these criteria and treated with placebo will deliver at term. Many women with persistent uterine activity who do not actually have PTL therefore receive treatment unnecessarily. False-negative diagnosis is also a significant problem. This poor diagnostic accuracy occurs because the symptoms and signs of early PTL are common in normal pregnancy, and because the digital examination of the cervix is imprecise. Symptoms of preterm labor are less severe than for labor at term, and include mild contractions, pelvic pressure, increased vaginal discharge, and menstrual-like cramps. Preterm labor contractions may be painful or painless, and differ from normal contractions of pregnancy (termed Braxton-Hicks) only by their persistence. Contraction frequency alone is a poor indicator of preterm labor because of wide variation in contraction frequency with both gestational age and time of day. Contractions are more frequent at night and after 24 weeks. Uterine contraction frequency decreases after maternal rest and increases after coitus. In early labor, small changes in dilation, effacement, and cervical consistency (soft or firm) are highly subjective and poorly reproducible. The presence in the vagina of fetal fibronectin, an extracellular matrix protein that functions as the "glue" that attaches fetal membranes to the maternal decidua, has been shown to improve diagnostic accuracy of early PTL. A positive fibronectin test in women with possible preterm labor is associated with a 10% to 30% risk of preterm birth for 14 days. More importantly, a *negative* fibronectin test in a symptomatic patient with cervical dilation less than 3 cm carries a negative predictive value of 99.5% for delivery within 1 week. Transvaginal ultrasonographic measurement of the cervix is another new test that may decrease the high false-positive rate of preterm labor diagnosis. A cervical length of greater than 30 mm indicates a very low chance of preterm birth; a length of less than 20 mm is

strong evidence that preterm labor is present. An alogorithm for PTL diagnosis is as follows:

1. Patient presents with signs and symptoms suggesting PTL or preterm PROM:
   - Persistent contractions (painful or painless)
   - Intermittent abdominal cramping, pelvic pressure, or backache
   - Increase or change in vaginal discharge
   - Vaginal spotting or bleeding
2. Sterile speculum examination for pH, fern, pooled fluid, cultures for group B streptococcus (outer one third of vagina and perineum), chlamydia (cervix), and *N. gonorrheae* (cervix), and fibronectin swab from the external cervical os and posterior fornix, avoiding areas with bleeding.
3. Transabdominal ultrasonographic examination for placental location, amniotic fluid volume, estimated fetal weight and presentation, and fetal well-being.
4. Digital examination (if preterm PROM is ruled out by above):
   - Cervix 3 cm or greater dilation: The diagnosis of PTL is confirmed. Tocolysis is appropriate.
   - Cervix 2 to 3 cm dilation: The diagnosis of PTL likely but not established. Send fibronectin and monitor contraction frequency. Repeat digital examination in 30 to 60 minutes. Administer tocolysis if any cervical change, contractions increase in frequency, cervical length is less than 30 mm, or if fibronectin is positive.
   - Cervix less than 2 cm dilation: The diagnosis of PTL is uncertain. Monitor contraction frequency, send fibronectin, and repeat digital examination in 30 to 60 minutes. Administer tocolysis if the cervical dilation changes by 1 cm or more, cervical length is less than 30 mm, or if the fibronectin is positive.
5. Treatment of symptomatic fibronectin-positive patients
   - Parenteral tocolysis
   - Steroids
   - Maternal transfer
   - Hospitalize for 3 to 7 days
   - Group B streptococcus prophylaxis
6. Treatment of symptomatic fibronectin-negative patients
   - Parenteral tocolysis begun and cervix 2 cm or greater dilated:
     Risk of delivery within 7 days is 1.7% to 3.5%.

Conclude course of tocolysis.
Reduced hospital stay.
- Tocolysis not begun
Risk of delivery within 7 days is 0% to 1.8%.
Observe in outpatient setting.
- Women whose fibronectin is negative and in whom cervical sonography shows a length of 30 mm or greater do not have preterm labor.

Treatment of Preterm Labor

The initial evaluation of PTL is focused on the risks and benefits of continuing the pregnancy. Potential causes of PTL should be sought not only in the initial evaluation of the patient, but should also be reassessed during the course of treatment. A cause of labor may be found that is best treated by delivery (e.g., abruptio placentae or amnionitis), that may influence the choice of tocolytic (e.g., a degenerating myoma is best treated with a prostaglandin inhibitor), or that may require adjunctive treatment (e.g., antibiotic for pyelonephritis or a therapeutic amniocentesis for polyhydramnios). Contraindications to tocolysis are shown in Table 2.

Tocolytic drugs are reasonably safe when used according to published protocols for 24 to 48 hours. The most commonly used agents are drugs that antagonize the effects of calcium (magnesium sulfate and the calcium channel blocker nifedipine), the beta sympathomimetic drugs (ritodrine and terbutaline), and prostaglan-

TABLE 2. Contraindications to Tocolysis

Maternal	Fetal

▸ Significant hypertension (eclampsia, severe pre-eclampsia, chronic hypertension)
 ▸ Cardiac disease
 ▸ Any medical or obstetric condition that contraindicates prolongation of pregnancy
 ▸ Hypersensitivity to a specific tocolytic agent
	▸ Gestational age ≥ 37 weeks
	 ▸ Advanced dilation/effacement
	 ▸ Demise or lethal anomaly
	 ▸ Birth weight ≥ 2500 g
	 ▸ Chorioamnionitis
	 ▸ In utero fetal compromise
	   • Acute: fetal distress
	   • Chronic: Intrauterine growth restriction or substance abuse

din inhibitors (indomethacin). Protocols for each are as follows.

Protocol for Magnesium Sulfate Tocolysis

1. Loading dose is 6 g magnesium sulfate in 10% to 20% solution over 15 minutes (60 mL of 10% magnesium sulfate in D_5 0.9 normal saline).
2. Maintenance dose is 2 g/hr (40 g of magnesium sulfate added to 1 L D_5 0.9 normal saline or Ringer's lactate at 50 mL/hr). The infusion may be increased by 1 g/hr until the patient has one contraction or fewer per 10 minutes or maximum dose of 4 g/hr is reached. While the patient is on magnesium sulfate, check deep tendon reflexes and vital signs hourly and intake and output every 2 to 4 hours. Magnesium levels may be checked if the infusion is greater than 4 g/hr or if there is clinical concern about toxicity.
3. When contractions are fewer than four per hour, maintain magnesium sulfate tocolysis for 12 to 24 hours, and then reduce the infusion by 1 g per hour each hour, discontinuing the infusion when the dose reaches 2 g per hour.
4. Maternal side effects include flushing, nausea, vomiting, headache, muscle weakness including diplopia and shortness of breath, and pulmonary edema. Neonatal complications are uncommon. Lethargy, hypotonia, and respiratory depression have been observed.

Protocol for Nifedipine Tocolysis

1. Administer 10 mg PO every 20–30 minutes up to maximum of three doses, then 10 to 20 mg PO every 4–6 hr.
2. Maternal side effects include a decrease in blood pressure and increased heart rate, rarely accompanied by significant hypotension, headache, flushing, dizziness, and nausea. Skeletal muscle blockade may occur when nifedipine is used in conjunction with magnesium sulfate.
3. Neonatal side effects are uncommon, and are secondary to maternal hypotension.

Protocol for Beta-Mimetic Tocolysis

Ritodrine

1. Begin intravenous infusion at 50 μg (0.05 mg) per minute, and increase by 50 μg every 20 minutes until contraction fre-

quency is six or fewer per hour, or a maximum dose of 350 µg per minute is reached.

2. When contractions are four or fewer per hour, maintain the infusion for 1 hour, and then decrease the dose to the lowest rate that maintains contractions at fewer than four per hour.
3. Continue this rate for 12 hours.

Terbutaline

Terbutaline may be given intravenously, but is more commonly administered subcutaneously.

1. A single dose of 250 µg (0.25 mg) via subcutaneous injection may be repeated every 3 to 4 hours for up to three doses.
2. A dose of subcutaneous terbutaline, 0.25 mg, may be given adjunctively with intravenous magnesium without increasing maternal or neonatal side effects. Continued treatment with more than one or two subcutaneous doses of terbutaline in combination with intravenous magnesium is associated with an unacceptable increase in side effects.

Side Effects of Beta-Mimetics

1. Maternal side effects include tachycardia, hypotension, arrhythmia, hyperglycemia, hypokalemia, hypocalcemia, nausea and vomiting, chest pain, jitteriness, pruritis, and pulmonary edema. Maternal deaths have occurred when beta-mimetics were given to patients with occult cardiac disease.
2. Most neonatal side effects are a consequence of the maternal side effects: tachycardia, neonatal hypotension, fetal hyperglycemia with subsequent neonatal hypoglycemia, and myocardial hypertrophy and ischemia.
3. There is preliminary evidence that beta-mimetic tocolytics may increase the incidence of serious neonatal intraventricular hemorrhage.

Protocol for Indomethacin Tocolysis

1. Use only before 32 weeks' gestation.
2. Loading dose of 100 mg rectally or 50 mg orally; may repeat in 1 hour if no decrease in contractions, followed by 25 to 50 mg PO every 4 to 6 hours for 48 hours.
3. Check amniotic fluid volume prior to initiation and at 48 to 72 hours.

4. Do not use the drug for longer than 48 consecutive hours.
5. Discontinue therapy promptly if delivery seems imminent.
6. Maternal side effects include nausea, heartburn, and vomiting. Rare but serious complications include gastrointestinal bleeding, alterations in coagulation, thrombocytopenia, asthma in aspirin-sensitive patients, and acute increases in blood pressure in hypertensive women. Prolonged treatment can lead to renal injury. Indomethacin may obscure a clinically significant fever. Maternal contraindications to indomethacin tocolysis include renal or hepatic disease, active peptic ulcer disease, poorly controlled hypertension, asthma, and coagulation disorders.
7. Three principal neonatal side effects have been reported, all of which occur rarely if at all when the duration of treatment is 48 hours or less: Constriction of the ductus arteriosus, oligohydramnios due to reduced urine production, and neonatal pulmonary hypertension. Fetal contraindications to indomethacin include growth restriction, renal anomalies, chorioamnionitis, oligohydramnios, ductal dependent cardiac defects, and twin-twin transfusion syndrome.

Adjunctive Care of Preterm Labor

Despite the various treatments for preterm labor, most women do not deliver at term. About 60% to 70% of women with preterm labor will deliver before 37 weeks. Two steps are among the most effective in perinatal medicine to reduce perinatal mortality and morbidity.

1. Medications given to the mother *before birth* to reduce the infant's chances of respiratory distress syndrome, intraventricular hemorrhage, and perinatal group B streptococcal infection. Administration of penicillin during labor (2 million units IV q 4 hours in labor) or an equivalent antibiotic is effective to reduce the incidence of neonatal group B streptococcal sepsis. When administered 24 or more hours before preterm birth, corticosteroids (12 mg of Celestone, a combination of 6 mg each of betamethasone phosphate and acetate) IM every 24 hr × 2 doses can reduce the incidence and severity of respiratory distress syndrome and intraventricular hemorrhage, and thereby also reduce the perina-

tal mortality rate in infants born before 34 weeks.

2. Maternal transfer to a tertiary care hospital with appropriate facilities for complicated maternal and neonatal care. Regionalization of perinatal care reduces perinatal morbidity by concentrating care for low birth weight and preterm infants in centers with appropriate facilities and experienced personnel.

Prostaglandin E₂ for Cervical Ripening

William F. Rayburn, MD

An induction of labor is defined as the stimulation of uterine contractions before the spontaneous onset of labor. Induction of labor is one of the most important and irrevocable interventions in obstetric practice. Between 10% to 20% of all pregnant women will undergo an induction, with approximately one half having an unfavorable cervix that requires ripening.

Cervical ripening refers to a prelabor change in the collagen fiber configuration of the uterine cervix to allow for greater compliance during labor. In most pregnancies, some degree of spontaneous cervical ripening is present near term, which generally precedes spontaneous labor. While natural cervical ripening is associated with successful labor induction, effects of iatrogenic ripening are less well defined. Methods of ripening the cervix include extraovular catheters, osmotic dilators, prostaglandins (E_1, E_2, $F_{2\alpha}$), and locally applied hormones such as relaxin and estrogens.

While various hormones have been implicated, prostaglandins are known to play a prominent role in the spontaneous maturation of the cervix. Histologically, changes in the cervix from low-dose topical prostaglandin E_2 (PGE_2) include a dissolution of the collagen bundles, an increase in the ground substance, an increase in the submucosal edema, and the presence of giant cells. These changes in cervical connective tissue in the term pregnancy are the same as those observed in early labor.

Methods of Drug Delivery and Doses

Most reports have described the delivery of PGE_2 intravaginally as a gel or an insert or intra-cervically as a gel. An intravaginal gel, compounded in hospital pharmacies by blending methylcellulose with a 20 mg PGE_2 suppository, has gained widespread use. Differences exist between product lots in terms of the effectiveness and adverse effects.

In December 1992, the US Food and Drug Administration approved a PGE_2 gel preparation for cervical ripening in women at or near term who have a medical or obstetric indication for inducing labor. The gel is available in a 2.5 mL syringe that contains 0.5 mg of dinoprostone (Prepidil, Pharmacia-Upjohn Company). The intracervical route offers the advantages of prompting minimal uterine activity and greater efficacy in the very unripe cervix.

A prostaglandin vaginal insert (Cervidil, Forest Pharmaceutical) was also approved by the US Food and Drug Administration in the summer of 1995. The vaginal insert provides 10 mg of dinoprostone at a 0.3 mg/hour rate of release over a 12-hour period. Similar to results with the 0.5 mg dinoprostone gel, clinical trials demonstrate that the vaginal insert shortens the interval from induction until vaginal delivery. The vaginal insert appears to have an advantage over the intracervical gel and the extemporaneous compounded intravaginal gel, because the insert can be removed. Should uterine hyperstimulation occur, the insert may be removed by pulling on the tail of the net surrounding it.

Clinical Effectiveness

The cumulative experience with an intracervical or intravaginal PGE_2 preparation, among more than 6000 pregnancies in more than 90 prospective clinical trials, supports the belief that PGE_2 is superior to a placebo or to no therapy in enhancing cervical effacement and dilation. Part of the prostaglandin-induced cervical ripening process often includes initiation of labor. When this occurs, the process is similar to that of spontaneous labor. When uterine-stimulating effects are not clinically apparent, PGE_2 may still function by enhancing the sensitivity to oxytocin.

Use of a low-dose PGE_2 preparation has been reported to increase the chances of successful induction, decrease the incidence of prolonged labor, reduce the total and maximal doses of oxytocin, and reduce the number of serial inductions. More than half of patients treated at term are expected to enter labor and to deliver within 24 hours. Effects of prostaglandin on the overall cesarean section rate have been inconsistent. Certain reports have shown a reduction, while most have not shown a statistically significant decrease.

Patient Selection

Anyone in whom the cervix is unfavorable and in whom labor is indicated would benefit from cervical ripening. The most common indication for induction of labor is postdates. With most current management protocols, however, significant perinatal morbidity or mortality in this group is too low to demonstrate any benefit from routinely ripening the cervix. In pre-eclamptic or hypertensive women with an unfavorable cervix, cervical ripening with PGE$_2$ can be accomplished safely. Oligohydramnios, either alone or in combination with another pregnancy complication, has become another common indication for induction at term.

Use of intravaginal PGE$_2$ in a patient with prolonged ruptured membranes at term may be safe and beneficial, although the agent is not approved for this indication using either commercially available product. An induction of labor for suspected fetal macrosomia alone is associated with a greater risk of cesarean delivery and has not been shown to be a valid indication. Despite reports of its successful use, the safety of PGE$_2$ therapy in grand multiparous patients has not been clearly demonstrated.

Monitoring Protocol

The patient should not have a fever, allergy to prostaglandins, or active vaginal bleeding. Other prerequisites to PGE$_2$ therapy include a complete explanation to the patient, a reassuring fetal heart rate (FHR) tracing (preferably a reactive nonstress test), and the absence of regular uterine contractions (every 5 minutes or less). There have been many methods described to assess the cervix, but the Bishop score technique (Table 1) has gained the widest acceptance. A Bishop score of 4 or less is considered to denote an unfavorable cervix. Use of prostaglandins in patients with

intermediate scores (of 5 to 6) has been shown to trigger labor more often without the need for subsequent oxytocin. A preinduction Bishop score of greater than 8 is associated with a vaginal delivery rate that is comparable whether the labor is induced or spontaneous.

The drug is inserted either at or near the labor and delivery suite, where continuous uterine activity and FHR monitoring are performed during either the first hour after gel instillation or during the first 2 hours after vaginal insert placement. An intravenous line or heparin lock is unnecessary. The time of day for drug insertion and pregnancy monitoring may affect health care costs, so this issue is deserving of consideration.

Intracervical instillation requires direct inspection using a speculum. After gel instillation, the patient is expected to remain recumbent for at least 1 hour. The drug is rapidly absorbed and has a short half-life (2.5 to 5.0 minutes). If the patient has no increase in uterine activity or change in the FHR pattern after this period, she may be transferred elsewhere. If contractions are recorded, they usually appear in the first hour and show peak activity in the first 4 hours. If any regular uterine contractions persist, electronic FHR monitoring should be continued and maternal vital signs should be recorded at least hourly for the first 4 hours. Minimum time intervals between sequential dosings of the gel or before beginning oxytocin have not been well determined but reflect the time necessary for the principal metabolite to clear. According to the manufacturer, this interval should be at least 6 hours, although we have published our experience with the successful infusion of low-dose oxytocin immediately after instillation of Prepidil. If insufficient cervical change (Bishop score change less than 3) or irregular uterine activity are found, sequential PGE$_2$ dosing may be considered, although any additional benefit has not been reported in term gestations. A second dose is given at least 4 to 6 hours after the first; prerequisites for the first dose also apply to the second. Even less is known about any additional value with more than two dosings.

The vaginal insert is placed by palpation,

TABLE 1. Bishop Scoring System

Score	Dilation (cm)	Effacement (%)	Station	Consistency	Position of Cervix
0	Closed	0–30	−3	Firm	Posterior
1	1–2	40–50	−2	Medium	Mid-position
2	3–4	60–70	−1,0	Soft	Anterior
3	>5	>80	+1,+2		

rather than by direct inspection, in a transverse position at the posterior vaginal apex. The tail of the net is left outside of the introitus. The manufacturer recommends continuous monitoring of FHR and uterine activity for 2 hours after dosing. The onset of uterine activity is often within the first hour, and peak contractions occur 3 to 5 hours after dosing. Unlike the gel, the sustained-release insert can stimulate contractions that persist, so prolonged monitoring is often necessary. The vaginal insert is intended for single dosing only, and oxytocin therapy may be instituted, if necessary, immediately after its removal.

Limitations
Uterine Hyperstimulation

Part of the cervical ripening process includes initiation of labor. Uterine hyperstimulation is present when the contraction frequency is more than five in 10 minutes (polysystole) or if a contraction exceeds 2 minutes in duration (tetany). The reported rate of uterine hyperstimulation for the sustained-release vaginal insert is 6% and for the intracervical gel less is than 1%. Because serious hyperstimulation is more common when PGE_2 is used with pre-existing labor, such use is not generally accepted.

Reversal of hyperstimulation is indicated in approximately half of affected cases when either the FHR becomes worrisome (e.g., repetitive decelerations or bradycardia) or the patient complains of persistent pelvic discomfort. Relief of hyperstimulation by irrigation of the gel near the cervix and vagina is not helpful, since PGE_2 is rapidly absorbed. By administering a β-adrenergic drug (e.g., terbutaline 250 μg intravenously or subcutaneously), prompt resolution of the worrisome hyperstimulation can be expected in 98% of cases without apparent untoward intrapartum effects. Removal of a vaginal insert is easily accomplished by pulling on the net. Reversal of hyperstimulation is expected in most circumstances without the need of a β-adrenergic drug.

Failed Induction and Cesarean Section

Reducing the need for cesarean delivery in cases requiring an induction of labor is a critical therapeutic endpoint. An approximate 10% prevalence of a failed induction (failure of the cervix to dilate to 4 cm) is to be expected after PGE_2 insertion and a minimum of 8 hours of adequate labor. Whether this is influenced by gestational age is unclear, but pretreatment Bishop scores of 0 to 2 are typically found in preterm gestations. The failed induction rate after vaginal insert use is unknown. Patients failing to respond may benefit from a cesarean section without a prolonged induction when imminent delivery is necessary.

Maternal Systemic Effects

Side effects from low-dose PGE_2 (fever, vomiting, diarrhea) are negligible. The manufacturers of the two commercially available preparations have recommended that practitioners exercise caution when using any PGE_2 product in patients with glaucoma, severe hepatic or renal impairment, or adult asthma. However, PGE_2 is a bronchodilator, and neither bronchoconstriction nor significant blood pressure changes have been reported after a low dose of PGE_2 gel. Such restrictions are understandable for conditions that exist rarely during pregnancy or in which full-dose therapy has been administered systematically. Physician discretion and individuality of patient care seem to be reasonable when a low-dose PGE_2 preparation is applied topically.

Special Considerations
Preterm Rupture of Membranes

Patients at term with premature rupture of membranes, especially nulliparous women with poor cervical scores, have a high cesarean delivery rate when labor is induced with oxytocin infusion or admission. Traditional teaching and reports from large retrospective studies point to an increased possibility of maternal and neonatal infectious morbidity with unlimited conservative management. Several authors claim that use of a single intravaginal dose of PGE_2 at admission results in more women establishing labor earlier, with a resultant reduction in the admission-to-delivery interval, compared with either no therapy or a placebo. The cesarean section rate would be expected to be similar, or perhaps lower, with PGE_2 therapy and with no differences in neonatal outcome.

Out-Patient Therapy

Both manufacturers recommend that their products be used on in-patients only. Despite this, much experience has been reported about the out-patient application of the PGE_2 gel. Most contractions are painless and infrequent. Unless there is a nonreassuring FHR pattern or an acute complication requiring hospitalization, cervical ripening may occur using a single dose of the gel rather than the sustained-release vaginal insert. By using the single-dose gel, the costs of hospital stays may be reduced. Furthermore, cervical ripening may take place without an absolute need for a scheduled induction. More clinical research is necessary.

Vaginal Birth after Cesarean Section

The most important means to reduce the cesarean section rate is to minimize repeat surgery. The use of PGE_2 on patients attempting a vaginal birth after a cesarean section for a previous pregnancy has gained more acceptance. The risk of a uterine rupture is not thought to be increased with PGE_2 treatment in cases with a single low transverse cesarean section. The physician should be willing to undertake such treatment as long as the patient understands the limitation written in the package insert, which states that the product is contraindicated in the presence of prior major uterine surgery.

Alternative Therapy

Cervical Dilators

Ripening by mechanical dilation may be effective for preinduction cervical ripening, although less experience has been reported than for PGE_2. Examples of dilators include an inflatable pediatric Foley catheter, an inflatable double-balloon catheter, and osmotic dilators such as *Laminaria japonicum* and various types of synthetic laminaria. As many osmotic cervical dilators as feasible (usually one to three) are placed in the endocervical canal without rupturing the membranes. Several small randomized trials have found that either inflatable catheters or osmotic cervical dilators are comparable in efficacy to PGE_2. Use of a speculum and, if necessary, a cervical retractor during insertion can often lead to temporary patient discomfort. The reduced need to monitor the uterus and fetus afterwards may result in greater convenience and reduced cost. Increased peripartum infections have not been consistently reported.

Misoprostol

The two commercially available PGE_2 products are expensive; the approximately cost per dose to the hospital for Prepidil is $75 and for Cervidil is $140. Use of a less expensive prostaglandin E_1 analogue (misoprostol; Cytotec, Searle) has been reported. This anti-ulcer medication, supplied as a 100 mg or as a 200 mg tablet, has been reported to be as effective as the other prostaglandin products to ripen the cervix when placed intravaginally. Limitations include the need for multidosing, the lack of Food and Drug Administration approval for this indication, the limited comparative investigations with insufficient safety information, and the manufacturer's discouragement of its product's being used in this manner.

Renal Disease in Pregnancy (Chronic)

Jane E. C. Milne

John M. Davison

Renal Alterations in Normal Pregnancy

Normal pregnancy is associated with substantial increments in renal hemodynamics, with both glomerular filtration rate and renal plasma flow increasing 50% to 70% above prepregnancy values, and decreases in the serum levels of urea and creatinine from mean nonpregnant values of 4.3 mmol/L (25 mg/dL) and 73 μmol/L (0.82 mg/dL), respectively, to mean pregnant values of 3.3 mmol/L (20 mg/dL) and 51 μmol/L (0.58 mg/dL), respectively. It should therefore be remembered that values of urea and creatinine that are acceptable in healthy nonpregnant women could be suspect during pregnancy. The serial assessment of renal function on the basis of serum creatinine values alone, particularly in the presence of renal disease, requires caution, as renal function can decline by up to 50% before serum creatinine increases to more than 130 μmol/L (1.45 mg/dL).

Renal volume increases by the third trimester of pregnancy because of enlargement of both the renal vascular volume and interstitial space, and 90% of women will show a marked dilatation (more prominent on the right) of the calyces, renal pelves, and ureters by the third trimester. These changes are important clinically because urine stasis within the ureters may be related to the tendency for pregnant women with asymptomatic bacteruria to develop frank pyelonephritis and contribute to errors in timed urine collections. The changes should not be mistaken for obstructive uropathy, and postpartum radiologic assessment of the renal tract should be delayed for at least 4 months until the changes have resolved.

Pregnancy in Women with Chronic Renal Disease

The degree of renal dysfunction and presence or absence of hypertension, rather than the underlying disease process, influence fertility and the incidence of maternal and fetal complications during and after pregnancy. Patients can be arbitrarily considered in three groups, the more severe the prepregnancy renal dysfunction, the worse the maternal and fetal prognosis (Table 1). *Minimal* renal dysfunction with absence of hypertension is usually associated with a successful obstetric outcome (perinatal mortality < 3%) and no adverse effect on the underlying disease process or basal maternal renal function. Unfortunately, this generalization does not hold true for certain diseases (Table 2). For instance, lupus nephropathy has a worse prognosis than primary glomerulopathies, particularly if a "flare" has occurred within 6 months of conception. Although the influence of pregnancy on the progression of immunoglobulin A (IgA) nephropathy, focal segmental glomerulosclerosis, membranoproliferative nephritis, and reflux nephropathy remains controversial, the consensus is that pregnancy does not adversely affect these disease processes. Pregnancy should be discouraged in women with active vasculitis (scleroderma and periarteritis nodosa, for example) where there is renal involvement because of the certainty of poor maternal and fetal prognosis.

Although fetal outcome is good in women with *moderate* renal dysfunction (about 90% of pregnancies are successful after spontaneous abortions have been excluded), the greatest concern is maternal health. Similarly, in women with *severe* renal dysfunction, there is significant risk of deterioration of renal function (that often fails to reverse after delivery), escalating and often life-threatening hypertension and/or acceleration of the underlying disease process with superimposed pre-eclampsia. Pregnancy counseling in these women needs considerable attention. In two recent analyses of 125 pregnancies in 97 women with moderate or severe renal insufficiency, there were fetal survival rates of greater than 90%, presumably reflecting specialist care in those centers and the fact that three quarters of the cases were undertaken after 1984. Again, however, anxieties for the mother were apparent with a pregnancy-related loss of renal function in almost 50%, with 10% to 23% of the total series rapidly progressing to end-stage renal failure within 6 months of delivery. These patients all had severe hypertension and heavy proteinuria before pregnancy.

Prepregnancy Counseling

In view of the risks, many practitioners would discourage pregnancy in women with serum cre-

TABLE 1. Severity of Renal Disease, Pregnancy Prospects, and Long-Term Sequelae*

	Prepregnancy Serum Creatinine (μmol/L)	Pregnancy Complications (%)	Successful Obstetric Outcome (%)†	Long-Term Sequelae (%)†
Preserved/mildly impaired renal function	≤125 (1.40 mg/dL)	26	96 (85)	<3 (8)
Moderate renal insufficiency (± hypertension)	≥125 (1.40 mg/dL)	47	90 (69)	25 (70)
Severe renal insufficiency (usually with hypertension)	≥250 (2.80 mg/dL)‡	86	75 (61)	53 (92)

*Estimates are based on 2477 women and 3602 pregnancies (1973–1997) and do not include collagen diseases.
†Numbers in parentheses refer to prospects when complications develop prior to 28 weeks' gestation.
‡Some authorities use 220 μmol/L (2.50 mg/dL) as the "cut-off" between moderate and severe renal insufficiency.

TABLE 2. Effect and Outcome of Pregnancy in Specific Renal Diseases

Disease	Effect
Chronic glomerulonephritis	Usually no adverse effect in absence of hypertension. Some consider glomerulonephritis may be adversely affected by coagulation changes of pregnancy. Urinary tract infections more frequent.
Immunoglobulin A nephropathy	Risks of uncontrolled and/or sudden escalating hypertension and worsening renal function.
Pyelonephritis	Bacteriuria in pregnancy can lead to exacerbation. Multiple organ system derangement may ensue, including adult respiratory distress syndrome.
Reflux nephropathy	Risks of sudden escalating hypertension and worsening renal function.
Urolithiasis	Infections more frequent, but ureteral dilatation and stasis do not seem to affect natural history. Limited data on lithotripsy, best avoided.
Polycystic disease	Functional impairment and hypertension usually minimal in childbearing years.
Diabetic nephropathy	Usually no adverse effect on renal lesion but increased frequency of infection, edema, and pre-eclampsia.
Systemic lupus erythematosus	Controversial, prognosis most favorable if disease in remission more than 6 months before conception. Steroid dosage should be increased postpartum.
Periarteritis nodosa	Fetal prognosis dismal and maternal death often occurs.
Scleroderma	If onset during pregnancy, rapid overall deterioration can occur. Reactivation of quiescent scleroderma may occur postpartum.
Previous urinary tract surgery	Might be associated with other malformations of the urogenital tract. Urinary tract infection common during pregnancy. Renal function may undergo irreversible deterioration. No significant obstructive problem but cesarean section often needed for abnormal presentation or to avoid disruption of continence mechanism if artificial sphincter is present.
Postnephrectomy, solitary kidney, and pelvic kidney	May be associated with other malformations of the urogenital tract. Pregnancy well tolerated. Dystocia seldom occurs with a pelvic kidney.
Wegener's granulomatosis	Limited information. Proteinuria (with or without hypertension) common from early in pregnancy. Cytotoxic drugs should be avoided if possible.
Renal artery stenosis	May present as chronic hypertension or recurrent isolated pre-eclampsia. Transluminal angioplasty can be undertaken during pregnancy if appropriate.

atinine greater than 125 μmol/L (1.40 mg/dL). Our policy, however, is to allow pregnancy in women with primary interstitial disease or a single kidney, or in transplant recipients with moderate but stable function (preferably for 2 years or longer) with serum creatinine of 180 μmol/L (2.00 mg/dL) or less. Furthermore, diastolic blood pressure prior to pregnancy should be 90 mm Hg or less because both first trimester hypertension and "uncontrolled" hypertension can be associated with considerable fetal loss. Pregnancy outcome can approach that in normotensive women if blood pressure is well controlled. Figure 1 depicts the various maternal outcomes when renal disease and pregnancy interact without emphasizing the time scale involved.

Management of Pregnancy

Pregnancy in women with chronic renal disease should be managed in tertiary care centers with the care coordinated by a fetomaternal specialist and a nephrologist. The hospital booking visit should be undertaken early in the first trimester (8–12 weeks' gestation) and should include an assessment of renal function as a baseline to allow subsequent early detection of deterioration or development of superimposed pre-eclampsia. The following parameters should be measured:

1. Serum creatinine, creatinine clearance, and 24-hour protein and albumin excretion (for monitoring of renal function)

2. Serum urea, albumin, and cholesterol (for monitoring of nephrotic complications)
3. Serum electrolytes (for assessment of osmolar, potassium, and acid-base homeostasis), urine analysis, and bacterial culture
4. Serum uric acid, aspartate and alanine transferases, lactate dehydrogenase, prothrombin time, partial thromboplastin time, and platelet count (for screening for superimposed pre-eclampsia).

Antenatal hospital visits should be every 2 weeks until 32 weeks' gestation and weekly thereafter. Renal parameters should be assessed every 4 weeks until 32 weeks' gestation and every 2 weeks thereafter, with more frequent assessment if necessary, depending on the level of renal dysfunction.

If renal function appears to deteriorate significantly at any stage of pregnancy, the rate of change of function should be determined by repeat testing, and reversible causes such as urinary tract infection as well as water or electrolyte inbalance should be sought and treated appropriately. Failure to detect a reversible cause for a confirmed significant deterioration in renal function is grounds for expediting delivery. It should be remembered that a decrease in creatinine clearance of 15% to 20% (with minimal alteration in serum creatinine), which occurs in normal pregnancy near term, is also permissible in women with chronic renal disease. The presence of persistent proteinuria, with normal blood pressure and maintained renal function, does not necessitate hospitalization of the patient and delivery. The pregnancy can be allowed to continue provided that the patient is closely monitored.

The true incidence of pre-eclampsia in women with chronic renal disease is unknown, as it can be difficult to differentiate from progression of the underlying disease in women with glomerular disease prone to hypertension and proteinuria. However, it is this superimposed pre-eclampsia to which most of the specific risks

of hypertension in pregnancy appear to be related. Although treatment of mild hypertension (diastolic blood pressure < 95 mm Hg in second trimester and < 100 mm Hg in third trimester) is not considered necessary in normal pregnancy, it should be treated in women with chronic renal disease with the aim of maintaining the diastolic blood pressure at 80 mm Hg. It is not known why pregnancy can exacerbate renal disease. It might be related to an increase in intraglomerular pressure as a mechanism to augment filtration and/or a superimposition of platelet and fibrin deposition onto the already damaged kidney along with the microvascular coagulation and endothelial dysfunction of the pre-eclamptic process.

Serial assessment of fetal well-being is essential because renal disease has a positive association with intrauterine growth retardation, and changes in the fetal status affect the timing of intervention and delivery when complications arise. Serial ultrasonographic studies with measurements of fetal growth and velocimetry as well as biophysical profiles should be commenced at 28 weeks' gestation, unless the maternal condition warrants earlier assessment.

Planned preterm delivery may be required if there are signs of significant fetal compromise and impending fetal demise, if renal function deteriorates significantly, or if hypertension becomes uncontrollable or eclampsia occurs.

Pregnancy in Women on Long-Term Dialysis

The true conception rate among women on long-term hemodialysis and peritoneal dialysis is unknown, owing to the high rates of early spontaneous miscarriage and therapeutic terminations. Although dialysis patients experience major changes in the hypothalamic-pituitary-ovarian axis as well as reduced libido, they are not infer-

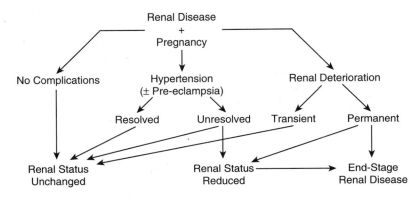

Figure 1. The interaction of renal disease and pregnancy.

tile, and conception rates of 1 in 100 are now quoted. It is therefore important that contraception is used to avoid pregnancy. Early diagnosis of pregnancy may prove difficult, as missed periods are often ignored because of menstrual irregularities associated with dialysis. In these women, even when urine is available, urine pregnancy tests are unreliable, so ultrasonography is needed to confirm and date pregnancy. A lack of responsiveness to her usual synthetic erythropoietin dosage may be the first clue suggesting pregnancy in an oligomenorrheic patient. Unfortunately, since pregnancy may not be suspected, women often do not present until pregnancy is advanced.

In comparison to renal allograft recipients (see Table 3), the livebirth rate is at best 40% to 50% (when terminations have been excluded), with the high rate of fetal wastage evident at all stages of pregnancy. Pregnancy in dialysis patients poses major risks to the mother, including volume overload, severe exacerbations of hypertension or superimposed pre-eclampsia, and polyhydramnios. Encouragement of pregnancy or its continuation when diagnosed is still not the consensus opinion. Nevertheless, more women on long-term dialysis are attempting to conceive, necessitating rigorous management protocols to optimize maternal and fetal outcomes.

Management of Pregnancy

The debate regarding the best route for dialysis during pregnancy continues. It has been argued that peritoneal dialysis should be the method of choice, as, theoretically, it maintains a more stable fluid and electrolyte environment and provides cardiovascular stability for the fetus. Whatever the route, however, dialysis usually requires a 50% increase in both duration and frequency and aims to do the following:

1. Maintain serum urea less than 20 mmol/L (120 mg/dL). Although successful fetal outcome has been achieved despite serum urea levels of 25 mmol/L (150 mg/dL), intrauterine death is more likely with urea

levels in excess of 20 mmol/L (120 mg/dL) and some would therefore advocate maintaining serum urea less than 15 mmol/dL (90 mg/dL).
2. Maintain meticulous control of maternal blood pressure, avoiding sudden fluctuations but particularly hypotension, which is damaging to the fetus. Supine posture should be avoided in late pregnancy, as hypotension may be aggravated by the pregnant uterus decreasing venous return.
3. Avoid rapid fluctuations in intravascular volume by limiting interdialysis weight gain to 1 kg until late pregnancy. This usually precludes the use of "high flux" technology.
4. Maintain meticulous control of electrolyte balance; in particular, calcium levels should be closely monitored to avoid hypercalcemia.
5. Monitor closely for preterm labor, as dialysis has a positive association with uterine contractions.

Dialysis patients have chronic anemia, which is invariably aggravated further in pregnancy. Synthetic erythropoietin is an effective treatment for the anemia and has been used successfully in pregnancy without any reported side effects. Transfusion may be required and should be undertaken with careful monitoring, as it can cause circulatory overload and exacerbate hypertension in spite of additional dialysis.

Vaginal delivery is not contraindicated and cesarean section should be reserved for obstetric indications only.

Pregnancy in Women with Renal Allografts

Approximately 1 in 50 women of childbearing age with a functioning renal allograft become pregnant. There is a high rate of early spontaneous miscarriage and therapeutic terminations with 30% of pregnancies not proceeding beyond the first trimester. However, 95% of pregnancies that do proceed beyond the first trimester have a successful outcome (Table 3).

TABLE 3. Pregnancy Implications for Renal Allograft Recipients°

Pregnancy Complications (%)	Successful Obstetric Outcome (%)†	Long-Term Sequelae (%)†
49	95 (75)	12 (25)

°Estimates are based on 4220 women and 5370 pregnancies (1961–1998) that attained at least 28 weeks' gestation.
†Figures in parentheses refer to prospects when complications develop prior to 28 weeks' gestation.

Couples should be encouraged to discuss all the implications regarding pregnancy from the initiation of treatment for renal failure and should be given information regarding the potential for optimal rehabilitation as well as maternal survival prospects if a pregnancy is embarked upon. Following successful transplantation, a delay of 18 to 24 months is recommended prior to conception to allow stabilization of graft function and reduction of immunosuppressive therapy to maintenance levels. It has been shown that if graft function is well maintained at 2 years, there is a high probability of graft survival at 5 years. Recent studies suggest that pregnancy does not necessarily compromise long-term renal prognosis.

Guidelines for successful pregnancy in women with renal allografts are as follows (relative not absolute criteria):

- Good general health for about 2 years after transplant
- Stature compatible with good obstetric outcome
- No or minimal proteinuria
- No hypertension
- No evidence of graft rejection
- No pelvicalyceal distension apparent on recent intravenous urogram or ultrasonography
- Stable renal function with serum creatinine < 180 μmol/L (2.00 mg/dL) and preferably < 125 μmol/L (1.40 mg/dL).
- Drug therapy reduced to maintenance levels: prednisolone ≤ 15 mg/day, azothiaprine ≤ 2 mg/kg/day, cyclosporin A < 5 mg/kg/day.

Most women with a renal allograft augment renal function during pregnancy and some experience a transient deterioration in function during late pregnancy (with or without proteinuria), but 12% to 15% will experience a permanent impairment in function of 10% to 20% following delivery. Despite a high rate of pregnancy complications, more than 90% have a successful obstetric outcome, but this is reduced to 70% if complications (hypertension, deteriorating renal function, and/or rejection) occur prior to 28 weeks' gestation. Overall there is a 30% risk of developing hypertension or pre-eclampsia. Intrauterine growth retardation affects at least 20% of pregnancies and the preterm delivery rate is 45% to 60%.

The allograft rarely causes dystocia and vaginal delivery is not contraindicated, reserving cesarean section strictly for obstetric indications.

From the data available, it seems that pregnancy does not compromise long-term renal outlook.

Neonatal complications (respiratory distress syndrome, leukopenia, thrombocytopenia, adrenocortical insufficiency, and infection) are rare, and maintenance levels of immunosuppressive agents appear to have no harmful effects on the fetus, but information regarding their intrauterine and neonatal effects remains limited.

Rheumatic Heart Disease: Safe Conduct in Pregnancy

Thomas F. Kelly, MD

Robert Resnik, MD

Rheumatic fever, while uncommon in the United States, is still prevalent in less developed countries despite the recognized treatment of Group A pharyngitis. The cardiovascular lesions complicating rheumatic fever include rheumatic pancarditis and endocarditis. The latter leads to the more commonly recognized valvular problems, particularly in the mitral and aortic valves. These cardiac sequelae of rheumatic fever remain the most common cause of valvular heart disease complicating pregnancy. This chapter deals primarily with the management of valvular sequelae of rheumatic heart disease in pregnancy and in intrapartum and postpartum periods. In addition, prevention of recurrences and management of complications of rheumatic heart disease are discussed.

Pregnancy Effects on Cardiac Function

Cardiac output increases up to 50% in pregnancy from a baseline of 3.5 L/min to a maximum of 6 L/min at term. While the majority of this increase occurs by 16 weeks' gestation, a small upward trend continues through the second trimester. Cardiac output may decline slightly in the late third trimester and is likely related to maternal position. Heart rate and stroke volume, the components of cardiac output, increase during pregnancy, with heart rate gradually rising to 5% to 32% above baseline by the third trimester. Increases in stroke volume are primarily responsible for the overall cardiac output rise seen in early pregnancy. The ventricles exhibit an increased end-diastolic volume and wall thickness.

Blood volume increases by approximately 45% above nonpregnant baseline by 30 to 34 weeks and then plateaus. The ventricles respond to the increased blood volume (thus preload) by increasing the cardiac output in a Frank-Starling fashion.

Approach to the Pregnant Patient with Rheumatic Heart Disease

The pregnant patient with valvular disease should be managed with a team approach, with consultative input from cardiology, anesthesiology, cardiovascular surgery, and nursing services. Preconception counseling and evaluation are desirable, since they may identify problems that are easier dealt with in the nonpregnant state.

For the patient with known valvular disease, identifying her functional status prior to or early in pregnancy is important prognostically. Women whose conditions fall into New York Heart Association class I (asymptomatic) or II (symptomatic with greater than normal activity) tend to have a favorable prognosis in pregnancy and a mortality rate of less than 1%. However, the condition of these well-compensated patients may deteriorate as gestation advances. Mitral stenosis with New York Heart Association class III or IV (symptoms with normal activity or rest, respectively) and mitral stenosis with atrial fibrillation and aortic stenosis are associated with mortality rates between 5% and 15%. Finally, patients with pulmonary hypertension approach a risk of mortality of 50%.

Pregnancy may unmask a previously asymptomatic cardiac condition, and the patient may initially present during late gestation. Complaints of orthopnea, paroxysmal nocturnal dyspnea, and fatigue with minimal activity should alert the physician to look for a potential cardiovascular problem.

Symptoms of normal pregnancy may be quite similar to those associated with valvular heart disease, however. Complaints of dyspnea on exertion and fatigue are common to both. Physical findings of concern include cyanosis, pulmonary wheezes or rales suggestive of pulmonary edema, cardiomegaly, and diastolic or harsh systolic murmurs. The current mainstay of diagnosis is echocardiography, which can make a more accurate assessment of the valvular process by estimating valve area from the half-life of time needed to eliminate the transvalvular gradient. An indirect assessment of pulmonary vascular pressures can also be made during this noninvasive study.

Prevention of recurrences of rheumatic fever is important. Recommended regimens include monthly intramuscular benzathine penicillin G, 1.2 million units, or daily oral penicillin, 200,000 units on an empty stomach. Prophylaxis is recommended for individuals less than 18 years of age, as well as for a minimum of 5 years for those over 18. Pregnancy, regardless of age, is a reasonable indication for prophylaxis.

Mitral Stenosis

Mitral stenosis (MS) is almost always due to rheumatic heart disease and is the most common rheumatic valve sequela in pregnancy. Pure MS accounts for 40% of patients with rheumatic heart disease. The normal mitral valve area ranges between 4 and 6 cm². Critical MS occurs when the valve area is less than 1 cm², where 25 mm Hg of left atrial pressure is required to maintain cardiac output. The stenotic area impairs filling of the left ventricle during diastole and results in a relatively fixed cardiac output. Problems associated with MS are twofold. First, the patient usually requires a higher left ventricular preload, which is reflected in elevated pulmonary arterial pressures. However, as the blood volume expansion of pregnancy occurs and blood return to the heart increases, the left ventricle is unable to respond by increasing stroke volume. The increases in central pressure are transmitted to the left atrium, where Starling forces are not operational. Since the increased volume does not result in increased output to the ventricle, higher pulmonary vascular pressure results, as does increased risk for pulmonary edema. Second, since the ventricle fills during diastole, anything that shortens this phase will decrease cardiac output. Thus, patients with MS respond poorly to tachycardia.

Pregnant patients with MS should limit their activity, and at times be placed on bedrest. With blood volume expansion, the asymptomatic woman may begin to experience symptoms and signs of pulmonary edema, and frequent assessments of her complaints and lung examinations are important. Diuresis, which may be necessary to reduce pulmonary congestion, can be accomplished with furosemide. However, one must watch the patient's electrolytes, blood urea nitrogen, and creatinine, and be careful not to deplete the patient's intravascular volume, which may further compromise cardiac output.

Anemia and systemic illness should be assessed and treated aggressively. Regular urine cultures should be done to screen for urinary tract infections. Digoxin is indicated to block the ventricular response in those with atrial fibrillation. Finally, liberal hospitalization for these patients is prudent when faced with either an infectious process or a question of early cardiac decompensation.

Patients with atrial fibrillation, mechanical valves, or an embolism require anticoagulation. Heparin is the mainstay for anticoagulation in the first and third trimesters because it does not cross the placenta. Coumadin may be used in the second trimester, when there is minimal fetal risk and maximum potential for patient compliance. Switching anticoagulants can be risky, however, particularly in those with mechanical heart valves, when any decrease in the anticoagulation may increase the patient's risk for clotting off the valve. Again, involving the cardiologist and pharmacy is most helpful.

Mitral Insufficiency

Mitral insufficiency is usually associated with other valvular problems and tends to be well tolerated in pregnancy. The major risks include the development of atrial enlargement and fibrillation, particularly during pre-eclampsia, when there is an increased afterload and a higher risk of pulmonary edema.

Aortic Stenosis

When resulting from rheumatic disease, aortic stenosis is usually associated with other valvular lesions. When the valve diameter is less than one third of the normal size, cardiac output becomes fixed. Patients usually tolerate pregnancy because of the blood volume expansion and subsequent increased left ventricular preload. Severe disease may be associated with deficits in coronary artery or cerebral perfusion. If the patient has pre-existing ischemic heart disease, she is at risk for myocardial infarction and death. Also, a transvalvular gradient greater than 100 mm Hg is of extreme concern. The patient is at the greatest risk during any event that predisposes her to hypovolemia (supine position, pregnancy termination, and delivery).

Intrapartum Management

Timing of delivery should be individualized, with consideration given to the maturity of the fetus, the degree of cardiovascular compromise, and the ripeness of the cervix. In the absence of

maternal decompensation, decisions regarding delivery timing and mode are made for standard obstetric indications after 38 weeks. If dates are uncertain, documentation of fetal pulmonary maturity is advisable prior to embarking on an elective induction. A planned delivery when the available support and consult services are available is preferable, rather than allowing the patient to present in labor, particularly if anesthesia may not be readily available.

Antibiotic prophylaxis for endocarditis, while controversial in the setting of an uncomplicated vaginal delivery without infection, is mandated for patients with prosthetic valves, a prior history of endocarditis, or surgical shunts. Because the risk associated with antibiotics is low, it is prudent to provide them to all patients with valvular heart disease. The recommended regimens from the American Heart Association include intravenous ampicillin, 2 g, and gentamicin 1.5 mg/kg (not to exceed 80 mg) 30 minutes prior to the procedure, followed by repeat doses 8 hours later. For penicillin-allergic patients, intravenous vancomycin, 1 g over 1 hour, may be substituted for ampicillin.

Certain principles apply to all patients. Management of the patient's fluids should be meticulous. Accurate recording of intake and output is mandatory. If a Foley catheter is utilized, one should regularly assess the patient for an ascending urinary tract infection. The patient should remain in a lateral recumbent position to optimize venous return and prevent decreases in cardiac output. Oxygen should be given. Use of epidural anesthesia is useful in most conditions. The obstetrician must be aware that cardiac output may increase by up to 50% by the second stage of labor, and that the normal fluid shifts that occur at delivery may be quite unpredictable. The patient may experience an autotransfusion with the release of the vena caval compression and from the return of blood to the systemic circulation from the newly contracted uterus. At the other extreme, she may suffer from a postpartum hemorrhage. These shifts, while easily tolerated in the normal patient, can result in cardiovascular decompensation in those with a fixed valve lesion or with pulmonary hypertension.

Anticoagulated patients represent an added challenge. For those who have had a recent embolic event, atrial fibrillation, or a mechanical heart valve, delivery planning is important. Usually, these patients are maintained on heparin in the third trimester because of the risk of spontaneous fetal bleeding associated with coumadin. There will be patients that will require coumadin even in the third trimester, and one must be familiar with the modalities to reverse the anticoagulation.

For the patient requiring full anticoagulation with subcutaneous heparin, discontinuing the medication in labor will usually allow her to deliver uneventfully. The major risk is episiotomy hematoma. Obtaining a partial thromboplastin time (PTT) on admission will be helpful, particularly when the need for epidural anesthesia or cesarean section is anticipated. If reversal of heparin anticoagulation is necessary, protamine sulfate is the drug of choice. Each milligram will reverse the effect of 100 units of heparin, and the dose must be calculated using plasma heparin concentration or titrated using the Lee-White clotting time. Particularly high-risk patients with mechanical heart valves may require a low level of intravenous heparin intrapartum because clotting can occur on the valve and lead to embolization or cardiovascular collapse. One must employ the advice of the cardiologist when making this decision.

For those anticoagulated with coumadin, reversal of anticoagulation is more difficult. The long duration of action (4–5 days) does not allow the physician to just discontinue the medication. Subcutaneous vitamin K will help regenerate maternal clotting factors within 12 hours. If factors are needed more quickly, fresh frozen plasma should be given. One must bear in mind that with coumadin the fetus will be anticoagulated and that there is a risk for spontaneous, including intracranial, bleeding.

After delivery, resumption of anticoagulation should occur within 6 hours of vaginal delivery and within 12 to 18 hours of cesarean section, usually with intravenous heparin. If prolonged anticoagulation is needed, coumadin may be begun after a stable prolonged PTT is obtained. Anticoagulation is more predictable and consistent with coumadin, and coumadin is easier for the patient to administer. The mother may breast-feed safely while taking coumadin.

Mitral Stenosis

The intrapartum and postpartum periods appear to be associated with the highest risk in patients with MS. In those with severe disease (valve area <1 cm²), those with a history of pulmonary edema or who require diuretics, or those with a history of pulmonary hypertension, a Swan-Ganz catheter is indicated. This will enable the physician to monitor pulmonary artery and pulmonary capillary wedge pressures as well as cardiac output. Patients often require a higher than normal preload to maintain cardiac output. However, pulmonary edema may occur if the wedge pressure is greater than 16 mm Hg, and a careful balance is required.

Tachycardia may lead to a decrease in cardiac output, since there is reduced filling time for the left ventricle. Investigation and treatment are of vital importance; beta-blockers are the treatment of choice for unexplained tachycardia. Since labor exertion and pain may be associated with increased heart rates, labor analgesia is recommended, particularly continuous lumbar epidural anesthesia. The block should be allowed to set up slowly, so the effects of the sympathectomy can be managed in a controlled fashion. A rapid onset of the block may cause hypertension and decreased blood return to the heart, resulting in decreased cardiac output. The catheter will allow appropriate doses for labor, delivery, and, if necessary, surgical anesthesia for cesarean section.

The second stage is ideally managed without the patient pushing. With epidural anesthesia in place, one can allow the uterine contractions to push the vertex to a position where a low forceps delivery may be performed, rather than attempting a more difficult mid-pelvic delivery. As is the norm in obstetrics, one must be prepared for an expedient delivery in cases of fetal distress. Preparing for cesarean section or a trial of forceps will take longer in individuals with MS than in a normal patient.

After delivery, fluid mobilization ensues immediately with the contraction of the uterus and decreased vena caval compression. Later the mobilization of extravascular fluid occurs. Both phases place the patient at risk for pulmonary edema because the stenotic valve does not transmit the increased preload. Maintenance of the wedge pressure below 16 mm Hg will reduce this risk, and gentle diuresis may be necessary.

Aortic Stenosis

The highest risk for patients with aortic stenosis appears to be at the time of delivery. Hypovolemia, or any condition that impairs venous return to the heart, will decrease cardiac output. These patients should be maintained in a relatively hypervolemic state, with wedge pressures approaching 18 mm Hg, to diminish the risk of a larger than normal blood loss. Death usually occurs secondary to myocardial infarction rather than from hemodynamic collapse. Vasodilators and beta-blockers should be avoided in these patients.

Potential Problems Associated with Rheumatic Heart Disease

Unfortunately, patients with long-standing MS may develop pulmonary hypertension. This represents a potentially dangerous situation for the pregnant patient, with mortality rates described as high as 50%. The two conditions affect both the pulmonary and the systemic circuits of the heart. The right heart requires an adequate preload to perfuse the pulmonary circuit to avoid hypoxemia. Unfortunately, this may lead to volume overload of the left atrium. Since the left ventricle cannot respond in a Frank-Starling fashion because of the stenotic mitral valve, pulmonary congestion and edema may occur. Diuresis needed to correct pulmonary edema may lead to decreased right ventricular preload and result in hypoxemia.

These patients are at highest risk in the intrapartum period. Central monitoring is crucial. An arterial pressure catheter and a transcutaneous oxygen saturation monitor can be quite helpful in management. As with MS, a carefully dosed continuous lumbar epidural will avoid the rapid sympathectomy that may result in decreased right ventricular preload. Epidural or intrathecal narcotics for labor analgesia, which further reduces the risk, have been used with good results. The principles of labor and delivery for the patient with MS apply here (uterine displacement, analgesia and the prevention of tachycardia, oxygen and second stage assistance). At delivery, the rapid autotransfusion from the uterus and relief of caval compression increase blood return to the heart and place the patient at risk of acute right heart failure and sudden cardiac decompensation. Alternatively, an intrapartum hemorrhage may decrease right ventricular preload and result in hypoxemia as well as decreased left ventricular output. These patients may be at risk for decompensation for upwards of 2 weeks postdelivery. Cardiovascular collapse can progress quickly, and one may be powerless in its management. Fluids should be given judiciously and not in large boluses. It is advisable to have the cardiologist close at hand to assist with the patient.

Atrial Fibrillation

The main concern with atrial fibrillation is the conduction of the arrhythmia to the ventricle, resulting in tachycardia. Digitalis is safe in pregnancy and can reduce the ventricular response. If fibrillation begins in labor, the patient must be treated expediently. Cardioversion can be used safely. Subcutaneous heparin is recommended for those patients with chronic atrial fibrillation.

Refractory Pulmonary Edema

In patients with MS, pulmonary edema may develop or worsen as the blood volume expansion occurs. In some instances, furosemide may not improve the patient's symptoms or signs. Closed mitral valvotomy, while it does not improve prognosis in those with little fractional impairment, can be quite dramatic in terms of alleviating severe intractable pulmonary congestion. The procedure in experienced hands is relatively safe (maternal mortality is approximately 3%) and should ideally be performed in the second trimester. Cardiac surgery and cardiopulmonary bypass can be performed, but the maternal and fetal mortality is higher. If it is necessary, monitoring the fetal heart rate during surgery is important, and monitoring for uterine activity may be helpful postoperatively.

Rheumatic Fever

Patients with rheumatic heart disease are at higher risk of recurrent bouts of rheumatic fever than those who escaped cardiac injury. Pregnant women appear to be at higher risk for developing rheumatic fever. Therefore, aggressive treatment of streptococcal pharyngitis and observation of the recommended prophylaxis protocols are important. If rheumatic fever occurs, management is similar to that proposed in the nonpregnant state.

Seizure Disorders in Pregnancy

James O. Donaldson, MD

Epilepsy is the most common major neurologic disorder that obstetricians encounter. Approximately once per year, an active obstetrician will manage an epileptic woman through her pregnancy. Although much has been learned about the complex interactions among the different types of epilepsy, anticonvulsant metabolism, birth defects, genetics, and socioeconomic and environmental factors, much of the immense literature is contradictory, and controversies abound. The following is my assimilation of that literature and my current approach to this clinical situation.

Pregestational Counseling

The management of epilepsy begins before gestation with counseling of the prospective parents. First, the diagnosis should be confirmed. Not infrequently, patients with syncope, panic attacks, hyperventilation, and sometimes more complex pseudoseizures have been mislabeled epileptics and treated inappropriately with anticonvulsant drugs. In other instances, the previous work-up of true seizures may not have been thorough enough to exclude a condition, such as an arteriovenous malformation, that could significantly alter management of both epilepsy and pregnancy.

I try to reassure women that the course and outcome of pregnancy will probably be unaffected by idiopathic epilepsy. Socioeconomic status, marital status, parity, regular prenatal care, and many other diseases are more important factors than maternal epilepsy in determining the outcome of pregnancy. Maternal epilepsy is not an indication for cesarean section unless either a seizure occurs during stage II labor or the patient cannot cooperate with vaginal delivery. Although the risk of almost any complication can be found to be increased in one survey or another, maternal epilepsy is not consistently associated with any obstetric complication of pregnancy, with the possible exception of third-trimester bleeding, which may be secondary to anticonvulsant-induced folate deficiency.

Birth Defects

Most women who seek pregestational counseling are concerned about the risk of birth defects. I stress that birth defects are not unusual and occur in 3% to 5% of all babies, depending on the population studied. The risk of some malformation approximately doubles for women with treated epilepsy. I cite the largest controlled series, a Norwegian study of 3879 infants in each group, in which the absolute risk increased from 3.5% to 4.4% if the mother was epileptic. Trimethadione and paramethadione are strongly teratogenic and are best avoided by teenagers and women with the potential for childbearing. Since the risk of birth defects increases with the number of anticonvulsants, monotherapy is preferred, if possible. The time to change medi-

cation is before conception. Probably one third of women on polytherapy who have come to me for prepregnancy counseling have been successfully converted to monotherapy. During pregnancy I change or add anticonvulsants if therapeutic doses of a proven regimen no longer work.

A fundamental problem in the interpretation of all studies in this field is that the risk of congenital malformation due to the severity of the maternal trait of epilepsy cannot be distinguished from the risk due to treatment. For instance, orofacial clefting is the most common major malformation that has been attributed by some to anticonvulsants, particularly phenytoin. However, a genetic link between epilepsy and orofacial clefts is suspected because epileptics have twice the expected incidence of orofacial clefts. Furthermore, epilepsy is more common than expected in the extended families of children with orofacial clefts. Thus, an important part of counseling is taking a detailed family history concerning diseases such as diabetes mellitus and congenital malformations—especially orofacial clefts, neural tube defects, and congenital heart disease.

In 1982, surveillance studies found a 1% to 2% risk of neural tube defects among infants exposed in utero to valproic acid, which was not predicted from animal studies. Avoiding high peak blood levels of valproic acid may lessen the risk of neural tube defects and can be accomplished by changing the customary twice-daily doses to smaller doses three or four times daily. More recently, a smaller risk has been reported due to carbamazepine. Fortunately, prenatal diagnosis of serious neural tube defects can be made in the second trimester. High-resolution ultrasonography at 18 to 19 weeks plus serum alpha-fetoprotein determination will be diagnostic in most instances. Quantitation of alpha-fetoprotein in amniotic fluid is preferred by some centers but the procedure carries a 1% risk of miscarriage.

Craniofacial dysmorphic features plus hypoplasia of fingertips and fingernails have been attributed to all major anticonvulsants. Distal digital hypoplasia and hypertelorism are most strongly associated with phenytoin exposure. It should be emphasized that, with the possible exception of hypertelorism, most babies grow out of these "minor malformations," which are regarded as typical of the fetal anticonvulsant syndrome. Some other reputed aspects of the fetal anticonvulsant syndrome reveal a genetic basis when families are studied. For instance, epicanthus in exposed infants is strongly associated with epicanthus in the mothers. Similar studies of head circumference and stature show genetics to be the major factor. The role of genetics in the "fetal anticonvulsant syndrome" is well illustrated by the remarkable case of heteroparental dizygotic twins simultaneously exposed to phenytoin throughout gestation. One baby had the syndrome; the other did not.

The increased risk of congenital malformations in the offspring of epileptic mothers is probably multifactorial. One mechanism could be an inherited deficiency of epoxide hydrolase which, in the case of phenytoin, could increase arene oxides. As discussed earlier, polytherapy can shift metabolism to potentially teratogenic pathways. For instance, the combination of valproic acid and carbamazepine plus phenobarbital appears to be associated with an exceptionally high rate of major congenital malformations.

A second proposed teratogenic mechanism is folate deficiency. Folate malabsorption is most commonly associated with phenytoin and phenobarbital but also occurs with carbamazepine and valproic acid. Therapy with multiple drugs causes the lowest folate levels. Folic acid supplementation before conception appears to decrease birth defects in children of epileptic and nonepileptic mothers. Folate deficiency could be one way in which socioeconomic status affects the malformation rate. The optimal dose of folate has not been determined, but 0.5 mg or 1 mg is reasonable. I measure red blood cell folate levels at counseling sessions. I recommend starting prenatal vitamins, which typically contain folate, before gestation occurs. Often women stop "the pill" and start on prenatal vitamins with folate.

Management During Pregnancy

The course of epilepsy during pregnancy can be best predicted from the seizure frequency beforehand. Almost all patients who experience more than one seizure per month can be expected to worsen during pregnancy. These patients and any others on polytherapy are ones which I, as a neurologist, see frequently during pregnancy. Women who have not convulsed in the 9 months before becoming pregnant have a 25% chance of convulsing during pregnancy. The risk drops further for patients who have been seizure free for 2 years.

The primary objective is to keep the prospective mother seizure free with the fewest drugs in the lowest effective dosage. Although a fetus almost always survives an isolated seizure without obvious ill effect, there is every reason to believe that a maternal convulsion accompanied by hypoxia and acidosis is not good for a fetus. Recurrent seizures in pregnant rabbits impaired development of fetal brain. Maternal status epilepticus is likely to cause fetal wastage. One Finnish study has shown learning disabilities to be more common at age 5 among children whose mothers convulsed during pregnancy.

Monotherapy is recommended if at all possible, as it is for approximately 85% of patients. A statistically significant comparison of the outcomes of pregnancies of epileptic mothers taking different anticonvulsant drugs in monotherapy would be a huge undertaking and has never been done. While I avoid benzodiazepines because they cause neonatal depression, I do not prefer any one of the front-line anticonvulsants—carbamazepine, phenytoin, valproic acid, and phenobarbital—just because pregnancy is contemplated. My first choice for an anticonvulsant drug is dictated by the type of seizure disorder and the patient's potential for compliance. For instance, juvenile myoclonic epilepsy is usually completely controlled by valproic acid in monotherapy, whereas polytherapy in several regimens is often unsuccessful. I recommend valproic acid in that instance, although women must understand that valproic acid is associated with a 1% to 2% risk of neural tube defects in their offspring in addition to the general risk of increased birth defects in the infants of treated epileptic mothers.

Because a major reason for an increase in seizure frequency during pregnancy is a decline in anticonvulsant blood levels, I monitor anticonvulsant blood levels approximately each month during pregnancy and attempt to keep the level in that patient's predetermined therapeutic range. Usually the blood is drawn during regular prenatal obstetric visits with the results sent to both the obstetrician and the neurologist. Actual visits to the neurologist can be infrequent for patients who have been completely controlled for years.

Free, protein-unbound anticonvulsant blood levels are preferred during pregnancy because protein binding decreases during pregnancy. Thus lower blood levels due to increased metabolism during pregnancy are partially offset by decreased binding and higher free drug levels. For instance, although total blood phenytoin may drop 56%, free phenytoin declines only 31%. The effect was not as great for carbamazepine, with a 42% decrease in total blood level accompanied by a 28% decrease in the protein-unbound amount. If the technology to assess free blood levels is not available, saliva anticonvulsant levels can be used because saliva concentrations approximately equal free anticonvulsant blood levels. Sputum production can be increased by having patients chew rubber bands.

Although not all agree, I recommend administration of vitamin K_1 during the last month of pregnancy as prophylaxis for a neonatal bleeding disorder reported with maternal use of phenytoin, phenobarbital, and primidone. Maternal coagulation studies are usually normal, although cord blood is deficient in vitamin K–dependent clotting factors. The optimal dose has yet to be determined, but it is known that 20 mg/day orally will prevent this disorder. Word of mouth has it that less is also effective.

Postpartum Management

If the dose of an anticonvulsant has been increased during pregnancy, I check blood levels at discharge from hospital and at 2 weeks and 6 weeks postpartum. In the case of phenytoin, blood levels increase quickly after childbirth. I usually discharge patients on their prepregnancy dose of phenytoin plus one-half of the increment added during pregnancy. The dose can be decreased again at 2 to 3 weeks postpartum. For example, a woman whose pregestational total daily dose of phenytoin was 300 mg and whose dose was increased during pregnancy to 700 mg would be discharged on 500 mg per day. About 2 weeks later the dose can probably be decreased to 400 mg per day. Because the rebound in carbamazepine and phenobarbital levels is slower, the first decrease in their dosage need not occur until 2 or 3 weeks postpartum. The pregnancy dosage is usually reestablished at the 6-week check-up.

If the woman wishes to breast-feed, I encourage her. All anticonvulsants are present in breast milk, but only in some instances with phenobarbital and benzodiazepines does the combination of the amount ingested plus slow neonatal metabolism produce sedation. Usually babies cannot ingest enough milk to cause any effect. Beginning about 1 week after birth, infants of women taking phenobarbital or primidone can experience withdrawal symptoms—hyperexcitability, tremor, high-pitched cry, feeding problems, and seemingly constant hunger.

Recurrent Spontaneous Abortion

Carolyn B. Coulam, MD

Spontaneous abortion is the expression of products of conception before 20 weeks' gestation. According to the World Health Organization (1992), 150,000 spontaneous abortions occur each day. Spontaneous abortion is the most common complication of pregnancy; it occurs among at least 75% of all women trying to become pregnant. Most of these losses are unrecognized and occur before or with expected menses. The remaining 15% to 20% are spontaneous abortions or ectopic pregnancies diagnosed after clinical recognition of pregnancy. As many as 5% of all couples conceiving experience two consecutive abortions, and 2% have three or more consecutive losses. The observed frequency of recurrent abortion is higher than that expected by chance (0.3%) implying an underlying cause contribution to the recurrent loss. All of these losses result in substantial physical and emotional pain and medical expense. Therefore, effective treatment is needed for couples experiencing recurrent abortion. Before effective treatment can be instituted, the cause of pregnancy loss must be determined. Although genetic, anatomic, hormonal, and immunologic factors have been implicated in the causation of recurrent abortion, the roles of anatomic defects and hormonal deficiencies have been questioned, leaving chromosomal abnormalities and immunologic factors as principal causes of recurrent abortion. Nonetheless, the tools currently used to facilitate the diagnosis of recurrent pregnancy loss include chromosomal analysis, examination of the uterine cavity, evaluation of endometrial receptivity, and immunologic tests (Table 1). Understanding the mechanisms involved in recurrent abortion allows a focused approach to treatment.

Genetic Factors

The most common genetic factor associated with recurrent spontaneous abortion is abnormal chromosomal analysis. Chromosomal analysis can be performed on peripheral blood leukocytes or on products of conception originating from couples experiencing recurrent spontaneous abortion.

TABLE 1. Evaluation for Recurrent Spontaneous Abortion

> Chromosome analysis
> > Parents
> > Products of conception
>
> Examination of uterine cavity
> > Hysteroscopy
> > Hysterosalpingography
> > Hysterosonography
>
> Evaluation of endometrial reception
> > Ultrasonography
> > Doppler flow
> > Integrins
> > Endometrial biopsy
> > Serum progesterone
>
> Immunologic evaluation
> > Autoantibodies
> > Antinuclear antibodies
> > Antiphospholipid antibodies
> > Lupus anticoagulant
> > Antithyroid antibodies
> > Reproductive immunophenotype
> > Embryotoxicity assay
> > Leukocyte antibody detection assay

Chromosomal Analysis from Parents

A parental chromosomal abnormality is present in 3% to 6% of couples presenting with recurrent miscarriage. The chromosomal abnormality is most commonly a balanced reciprocal or robersonian translocation. In 4.4% of couples with a history of two spontaneous abortions, one of the parents will prove to be a carrier of a balanced structural abnormality. The frequency increases to 4.7% after three spontaneous abortions. Identification of this small group is necessary to allow appropriate genetic counseling. Chromosomal translocations and inversions are associated with pregnancy wastage and are an indication for prenatal diagnosis in subsequent pregnancies.

Chromosomal Analysis from Products of Conception

It has been recognized for some time that products of at least 50% of early spontaneous abortions are cytogenetically abnormal. This figure contrasts markedly with the prevalence of chromosomal abnormalities observed among stillbirths (5%) and livebirths (0.5%). The most plausible explanation for the large number of chromosomal abnormalities among lost pregnancies is that most chromosomal abnormalities result in disordered development incompatible with prolonged intrauterine survival. The extent

to which chromosomal abnormalities contribute to recurrent abortion was previously thought to be relatively low (5%). Current data indicate that 60% of all abortuses from women experiencing recurrent abortion are chromosomally abnormal. Compared with a control group, aneuploid conceptions occur more frequently in couples experiencing recurrent spontaneous abortion (0.3% vs 1.6%). The frequency of disordered development may be increased in pregnancies from a subset of women experiencing recurrent pregnancy loss.

The results of a chromosomal analysis performed on the products of conception of a lost pregnancy can help predict subsequent pregnancy outcome. A history of a previous trisomy is a risk factor for another trisomy. The risk of spontaneous abortion in a subsequent pregnancy is increased when a normal embryonic karyotype is found in abortus material. Thus with a history of recurrent spontaneous abortion, demonstration of normal embryonic karyotype may be the most important indication for diagnostic evaluation and possible treatment of women experiencing recurrent spontaneous abortion. At this time, the only way to identify such women is to have the results of chromosomal analysis of previous pregnancy losses available.

Anatomic Factors

Anatomic uterine abnormalities have been more closely associated with late pregnancy loss than first trimester abortions. Congenital uterine anomalies have been reported to be increased among women with recurrent spontaneous abortion. However, in a study of 680 parous women with a normal reproductive history, 3% had müllerian duct anomalies, of which 90% were septate uteri and 5% bicornuate uteri. This frequency of congenital uterine anomalies is similar to that reported in a series of 500 women with recurrent abortion.

Techniques used to evaluate the uterine cavity include hysteroscopy, hysterosalpingography, and hysterosonography. When the results of these methods have been compared, hysterosonography has been shown to be the most accurate method of detection and evaluation of size, intracavitary growth, and location of intrauterine lesions. In a study of 600 women undergoing hysterosonography for evaluation of recurrent pregnancy loss and infertility, 499 (83.7%) had normal findings and 101 (16.8%) had abnormal findings. The abnormalities were müllerian duct anomalies (11), endometrial polyps (40), uterine synechiae (31), submucous fibroid (17), T-shaped uterus (1), and retained intrauterine device (1).

Although reports have shown a marked improvement in fetal salvage rates after metroplasty among women with müllerian duct defects and a history of recurrent spontaneous abortion, live birth rates were the same when the women with the same uterine anomaly who did not have surgery were followed for the same period of time. Because uterine surgery has been shown to be associated with significant postoperative infertility, justification for surgical intervention has been questioned.

The association between endometrial polyps, submucous myoma, intrauterine adhesions, and intrauterine diethylstilbestrol exposure and recurrent spontaneous abortion is presently unclear.

Endocrine Factors

Traditionally, an underlying endocrinopathy has been ascribed to many women experiencing recurrent spontaneous abortion. Luteal phase defect (defined as an inadequate secretion or effect of progesterone by the corpus luteum in the luteal phase and early pregnancy) is estimated to occur in 23% to 60% of women with recurrent abortion. Since there is no reliable method to diagnose inadequate luteal function in the pregnant woman, the diagnosis has been based on serum progesterone concentrations and endometrial biopsies in nonconception cycles. "Out of phase" endometrial biopsies were found to be higher in frequency in the fertile control population than in women with recurrent spontaneous abortion. Low serum progesterone concentrations after implantation may be the result of insufficient human chorionic gonadotropin "rescue" rather than the cause of the abortion. Furthermore, hormonal profiles in the preimplantation period of pregnancies ending in early abortion do not differ from profiles of a successful conception cycle in the same women. A meta-analysis of six trials in which exogenous progesterone was administered after conception failed to show any benefit from this treatment.

Although the role of hormonal factors has been questioned as a cause of recurrent pregnancy loss, the role of hormones has been implicated in infertility. Studies have correlated ultrasonic patterns of the endometrium with hormonal stimulation and subsequent pregnancy rate. The sonographic findings of endometrial thickness of more than 6 mm, a triple line echogenic pattern, and pulsatility index of uterine arteries less than 3.3 in the late follicular phase have been used to predict successful implantation.

Immunologic Factors

A body of literature is accumulating that suggests that immunologic mechanisms provide an explanation for a large proportion of recurrent spontaneous abortions that were heretofore unexplained. It is not surprising that a large proportion of unexplained recurrent pregnancy loss could result from immunologic maladaptation to the pregnancy, since the conceptus is both an autograft and an allograft to its host mother. If the maternal immunologic response to the conceptus is not appropriate and the problem involves a maternally derived target antigen, an autoimmune cause of recurrent spontaneous abortion is diagnosed. Alternatively, if an inappropriate response to a paternally derived antigen is found, an alloimmune cause of recurrent spontaneous abortion is diagnosed. Laboratory tests used to identify autoimmune causes of recurrent pregnancy loss have included antiphospholipid, antinuclear, and anthyroid antibodies. Laboratory tests used to identify alloimmune causes include quantitation of circulating natural killer (NK) or CD56+ cells and detection of circulating embryotoxins. The leukocyte antibody detection assay can identify individuals less likely to respond to white blood cell immunization therapy. That autoimmune and alloimmune mechanisms are causes of recurrent pregnancy loss is supported by basic laboratory studies as well as results of clinical trials using various forms of immunotherapy for treatment.

Autoantibodies

The association of autoantibodies and recurrent pregnancy loss has been known for over a decade. A number of clinical trials have shown that women with the presence of circulating antiphospholipid and antinuclear antibodies respond to treatment with low-dose aspirin and heparin or prednisone as well as intravenous immunoglobulin (IVIg). The overall live birth rate is similar (70–85%) after treatment with heparin and aspirin, prednisone and aspirin, and IVIg among women with recurrent spontaneous abortion associated with antiphospholipid antibodies. Treatment with low-dose aspirin alone is associated with half the live birth rate (45%). The usual doses are aspirin 80 mg orally daily, heparin 5000 to 10,000 U subcutaneously twice daily, prednisone 10 to 60 mg orally daily, and IVIg 400 to 1200 mg/kg every 3 to 4 weeks. Live birth rates are higher when therapy is begun preconceptually compared with postconceptually (44% vs 76%).

Natural Killer Cells

Natural killer cells express the cell surface antigen CD56+. Mononuclear cells that express CD56+, present in early pregnancy decidua, have been associated with successful pregnancy outcome. A deficiency of these CD56+ cells have been observed in placentae from women with incipient miscarriage. Animal studies have demonstrated a role of CD56+ cells in the prevention of abortion. Other studies have proposed that the systemic regulation of lymphocine activated killer cells determines reproductive success. Peripheral NK cells from women with recurrent spontaneous abortion have cytotoxic actions to autologous placental extracts. A study of peripheral circulating NK cells in women with recurrent spontaneous abortion has reported NK cells to be significantly elevated as compared with those in normal fertile control subjects. The concentration of circulating NK cells has been shown to be correlated with pregnancy outcome in pregnant women carrying singleton gestation and in women with an obstetric history of recurrent pregnancy loss. A significantly higher proportion of women with CD56+ cell levels greater than 12% who received IVIg had viable pregnancies than did those who did not receive IVIg ($p = 0.0002$).

Embryotoxic Factors

Cells secrete cytokines. A number of cytokines have been shown to be embryotoxic. Hill and colleagues reported that embryotoxic factors were produced by activated leukocyte cultures from 90% of 180 women with recurrent spontaneous abortion. Other studies have identified embryotoxic factors in 24% to 60% of women experiencing recurrent spontaneous abortion. Successful pregnancies have been observed in these women following IVIg therapy or progesterone supplementation. However, none of these studies reported control results. Randomized controlled clinical trials of immunotherapy for the treatment of recurrent spontaneous abortion associated with circulating embryotoxins are required to determine efficacy.

Unexplained Recurrent Spontaneous Abortion

Management of unexplained recurrent spontaneous abortion has been controversial. Results of meta-analysis and randomized clinical trials have provided evidence for successful treatment of recurrent spontaneous abortion using immunotherapy in the forms of immunization with allogenic monocytes and IVIg.

Allogeneic Mononuclear Cell Immunotherapy for Recurrent Spontaneous Abortion

Clinical trials evaluating allogeneic monocyte immunization have both supported and challenged the efficacy of immunotherapy for treatment of recurrent spontaneous abortion. To address the uncertainties caused by these conflicting results, a worldwide collaborative observational study and meta-analysis was performed (Fig. 1). Fifteen collaborating centers participated in the study. Nine randomized trials (seven double-blinded) were evaluated independently by two data analysis teams to ensure that conclusions were robust.

Although the independent analyses used different definitions and statistical methods, the results were similar. The percent live birth ratios (ratio of live births in treatment and control groups) with 95% confidence intervals were 1.16 (range, 1.01–1.34; $p = 0.03$) and 1.21 (range, 1.04–1.37; $p = 0.02$). The absolute differences in live birth rates between treatment and control groups were 8% and 10%. When the analysis was restricted to patients who became pregnant after intervention, similar results were obtained.

Intravenous Immunoglobulin Therapy for Treatment of Recurrent Spontaneous Abortion

Because of the low treatment effect of allogeneic mononuclear cell immunization, other treatments for recurrent spontaneous abortion were sought. Three randomized controlled trials of IVIg for treatment of recurrent spontaneous abortion have been published (Fig. 2). A European-based study showed a positive trend but did not achieve statistical significance because too few patients were enrolled for adequate statistical power, given the magnitude of the effect. However, a second US-based trial did show a significant benefit. This prospective, randomized, placebo-controlled trial showed the difference in live birth rates between women receiving IVIg (62%) and placebo (34%) ($p = 0.04$). As the US-based trial did not have larger numbers than the European-based trial, the positive result was due to an effect of greater magnitude. Based on the magnitude of the effect in the US-based trial, one needs to treat four women to achieve one

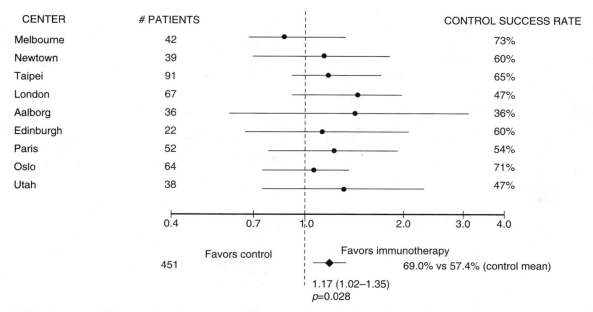

Figure 1. A cumulative meta-analysis of randomized trial results from the worldwide collaboration study on paternal leukocyte immunotherapy for treatment of recurrent spontaneous abortion. The horizontal axis shows relative risk of live birth versus repeat abortion. For each center, mean (●) and 95% confidence interval (CI) is shown. The result of combined analysis is given below, total number of patients to the left, and overall risk ratio and 95% CI to the right.

additional live birth, making IVIg therapy more effective than mononuclear cell immunization in the treatment of recurrent spontaneous abortion. The greater magnitude of effect in the US-based study compared with the European-based trial could have arisen by use of a different study design. One of the potentially significant differences in study design between the two trials was timely initiation of treatment. Patients began IVIg treatment prior to conception in the US-based trial. By waiting until 5 to 8 weeks of

gestation (for diagnosis or pregnancy) women with pathology related to NK cells occurring earlier would be excluded and best prognosis pregnancies would be included, providing an opportunity for selection bias. Studies using other forms of immunotherapy have shown a significant increase in live birth rates when treatment was begun preconceptually compared with postconceptually. A third study treated only patients with secondary recurrent spontaneous abortion, a group that showed no significant benefit to

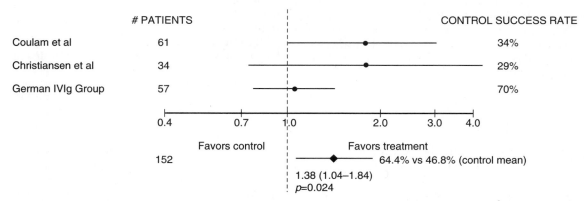

Figure 2. A cumulative meta-analysis of published randomized clinical trials using intravenous immunoglobulin (IVIg) for treatment of recurrent spontaneous abortion. The horizontal axis shows relative risk of live birth vs repeat abortion. For each center, mean (●) and 95% confidence interval is shown. The result of combined analysis is given below, total number of patients to the left, and overall risk ratio and 95% confidence interval to the right.

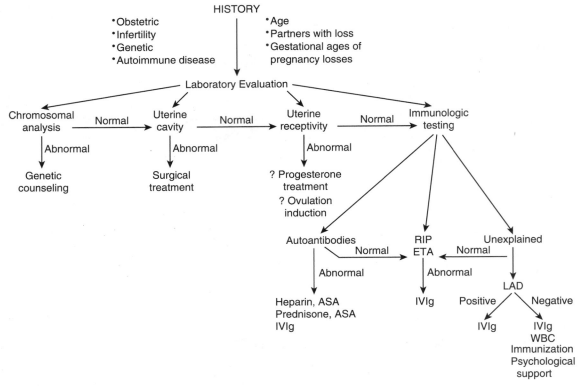

Figure 3. Algorithm for management of couples experiencing recurrent spontaneous abortion. ASA, aspirin; ETA, embryotoxicity assay; IVIg, intravenous immunoglobulin; LAD, leukocyte antibody detection assay; RIP, reproductive immunophenotype; WBC, white blood cell.

treatment using leukocyte immunization. A non-controlled study by the same investigators using IVIg to treat 11 women who had four to eight unexplained pregnancy losses reported a live birth rate of 855 per 1000. A meta-analysis of the randomized controlled studies using IVIg for treatment of recurrent spontaneous abortion revealed an overall relative risk of 1.38 (95% CI, 1.04–1.84; $p = 0.02$). While these results show IVIg to be effective in the treatment of recurrent spontaneous abortion, it still is not clear what the ideal dosage is and how frequently and for how long IVIg therapy should be given.

Conclusion

Recurrent spontaneous abortion is a health care concern. Safe and effective treatments are necessary. Since women experiencing recurrent spontaneous abortion are a heterogenous population, specific markers are necessary to identify those who will respond to various treatments. An algorithm for management of couples experiencing recurrent spontaneous abortion is presented in

Figure 3. Diagnostic tests have been used to identify putative causes of recurrent spontaneous abortion, including genetic, anatomic, endocrinologic, and immunologic factors. The tests to identify anatomic and endocrinologic causes that have been accepted as practice and are routinely used merit re-evaluation to determine whether the result of the test affects the outcome of pregnancy. Immunologic tests not yet accepted as routine merit further validation by wider usage.

Recent data obtained by early sampling and karyotyping of chorionic villus tissue from failing pregnancies have shown a substantial proportion (average 60%) to have chromosome anomalies. Peripheral blood NK cell levels tend to be elevated in those patients aborting karyotypically normal embryos. Active immunotherapy with paternal mononuclear cells and passive immunotherapy with IVIg appear able to increase the probability of a live birth among affected couples. These inferences have been based on level I evidence (meta-analysis of sufficient power to avoid type II error, using primary patient data from published and unpublished trials subject to two independent analyses and randomized placebo controlled trials).

Systemic Lupus Erythematosus in Pregnancy

Rebecca Shiffman, MD
John B. Josimovich, MD

Systemic lupus erythematosus (SLE) is a rare collagen autoimmune disease that primarily affects women of reproductive age. It has a 10:1 female to male prevalence ratio and is thought to affect 1 in 1660 pregnancies. It is possible that many milder cases have gone undetected in the past and that more sensitive assays may reveal a much greater incidence of SLE complicating pregnancy.

The diagnosis of SLE is based on demonstrating four or more of 11 criteria listed in the 1982 revised criteria by the American College of Rheumatology (formerly known as the American Rheumatism Association) (Table 1).

The many manifestations of this disease seem to be due to immune complex deposits in various organ systems. These include malar rash, fever, arthritis, and lupus nephritis.

The most common positive serologic tests in-

TABLE 1. 1982 Revised Criteria for Classification of Systemic Lupus Erythematosus Suggested by the American Rheumatism Association

1. Malar rash
2. Discoid rash
3. Photosensitivity
4. Oral or nasopharyngeal ulcers
5. Nonerosive arthritis involving two or more peripheral joints
6. Serositis: Either pleuritis or pericarditis
7. Renal disorder: Either proteinuria >0.5 g/day or cellular casts
8. Neurologic disorder: Either psychosis or convulsions
9. Hematologic disorder. One of the following:
   a. hemolytic anemia
   b. leucopenia
   c. lymphopenia
   d. thrombocytopenia
10. Immunologic disorder. One of the following:
    a. positive LE cell preparation
    b. antibody to native DNA in abnormal titer
    c. antibody to smooth muscle antigen
    d. chronic false positive syphilis serology for 6 months
11. Antinuclear antibody in abnormal titer

---

clude antinuclear antibodies (ANAs) which are present in 98% of patients. Other autoantibodies include anti-double and anti-single stranded DNA and RNA and antiplatelet antibodies. More recent attention has been focused on phospholipid antibodies, anticardiolipin antibodies (ACA) and lupus anticoagulant (LAC), and their association with early pregnancy losses. In addition, anti-Ro (SS-A), an antibody to soluble ribonucleoprotein antigen, has been associated with congenital heart block.

Effects of Pregnancy on Systemic Lupus Erythematosus

When evaluating a chronic condition during pregnancy, one needs to look at both the effects of pregnancy on the disease and the effects of the disease on the pregnancy. Most of the evidence indicates that pregnancy does not alter the long-term prognosis of SLE. Because SLE is a condition characterized by exacerbations and remissions, the effect of pregnancy on the frequency of exacerbations is difficult to assess. Older data indicate that flare-ups were relatively rare during pregnancy, but more recent evidence indicates that relapses may be more common in pregnant than in nonpregnant patients. The incidence of exacerbations during pregnancy correlates with the presence or absence of active disease at the time of conception and 6 months prior. Hence, preconception counseling and careful planning of pregnancy is crucial to improve perinatal outcome.

Most studies agree that there is roughly a 20% increase in flare-ups in the postpartum period. These relapses can occur even after a therapeutic abortion. Pregnancy termination is not advised purely on the basis of disease activity; maternal mortalities have occurred in patients after an abortion induced because of active SLE disease.

Effects of Systemic Lupus Erythematosus on Pregnancy

Fertility rates do not appear to be affected by SLE, except for patients with lupus nephritis and a serum creatinine of 2 mg/dL or greater. These women may have difficulties conceiving.

The major effect of SLE is on pregnancy outcome. Early pregnancy losses of 25% to 40% have been reported. The incidence is even higher when antiphospholipid antibodies are present. Often these early pregnancy losses precede the diagnosis of SLE; therefore, ANA, LAC, or ACA testing must be a part of the evaluation for recurrent pregnancy loss. When the disease is relatively quiescent during pregnancy, there is a 90% chance of a live birth. When pregnancy is punctuated by active disease, the chances for a successful pregnancy outcome are reduced to 65%. The prognosis is markedly reduced in the presence of hypertensive renal disease, and perinatal mortality is close to 50%. Women with nephrotic syndrome without hypertension or with renal transplants and normal kidney function may expect a favorable outcome if they have been in remission prior to conception.

Management

The management of pregnancy complicated by SLE requires a team approach and close cooperation between rheumatologist and perinatologist.

As mentioned earlier, preconception planning is extremely important, since conception during a period of quiescence is more likely to result in a live birth.

The initial work-up should include ANA levels, complement levels, LAC, ACA, anti-Ro (SS-A), 24-hour urine for evaluation of renal function, complete blood count and platelet count, antiplatelet antibodies, and thyroid function tests. If a patient is on chronic corticosteroids, a glucose challenge test (GCT) should also be performed (Table 2).

The usefulness of complement levels during pregnancy to follow disease status is controversial. Complement levels (C_3, C_4) are known to be elevated in pregnancy. A decrease in values may indicate a flare-up.

We usually repeat ANA, complement levels,

TABLE 2. Initial Evaluation of Systemic Lupus Erythematosus in Pregnancy

Complete blood count with platelets
Antinuclear antibodies
Lupus anticoagulant
Cardiolipin antibody
Anti-Ro (SS-A) antibodies
C_3 and C_4
SMA 18
Thyroid-stimulating hormone, thyroxine, and triiodothyronene
Antiplatelet antibodies
24-hour urine for total protein and creatinine clearance
Glucose challenge test

and 24-hour urine every 4 to 6 weeks. Other tests are repeated as indicated by the patient's condition. Fetal surveillance includes ultrasonography for early pregnancy dating. We usually perform a sonogram at 18 to 20 weeks for a complete anatomical survey.

If anti-SSA (Rho) antibodies are present we usually will perform a thorough fetal cardiac evaluation, since these antibodies have been associated with complete congenital fetal heart block due to deposits of immune complexes in the fetal conducting system. Over 80% of fetuses affected require a neonatal pacemaker.

Because the risks of intrauterine growth restriction (IUGR) and preterm birth are increased in SLE, serial sonograms every 4 weeks are recommended to monitor fetal growth. Electronic fetal monitoring (non-stress testing) should be started at 26 to 28 weeks' gestation. Antepartum surveillance also includes umbilical velocimetry in cases in which IUGR is suspected. Amniotic fluid volume should be assessed weekly from 32 to 34 weeks, or earlier if IUGR is present.

Systemic Lupus Erythematosus and Pre-Eclampsia

Pre-eclampsia and lupus nephritis may be indistinguishable, as both produce hypertension, edema, and proteinuria. Since patients with renal disease are also more prone to develop pre-eclampsia, it is very important to make the distinction, particularly if symptoms occur early in gestation. The treatment for lupus nephritis includes immune suppressants (glucocorticoid steroids and possibly azathioprine), whereas the treatment of pre-eclampsia may require delivery. If pre-eclampsia occurs early in gestation, premature delivery may result in increased perinatal morbidity and mortality. Increasing ANA titers and falling C_3 and C_4 levels may be valuable in differentiating between a lupus flare-up and pre-eclampsia. Uric acid levels, thrombocytopenia, or elevated liver enzymes may not be useful, since these can be altered due to SLE manifestations, as well as pre-eclampsia.

Therapy

The treatment of SLE during pregnancy poses many difficult problems for both the patient and the physician team.

The most common medications used are glucocorticosteroids. These may be associated with decreased neonatal weight, although it is difficult to separate the effects of glucocorticosteroids from the potential effects of the disease itself in causing IUGR. Prednisone crosses the placenta very poorly and is the preferred drug for the mother. If a patient is on prednisone prior to conception, we continue this medication on the lowest dose possible.

Serum glucose must be monitored because of the potential development or worsening of glucose intolerance with corticosteroids. We usually obtain a 50 g GCT at the first visit, at 24 to 28 weeks, at 30 to 32 weeks, and at 34 to 36 weeks. If the GCT is 135 mg/dL or greater, a 3-hour glucose tolerance test is done, and, if abnormal, the patient is treated as a gestational diabetic and controlled with either diet or insulin.

During an exacerbation, the dose of prednisone is increased as necessary (60 to 200 mg/day) until a clinical response is achieved, and then the dose is gradually tapered off to the original "baseline" level.

We also give an acute dose of 100 to 200 mg hydrocortisone parenterally during the peripartum period, even if the patient has been in remission.

Other Immunosuppressants

Azathioprine may occasionally be required during pregnancy to control a flare. Azathioprine crosses the placenta, although it appears to be inactivated by placental metabolism. No teratogenic effects have been described so far. The possibility of fetal/neonatal immune suppression needs to be kept in mind, and it is advisable to decrease maternal dose after 32 weeks to minimize fetal immunosuppression. While the use of azathioprine is associated with IUGR, the effect of the drug versus the effect of underlying renal insufficiency of SLE cannot be determined. Side effects, including bone marrow depression, fever, and alopecia, are the same as in the nonpregnant patient. The dose is 1 to 2 mg/kg/day.

Cyclophosphamide is occasionally used in conjunction with prednisone. Animal studies have shown cyclophosphamide to be fetotoxic in a dose- and time-dependent manner. In humans, digital anomalies have been reported. Hence, the risk to the fetus must be weighed against the risk of the disease to the mother. When possible, cyclophosphamide should be avoided in the first trimester.

Breast-feeding is not recommended with either cyclophosphamide or azathioprine.

The recent literature is replete with articles praising the benefits of low-dose aspirin (80 mg PO qd). Low-dose aspirin has been reported to decrease the incidence and severity of preeclampsia and to improve pregnancy outcome in the presence of the phospholipid antibodies. Since patients with SLE are at risk for both of these conditions, we usually advise prophylactic low-dose aspirin to all our patients with SLE, unless otherwise contraindicated. A recent study has shown an increased incidence of abruptio placenta in a group of low-risk patients treated with low-dose aspirin. Although the incidence of abruptio placenta in this group was lower than that reported in the general population, the benefits of aspirin for prophylaxis need to be weighed against the potential risks. The use of heparin in the management of phospholipid antibodies remains controversial.

Labor and Delivery

The timing of delivery in patients with SLE should be individualized, depending on patient and fetal condition. As mentioned earlier, the onset of pre-eclampsia or severe IUGR may mandate early delivery. The mode of delivery should be for purely obstetric considerations, and, when possible, one should strive for vaginal delivery.

If the cervix is unfavorable for induction, prostaglandin gel may be used for cervical ripening. As mentioned earlier, the patient should receive parenteral corticosteroids during the peripartum period. If a patient undergoes cesarean section, we usually continue steroids for 48 hours postoperatively, and then gradually taper them off.

Neonatal Complications

In addition to the complications related to IUGR and prematurity, the fetus of a mother with SLE may develop a neonatal lupus syndrome, including thrombocytopenia, presumably due to the presence of lupus erythematosus cells in the umbilical circulation. This usually tends to be transient. A more serious complication is congenital heart block due to the deposit of anti-SSA antibodies in the fetal conducting system. This results in permanent damage and requires a pacemaker in 80% of cases. The genetic susceptibility to SLE has not been clearly demonstrated.

Family Planning

The most favorable prognosis for a successful pregnancy outcome occurs in patients who have been in remission for 6 months prior to conception. Thus, patients must be advised regarding contraceptive methods.

Because oral contraceptives contain hormones that might affect SLE and intrauterine devices may predispose to infection in the immune-suppressed patient, we recommend barrier methods at present. Norplant, a subdermal progestin implant, should theoretically be a useful contraceptive method, although its use in patients with SLE has not been fully evaluated and the potential for thrombotic complication warrants caution in patients prone to thromboemboli. Once childbearing is completed, tubal ligation should be considered.

In summary, pregnancy complicated by SLE poses a challenge to the obstetrician and rheumatologist. Although perinatal morbidity and mortality are markedly increased in patients with lupus nephritis and hypertension and in patients whose pregnancy is complicated by repeated lupus flare-ups, with a careful team approach to SLE in pregnancy, preconception counseling, timely planning of conception, and close follow-up by a perinatologist and rheumatologist, a successful pregnancy outcome can be achieved.

Therapeutic Abortion

William Benbow Thompson, Jr, MD

To start this section, it is important to understand the terminology involved. Abortion is the expulsion or removal of the products of conception before the period of viability. The term *weeks* is used to mean time dated from the last menstrual period, in contradistinction to *gestational age*, which dates pregnancy from conception. In the past, abortion was either *therapeutic* or *criminal*. The adjective *therapeutic* remains even though most abortions are performed for socioeconomic reasons rather than to preserve the health and well-being of the mother. It should probably be termed *termination of pregnancy* rather than *therapeutic abortion*. The Centers for Disease Control and Prevention (CDC) simply use *abortion* or *legal abortion*. *Partial birth abortion* is a political description used by anti-abortion activists to vilify the procedure. It is not truly an abortion and the description is of a fetal destructive procedure almost never performed in modern obstetrics.

The CDC has been issuing reports on abortion for over 20 years. The last such survey was published on December 5, 1997, and included data for calendar year 1995. In this period, 1,210,883 abortions were reported, representing a 4.5% decrease from 1994. The abortion rate, the number of abortions per 1000 women aged 15 through 44 years, also fell to 20 from 21. As in the past, over half of the abortions were performed prior to the tenth week, and almost 20% were performed at less than 6 weeks. Over 80% were performed in the first trimester; more than half the women seeking abortion were less than 25 years of age.

Induced abortion remains one of the safest operative procedures performed in the United States, a far cry from the years before the Supreme Court decision on abortion, when abortion was one of the leading causes of maternal death, at 6.8 per 1000 live births. The accumulation and distribution of data by the CDC have played an important role in the reduction of risk. Factors that affect risk fall into three general categories: the experience of the surgeon, the gestational age, and the sophistication of the equipment. Equipment is discussed under Procedure as it relates to weeks of pregnancy. I have been predicting that RU 486, mifepristone, would be released, but this has not occurred. Nonetheless, the dosage and administration are given in the event that it does become available soon. It is being tested under the auspices of the Population Council of New York and would be an alternative to operative abortion for close to 20% of women seeking abortion.

Procedure

For all patients undergoing abortion certain laboratory data should be obtained: hemoglobin and hematocrit, urinalysis, blood group, and Rh status. Patients with gestations under 12 weeks can be protected from Rh sensitization by MICRhoGAM, which need not be cross-matched. Midtrimester patients require a full therapeutic dose of RhoGAM.

Four to Six Weeks' Gestation

Early in the first trimester is the ideal time for RU 486, a single oral dose of 600 mg of mifepristone. Studies done in the United States have confirmed the efficacy of the procedure, which offers a 90% +/− 4% chance of successful complete abortion. The patients have preliminary lab work, including CBC, HCG, UA; then after an overnight fast take twelve (12) tablets of mifepristone (RU 486). Abortion usually follows within one week. The efficacy can be enhanced by giving a small intramuscular dose of prostaglandin on day three or four. If the use of mifepristone is indeed this effective in general usage, the earliest abortions will be considerably less costly. The failures are increased with increasing gestational age so six weeks is about the limit.

The use of "menstrual extraction" will probably continue to have advocates since there is no waiting period for completion. One needs a vacuum pump capable of 0.5 atm of negative pressure to accomplish termination. A simple electrical pump will suffice. Caution: these pumps are not designed for this purpose and thus have a positive as well as a negative pressure port. The positive pressure port should be modified to prevent the inadvertent misapplication of the tubing. A locking 30 to 50 mL syringe can also be used. A disposable tubing and 6 mm vacurette is available in sterile pack. Paracervical block provides adequate anesthesia and is safe.

The procedure is safe, inexpensive, and practical in most office settings. A procedure room that is scrubbed regularly should be used. If this is not available, a surgicenter or a hospital facility using standard equipment is acceptable. The patient should be prepared as for any other vaginal surgical procedure. In an office setting, it is important to question the patient about food allergies, in particular, since an iodine preparation is generally used, and people allergic to shellfish frequently exhibit an acute iodine sensitivity. Laminaria should be used preoperatively in most nulliparous patients. It greatly reduces the pain associated with the dilation of the cervix and prevents a large number of cervical injuries that may occur with attempted rapid dilation of the cervix.

Potential problems in this early stage are minor but frequent. Other than those that are common to all abortions, the major problem in menstrual extraction is failure to substantiate that abortion indeed has been performed. All tissue should be sent to the laboratory, since ectopic pregnancies may well be missed, subjecting the patient to an additional hazard. In addition, the pregnancy itself may be missed early in gestation. The amount of tissue removed from an ectopic pregnancy is noticeably smaller in amount than that removed from a normal uterine gestation. Histological identification of villi is important and may be obtained by frozen section in a surgicenter or hospital evacuation.

The second problem that is common in menstrual extraction is retention of products. This occurs much more frequently after the fifth week; for this reason menstrual extraction or office evacuation is not usually attempted beyond this date. A second reason for maintaining the 5-week limit is the discomfort of the patient, who must be dilated up to eight Hegar to assure adequate size cannula. Major hemorrhage is infrequent but continued bleeding following evacuation is a sign of incomplete evacuation.

Seven to Twelve Weeks' Gestation

A hospital or surgicenter is the advisable location for the procedure during this stage. A nonreversible pump capable of at least 1.0 atm of negative pressure is needed. The pump should be so constructed that it is not possible to reverse the flow. General or local anesthesia is satisfactory. Patients should have an intravenous line with at least a 20-gauge needle. As a rule of thumb, the vacurette should be 1 mm larger than the week of gestation. The more advanced the pregnancy, the more advisable general anesthesia is. Oxytocin should be added to the intravenous solution at the beginning of the procedure. One should expect blood loss of 250 to 300 mL. Nulliparous patients should have laminaria inserted the day before the procedure; this greatly reduces the possibility of cervical injury and facilitates the dilatation. Frozen section should be requested when it is apparent that not enough tissue has been obtained. Women with ectopic pregnancies also request abortion before the diagnosis is obvious.

Thirteen to Fifteen Weeks' Gestation

At 13 to 15 weeks, dilatation and evacuation (D&E) is performed using large-diameter tubing, 18 to 20 mm, and a 16 mm vacurette. A clot should be drawn for cross-match if needed. Ultrasonography should be available for preliminary screening and for evaluation of the uterus at the end of the procedure. This may show that a portion of the products has not been evacuated and thus prevents a complication. Preparation of the patient is important. Laminaria should be used to achieve at least 15 mm dilatation. This can be done by serial insertions of laminaria, or in multiparous women it is often possible to insert two or three laminaria simultaneously. The laminaria are removed before the internal preparation is done. One must be prepared to remove fetal parts with ovum or Sopher forceps. Instillation procedures with hypertonic saline or prostaglandin $F_{2\alpha}$ may be used, but it is easier at a more advanced stage, 16 to 18 weeks. However, complications are greater with instillation procedures.

Sixteen to Eighteen Weeks' Gestation

A D&E using large-diameter vacurette and tubing is the safest procedure. This is not a procedure for the occasional abortionist. Ultrasonographic confirmation of gestational age and localization of the placenta are advisable. Our preference is continuous observation during the procedure. Perforation of the uterus when using large-diameter tubing and high-pressure vacuum is catastrophic. Blood should be available, as blood loss is frequently in excess of 500 mL. If you are not familiar with this procedure, do not attempt it; send your patient to a facility where late abortion is commonplace. If this is not possible, instillation of hypertonic saline is safer in the hands of a novice than surgical evacuation. The procedure is similar to amniocentesis for other indications. Ultrasonography should be used to locate a good window, and a Toohey needle should be introduced. The needle should be inserted at a point about halfway between the pubis and the fundus. It should be directed cephalad, so that fluid loss does not extract the needle. Amniotic fluid is removed in 50 to 100 mL increments and replaced with hypertonic saline with or without prostaglandin. The total volume using hypertonic saline should be 200 to 250 mL. Abortion usually follows within 24 hours.

Nineteen to Twenty Weeks' Gestation

A D&E is still statistically safer, but instillation is almost as safe. Experience of the operator should dictate the procedure. If instillation is selected, the patient should be an inpatient. Use of prostaglandin E enhances the efficacy of instillation procedures. Cross-matching is advised.

Twenty-one to Twenty-four Weeks' Gestation

A D&E as an in-hospital procedure remains the safest way to deal with advanced mid-trimester pregnancy. Instillation using hypertonic saline has about the same risk. Even induction with prostaglandin E_2 suppositories is acceptable. D&E should be contemplated only by those practitioners accomplished in this procedure. Preoperative laminaria, typing and cross-matching, and general anesthesia are needed. Prophylactic antibiotics are advisable.

Complications

The most common complications for all types of abortion are perforation, hemorrhage, and infection.

Perforation may be of little or major consequence. The larger the instrument producing the perforation, the more likely it is that serious damage has been inflicted. Perforation from a uterine sound is of no significance. The procedure should be stopped and the patient placed on prophylactic medication, and the procedure should be rescheduled in a few days. The patient should be observed for 2 to 3 hours and then allowed to go home. If it is deemed necessary to complete the abortion in the presence of a perforation, a second surgeon should observe the procedure via laparoscope to ensure that further damage is not inflicted. If the perforation is caused by a large vacurette and suction has been applied, it is mandatory that exploration be carried out by either laparoscopy or laparotomy. Severe injuries to the intestines have been reported and require prompt attention to avoid more serious consequences, including death. Hemorrhage is less of a problem, but one must be prepared for it. Typing and cross-matching should be routine for patients with gestation beyond 17 weeks. "Type and hold" for earlier midtrimester patients. Infection is relatively rare, probably because it is anticipated in mid-trimester and prevented by judicious use of prophylaxis.

What Next?

The future of pregnancy termination remains somewhat tenuous. It is likely that restrictions will continue to be imposed by the states. I think it is probable that mifepristone will be available in the coming years. Hopefully the concept that women may control their destinies will not be reversed.

Third-Trimester Bleeding

Fernando Arias, MD, PhD

Differential Diagnosis

In the majority of cases, the first step in the management of patients with third-trimester bleeding is to decide whether the patient has placenta previa, abruptio placentae, or other causes of bleeding. Rarely, bleeding is so profuse that life-saving measures are necessary before any time can be spent in the differential diagnosis.

Placenta previa and abruptio placentae are serious obstetric complications with significant fetal and maternal mortality and morbidity. Other causes of third-trimester bleeding are less ominous, although they are also associated with preterm delivery and fetal and neonatal morbidity.

The diagnosis of placenta previa is made by ultrasonographic examination with endovaginal probe. The positive and negative predictive value of this technique for the diagnosis of placenta previa is 93.3% and 97.6%, respectively. A total previa covers the internal cervical os; in a partial previa the low border is within 3 cm of the internal os.

The diagnosis of abruptio placentae is based on clinical and laboratory evaluation. Vaginal bleeding, history of cocaine abuse, uterine tenderness, uterine hypertonicity, symptoms of hypovolemia, and fetal demise are the most common clinical findings. Anemia and coagulation abnormalities, particularly an elevated concentration of D-dimer, are the predominant laboratory findings. Ultrasonography has limited value for the diagnosis of this condition.

Placenta Previa

In managing bleeding because of placenta previa, the obstetrician must first estimate the severity of the bleeding and the gestational age. A massive hemorrhage threatening maternal life requires interruption of the pregnancy regardless of the maturity of the fetus. Moderate to mild bleeding episodes in patients at term should also be managed by operative delivery. When the bleeding is not an immediate threat to the mother's life and the pregnancy is preterm, expectant management is indicated.

Another important factor in the management of these patients is the ability of the hospital nursery to handle preterm infants. If the neonatal care facilities are inadequate for preterm babies the mother should be transferred to a perinatal center where a high proportion of normal neonatal outcomes follow preterm delivery.

Evaluation of the Severity of Bleeding

In pregnant patients, it is sometimes difficult to make an adequate evaluation of the severity of a bleeding episode. In fact, the pulse rate and the blood pressure may remain within normal limits despite considerable blood loss because of the tolerance for bleeding generated by the intravascular volume expansion of pregnancy. Also, hematocrit and hemoglobin concentrations may be within normal ranges because of compensatory vasoconstriction. We have found the following clinical criteria useful to classify the severity of a bleeding episode:

Mild bleeding (the patient has lost less than 15% of her intravascular volume):
- No change in vital signs
- No postural hypotension
- Normal urinary output
- No evidence of circulatory volume deficit

Moderate bleeding (the patient has lost between 15% and 30% of her blood volume):
- Changes in pulse rate (increase of 10 to 20 bpm) and in diastolic blood pressure (drop of 10 mm Hg or more) when moving from the supine to the upright position
- Evidence of circulatory volume deficit (dyspnea, thirst, pallor, clammy extremities, apathy, or agitation)

Severe bleeding (the patient has lost more than 30% of her blood volume):
- Patients in shock or with decreased blood pressure
- Oliguria or anuria
- Persistent loss of fresh blood from the vagina
- Fetus dead or showing signs of distress

Management of Patients with Severe Bleeding

In cases of severe bleeding it is obvious that a catastrophic event is present and that maternal and fetal life are in danger. The objectives of management in these patients are to restore the maternal intravascular volume, to improve her oxygen-carrying capacity, and to prepare for interruption of pregnancy. These objectives are achieved by administration of intravenous fluids, transfusion therapy, assessment of renal function and intravascular volume, fetal monitoring, and delivery.

A large-bore cannula, at least 18 gauge, should be inserted for the rapid administration of lactated Ringer's solution. If the patient is in shock it is better to start two intravenous lines. When the intravenous lines are being established, blood samples should be obtained for complete blood count, type and screen of at least 4 units of packed red cells, electrolytes, glucose, creatinine, and disseminated intravascular coagulation (DIC) profile, which includes the prothrombin time, partial thromboplastin time, D-dimer, platelet count, and quantitative fibrinogen determination.

In most cases of severe obstetric bleeding, the blood bank can type and screen the patient's blood while her intravascular volume is being expanded with crystalloid solutions. However, if there is no time to wait for type-specific blood the patient should be given type O, Rh-negative cells. If Rh-negative cells are not available, type O Rh-positive cells should be used. The possibility of Rh isoimmunization if the patient is Rh negative and receives Rh-positive blood should not be an obstacle to transfusion in the patient with massive obstetric hemorrhage.

Usually there is a response to volume expansion with crystalloids and it is possible to wait 15 to 30 minutes for type-specific blood or even 40 to 60 minutes for a complete crossmatch. Transfusion of type O or type-specific noncrossmatched blood is justified only in extreme emergencies.

As blood is being used, it is necessary to have more units crossmatched so as to have 4 units available all the time. The need for massive blood replacement (10 or more units in 24 hours) occasionally occurs in patients with placenta previa, particularly those with placenta previa and accreta. A common problem with massive transfusion is platelet depletion requiring platelet transfusion. Deficiency in clotting factors is uncommon, but it is recommended to give 1 unit of fresh frozen plasma for every 4 units of packed red cells.

The majority of long-term complications of severe bleeding are related to hypoperfusion of vital organs. Particularly, acute tubular and cortical necrosis are relatively common complications of obstetric shock. For this reason observation of the urinary output is critical. A patient with severe obstetrical hemorrhage needs a Foley catheter and aggressive therapy for decreased urine output. The intravascular volume should be expanded to maintain a urine output of 30 ml/hr. This reflects a blood perfusion adequate to protect the kidney from severe damage.

With the initial steps to restore maternal blood volume and oxygen-carrying capacity, it is necessary to begin fetal heart rate monitoring. Also, as soon as possible, an ultrasonographic examination should be performed to determine fetal number, position, and weight, and to determine the placenta location.

Patients with placenta previa and massive bleeding should be delivered by cesarean section. The anesthesia of choice is general with endotracheal intubation. A transverse uterine incision is usually adequate but when the low uterine segment is not developed and the baby is preterm or when the presentation is transverse it is better to use a vertical uterine incision. In patients with previa and prior cesarean section, the possibility of placenta accreta is substantial and the obstetrician should be prepared to perform a cesarean hysterectomy.

Management of Patients with Moderate Bleeding

The management of patients with moderate bleeding is dictated by the gestational age and the maturity of the fetal lungs. The pregnancy should be interrupted if the gestational age is 36 weeks or more. Patients between 32 and 36 weeks should undergo amniocentesis to assess fetal pulmonary maturity, and the pregnancy should be interrupted if amniocentesis reveals adequate fetal pulmonary maturity. We use the surfactant to albumin ratio (S/A) rather than the lecithin to sphingomyelin (L/S) ratio for the assessment of fetal lung maturity. An S/A ratio of 0.7 or greater basically rules out hyaline membrane disease (HMD).

If the baby's lungs are immature, the patient with previa and moderate bleeding should remain under intensive monitoring in labor and delivery until stabilization or delivery. The hemoglobin should be maintained at a level of 11 to 12 g/dL by means of transfusions. Tocolytic agents should be used with caution to keep the uterus quiet. Steroids (betamethasone 12 mg daily, intramuscular, two doses, 24 hours apart) should be given to accelerate fetal lung maturity. If the patient's condition becomes stable, she should be transferred to a high-risk antepartum ward and managed expectantly until delivery.

The obstetrician should not hesitate to interrupt pregnancy if the mother remains unstable, that is, losing blood steadily in moderate amounts and requiring transfusions two or three times per week. In these cases it is better to take the risk of neonatal HMD than to continue expectant management. It is important to remember that the outcome of preterm neonates with HMD has changed dramatically with the advent of surfactant therapy.

Management of Patients with Mild Bleeding

The management of patients with placenta previa and mild bleeding is also dictated by the gestational age and the maturity of the fetal lungs. Immediate delivery is the best course of action when the gestational age is 36 weeks or more or when the baby's lungs are mature. Expectant management is the best course of action if the fetal lungs are immature or the gestational age is less than 36 weeks.

Some investigators have postulated criteria for out-patient expectant management of patients with placenta previa. However, continued hospitalization seems to be the best alternative. The patients are kept on bedrest with bathroom privileges. During their stay in the hospital we treat these patients with nifedipine to avoid uterine contractions, steroids to accelerate the maturity of the baby's lungs, and ferrous sulfate to replenish their iron stores. We also give them vitamin K_1 and phenobarbital, if they are at less than 30 weeks, for the prevention of intraventricular bleeding. Although the use of these medications is controversial, their potential advantages clearly outweigh the minimal risks associated with their administration. In the absence of complications, patients are delivered when they reach 37 weeks or when the fetal lungs are mature.

We have used cervical cerclage as a temporary measure in patients with placenta previa who start bleeding before 28 weeks and are at significant risk of requiring preterm delivery. The rationale behind this approach is that a cervical cerclage limits the development of the low uterine segment and avoids the partial detachment of the placenta that is the most likely cause of bleeding. The results we have obtained are excellent: patients undergoing cerclage reach more advanced gestational age and larger birth weight and have fewer neonatal complications than patients treated with expectant management alone.

Abruptio Placentae

All patients with abruptio placentae require aggressive measures to treat or prevent hypovolemia. When the abruptio is severe, it is necessary to anticipate the need to give large amounts of intravenous fluids. Therefore, establishment of adequate venous access is a priority. Samples for blood cell count, type, and screen of several units of blood, and DIC profile should be obtained at the time that venous access is achieved. Simultaneously or immediately after establishing intravenous lines it is necessary to determine whether the fetus is alive. Fetal life is an indirect index of the size of the retroplacental clot, the probability of coagulopathy, and the approach to delivery. If the fetus is dead, placental detachment is

greater than 50%, and approximately 30% of the patients will develop coagulopathy. Vaginal delivery will then be the management of choice. If the fetus is alive, the extent of the placental separation is usually less than 25%, and the chances of developing coagulopathy are under 5%. In these cases, the probability of fetal distress during labor and cesarean delivery is high.

Management of Patients with a Dead Fetus

With the loss of fetal life, the objective of management becomes to decrease maternal mortality and morbidity. To achieve this objective, it is necessary to replace blood volume losses and avoid organ perfusion deficits, manage the coagulopathy when present, and deliver the fetus in the most advantageous way for the mother.

When the abruptio is severe enough to cause fetal death the average blood loss, mostly retroplacental, is 2,500 cc. Despite their substantial blood loss these patients frequently present with normal vital signs and with blood counts within normal range. Thus, blood loss may be underestimated. Therefore, immediate transfusion of at least 2 units of blood should be instituted regardless of the normality of the admitting vital signs and the initial result of hemoglobin/hematocrit determinations.

The guidelines for the administration of packed red cells and intravenous fluids is to keep the hematocrit above 30 per cent and the urinary output above 30 mL/hr. These two criteria are of fundamental importance and indicate that oxygen-carrying capacity and effective intravascular volume are adequate to maintain the perfusion of vital organs.

Alterations of the coagulation system occur frequently in patients with abruptio and should be evaluated with the DIC profile. The presence of abnormal laboratory results is not necessarily an indication for therapy since the coagulopathy will resolve within hours following delivery. In particular, the belief that the presence of DIC in patients with abruptio is an indication for cesarean is unfounded. The opposite is true, and in the presence of a generalized hemostatic disorder operative interventions should be avoided, if at all possible. The best management of coagulopathy in these patients is to avoid administration of blood products unless there is excessive bleeding thought to be secondary to a specific coagulation factor deficiency. If the patient has marked depletion of fibrinogen (less than 100 mg/dL) and platelets (less than 40,000/mm³) it is adequate to replace these factors at the time of delivery to avoid excessive blood loss.

Unless there is a transverse lie, every effort should be made to achieve vaginal delivery in patients with abruptio and fetal death. Amniotomy should be performed shortly after admission and oxytocin infusion started unless the intrauterine pressure catheter shows the presence of spontaneous labor. The rigidity of the uterus, the presence of an unfavorable cervix, and the presence of elevated basal intrauterine pressure should not be deterrents to the administration of oxytocin or prostaglandin E_2. In most patients the cervix starts to change rapidly following induction and the progress in labor is rapid.

There is not an absolute time limit for obtaining a vaginal delivery in patients with abruptio and fetal death. With appropriate maintenance of their intravascular volume and oxygen-carrying capacity the time for obtaining a vaginal delivery may be extended safely to 24 hours.

Management of Patients with a Live Fetus

Pregnancy should be interrupted when the diagnosis of abruptio is made and the fetus is alive. The question is whether delivery should be accomplished by cesarean or vaginally. An important help in this decision is the situation of the uterus. If the uterus is rigid the abruptio most probably is large, although less than 50%, and the probability of fetal distress during labor is 90%. Alterations of the hemostatic system are uncommon when the baby is alive but when they are found it is usually in patients with hypertonic uterus. In this situation the patient should be delivered by cesarean.

When the uterus is soft vaginal delivery may be attempted under close surveillance. If the uterus becomes hypertonic or there are suggestions of fetal distress, cesarean should be performed immediately. The majority of patients with a live fetus and soft uterus will deliver vaginally uneventfully.

Other Causes of Third-Trimester Bleeding

In patients with third-trimester bleeding, the most common diagnosis, after excluding placenta previa and abruptio placentae, is marginal placental separation, also called marginal sinus bleeding. Unfortunately it is not possible to make a positive diagnosis of this condition before birth,

and therefore, very little is known about its natural history. It is assumed to be a benign condition. However, patients with third-trimester bleeding of unknown origin have an incidence of preterm labor of 17% and increased perinatal mortality.

Twin Pregnancy

Adam F. Borgida, MD
John F. Rodis, MD

Most families are overjoyed at the identification of a twin pregnancy. For the obstetrician, however, a twin gestation is more complex and requires careful management and delivery. The delayed onset of reproduction and increased use of fertility medications have increased the frequency of twin pregnancies. Patients must be counseled as to the increased maternal and fetal complications associated with twin pregnancies.

Incidence

The incidence of monozygotic twins is relatively consistent at 1 per 250 births across different populations. The incidence of dizygotic twinning varies widely. The occurrence of twins in the United States is approximately 1% to 2% of all pregnancies. The incidence increases with age, parity, and the use of fertility drugs. The incidence is highest in African-Americans and lowest in Asians.

Diagnosis

While the diagnosis of twins is relatively straightforward with the modern use of ultrasonography, zygosity is not as easy to determine. If an early ultrasonographic examination is performed, it is important to note the number of embryos, the number and location of placentas, and the presence and character of a dividing membrane. Separate placentas do not ensure dizygotic twins, but one placenta or one amniotic sac confirms monozygosity.

Dizygotic twins are always diamniotic and dichorionic; however, monozygotic twins can have a variety of placentas. When the twinning event occurs within the first 72 hours after conception, dichorionic, diamniotic twins result. This accounts for 20% to 30% of monozygotic twins. The most common type of placentation in monozygotic twins is monochorionic, diamniotic. This accounts for 60% to 70% of monozygotic twins and results from division between 3 and 8 days after conception. On ultrasonographic examination, typically, there is one placenta, a very thin dividing membrane, the membrane has no peak sign, and the fetuses have the same sex. One study has reported that zygosity can be determined with greater than a 90% positive predictive value using ultrasonographic features. Monoamniotic twins result when twinning occurs between days 8 and 13 after conception and accounts for 1% of monozygotic twins. Monoamniotic twins carry a great deal of risk, as will be discussed later.

Twinning that occurs 13 days or more after conception results in conjoined twins. The incidence is 1 in 50,000 deliveries. Ultrasonography is key in determining the site of joining and the possibility of shared organs. Several ultrasonographic features suggest conjoined twins. These include no change in the relative positions of the twins on successive examinations, hyperextension of the cervical spine, a single inseparable trunk, more than a three-vessel cord with one insertion, or the identification of shared organs.

Acardiac twins are another very unusual form of twinning. This occurs in less than 1% of monozygotic twins and, as with conjoined twins, has a very high pregnancy complication rate. Ultrasonographic features are the identification of a mass in the amniotic cavity with a variable degree of differentiation and no identifiable heart activity. The most frequent complications are preterm labor (80%), polyhydramnios (50%), and intrauterine fetal death of the normal twin (25%). If an acardiac twin is identified early in gestation several treatment options exist. Selective delivery, tamponade of the cord, laparoscopic clipping of the cord, and thrombus-inducing injections into the cord have all been performed on the acardiac twin with survival of the normal twin.

Complications

Twin gestations have an increased risk for maternal and fetal complications compared with singletons. Major complications include a higher rate of preterm labor and preterm birth, an increased risk for pre-eclampsia, and an increased incidence of gestational diabetes. Other complications that are increased in twin pregnancies are anemia, hyperemesis gravidarum, and spontaneous abortion.

Preterm birth is common with twin pregnancies. While the average gestational age of twin births is 35 to 36 weeks, 70% deliver after 37 weeks. Several factors contribute to the increased risk for preterm delivery. Preterm labor is more frequent, possibly because of uterine overdistention or polyhydramnios related to twin-to-twin transfusion or fetal anomalies. Iatrogenic preterm birth is also more common owing to the increased risk of other complications with twin pregnancies, such as pre-eclampsia and diabetes. Pre-eclampsia occurs about three times more frequently in twin pregnancies than in singletons; more importantly, it can occur earlier and more severely in twin pregnancies. This contributes to the increased risk of fetal complications as well as preterm birth.

Fetal complications are also increased in twin gestations. An increased incidence of anomalies, growth and fluid disturbances, twin-to-twin transfusion syndrome, and perinatal mortality are the most critical concerns in twin pregnancies. Fetal anomalies occur with twice the frequency in twin pregnancies compared with singletons, with an even higher risk in monozygotic twins. Three categories of anomalies have been described: those resulting from the teratogenic event that caused the twinning; those resulting from the vascular interchange between monozygotic twins; and deformations resulting from intrauterine crowding. Ultrasonography is essential in detecting fetal anomalies, and an anatomic survey at approximately 18 weeks is recommended.

Twin gestations, especially monozygotic twins, have an increased incidence of growth disorders. Serial ultrasonograms can detect discordant fetal growth and intrauterine growth restriction of one or both fetuses. Percent discordance is determined by subtracting the estimated fetal weight of the smaller from the larger twin, dividing by the estimated fetal weight of the larger twin, and multiplying by 100. Intrauterine growth restriction is diagnosed by a growth fall-off from an established twin growth curve over time. This can occur in either the larger or the smaller twin. Intervention is indicated if no fetal growth occurs in either twin after an adequate period of observation, usually at least 10 to 14 days.

Twin-to-twin transfusion syndrome is a unique situation in which vascular connections between monozygotic twins lead to preferential fetal blood flow in favor of one twin. This can result in polyhydramnios associated with one twin and oligohydramnios, or "stuck twin," with the other. The stuck twin typically has intrauterine growth restriction as well. When confronted with a stuck twin, one should not immediately conclude the diagnosis of twin-to-twin transfusion syndrome. A careful ultrasonogram to diagnose fetal anomalies is needed, as several have been reported to cause the stuck twin phenomenon. If the diagnosis of twin-to-twin transfusion syndrome is confirmed by excluding other possible causes, therapy is needed, since the pregnancy loss rate approaches 70% to 90% without intervention.

Therapeutic amniocentesis is the preferred method of treatment for twin-to-twin transfusion syndrome at this time. Withdrawal of fluid from the amniotic sac of the twin with polyhydramnios can alleviate the oligohydramnios of the stuck twin and fetal growth can equilibrate. Often one therapeutic amniocentesis is sufficient, but several attempts may be required (rarely more than three). Removal of enough amniotic fluid to completely resolve the polyhydramnios is most effective at normalizing the fluid volumes between the twins and minimizing the number or needed interventions. Serial ultrasonograms are necessary to evaluate the effectiveness of the treatment and for timing of serial procedures. Utilizing therapeutic amniocentesis, the survival rate of both twins can be improved to nearly 75%.

Perinatal mortality is five to 10 times higher in twin pregnancies compared with singletons. Monochorionic twins have a two to three times higher perinatal mortality rate than dichorionic twins. Monoamniotic twins have the highest rate of all twins, reported to be as high as 50%. Besides the increased complications mentioned earlier, low birth weight contributes greatly to the increased mortality rate in twins. Low birth weight is an end result of prematurity and intrauterine growth restriction, both more frequent in twins than singletons.

The death of one twin represents an uncommon complication in twin pregnancies, although very early losses may be more frequent (approximately 30%) and never recognized at delivery (vanishing twin). Fetus papyraceous has been described after death of one twin. Acquired coagulation defect is the most serious complication after the death of one twin. Heparin therapy has been used to successfully reverse maternal hypofibrinogenemia associated with disseminated intravascular coagulopathy (DIC) after the death of one twin. Close monitoring of the surviving twin is essential, especially for monochorionic twins in whom vascular connection may be present. This can lead to reverse twin-to-twin transfusion or DIC in the surviving fetus owing to embolization of thromboplastic material from the dead twin.

Management

Since twin pregnancies have an increased incidence of maternal and fetal complications, close management of all twin pregnancies is warranted.

Ultrasonography

We advocate several ultrasonographic examinations for all twin pregnancies. An early examination is especially helpful in determining placentation and possible zygosity. Owing to the increased risk of congenital anomalies in twins, a targeted scan approximately at 18 weeks is important. Fetal echocardiography may be performed at 20 to 22 weeks, since congenital heart disease is the most common major birth defect.

Ultrasonography is the key in diagnosing growth discordance or intrauterine growth restriction in twin pregnancies. For twin pregnancies that appear to be dichorionic or dizygotic, examination every 4 weeks is recommended. If discordance or intrauterine growth restriction is suspected, scans can be performed every 2 weeks. For pregnancies with one placenta and like-sex twins (monochorionic), more intensive monitoring is warranted, especially at 20 to 24 weeks when twin-to-twin transfusion syndrome may become evident. Growth scans every 3 to 4 weeks are acceptable if fetal growth is normal and amniotic fluid volumes appear to be similar. In the presence of abnormal fetal growth, more frequent scans are indicated. Each ultrasonographic examination should include a review of the dividing membrane and amniotic fluid. Detection of the stuck twin or twin-to-twin transfusion syndrome should prompt rapid therapy.

Antepartum Testing

The non-stress test (NST) is the standard test used for antepartum fetal surveillance. We recommend twice-weekly NSTs starting at 32 weeks in all twin pregnancies to reduce perinatal mortality. In complicated twin pregnancies, NSTs may be started at an earlier gestational age. The biophysical profile can be used efficaciously as a follow-up to nonreactive NSTs in twin pregnancies. Doppler velocimetry may be useful in identifying pregnancies at high risk for growth disturbances and discordance.

Intervention

Since the fetal death rate is significantly higher in twin pregnancies than singletons, antepartum testing must be relied on to warrant intervention. Severe fetal growth abnormalities may be an indication for early delivery. Nonreassuring fetal heart rate testing and biophysical profiles can also be used to guide early delivery.

Genetic Testing

The use of assisted reproductive technologies has allowed more women of advanced maternal age the opportunity for pregnancy. This in turn has increased the need for genetic testing in twin gestations. Amniocentesis and maternal serum screening are both used for the identification of aneuploidy in twin pregnancies. Slight modifications are required for genetic amniocentesis in twin pregnancies. Two separate needle insertions are performed with continuous ultrasonographic guidance. After aspiration of amniotic fluid, indigo carmine dye (2 mL) must be injected into the first sac to ensure the two different sacs are aspirated. Attempting to sample both sacs with one needle insertion should be avoided, since this may cause disruption of the membrane creating "monoamniotic" twins.

Chorionic villus sampling can be performed in twin pregnancies. The approach needs to be individualized for each patient. Often, one twin can be approached transcervically while the other is sampled transabdominally. Great care must be taken in the initial ultrasonogram. Explicit descriptions of the placental and fetal locations are required for proper interpretation of results, since selective termination may be an option in cases of discordant aneuploidy.

While maternal age of 35 years at the time of expected delivery has been the historic cut-off for advanced maternal age, a younger age cut-off (approximately 32 to 33 years of age) may be appropriate. Maternal serum screening can also be performed in twin pregnancies to identify women with an increased risk for aneuploidy. Maternal serum alpha-fetoprotein has been used for this purpose. Currently, there may not be enough data on multiple serum markers for use in twin pregnancies.

Selective Termination

When one fetus in a twin pregnancy is noted to have a major structural defect or genetic abnormality, selective fetocide has been performed. There are risks to the normal surviving twin arising from the procedure that still make the pregnancy more complicated than a singleton gestation. Most important in the evaluation and work-up of twin gestations discordant for anomalies is the counseling of the patient and proper informed consent. There is an increased risk of preterm delivery, preterm labor, preterm premature rupture of membranes, and low birth weight in surviving twins when selective termination is performed after 20 weeks' gestation.

Monoamniotic Twins

The rare diagnosis of monoamniotic twins deserves special mention. The incidence of monoamniotic twins is only 1% to 2% of monozygotic twins and has been reported to have a perinatal mortality rate as high as 50%. We have managed our monoamniotic twins with intensive antepartum fetal testing, with excellent survival for both twins. We recommend at least three serial ultrasonographic examinations to be sure that a dividing membrane does not exist. Once the diagnosis is established, serial scans for growth are needed owing to the high incidence of twin-to-twin transfusion syndrome and discordant fetal growth. We begin daily fetal heart rate testing at viability in an effort to reduce the perinatal mortality rate. Experience with Doppler ultrasonography is building and may be promising for the early prediction of vascular accidents secondary to cord entanglement. Since cord entanglement is universal in cases of monoamniotic twins, we recommend planned cesarean delivery once fetal lung maturity is documented. This will prevent any iatrogenic cord accidents or twin exsanguination. With intensive antepartum testing and cautious delivery, the perinatal mortality rate can be drastically reduced.

Delivery

The labor and delivery of a twin pregnancy is more complicated than a singleton birth and experienced obstetric attendants and support staff are required. We recommend continuous fetal monitoring of both twins during the labor and delivery process. It is vital to monitor the fetal heart rate tracing of both twins and to pay particular attention to the second twin during and immediately following the birth of the presenting twin.

There is an increased risk for malpresentations, premature separation of the placenta, vasa previa, and cesarean section associated with twin deliveries. A team approach is required to safely complete the birth of twins. Proper arrangements need to be made so that an emergency cesarean section can be performed and to have the required neonatal staff present for resuscitation of two infants.

With only approximately 40% of twins both presenting cephalic, the need for an approach to malpresentations is important. Many studies have shown that the breech delivery of the second twin is very safe; however, many obstetricians are no longer well trained in assisted breech deliveries. Also, external cephalic version of the second twin has recently been shown to have more morbidity than breech delivery. The mode of delivery for twins, therefore, must be a well-informed decision between the obstetrician and the patient, taking into account the experience of the physician and the comfort of the patient. Planning ahead and proper counseling are key. There is little controversy that vaginal delivery should be attempted when the twins are presenting vertex-vertex. Conversely, if the presenting twin is breech, a planned cesarean is our usual mode of delivery. The decision over the mode of delivery for a cephalic-presenting twin and malpresenting second twin must be left up to the individual obstetrician and the patient.

Anticipating the complications that may occur while attempting the birth of the second twin must be stressed. Experienced assistants, nursing staff, and anesthesia support are required. We recommend having an ultrasonography machine present at the birth of all twins to diagnose malpresentations and assist in the delivery process. This is especially important if external cephalic version of the second twin is anticipated. Additionally, an intravenous line and proper maternal analgesia are important.

In conclusion, the incidence of multiple gestations is increasing with the increasing use of ovulation-inducing agents. Widespread use of serum screening for birth defects and ultrasonography has led to most twin pregnancies being identified prior to birth. With close surveillance and appropriate testing and intervention when necessary, successful outcomes can be anticipated in the majority of cases.

Venous Thromboembolic Disease in Pregnancy

Daniel L. Clarke-Pearson, MD

Because of physiologic changes in pregnancy, a pregnant woman is at significantly increased risk to develop deep vein thrombosis and pulmonary embolism. This is most dramatically evidenced by the fact that pulmonary embolism is one of the leading causes of maternal mortality in the United States and other industrialized nations. To reduce maternal mortality and morbidity associated with deep vein thrombosis and pulmonary embolism, the obstetrician must be able to identify particularly high-risk patients, utilize prophylactic methods wisely, and diagnose and treat deep vein thrombosis and pulmonary embolism in an effective and expedient manner.

Risk Factors

Pregnancy alters many of the parameters of Virchow's triad, resulting in an increased risk of deep vein thrombosis or pulmonary embolism. Hypercoagulability is recognized in pregnancy with increasing levels of fibrinogen, factors VII, VIII, IX, and X, and fibrin split products. This thrombotic tendency is further compounded by diminished fibrinolysis due to a decrease in activity of factors XI and XII and of antithrombin III. Enhanced coagulation and diminished fibrinolytic activity shift the balance in favor of thrombosis.

Venous stasis and increased venous distensibility are well-recognized components of normal pregnancy. Lower extremity edema and worsening varicose veins are evidence of the venous stasis associated with an advancing gestation. Vessel wall injury is increased by difficult obstetric deliveries, cesarean section, endometritis or pelvic cellulitis, and leg trauma from unpadded or poorly positioned lithotomy stirrups.

The single most important clinical risk factor associated with the development of venous thromboembolic complications is a past history of deep vein thrombosis or pulmonary embolism. In women with such a history, the risk of recurrent venous thromboembolism in a subsequent pregnancy is estimated to be between 4% and 20%. Other factors thought to increase the risk of venous thromboembolism include pre-eclampsia, cesarean section, prolonged bedrest, obesity, diabetes, cardiac disease, high parity, advanced maternal age, or severe varicose veins. However, the exact degree of increased risk to develop venous thromboembolism from these factors is not known. Patients with a family history of hypercoagulable syndromes including antithrombin III deficiency, pregnancy-specific protein PAPP-A, protein C or S, or prostacyclin deficiency are also at increased risk. Elevated levels of lupus anticoagulant also appear to increase the risk of developing deep vein thrombosis.

The recognition of factors associated with venous thromboembolism in obstetric patients should allow the clinician to stratify patients into low-risk and high-risk groups and thereby apply appropriate prophylactic methods while not exposing low-risk patients to the potential complications and expense of some treatment regimens.

Prevention of Venous Thrombosis

Over the past two decades there have been extensive prospective trials investigating a variety of methods to prevent the occurrence of postoperative deep vein thrombosis and pulmonary embolism. Unfortunately, prospective randomized trials in obstetric patients are limited. Therefore, recommendations regarding the use of prophylactic methods in high-risk patients are based on extrapolation from surgical trials and empiric experience in nonrandomized obstetric studies. Low-dose heparin is the most commonly utilized prophylactic agent in obstetric patients. When a high-risk patient (such as a patient with a past history of deep vein thrombosis or pulmonary embolism) is recognized to be pregnant, we initiate low-dose heparin therapy. Several low-dose heparin regimens have been proposed. Our general approach is based on the observation that, as pregnancy progresses, patients become increasingly hypercoagulable and have increasing stasis. Further, there is an increasing need for heparin later in pregnancy. We initiate low-dose heparin therapy with 5000 units subcutaneously every 12 hours the first 13 weeks of pregnancy. Between the 13th and 29th week of pregnancy, the heparin dose is increased to 7500 units every 12 hours and, between 30 weeks and the onset of labor, heparin is administered 10,000 units subcutaneously every 12 hours. Because the patient remains at increased risk during the postpartum period, low-dose heparin is reinitiated postpartum (5000 units subcutaneously every 12 hours). Other regimens that adjust heparin dose to achieve a plasma concentration of 0.08 to 0.15 IU per milliliter or that use once-daily low

molecular weight heparin (LMWH) have been recommended, but none have been evaluated in prospective randomized trials.

The risks of low-dose heparin therapy include bleeding, thrombocytopenia, and osteoporosis. In the only randomized trial of low-dose heparin in pregnancy, Howell showed no increase in the risk of bleeding complications or premature labor in patients receiving low-dose heparin. While it has been suggested that LMWH might result in fewer bleeding complications, that has not been proved in clinical practice. The risk of osteoporosis has been recognized in case reports. Osteoporosis associated with prolonged heparin use usually presents with particularly painful compression fractures. The risk of osteoporosis seems to be increased when the daily dose of heparin is in excess of 15,000 units per day and is associated with prolonged therapy. Clearly, well-designed, multicentered clinical trials are needed to evaluate the many issues associated with low-dose heparin prophylaxis therapy in pregnancy.

Alternative methods of venous thrombosis prophylaxis might include mechanical methods, such as graded compression stockings or intermittent pneumatic compression. Graded compression stockings are certainly helpful in patients with venous stasis changes, edema, and symptomatic varicose veins. Their value in preventing deep vein thrombosis during pregnancy is not established; however, because of the lack of side effects and the minimal expense, we recommend them in patients with evidence of venous disease or past history of venous thromboembolic complications. External pneumatic calf compression has been found to be effective in reducing the incidence of postoperative deep vein thrombosis in patients who are not ambulatory. This prophylactic method might be seriously considered in patients who are placed on bedrest during pregnancy, although it is probably not practical for the ambulatory patients at high risk. Pneumatic compression might also be considered for prophylaxis in the peripartum period to reduce potential bleeding at the time of delivery and to allow for the use of epidural anesthesia for a vaginal delivery or cesarean section. (In most cases, anesthesiologists are loathe to use conduction anesthesia in patients receiving low-dose heparin.)

Diagnosis

The clinical diagnosis of deep vein thrombosis in pregnancy is often fraught with error. A number of conditions during pregnancy mimic deep vein thrombosis, including dependent edema of pregnancy, gastrocnemius muscle rupture, symptomatic varicosities, superficial thrombophlebitis, and Baker's cyst. Since the clinical diagnosis of deep vein thrombosis is in error at least 50% of the time, an objective method should be employed to evaluate the patient with symptoms of deep vein thrombosis to establish a definite diagnosis. While ascending contrast venography has been the gold standard diagnostic technique, the risk of venography (including intravenous iodinated contrast load, pain, anaphylaxis, and radiation exposure) may be avoided by using one or more of the noninvasive diagnostic techniques. All of these techniques have 90% to 95% accuracy when evaluating symptomatic patients. The most commonly available noninvasive diagnostic methods is duplex Doppler scanning of the deep veins from the popliteal region to the inguinal ligament. If a thrombus is visualized in the deep venous system, it is our feeling that no further diagnostic evaluation is required. Likewise, if the deep venous system appears normal, the chance of missing a clinically significant thrombus is rare. Impedance plethysmography is also a very accurate noninvasive method for diagnosing deep vein thrombosis. Because impedance plethysmography measures changes in venous blood volume and flow, false-positive test results are occasionally encountered if the gravid uterus causes extrinsic compression on the common iliac vein or vena cava. Most of these false-positive results may be rectified by performing the impedance plethysmogram examination in the lateral recumbent position.

Magnetic resonance imaging (MRI) also appears to demonstrate thrombi with good accuracy in symptomatic patients. MRI may be useful in diagnosing suspected ovarian vein or pelvic venous thrombosis. Because of the expense and time involvement in performing an MRI examination of the legs, we would recommend duplex Doppler scanning or impedance plethysmography as our initial diagnostic test in the evaluation of the patient with symptoms of deep vein thrombosis. These studies might also be considered in patients with symptoms of pulmonary embolism, as most pulmonary emboli will arise from the deep veins of the lower leg. Therefore, in a patient with symptoms of pulmonary embolism and evidence of deep vein thrombosis by noninvasive studies, the diagnosis of venous thromboembolism can be established and therapy initiated.

The symptoms associated with pulmonary embolism are also often incorrectly diagnosed, and it is therefore prudent to fully evaluate the patient to establish proper diagnosis before committing to prolonged anticoagulant therapy. Dyspnea, pleuritic chest pain, hemoptysis, and tachycardia are the most common signs and symptoms of pulmonary embolism. However, these symptoms may also be present in myriad other pulmonary and cardiovascular diseases. Therefore, a thorough evaluation including arterial blood gas, chest radiograph, and electrocardiogram should be initiated immediately. A ventilation-perfusion lung scan should be strongly considered when the diagnosis remains in doubt, as the risks of not diagnosing pulmonary embolism clearly outweigh the risk of minimal radiation exposure to the fetus. Finally, selected pulmonary arteriography should be employed when the diagnosis of pulmonary embolism cannot be confirmed or excluded by other methods.

Treatment

The treatment of deep vein thrombosis should be initiated in the hospital utilizing intravenous heparin therapy beginning with 5000 units intravenous push and then a continuous heparin infusion starting at 1000 units per hour. Activated partial thromboplastin time (APTT) should be monitored and the heparin dose adjusted, attempting to achieve an APTT of approximately 1.5 to 2 times the control value. Patients should be placed at bed rest for 2 days until her anticoagulant status is fully established. Thereafter, she is allowed to ambulate. Stool softener and excellent hydration are also employed to minimize constipation and contracted intravascular volume. In the nonpregnant patient, maintenance therapy with warfarin (Coumadin) is usually initiated on the second day of heparin therapy with a plan of switching to maintenance anticoagulant therapy using Coumadin on about the fifth day of anticoagulation. However, Coumadin is contraindicated in pregnancy because of increased risk of warfarin embryopathy and fetal hemorrhage. Therefore, heparin anticoagulant therapy should be continued throughout the pregnancy while the patient remains at risk for a recurrent venous thromboembolism. We switch the patient on the fifth day of intravenous heparin therapy to maintenance heparin therapy with subcutaneous injections. The heparin dose is administered every 12 hours with a goal of achieving a dose sufficient to prolong the APTT to approximately 1.5 to 2 times control value 6 hours after the subcutaneous heparin administration. Once a dose of heparin is established, the patient may be discharged from the hospital to administer

TABLE 1. Anticoagulant Treatment of Deep Vein Thrombosis and Pulmonary Embolism in Pregnancy

Stage	Treatment
Initial treatment (antepartum)	1. Intravenous heparin 5000 U IV bolus ≈1000 U IV/hr (Adjust dose to APTT 1.5–2× control × 5–7 days) 2. Subcutaneous heparin q 12 h (Adjust dose to have APTT 1.5–2× control @ 6 hr after last dose)
Onset of labor	Stop heparin (Protamine sulfate if APTT prolonged or bleeding)
Postpartum	Subcutaneous heparin q 12 h (Same as antepartum) *or* Oral warfarin (INR 2–2.5 × control) Continue at least 6 weeks postpartum

APTT, activated partial thromboplastin time; INR, international normalized ratio.

subcutaneous heparin throughout the remainder of her pregnancy. Periodic checks of the APTT time (6 hours after heparin administration) should be obtained to ascertain the need for adjusting the dose of heparin as pregnancy progresses. Low-molecular-weight heparin has also been used in pregnancy for therapy of deep vein thrombosis or pulmonary embolism. Limited clinical experience, to date, shows similar rates of rethrombosis and bleeding and probably equal efficacy.

Heparin should be withheld at the onset of labor. (If bleeding is caused by heparin, it may be reversed with protamine sulfate.) Heparin should be restarted postpartum and continued for at least 6 weeks. Warfarin may be used postpartum instead of heparin (Table 1).

As noted previously, heparin therapy increases the risk of bleeding as well as the occurrence of thrombocytopenia and osteoporosis, and patients should be monitored carefully for evidence of hematuria, easily bruisability, and any evidence of progressive osteoporosis. Platelet count should be monitored at 2- to 3-week intervals to ascertain evidence of thrombocytopenia.

The general management of the patient with pulmonary embolism in pregnancy should follow the same guidelines as those listed earlier. In addition, acute pulmonary embolism may require intensive care, ventilatory support, nasal oxygen therapy, and other supportive measures, depending on the patient's pulmonary status and blood gases.

The placement of inferior vena cava filters to prevent pulmonary embolism has been used safely in pregnancy. The primary indication for placement of an inferior vena cava filter is (1) recurrent pulmonary embolism, (2) serious complications of anticoagulant therapy, or (3) when anticoagulation is contraindicated.

Thrombolytic drugs should be avoided in pregnancy except in the most life-threatening cases.

Fetus, Placenta, and Newborn

Antepartum Fetal Surveillance

Lawrence D. Devoe, MD

Antepartum evaluation of fetal wellbeing plays a significant role in the management of complicated pregnancies. Current fetal surveillance addresses five major goals:

1. Prevention of antepartum stillbirth
2. Prevention of major neonatal morbidity
3. Identification of fetuses at high risk for point 1 or 2
4. Detection of deterioration in the health of a high risk fetus
5. **Avoidance of unnecessary antepartum intervention**

While one could argue the equal importance of these goals, most infants screened or assessed by antepartum tests will not be moribund during their actual testing sessions. The proper interpretation and application of the tests described in this section are vital to ensuring the best outcome. Further, the physiologic principles underlying the tests themselves should be understood to avoid inappropriate responses to normal variants (eg, nonreactive non-stress test during fetal sleep). Finally, the limitations of test performance, both false-negative and -positive results, must be accepted in the scheme of antepartum management. As the rationale for applying antepartum surveillance is developed in this section, it is important to use a phased and interdependent approach to obtain the best utility (Fig. 1).

Fetal Movement Counting

The oldest, most frequently used fetal surveillance modality, applicable to all patient settings, is maternal registration of fetal movements. The basis for movement counts has been supported experimentally by the correlation of fetal oxygenation levels and motor activity blocks. Healthy, well-oxygenated infants move frequently, while those whose oxygenation is being compromised

will adapt to conserve energy by decreasing absolute quantity of movements as well as time of the day spent in moving.

Various schemes for tabulating fetal movements have been reported, differing only in the absolute number of "kicks" or movements required for a reassuring session. The role of maternal perception of fetal movements has yet to be established in routine antenatal care. However, both controlled and uncontrolled prospective studies show it is associated with lower stillbirth rates in high-risk populations. At the Medical College of Georgia, we instruct mothers to establish baseline counts of fetal movements over a period of several sessions, divided between morning and evening. Each counting session lasts for 30 minutes. Any session in which

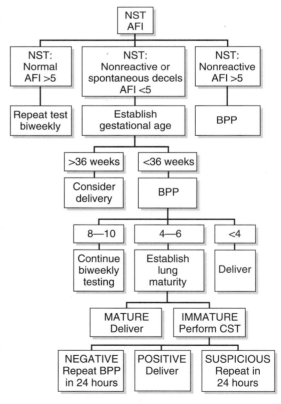

Figure 1. Standard decision-tree algorithm for fetal assessment.

there has been a 50% decrease in activity from the previous session or in which fetal movement is absent is extended for an additional 30 minutes. If no improvement occurs, the mother presents to the office or hospital for additional monitoring. The typical next step in fetal surveillance is non-stress testing.

Fetal movement counting is the least expensive means of fetal surveillance and engages the mother in her own care. It is also the least accurate and often engenders additional testing for false-positive results. Moreover, not all patients, as shown by correlative realtime ultrasonographic studies, have suitable observational skills to track the activity of their fetuses.

Non-Stress Test

The non-stress test (NST) is the most commonly performed laboratory test of fetal well-being. Physiologically, the association of transient fetal heart rate (FHR) accelerations with fetal movements has enabled this test to be a surrogate for fetal movement counting. In third trimester fetuses, FHR accelerations have a 90% linkage with fetal movements, and their amplitude and duration increase with gestational age. By convention, a qualifying acceleration exceeds the pre-established FHR baseline by at least 15 bpm with a total duration greater than 15 seconds. Testing conventions require that at least one such acceleration occurs in a 10-minute window with typical standards being counts of two accelerations in 20 minutes or three accelerations in 30 minutes. NSTs not meeting these criteria are considered nonreactive and require follow-up to exclude physiologic sleep states by extending the testing period for as long as 90 minutes or until a qualifying 20- or 30-minute window occurs, whichever comes first. Persistently nonreactive NSTs, especially in term fetuses, are presumptive evidence of fetal compromise and should be promptly corroborated by a biophysical profile (BPP) or contraction stress test (CST) (see Fig. 1).

Vibroacoustic Stimulation

Vibroacoustic stimulation (VAS) is a modification of the NST that results from the application of a vibroacoustic signal generator (a modified electronic artificial larynx) to the maternal abdomen over the fetal head or body to obtain a brief acceleration (positive VAS test). The vibratory component of this device is probably the dominant stimulus and, in response subjects, causes FHR accelerations through reflex stimulation pathways stemming from Meissner's corpuscles to the medullary cardiorespiratory control center. A typical acceleration following a 3-second signal occurs within 10 seconds and may last as long as 5 to 10 minutes. While most healthy fetuses will respond in this manner, occasionally a well-oxygenated fetus in active sleep will fail to respond or will demonstrate a brief decelerative response before converting to wakefulness; rarely, a healthy fetus will exhibit a sustained tachycardia following VAS. VAS testing has been shown to shorten the testing time required to achieve reactivity with no increase in the rate of falsely reassuring tests. Although long-term studies on method safety are lacking, no short-term follow-ups have shown any adverse effects on fetal hearing.

Actocardiotocography

Recently, application of noninvasive Doppler transducers coupled with specially adapted algorithms for selective processing of low-frequency Doppler signals has enabled the development of antepartum monitoring systems that exhibit simultaneous FHR and fetal movement signals. This augmented version of non-stress testing allows the discrimination of nonreactive tests due to fetal sleep state (no accelerations, sporadic isolated, low amplitude movements) from those due to hypoxia (prolonged absence of accelerations and movements). This modality is currently considered as investigational, since clinical trials of its efficacy relative to standard non-stress testing or biophysical testing are limited.

Contraction Stress Test

The original FHR testing method in the United States, the CST is a simulation of the conditions associated with repetitive uterine contractions during labor. The physiologic basis of this test is that the expected normal response of a well-oxygenated fetal myocardium exhibits no decelerations following uterine contraction peaks, while the marginally oxygenated or hypoxic fetus will exhibit late decelerations due to myocardial depression. In the testing center, uterine contractions of adequate frequency and intensity (strong to palpation, at least every 3 minutes) can be induced with either intravenous oxytocin or maternal nipple massage, resulting in successfully completed CST in 30 to 60 minutes. Tests may be classified as negative (no late decelerations), positive (late decelerations present with most contractions), equivocal or suspicious (occasional, nonrecurrent late decelerations, variable decelerations), hyperstimulation (excessive uterine activity with reflexive bradycardia), and unsatisfactory (failure to achieve adequate uterine activity pattern).

Recommended management after a negative CST is to continue surveillance at intervals ranging from 3 to 7 days, depending on test indication. Following a suspicious test, a followup CST should be performed within 24 hours, whereas after a positive CST, the fetus should be evaluated for delivery. Hyperstimulation is unusual but generally invalidates the use of the CST until adequate recovery has occurred preceding repetition. An unsatisfactory test mandates either extending the observation until an adequate uterine activity pattern has occurred or, if due to early third trimester gestational age, another modality such as the BPP must be selected.

Biophysical Profile

During the past decade, BPP testing has become an important addition to antenatal testing schemes. The BPP is supported by sound physiologic observations that fetal adaptation to progressive hypoxemia and acidosis can be detected by alterations in dynamic fetal behavior (FHR accelerations, fetal body movements, fetal breathing, fetal reflex activity) and gradual decline in amniotic fluid volume. The most popular criteria for rating the BPP are shown in Table 1.

The BPP may be affected by length of observation, maternal medications (sedatives, beta blockers), time of day, time the mother last ate, and circadian rhythms, so it is vital that this test be performed under optimal conditions to avoid environmental artifacts. At the Medical College

of Georgia, we standardize BPP testing with the following criteria:

1. Maternal rest for at least 1 hour
2. Two hours postprandial state
3. Avoidance of central nervous system depressants (unless vital)
4. Scheduled for morning to early afternoon hours
5. Minimum test duration of 30 minutes

Although the five variables listed in Table 1 are generally rated equally, further experience with correlation of BPP scoring and clinical outcomes suggest that their individual importance should be weighted. As the fetus becomes progressively hypoxic, there is a sequential loss of FHR reactivity, followed by fetal breathing movements, fetal body movements, and finally reflex activity. Further, there is a significant increase in risk for birth asphyxia and cerebral palsy once BPP scores fall below 6. Figure 1 suggests appropriate clinical management related to BPP score.

Clinical management of the BPP results should consider not only BPP scores but also the nature of the variables that are abnormal. At term, the most important combination of abnormal BPP elements is the combination of decreased amniotic fluid (whether measured by single deepest pocket or amniotic fluid index) and prolonged nonreactive NST, as this reflects both a long-standing adaptation to hypoxia (oligohydramnios) and acute hypoxemia (nonreactivity). This has led to the adoption of a less labor-intensive or modified BPP that incorporates the NST and amniotic fluid volume assessment. This approach, the current first tier of fetal testing at the Medical College of Georgia, has decreased the need for full BPP testing, which, in the course of a year, reflects a savings in personnel time and effort (see Fig. 1).

TABLE 1. Conventional Fetal Biophysical Profile Scoring System

Biophysical Variable	Normal (Score = 2)	Abnormal (Score = 0)
Non-stress test	Reactive (two accels/20 min)	Nonreactive (<two accels/20 min)
Fetal breathing movements	At least one episode of 30 sec continuous breathing/30 min	Absent or no qualifying breathing episodes
Fetal body movements	At least three body or limb movements in 30 min	Fewer than three body or limb movements in 30 min
Fetal tone	At least one episode of flexion/extension in 30 min	Absent flexion/extension episodes during observation
Amniotic fluid volume	Four-quadrant amniotic fluid index > 5	Four-quadrant amniotic fluid index ≤ 5

Umbilical Artery Doppler Velocimetry

Doppler insonation of the fetal umbilical arteries has been investigated extensively during the past decade. The physiologic basis for this assessment modality is derived from the relationship of the umbilical-placental vasculature tree as it evolves during the last half of pregnancy. Since the major cotyledonary divisions of the placenta are essentially fixed after 4 months' gestation, the most significant change in the flow dynamics of this circulatory system stem from the dramatic expansion of the tertiary villous capillary network. This leads to a progressive and obvious decrease in blood flow impedance, which can be represented as decline in the ratio between systolic peak and diastolic trough velocities. Conventionally, this relationship is expressed as a systolic to diastolic ratio.

When villous capillary counts are reduced due to placental deterioration (maternal hypertension) or intrinsic hypocellularity (aneuploidy), systolic to diastolic ratios rise or fail to decline with advancing gestation. In the most extreme scenarios, the diastolic waveform will disappear (absent end-diastolic velocity) or appear on the opposite side of the time axis (reversed end dia-

stolic velocity). Reports of these latter cases associate them with severe intrauterine growth restriction as well as a higher risk for in utero fetal death. However, the time frame leading from test result to fetal demise is neither clear nor readily determinable for individual cases.

Although umbilical arterial Doppler velocimetry is arguably the most rigorously evaluated method of fetal assessment during this epoch, the role of this test in the prospective strategy of high-risk fetal management remains controversial.

Test Indications and Test Initiation

It is now well appreciated that a relatively short list of common and less frequent medical and obstetric complications can and should provoke the use of antepartum suveillance tests. The common indications are listed in Table 2.

The rationale for differentiating both onset and intensity of testing in these various disorders stems from the differential impact that they exert on fetal outcome. In essence, disease states more likely to result in fetal growth restriction, accelerated placental senescence, or abruptio placentae

TABLE 2. Common Test Indications and Recommended Approaches

Test Indication	Onset of Testing	Frequency of Testing (days)
Medical Problems		
Hypertension (chronic)		
Mild	36 weeks	1–2
Moderate-severe	26–28 weeks	2–7
Pre-eclampsia	At time of diagnosis	Daily (if hospitalized)
Diabetes		
Class A1	40 weeks	2
Class A2	32 weeks	2
Class B-R	26–32 weeks	2–3
Cardiac disease	At onset of maternal decompensation or IUGR	2
Collagen vascular disease	26–32 weeks (severity dependent)	2–3
Renal disease	Similar to chronic hypertension	Similar to chronic hypertension
Obstetric Problems		
IUGR	At diagnosis in third trimester	2 or more°
Postdatism	41 weeks	2
Oligohydramnios	At diagnosis in third trimester	2 or more°
Polyhydramnios	At diagnosis in third trimester	2 or more°
PPROM	At diagnosis	Daily
Multiple gestation	At diagnosis of discordance	2 or more°
Rh-sensitization	26+ weeks	2 or more°

IUGR, intrauterine growth restriction; PPROM, preterm premature rupture of membranes.
°Depending on severity of condition.

mandate early and more intense testing schemes. Conditions in which risk accrues either late in pregnancy (postdatism, by definition) or in which cord problems are more probable (oligohydramnios, premature rupture of membranes, postdatism, polyhydramnios) should begin with initial diagnosis. For most of the latter conditions, optimal frequency is yet to be determined but must be gauged on the apparent severity of the clinical problem.

Contextual evaluation of all test results is vital. Response to mildly abnormal biophysical testing in a fragile fetus (eg, severe intrauterine growth restriction with score of 6) should prompt as brisk a response as that engendered by more abnormal testing (postdatism with score of 2). Intervention for suspicious, intermediate or equivocal tests should always be tempered by a firm grip on gestational dating and maturity assessment, since iatrogenic prematurity can be more devastating than minimal, well-tolerated hypoxemia.

Conclusion

Current methods of fetal assessment now permit a logical, phased, and well-structured approach to antepartum management of high-risk pregnancy. At the Medical College of Georgia, such approaches have reduced preventable antepartum stillbirths to nearly zero per 1000 births, as well as avoiding unnecessary interventions for false-positive test results in the preterm population. Considering context and proceeding in an orderly objective manner, most high-risk pregnancies can be maintained to the ideal goal, achieving term gestational age in intact condition.

Biophysical Profile

Luanna Lettieri, MD

Anthony M. Vintzileos, MD

David J. Nochimson, MD

Antepartum fetal assessment has long been a diagnostic challenge. With the advent of electronic fetal heart rate monitoring, the non-stress test (NST) and the contraction stress test (CST) were developed to identify fetuses at risk for asphyxia. Both the NST and the CST have low false-negative rates and high false-positive rates,

which indicates that these tests are useful in detecting nonasphyxiated fetuses but do poorly in detecting fetal asphyxia. A disadvantage of the CST is that it can only be used on a limited number of patients due to its contraindication in patients with preterm premature rupture of membranes, preterm labor, vaginal bleeding, multiple gestation, and so on. Manning in 1980 first proposed the use of fetal biophysical parameters to detect fetal well-being. The biophysical profile (BPP) was subsequently developed to examine multiple biophysical parameters to assess fetal well-being in much the same manner that Apgar scores or vital signs give information about the neonate or adult patient. In 1983, Vintzileos developed a scoring system for the BPP using six components: NST, fetal breathing movements, fetal movements (FM), fetal tone (FT), amniotic fluid volume, and placental grading (Table 1).

Pathophysiology

The biophysical profile is essentially a detailed examination of the fetus. The individual components of the examination will vary according to gestational age, fetal well-being normal periodic cyclicity, and maternal drug or medication ingestion. The individual components are a combination of acute and chronic markers of fetal well-being. The acute markers are the fetal heart rate (FHR) reactivity (NST), breathing movements, fetal movements, and fetal tone; the chronic markers are the amniotic fluid and the placenta.

Vintzileos has proposed that the acute markers are controlled by different central nervous system (CNS) centers and accordingly develop at different stages in gestation. Fetal tone is the earliest to develop and occurs at 7½ to 8½ weeks' gestation, followed by fetal movements at 9 weeks. Regular breathing movements occur by 21 weeks and fetal heart rate reactivity is observed by the end of the second or the beginning of the third trimester. The "gradual hypoxia concept" also proposed by Vintzileos suggests that the CNS centers that control each individual parameter are unequally affected by fetal hypoxia and acidemia. This concept also proposes that the biophysical parameters that develop first are the last parameters to disappear during fetal asphyxia. Therefore, one would expect to see FHR reactivity and breathing movements disappear initially, followed by fetal movement and tone. This is evidenced by the umbilical artery pH at which the biophysical parameters are inhibited: FHR reactivity and fetal breathing movements at a cord arterial pH less than 7.20, compromised

TABLE 1. Criteria for Scoring Biophysical Variables According to Vintzileos and Colleagues°

Non-stress test
> Score 2 (NST 2): five or more FHR accelerations of at least 15 bpm in amplitude and at least 15 seconds' duration associated with fetal movements in a 20-minute period.
> Score 1 (NST 1): two to four accelerations of at least 15 bpm in amplitude and at least 15 seconds' duration associated with fetal movements in a 20-minute period.
> Score 0 (NST 0): one or fewer accelerations in a 20-minute period.

Fetal movements
> Score 2 (FM 2): At least three gross (trunk and limbs) episodes of fetal movements within 30 minutes. Simultaneous limb and trunk movements were counted as a single movement.
> Score 1 (FM 1): one or two fetal movements within 30 minutes.
> Score 0 (FM 0): absence of fetal movements within 30 minutes.

Fetal breathing movements
> Score 2 (FBM 2): at least one episode of fetal breathing of at least 60 seconds' duration within a 30-minute observation period.
> Score 1 (FBM 1): at least one episode of fetal breathing lasting 30 to 60 seconds within 30 minutes.
> Score 0 (FBM 0): absence of fetal breathing or breathing lasting less than 30 seconds within 30 minutes.

Fetal tone
> Score 2 (FT 2): at least one episode of extension of extremities with return to position of flexion, and also one episode of extension of spine with return to position of flexion.
> Score 1 (FT 1): at least one episode of extension of extremities with return to position of flexion, or one episode of extension of spine with return to position of flexion.
> Score 0 (FT 0): extremities in extension; fetal movements not followed by return to flexion; open hand.

Amniotic fluid volume
> Score 2 (AF 2): fluid evident throughout the uterine cavity. A pocket that measures 2 cm or more in vertical diameter.
> Score 1 (AF 1): a pocket that measures less than 2 cm but more than 1 cm in vertical diameter.
> Score 0 (AF 0): crowding of fetal small parts; largest pocket less than 1 cm in vertical diameter.

Placental grading
> Score 2 (PL 2): placental grading 0, 1, or 2
> Score 1 (PL 1): placenta posterior difficult to evaluate
> Score 0 (PL 0): placental grading 3

AF, amniotic fluid; bpm, beats per minute; FBM, fetal breathing movements; FHR, fetal heart rate; FM, fetal movements; FT, fetal tone; NST, non-stress test; PL, placental grading.
    °Maximal score 12; minimal score 0.
    From Vintzileos AM, Ingardia CJ, Nochimson DJ: Congenital hydrocephalus: A review and protocol for perinatal management. Obstet Gynecol 1983;62:271–278. Reprinted with permission from the American College of Obstetricians and Gynecologists.

FM and FT at a pH 7.10 to 7.20, and absent FM and FT at a pH less than 7.10.

The two chronic markers of fetal well-being are amniotic fluid volume and placental grading. It is well known that with chronic fetal hypoxia, blood is shunted away from nonvital organs such as the kidneys and the lungs toward the more vital organs (heart and brain). As the kidneys receive less blood supply, they produce less urine, which ultimately results in oligohydramnios. Therefore, the amniotic fluid volume is an indicator of fetal status over long periods of time. The placenta itself obviously is not a fetal biophysical marker. It has been included in the biophysical profile, however, because grade 3 placentas have been associated with an increased incidence of abnormal fetal heart rate patterns and abruption during labor. The presence of a grade 3 placenta by itself does not increase the antepartum risk and therefore does not change obstetric management. Thus, placental grading has been abandoned by many clinicians.

Method

An NST is performed first and is graded on its reactivity. The NST is performed for a maximum of 20 minutes during which the number of FHR accelerations associated with fetal movements are noted. An ultrasonographic examination is then performed to obtain the remaining biophysical parameters. Each parameter is given an individual score out of three possibilities: zero, one, or two (Table 1). The examination is complete when each of the biophysical parameters meets the maximum score (2) or when 30 minutes of real-time scanning have elapsed.

When scanning, it is important to view the fetus in a longitudinal or transverse plane so that breathing, limb, and body movements can be observed simultaneously. Otherwise it is necessary to continually reposition the transducer so that body, limb, and breathing movements can be observed. To obtain credit for the fetal movement parameter, the fetus must move its trunk. Isolated movements of limbs or hands do not meet the criteria. Fetal breathing movements consist of a downward movement of the diaphragm with a return to its original position. An easy way to observe breathing movements is to obtain a transverse or longitudinal view of the lower abdomen. As the diaphragm moves, the abdominal organs, in particular the kidneys, can also be observed to move in a similar manner. Evidence of fetal tone consists of extension and flexion of the extremities or the spine. A persistently open fetal hand indicates poor tone. Amniotic fluid is scored according to the largest vertical pocket. The placental score is based on placental grading. If the placenta is difficult to evaluate due to a posterior position, a score of 1 is given.

Management of High-Risk Pregnancies with Intact Membranes

We perform biophysical profiles as early as 23 weeks' gestation or at the age of fetal viability. As previously stated, some of the biophysical parameters are gestational age–dependent. NSTs become consistently more reactive after 32 weeks' gestation, and grade 3 placentas are also more common after 32 weeks. Breathing movements and amniotic fluid volume are both decreased after 40 weeks. Fetal tone and movement remain relatively unchanged throughout pregnancy. However, the frequency of reassuring BPPs (a score of 8 or greater) is unchanged across gestation.

It has been shown that an abnormal biophysical profile correlates well with adverse fetal and neonatal outcomes, in particular, fetal distress, abnormal FHR patterns in labor, meconium, and an increased perinatal mortality rate. A BPP score of 8 or more by both Vintzileos's and Manning's criteria is predictive of a good pregnancy outcome in virtually 100% of cases. A score of 4 or less indicates a high probability of fetal acidemia and distress. It has become evident that the individual components of the BPP do not contribute equally to its predictive value for fetal well-being. Each of the parameters is predictive of different fetal states. A nonreactive NST is the

best predictor of meconium in labor (33%). The best predictor of abnormal FHR patterns in labor is absent fetal movements (80%), whereas oligohydramnios is the best parameter for predicting fetal distress (37.5%). Absent fetal tone is the best predictor of fetal death (42.8%).

Therefore, it is important to consider each of the individual components rather than the total score of the biophysical profile. It is equally important to consider the clinical situation and to make decisions regarding the fetal status based on that situation, the BPP, and any other laboratory tests or data available.

Our present management of fetal biophysical assessment centers on the analysis of each of the biophysical parameters (Fig. 1). The NST is performed first. If the NST is reactive, fetal acidemia is ruled out and the remainder of the BPP can be abandoned, provided the amniotic fluid volume is normal. The amniotic fluid status should always be assessed regardless of whether the remainder of the BPP is performed. If the NST is nonreactive, the ultrasonographic portion of the BPP is performed. If fetal breathing is observed for at least 30 seconds, fetal acidemia is again ruled out. The biophysical profile can be halted at that time.

If the NST is nonreactive and no fetal breathing movements are noted after 30 minutes of scanning, and the remainder of the parameters are present and normal (including amniotic fluid volume), we initiate extended fetal heart rate monitoring for 2 hours to differentiate between a fetal sleep cycle and fetal asphyxia. If the extended monitoring shows fetal heart rate reactivity, the biophysical assessment is considered complete and is regarded as reassuring. If the extended FHR monitoring is nonreactive and a repeat ultrasonographic assessment is not reassuring, delivery is considered, owing to persistent nonreassuring fetal biophysical parameters. If fetal movement or tone is impaired or absent, prompt delivery is recommended. Oligohydramnios is an abnormal biophysical parameter and delivery should be considered to avoid in utero death from cord compression, even in the presence of a reactive NST or fetal breathing, especially if fetal growth retardation has occurred.

Common mistakes involving the biophysical profile include (1) considering the total score without regard to the individual components or the clinical situation, (2) inappropriate scoring of the parameters, (3) failing to act promptly on abnormal test results, and (4) inappropriate intervals between testing. The interval for retesting is based on the individual situation. In general, fetal testing is performed twice weekly. The use

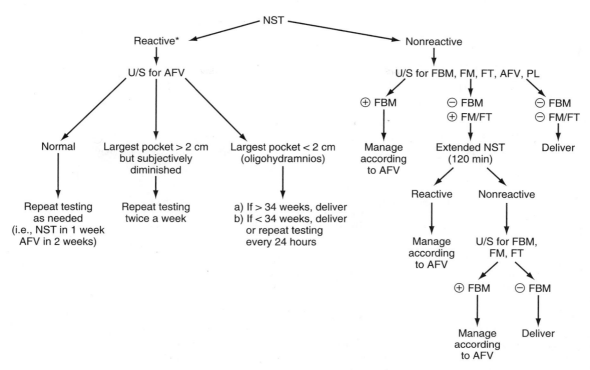

Figure 1. Protocol of antepartum fetal evaluation in pregnancies with intact membranes. °In the presence of variable decelerations and oligohydramnios, consider delivery; in the presence of variable decelerations and normal AFV, consider extended (120 minutes) or repeat NST within 24 hours. NST, non-stress test; U/S, ultrasonography; AFV, amniotic fluid volume; FBM, fetal breathing; FM, fetal movement; FT, fetal tone; PL, placental grading; +, present/normal; −, absent/abnormal. Reprinted with permission from Am J Obstet Gynecol 1987;157:627–631.

and misuse of the fetal biophysical profile has been extensively described by Vintzileos et al.

Management of Premature Rupture of Membranes in Preterm Gestation

The preterm patient with premature rupture of membranes (PROM) is at risk for the development of chorioamnionitis, fetal infection, fetal distress, and cord accidents secondary to oligohydramnios. Fetal testing is very important in these patients, and a protocol designed for PROM is recommended. The interpretation of the BPP and subsequent management in patients with PROM is different than for patients with intact membranes. Studies have indicated that there is an increased incidence of absent fetal breathing, decreased amniotic fluid volume, and reactive NSTs in patients with PROM versus intact membranes, across all gestational ages. Interestingly, though, the biophysical profile of healthy fetuses is not altered by the presence of PROM.

Abnormal BPPs in patients with PROM corre-

late well with fetal infection. A nonreactive NST and absent breathing movements are the first signs of fetal infection, whereas poor or absent fetal tone and movement are late indicators. Therefore, in cases of preterm PROM, a nonreactive NST or absent fetal breathing should not be attributed to fetal immaturity until fetal/maternal infection has been ruled out and other signs of fetal well-being are present.

As is the case with intact membranes, oligohydramnios is correlated with pregnancy outcome. In PROM, increasing severity of oligohydramnios is associated with an increased incidence of fetal infection. In patients with severe oligohydramnios (<1 cm vertical pocket), the incidence of chorioamnionitis is 47% and neonatal infection (possible neonatal sepsis and/or neonatal sepsis) is over 50%.

Our management protocol for patients with preterm PROM includes the use of daily NSTs or biophysical profiles. It is our practice to review the NSTs daily not only for reactivity, but also to compare them to the previous NSTs. Often before the NST becomes nonreactive, the fetal

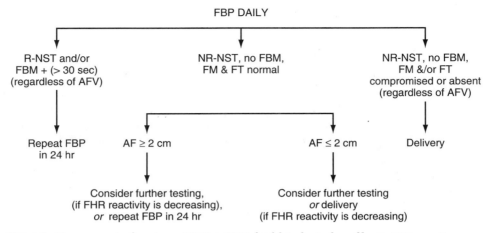

Figure 2. Management of preterm PROM. FBP, fetal biophysical profile; R-NST, reactive non-stress test; NR-NST, nonreactive non-stress test; FBM+, fetal breathing present; FM, fetal movements; FT, fetal tone; AFV, amniotic fluid volume; AF, amniotic fluid (largest vertical pocket); FHR, fetal heart rate.

heart rate tracing becomes progressively less reactive (over a span of hours or days), although it may meet the criteria for reactivity. This may be the earliest sign of impending fetal infection or distress, although no formal studies have been performed addressing this issue. The conversion of reactive to nonreactive NST in longitudinal follow-up is associated with infection in approximately 90% of the cases.

If the NST is reactive or 30 seconds of fetal breathing is present, the test is repeated in 24 hours regardless of the amniotic fluid status. If those two parameters are absent and the amniotic fluid pocket is greater than 2 cm, extended monitoring is undertaken if the NST had previously been reactive. Otherwise the BPP is repeated in 24 hours. If the AF amniotic fluid is less than 2 cm, the patient is delivered or undergoes extended monitoring depending on the clinical situation and previous testing results. If all of the biophysical parameters are impaired or absent, the fetus is delivered regardless of the amniotic fluid volume. Our management protocol for patients with preterm PROM is illustrated in Figure 2.

Summary

The biophysical profile is a detailed physical examination of the fetus and allows the clinician the opportunity to assess fetal well-being. The BPP is easy to perform and provides valuable information regarding the status of the fetus at the time of testing. The individual fetal biophysi-

cal parameters are controlled by different CNS centers that are affected unequally by fetal hypoxia and acidemia. Therefore, the correct interpretation of the BPP must take into account the status of the individual parameters and the clinical situation rather than the total score.

Congenital Anomalies of the Neonate

Nancy Hansen, MD
Daniel L. Coury, MD

Approximately 2% of newborn infants have a major congenital malformation that requires surgical intervention for functional or cosmetic reasons or results in lifelong disability. Congenital anomalies (malformations) are the second leading cause of death in the first year of life, second only to complications arising in the perinatal period such as extreme prematurity or birth asphyxia. Advances in prenatal diagnosis such as amniocentesis, maternal alpha-fetoprotein screening, and fetal ultrasonography have lessened the likelihood of delivery of an infant with an unexpected severe congenital anomaly, but up to one half of all infants with major anomalies do not have significant prenatal risk factors that would lead to prenatal diagnosis. Furthermore, an etiologic determinant (such as a single gene defect or chromosomal abnormality) has been identified for only a minority of the thousands of described syndromes of congenital malformations. In this chapter, the various causes of congenital malformations are reviewed, followed by suggestions for a systematic diagnosis and treatment plan.

The initial step in evaluation of the dysmorphic neonate is to determine whether there is a single primary defect in morphogenesis or whether there are multiple organ systems involved. Three basic mechanisms result in primary or isolated defects during fetal development. *Malformation* causes a primary structural defect secondary to an intrinsic developmental abnormality in the cells of an affected tissue, such as occurs with congenital heart disease or cleft lip. *Disruption* is a structural defect resulting from the destruction of a normal formed body part, as is seen in amniotic band anomalies. *Deformation* occurs when mechanical forces act upon normally developed tissue and result in abnormal form or shape of a body part (cranial molding or clubfoot secondary to oligohydramnios). It is extremely important to differentiate between these three mechanisms, as they determine the potential outcome of the anomaly and its recurrence risk. The recurrence risk is extremely low for disruptions, whereas most malformations and polygenically determined deformations (congenital hip dislocation or talipes equinovarus) have recurrence risks in the range of 2% to 5% (Table 1). The potential for reversibility is good for those deformations that are secondary to the uterine constraint of growth that often occurs during the third trimester, whereas malformed and/or disrupted tissues are usually irreversibly affected unless surgical intervention is an option.

Etiology

The most common cause of genetic dysmorphogenesis is *multifactorial* or *polygenic inheritance* (variation), which affects approximately 5% to 10% of all individuals. These disorders result from the cumulative effects of multiple genes and their interactions with environmental factors. Polygenic variation is thought to be the mechanism responsible for the majority of congenital structural malformations (eg, cleft lip, neural tube defect) as well as other common disorders with familial tendency such as diabetes mellitus. Environmental influences often play a major role in the determination (or expression) of the potential malformation associated with polygenic disorders. These disorders cannot currently be detected by chromosomal analysis. After the birth of one child with a polygenic disorder, the recurrence risk for future pregnancies is usually 3% to 5%.

Morphogenesis (and dysmorphogenesis) is ultimately genetically controlled, although the environment has varying effects on the expression of an individual's genetic potential. There are three basic *genetic causes* for abnormal morphogenesis. The least frequent but most commonly recognized is *genetic imbalance* due to a chromosomal abnormality. Chromosomal abnormalities affect at least 4% of all pregnancies, although the majority of these pregnancies end in spontaneous abortions. Only 0.5% of pregnancies result in the delivery of a liveborn baby with a chromosomal abnormality. The most common chromosomal abnormality noted at birth is trisomy 21. Trisomy 13 and 18 are the other two trisomies that are commonly recognized at birth. The sex chromosome abnormalities (eg, XO, XXY, XYY) are not usually diagnosed in the neonatal period.

A second genetic cause for multiple malformations is *individual gene mutations*. Human genes normally occur in pairs except for those carried on the sex chromosomes. Thus, an individual usually has one gene inherited from the father and one gene inherited from the mother. Approximately 1500 individually rare disorders have been described that are caused by single gene mutations, with an overall frequency of these disorders of approximately 1%.

During the last several years, advances in molecular genetics have led to the ability to detect many single gene disorders by linkage analysis, DNA probes, or gene product determination. Thus, for many relatively rare disorders, it is now possible to accurately diagnose gene disorders via fetal blood sampling and DNA analysis.

Multiple malformation syndromes may be caused by environmental factors. Included in this group are teratogenic drugs and substances such as alcohol and maternal anticonvulsants, congenital intrauterine infections such as rubella and cytomegalovirus, and physical agents such as radiation and thermal exposure. Generally, environmental factors are most devastating when exposure occurs during the early portions of pregnancy and fetal organogenesis.

For many well-described multiple malformation syndromes, the underlying mechanism of dysmorphogenesis is currently unknown. Generally, the recurrence risk for such disorders is low. It is important, however, to attempt to make a syndrome diagnosis, as this often gives the family and managing physician important information regarding long-term prognosis.

TABLE 1. Categorization of the Newborn with Congenital Anomalies

	Isolated Defect or Sequence of Related Defects			Multiple Defects			
				Genetic			
	Malformation	Deformation	Disruption	Chromosomal	Gene Mutation	Teratogen	Unknown
Incidence	1–2%	1–2%		0.5%	1% (in total) < 1/3000 (individually)		1–2% (in total) < 1/1000 (individually)
Recurrence	2–5%	2–5%	Extremely low	Varies (see text)	Varies	Low if causative agent not present in subsequent sequences	Low
Examples	Cleft lip/palate Neural tube defect Pierre Robin sequence Neural tube defect sequence	Congenital dislocation Clubfeet Breech deformation sequence	Gastroschisis Amniotic band sequence	Trisomy 21 18	Achondroplasia Hemophilia A	Fetal alcohol syndrome Rubella syndrome	CHARGE association Cornelia de Lange's syndrome

Diagnostic Evaluation of the Infant with Malformations

Historical Data

A detailed pregnancy and delivery history is the first step in evaluating the dysmorphic infant. Pertinent information regarding the pregnancy includes the length of gestation and fetal growth patterns. Information about historical factors such as maternal acute or chronic illnesses, medication intake, smoking, alcohol intake, and the use of street drugs should be obtained, as they are the leading causes of environmental teratogenesis. Experimental animal data suggest that radiotherapy or maternal hyperthermia in the first trimester may lead to fetal dysmorphogenesis. Thus, history of fever, sauna or hot tub usage, and radiation exposure, especially during the first trimester, should be sought. If this is not the first pregnancy, it is often helpful to ask the mother to qualitatively rate the baby's activity in utero compared to other pregnancies, as infants with central or peripheral nervous system anomalies often have decreased fetal movement.

Important information regarding the labor and delivery process includes the presentation of the infant as well as the mode of delivery. For example, full-term infants with growth retardation, presenting in the breech position, are in a high risk category for congenital anomalies. An estimate of the volume of the amniotic fluid is helpful, as both polyhydramnios and oligohydramnios are associated with serious congenital malformations. The Apgar scores are also important. Respiratory depression at birth in the absence of any clinical evidence of birth asphyxia suggests an intrinsic central nervous system or peripheral nervous system deficit such as a primary myopathy or neuropathy. The family history should also be obtained and should include information regarding previous pregnancies (especially important is a maternal history of repetitive miscarriages). Advanced maternal and paternal age are known risk factors for chromosomal or genetic abnormalities. Finally, information should be sought regarding previous congenital malformations in family members. The majority of single or isolated malformations are inherited in a multifactorial or polygenic fashion and there is a 5% to 10% recurrence risk for most of these disorders. Examples of polygenic inherited disorders include cleft lip and palate, neural tube defects, congenital heart disease, clubfoot, congenital hip dislocation, and pyloric stenosis.

Historical data should also include information on antenatal diagnosis of structural malformations by ultrasonography and/or chromosomal or metabolic diagnostic evaluation done on amniotic fluid or chorionic villus sampling. If possible, the placenta should be submitted to pathology for examination for evidence of vascular malformations or amniotic bands.

Physical Examination

Evaluation of the infant with congenital anomalies should proceed in a systematic manner. One of the major goals of examination of an infant with congenital anomalies is to detect a recognizable pattern of malformations so that a specific etiologic diagnosis or syndrome identification may be made. It is important to differentiate between major and minor malformation. Minor malformations are considered phenotypic (normal) variations but are important in that when multiple minor variations occur in a single infant, the likelihood of that infant also having a major malformation is increased dramatically. Approximately 2% of newborns have a single minor anomaly and less than 2% of these infants have a major malformation (no higher than the background rate for major malformations). However, if three or more minor anomalies are found in a single infant, there is a greater than 90% chance that the infant has at least one major malformation. Only 0.5% of liveborn infants have three or more minor malformations.

Size and Gestational Age

The initial step in the physical examination is to estimate the infant's gestational age based on the maternal dates and/or the infant's physical and neurologic characteristics and to determine whether the infant is appropriately grown for his or her gestational age. If the infant is small for gestational age, it is important to note whether the growth retardation is symmetric (head circumference, length, and weight diminished to a similar degree) or asymmetric (weight being more severely affected than either the head circumference or length). Asymmetric growth retardation is most commonly seen during the third trimester secondary to placental insufficiency and is usually not associated with an increased risk of congenital malformations. Symmetric growth retardation implies either severe placental insufficiency during the early third trimester or an intrinsic fetal problem such as an intrauterine infection or possibly a chromosomal disorder.

Examination of the Head

Careful measurement of the head circumference should be made, noting the size of the anterior and posterior fontanelles. Macrocephaly may be indicative of congenital hydrocephalus or other disorders such as achondroplasia or familial macrocephaly. Microcephaly may also be familial but is particularly associated with neurologic disorders and/or congenital infections. Large fontanelles may be found in infants with chromosomal trisomies as well as congenital hydrocephalus. The overall shape of the skull should be noted, but caution should be taken in diagnosing malformations such as craniosynostosis. Cranial molding and deformation of the skull are extremely common after birth and usually resolve within several months.

Neural tube defects affecting the cranium are usually quite obvious. These include anencephaly with absence of both the skull and cerebral hemispheres' encephalocele with herniation of brain tissue and meninges through a skull defect, and a cranial meningocele with herniation of only meninges. Meningoceles have a much better prognosis than either of the other two defects.

The distribution of hair on the head may be an important clue for diagnosis. Hirsutism, especially of the eyebrows, is very typically seen in Cornelia de Lange's syndrome as well as fetal alcohol and fetal hydantoin syndromes. Abnormal scalp hair patterns may also be indicative of an underlying brain malformation. Scalp defects are commonly seen with trisomy 13.

Examination of the Face

Examination of facial structures is extremely important and should be viewed in terms of overall embryogenesis (malformation) as well as considering intrauterine molding and/or post-traumatic swelling from delivery (deformation). The facial structures are formed from the frontal nasal processes (central nervous system [CNS]) as well as the lateral brachial arches. Midline facial defects involving the eyes and nose have a strong association with CNS anomalies. In contrast, the facial defects associated with failure of fusion of the brachial arches such as cleft lip and cleft palate may be isolated major congenital anomalies.

Examination of the Ears

The external ear is commonly affected by deformational forces in utero. However, true ear anomalies (malformations) are important to note, as they may be associated with other congenital malformations and/or anomalies of the middle or inner ear with associated hearing loss. In particular, any infant with a preauricular tag should be carefully examined for evidence of other brachial cleft closure defects or cysts.

Examination of the Nose

The nose should be symmetric in shape with two patent nares. Like the external ear, the nose shows great individual variation and is especially prone to transient deformational changes resulting from in utero crowding.

Examination of the Mouth

Examination of the mouth includes both external contour and internal structure. The most obvious abnormality involving the mouth is failure of closure of brachial clefts resulting in cleft lip and/or palate. An abnormally small mouth may be associated with trisomy 18. Macroglossia is seen in conjunction with Pierre Robin syndrome, in which the tongue is normal in size but, owing to a hypoplastic mandible, protrudes from the mouth. It may also be caused by disorders such as congenital hypothyroidism, Beckwith-Wiedemann syndrome, and rare disorders of mucopolysaccharide metabolism.

Examination of the inside of the mouth should include careful investigation of both the hard and the soft palate for clefts. High arched palates are seen in many syndromes and are generally indicative of abnormal oral motor function in conjunction with CNS dysfunction, which results in poor sucking and swallowing.

Examination of the Eyes

Examination of the eyes should include measurement of the interpupillary distance. Comparison to established standards determines whether the infant has hypotelorism, which is commonly associated with CNS anomalies such as holoprosencephaly and trisomy 13. Hypertelorism, or widely spaced eyes, is seen in association with other malformation syndromes but is usually not related to underlying brain malformation. The presence of a fold of skin over the inner canthus of the eye (epicanthal skin fold) should be noted and may be seen in association with trisomy 21 as well as other malformation syndromes, including fetal alcohol syndrome. The external eye should be carefully examined for colobomas, which are fusion defects affecting both the retina and the eyelid. Colobomas may be isolated anomalies but are also seen in association with various syndromes, including Goldenhar's syndrome and the CHARGE association. Blue sclera may be associated with connective tissue disorders such as osteogenesis imperfecta, although premature infants may have faintly blue sclera as a normal finding. The corneas should be examined for any cloudiness as well as for symmetry in size. Corneal cloudiness or an enlarged cornea is indicative of congenital glaucoma. Other important components of the eye examination include elicitation of a red reflex to search for congenital cataracts. Finally, any infant with multiple major malformations should have a careful eye examination performed by a neurologist and/or ophthalmologist, as retinal abnormalities are frequently seen in conjunction with CNS malformations and may be an important diagnostic clue in syndrome identification.

Examination of the Neck

The newborn infant's neck is normally short and may be somewhat difficult to examine. Redundant skin folds are seen in association with trisomy 21 as well as Turner's syndrome (XO). In addition, brachial cleft remnants such as cystic hygromas are seen in the neck and may be associated with other facial abnormalities.

Examination of the Chest

Chest examination includes evaluation of the external thoracic cage as well as examination of the lungs and heart. External abnormalities include supernumerary nipples, minor malformations that are inherited in an autosomal dominant fashion. Hypoplasia of the thoracic cage is seen in association with several skeletal dysplasias and usually results in pulmonary hypoplasia with severe respiratory distress after birth. Lung hypoplasia may also be secondary to either a diaphragmatic hernia that compresses the lung during development or primary pulmonary hypoplasia in association with the oligohydramnios sequence.

Heart murmurs are frequently heard during the first 48 hours of life in normal newborns. However, congenital heart malformations occur in many malformation syndromes, including chromosomal trisomies 21, 13, and 18.

Examination of the Abdomen

External abdominal wall defects may be categorized as either a gastroschisis or an omphalocele. Omphaloceles are midline and involve the umbilical cord, whereas a gastroschisis is laterally placed with a normal insertion of the umbilical cord. It is important to differentiate these two entities, as additional malformations are seen in one third of infants with omphaloceles, while gastroschisis occurs as an isolated anomaly owing to disruption of blood supply to the abdominal wall in utero. The umbilical cord itself should be carefully inspected for the number of vessels. Single umbilical arteries are seen in 1% of normal newborns but may also be seen with urinary tract anomalies and the VATER association. Hypoplasia of the abdominal musculature resulting in the prune belly syndrome is the result of in utero bladder obstruction. The abdomen should be carefully palpated for masses, which are usually of urinary tract origin.

Examination of the Anus

Imperforate anus may occur in association with other congenital malformations, such as the VATER association. It is also seen in the caudal regression syndrome observed in conjunction with maternal diabetes.

Examination of the External Genitalia

Female genitalia should be examined for abnormalities such as imperforate hymen or masses in the groin or labial area. Groin masses in a female infant most commonly represent inguinal hernias but may be secondary to an ectopic gonad. The urethral opening in the female infant is usually difficult to visualize unless the infant is seen voiding. There are marked gestational age differences in the external genitalia between the extremely premature infant and the term female infant. In the female infant born prior to 32 weeks' gestation there is little fat deposition in the labia majora, and the clitoris and labia minora may appear abnormal to the inexperienced examiner.

The male genitalia should be inspected for abnormal positioning of the urethral meatus. The dorsal displacement of the urethral opening is called epispadias and is often associated with exstrophy of the bladder. Normally, the foreskin is tightly adherent over the glans penis and the meatal opening is usually not visible. A visible meatal opening on the tip of the glans with an incomplete foreskin implies first-degree hypospadias. Second-degree hypospadias describes the urethral opening ventrally displaced to the mid-shaft of the penis, and third-degree hypospadias occurs when the urethral opening is at the base of the penis. All infants with third-degree hypospadias need further evaluation for ambiguous genitalia. The scrotum should be palpated to identify two descended testes. Circumcision is contraindicated in any infant with bilateral undescended testes, hypospadias, bifid scrotum, or micropenis, as these conditions may be associated with ambiguous genitalia.

Ambiguous Genitalia

Infants with ambiguous genitalia present an immediate problem to the managing physician. The parents of such infants should be told initially that there is a problem with genital development and that further studies need to be performed to determine the baby's sex. An infant with male-appearing genitalia who has third-degree hypospadias, bilateral undescended testes, or micropenis falls into this category. Similarly, a female infant who has palpable inguinal masses needs evaluation for ambiguous genitalia. An infant with female-appearing genitalia who has posterior labial fusion or clitoromegaly may have congenital adrenal hyperplasia.

Examination of the Skeletal System

Neural tube defects are the most common anomalies of the spine and range from open defects (meningomyelocele) to closed meningoceles in association with spina bifida. The lower spine should be carefully examined for hair tufts or deep sacral dimples, which may be indicative of significant deeper spinal defects.

The extremities should be inspected for symmetry as well as full mobility around the appropriate joints and digits. The extremities are commonly involved in amputations associated with amniotic bands (disruption sequence). Abnormal shortening of the extremities occurs in a number of skeletal dysplasias. The upper extremities are considered to be abnormally short when the fingertips do not extend beyond the hip joint when the arm is lying in approximation to the thorax. The entire upper extremity, including the hands, should be carefully examined for asymmetry between the two sides as well as range of motion. Asymmetry in extremity size may be seen in

association with neurofibromatosis, Beckwith-Wiedemann syndrome, or Wilms' tumor. Enlargement of the hands and feet may be the result of lymphedema, which is seen in association with Turner's and Noonan's syndromes. Hypoplastic fingernails may be due to environmental teratogens such as fetal alcohol syndrome or maternal anticonvulsants. Examination of the lower extremities should include evaluation for congenital hip dislocation and evaluation of the feet for positional malformations as well as true congenital deformities such as a clubfoot. Rocker-bottom feet are seen in association with trisomy 18.

Absence deformities of the extremities are most often the result of disruption (amniotic bands) but may be seen in association with other syndromes such as thrombocytopenia/absent radius (TAR) syndrome or Cornelia de Lange's syndrome. Polydactyly is the most common hand malformation. Postaxial or ulnar polydactyly is the most common type and is usually inherited as an autosomal dominant trait, especially in African-Americans. Polydactyly is also seen in association with various multiple malformation syndromes. Syndactyly (fusion of the skin or bones) of the hand or foot is another autosomal dominant trait but may be seen in association with multiple malformation syndromes such as Apert's syndrome. Brachydactyly (shortening of the digits) is associated with achondroplasia as well as shortening of the proximal portion of the extremity. Arachnodactyly (elongation of the digits) may be seen with Marfan's syndrome or homocystinuria.

Joint deformities may be isolated (as in clubfoot) or more generalized as in arthrogryposis (multiple congenital joint contractures). Arthrogryposis may result from a neurologic defect in either the central or peripheral nervous system, from a primary muscle disorder, or from severe fetal constraint secondary to either multiple births or oligohydramnios. Infants with arthrogryposis need careful evaluation for other congenital abnormalities and detailed neurologic and skeletal evaluation for proper diagnosis and treatment.

Examination of the Skin

Skin lesions can be categorized as hyperpigmented, hypopigmented, or vascular. Hyperpigmented skin lesions include the commonly observed mongolian spots (large grayish blue pigmented areas in the lumbosacral or lower extremities) of dark-skinned individuals. Cafe au lait spots are smaller brownish patches and, when larger than 6 cm in size or more numerous than five, may signify neurofibromatosis. Pigmented nevi are important to note, as they may predispose the infant to development of malignant melanoma at a later age. Hypopigmented lesions (ash leaf spots) are one manifestation of tuberous sclerosis. Erythematous lesions (hemangiomas) in the distribution of the trigeminal nerve may be part of the Sturge-Weber syndrome and have associated intracranial vascular malformations. Raised hemangiomas (strawberry hemangiomas) are usually not present at birth but appear during the first month of life. Faint pink capillary hemangiomas (nevus flammeus or "stork bite") on the head are extremely common and are not associated with any specific syndromes.

Neurologic Examination

Significant information to be obtained from the neurologic examination pertains to the infant's general state of consciousness and assessment of underlying muscle tone. Infants who are extremely lethargic or unresponsive or who are excessively irritable and jittery may have underlying CNS disorders or inherited metabolic disorders. Infants with extreme hypotonia may have CNS deficits or peripheral nervous system problems such as congenital muscle disorders or neuropathies. Hypotonia is commonly seen with trisomy 21 as well as many other syndromes.

Management of the Infant with Congenital Malformations

Aggressive supportive care is indicated in all infants with life-threatening major malformations until a specific diagnosis and prognosis have been determined. In situations in which prenatal diagnosis of chromosomal abnormality or life-threatening malformation has been made, it is important to respect the parent's wishes regarding the aggressiveness of intervention after birth. In the event of an unanticipated malformation, a general management plan should first delineate the severity of the primary malformation and determine any additional malformations to attempt to make a diagnosis. Once a diagnosis is made or a syndrome is identified, the infant's prognosis and management plan as well as future genetic counseling can be discussed with the parents.

During the initial days following the birth of a child with a major malformation, it is important to remember that, owing to severe emotional shock, parents will comprehend and retain only part of the information presented. It is preferable to talk to both parents together and to understand that basic information regarding their infant may have to be repeated several times. If an infant has a malformation that severely limits its capacity to survive, parental counseling may include the option of no medical intervention. Congenital defects falling into this category include anencephaly, holoprosencephaly, and trisomies 13 and 18. In contrast, infants with a repairable structural disorder such as a positional deformation (talipes equinovarus) or primary malformation defects such as cleft lip, polydactyly, or uncomplicated cardiac defects, should have their normalcy emphasized along with information regarding later surgical options. Remember that parents react differently in crises and what may be seen as a minimal malformation to the physician may, in some families, result in a period of intense grieving for their lost "ideal" infant. It takes varying amounts of time for parents to accept and understand the nature of their infant's problems.

Perinatal Death in the Infant with Congenital Abnormalities

In the event of a stillbirth or neonatal death in an infant with identified congenital malformations, it is important to perform a thorough diagnostic work-up to answer questions regarding the outcome of the pregnancy and the infant's problems as well as for parental planning for later pregnancies. A thorough diagnostic work-up would in most cases include an autopsy with examination of both the infant and placenta. Permission for autopsy ideally should be requested by the physician who managed either the pregnancy or the newborn's care. Infants with major or multiple malformations should also have blood samples or tissue samples submitted for cytogenetic evaluation. In some situations, such as with a severely growth-retarded infant, one should obtain bacterial and viral cultures. The importance of this diagnostic evaluation, including the autopsy, should be explained to the parents in terms of answering later questions and obtaining a definitive diagnosis for future genetic counseling. Most parents experiencing perinatal death will benefit from bereavement counseling, both at the time of the death and at a meeting some months later to discuss autopsy findings or the events surrounding the death. It is important to remember that the grief process includes the emotions of disbelief, anger, and hostility prior to resolution of the event. It takes parents varying amounts of time to cope with the death of an infant or the birth of a child with major malformations.

Finally, parents should be encouraged and supported to hold their deceased infant in a quiet place. In the event that the parents do not wish to see their infant, it is important to obtain pictures and remembrances such as arm identification bands or locks of hair, as parents may want these mementos at a later date.

Summary

The birth of a dysmorphic child can be a source of confusion for the physician and disappointment for the family. Awareness of the more common major and minor malformations, their associated syndromes and complications, and their significance can help the physician develop a diagnostic plan. Once a diagnosis is reached, an appropriate course of management can be planned with input from the parents. Parents experiencing the birth of a child with a serious congenital malformation will appreciate a later counseling session with their obstetrician to discuss the possible etiologic basis for the congenital malformations, including autopsy findings as applicable. At that time possible diagnostic tests for future pregnancies can be reviewed (e.g., amniocentesis, fetal ultrasonography) and referral made for genetic counseling, if appropriate. At all times the physician must be aware of the emotional effects on the family, as these early days have a tremendous impact on the parents' ability to cope with this child and to grow and develop as a family.

Doppler Velocimetry in Fetal Surveillance

Dev Maulik, MD, PhD

The primary aim of antepartum fetal surveillance is timely recognition of fetal stress and compromise so that appropriate intervention may improve the perinatal outcome. Doppler velocimetry enables us to investigate fetal circulatory response to chronic stress and compromise, and thus provides a powerful fetal monitoring tool. There is a considerable amount of information available on the diagnostic efficacy of umbilical arterial Doppler in predicting adverse perinatal outcome in high-risk pregnancies. More significantly, the efficacy of umbilical arterial (UA) Doppler investigation in reducing perinatal mortality in high-risk pregnancies is substantially supported by randomized clinical trials. In contrast, in low-risk pregnancies UA Doppler velocimetry has been shown to be an ineffective screening tool. Furthermore, evidence for an improved outcome is not yet available in relation to Doppler investigation of other fetal or uteroplacental circulations, although valuable insight into fetal compromise may be obtained from its use. It is noteworthy that our current standards of antepartum fetal monitoring, non-stress test (NST) and biophysical profile (BPP), are not based on any affirmative evidence from randomized clinical trials. As Doppler velocimetry, NST and BPP reveal inter-related but differing aspects of fetal pathophysiology, no single testing modality should be regarded as the exclusive choice for fetal surveillance. This chapter presents the rationale and evidence-based practical guidelines for the use of UA Doppler sonography in conjunction with other fetal surveillance tests in a high-risk obstetric practice and briefly examines the utility and limitations of Doppler velocimetry of fetal middle cerebral and uterine arteries.

Rationale for Doppler Fetal Surveillance

Antepartum challenge to fetal well-being may arise from chronic nutritive and respiratory deprivation. A spectrum of obstetric complications including fetal growth restriction and hypertension may expose the fetus to such risks. Although an immense amount of information is available on acute and subacute fetal respiratory deficit, the pathophysiologic mechanism of chronic fetal stress has been less clear. Significant advances have been made recently, providing considerable insight into the mechanisms of fetal compensation and decompensation. There is emerging evidence that encountering sustained stress, the fetus appears to mobilize a spectrum of defensive responses that include preferential preservation of fetal growth over placental growth, changes in fetal movement pattern, and the eventual deceleration of the fetal growth rate.

In the face of continuing deprivation, compensation gives way to decompensation. For example, growth-restricted human fetuses have been shown to develop chronic hypoxia and acidosis. A critical component of fetal homeostatic response involves flow redistribution that favors perfusion of the vital organs (the brain, heart, and adrenals) at the expense of flow to muscle, viscera, skin, and other less critical tissues and organs. Underlying this phenomenon are the diverse changes in blood flow impedance in fetal regional circulations. The ability of Doppler indices to reflect changes in flow impedance has been conclusively demonstrated. It also has been shown that fetoplacental or uteroplacental vaso-obliterative pathology results in an increase in the arterial impedance, which is reflected by the abnormal Doppler indices. Doppler velocimetry thus elucidates these circulatory changes associated with fetal compromise and allows perinatal prognostication. This constitutes the rationale for using Doppler ultrasonography for fetal surveillance in complicated pregnancies.

Indications

Doppler velocimetry is indicated in pregnancies in which the fetus is at risk for chronic nutritive and respiratory stress. A variety of pregnancy complications such as intrauterine growth restriction (IUGR) and hypertensive disease can cause such stress. Common indications for performing Doppler surveillance of the fetus are listed in Table 1 and discussed subsequently.

Umbilical arterial Doppler velocimetry is predictive of adverse perinatal outcome in well-defined high-risk pregnancies including IUGR, preeclampsia, and the concurrence of both. Although umbilical arterial Doppler has been recommended in the past for identifying a small for gestational age (SGA) infant, sonographic measurement is the better predictor of fetal size. Unless the fetal hemodynamic state is compromised from stress, the Doppler indices will not change. Consistent with this, it has been shown that in high-risk pregnancies, abnormal umbilical arterial Doppler indices correlate with antepartum fetal asphyxia. The indices, therefore, may be helpful in distinguishing a growth-restricted and compromised SGA fetus from a constitutionally SGA fetus. Finally and most importantly, randomized trials have shown significant improvement in perinatal mortality from the use of UA Doppler in managing pregnancies complicated with clearly defined IUGR and hypertension.

Doppler velocimetry is also useful in managing pregnancies affected by autoimmune disorders, including systemic lupus erythematosus and antiphospholipid syndrome. Similarly, umbilical arterial Doppler is helpful in recognizing fetal compromise in multiple pregnancies, particularly in those with discordant growth and twin transfusion syndrome. Doppler is also recommended for fetal surveillance in pregnancies with pregestational diabetes, especially when vasculopathy is present; however, it should not be used to assess the quality of glucose control. Finally, there is no evidence that umbilical arterial Doppler is efficacious in managing postdated pregnancies.

Procedure of Umbilical Arterial Doppler Sonography

Before Doppler examination, the patient is appropriately counseled regarding the reason for the test, the nature of the information generated by the device, its reliability and safety, and other relevant issues. Similar to the procedure in fetal heart rate monitoring, the patient lies in a semi-recumbent position with a slight lateral tilt to minimize the risk of significant caval compression. Examination should be conducted only during fetal apnea and in the absence of fetal hiccup or excessive movement. Doppler insonation of the umbilical arterial circulation can be performed by either a continuous wave Doppler device or a pulsed Doppler duplex system.

Continuous wave Doppler interrogation of the umbilical arteries is a relatively simple procedure and can be performed in the office using a free-standing Doppler instrument. The transducer is usually a pencil-shaped probe with an operating frequency of 2 to 4 MHz. The transducer is placed on the patient's abdomen overlying the fetus with an acoustic coupling jelly intervening between the transducer face and the maternal abdominal skin. The method is similar to that used for listening to fetal heart tones with the simpler Doppler devices. The transducer is systematically manipulated to obtain the characteristic Doppler frequency shift waveforms from the umbilical arteries, which is seen in the device

---

TABLE 1. Indications for Umbilical Arterial Doppler Velocimetry

Small for gestational age fetus (<10th percentile)
Pre-eclampsia (primary and superimposed)
Secondary hypertension
Maternal renal disease
Autoimmune vascular disease
   Systemic lupus erythematosus
   Antiphospholipid antibody syndrome
   Other
Pregestational diabetes mellitus
Sickle cell disease
Multiple gestation

display screen. The process of identification is also facilitated by listening to the typical audible sound of the UA Doppler shift. Complete Doppler insonation of the artery is ensured by obtaining the umbilical venous Doppler signals simultaneously with the arterial signals.

With a pulsed wave duplex Doppler system, an obstetric scan is initially performed, and loops of the umbilical cord are identified. Unlike the continuous wave mode, the pulsed wave Doppler insonation permits selection of the location in the umbilical cord for interrogation. Usually, a free-floating loop of the cord is insonated. The cursor line representing the beam path is aligned to intersect the umbilical vessels at the selected location and the Doppler sample volume is placed in that location. The Doppler mode is then activated and the Doppler waveforms are recorded and analyzed.

Doppler Indices

Analysis of the Doppler waveforms predominantly consists of determination of the indices and visual assessment of the presence or the absence of the end-diastolic velocity. Most indices are calculated from the peak systolic and the end-diastolic values of the Doppler waveform. The indices measure pulsatility of the waveforms in an angle-independent manner. Of the numerous indices described in the literature, the systolic to diastolic (S:D) ratio, the resistance index (RI) and the pulsatility index are most commonly used in clinical practice. Although the RI is superior to the S:D ratio, the latter remains the most widely used Doppler index for fetal surveillance. This may be attributable to the apparent simplicity of the S:D ratio and its familiarity to the obstetric community. In practice, the choice of a specific index may not significantly affect the clinical efficacy of UA Doppler investigation.

Interpretation of the Umbilical Arterial Doppler Indices

Of the various characteristics of the UA Doppler waveform, the end-diastolic velocity is of primary hemodynamic and clinical significance. The end-diastolic velocity continuously increases with advancing gestation, which is related to the progressive decline of the fetoplacental flow impedance. This is reflected in the Doppler indices such as the S:D ratio and the RI, which continuously decline as pregnancy progresses. These changes are prognostically reassuring. In contrast, any decrease in the end-diastolic velocity with the consequently rising Doppler indices indicates rising impedance in the fetoplacental vascular bed and signifies worsening prognosis.

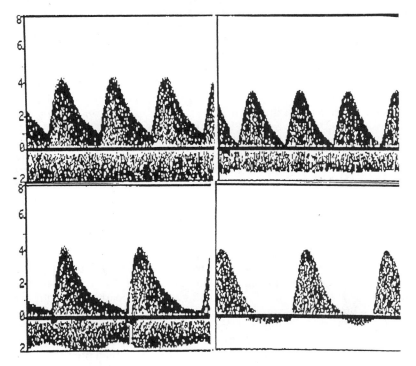

Figure 1. Progressive disappearance of the end-diastolic frequency shift in the umbilical arterial Doppler waveforms from a pregnancy complicated with severe fetal growth restriction at 33 weeks' gestation. *Top left,* Presence of the end-diastolic frequency shift, although the Doppler indices were high for the gestational age (systolic/diastolic ratio, 5; resistance index, 0.8). *Top right,* Absence of the end-diastolic frequency shift. *Bottom left,* Spontaneous deceleration with prolongation of the diastolic phase and the appearance of umbilical venous pulsation. *Bottom right,* Progression to the reversal of the end-diastolic frequency shift. (From Maulik, D: Absent end-diastolic velocity in the umbilical artery and its clinical significance. In Maulik, D [ed] Doppler Sonography in Obstetrics and Gynecology. New York: Springer-Verlag, 1997.)

For the umbilical arteries, an S:D ratio greater than 3.0 is considered abnormal after 27 weeks of pregnancy. A more appropriate approach would be to use a gestational age–specific nomogram of the Doppler index; however, there has been no standardization of such a nomogram. An initially high S:D ratio may progressively decline with the advancing gestation, signifying improved prognosis. In contrast, a rising S:D ratio reflects continuing fetal hemodynamic compromise and implies adverse prognosis. With further deterioration of impedance, the end-diastolic velocity eventually becomes absent and even may be reversed (Fig. 1). Such a development is ominous and results in very high perinatal mortality and morbidity (Table 2). In addition to those listed, the risks of cerebral hemorrhage, anemia, and hypoglycemia may also increase.

The frequency of absent end-diastolic velocity (AEDV) varies according to the obstetric risk, the gestational age, and the technique of Doppler examination. The incidence is approximately 2% in well-defined high-risk pregnancies and may be as low as 0.3% in a general obstetric population.

The appearance of AEDV does not necessarily lead to immediate fetal demise. Days to weeks may pass before the emergence of other ominous signs of fetal jeopardy that would necessitate delivery. In some cases, the end-diastolic velocity may return, which may suggest diminished fetal risks; however, this seems to be a rare occurrence. To increase the reliability of diagnosing AEDV, appropriate Doppler procedure should be used, ensuring a low filter setting (50 Hz or below) and a consistent sampling site in the cord if a pulsed duplex system is used. The use of a high filter setting or different sampling sites may lead to erroneous diagnosis of disappearance or reappearance of the end-diastolic velocity.

TABLE 2. Absent End-Diastolic Velocity in the Umbilical Artery and Perinatal Outcome

Perinatal mortality	45%
Mean gestational age at delivery	32 weeks
Mean birth weight	1000 gms
Small for gestational age	68%
Cesarean section for fetal distress	73%
Apgar score at 5 min <7	26%
Admission to neonatal intensive care unit	84%
Congenital anomalies	10%
Aneuploidy	6%

Modified from Maulik D: Absent end-diastolic velocity in the umbilical artery and its clinical significance. In Maulik D (ed): Doppler Sonography in Obstetrics and Gynecology. New York: Springer-Verlag, 1997.

Doppler Sonography of the Fetal Cerebral and the Uteroplacental Circulations

Considerable insight into fetal circulatory response to stress can be obtained from the Doppler investigation of the fetal middle cerebral artery (MCA). MCA Doppler indices decline with fetal stress, indicating cerebral vasodilation consequent to fetal circulatory redistribution. Further progression of fetal compromise leads to disappearance of this response, which is reflected in the rise in the MCA indices. Moreover, MCA Doppler may be used in conjunction with the UA Doppler indices as an index for fetal circulatory redistribution. Further investigation is needed to define the benefits of utilizing fetal cerebral Doppler in clinical practice.

Doppler waveforms of the uteroplacental arteries demonstrate a substantial increase in the end-diastolic velocity during the second half of pregnancy. The diastolic notch, which is present in the uterine arterial waveform in early pregnancy, disappears between 24 and 26 weeks of gestation. Increased pulsatility of the uterine arterial Doppler waveform, persistence of the notch and significant difference between the right and the left uterine arteries have been associated with IUGR, pre-eclampsia, and adverse perinatal outcome. It has also been suggested that a combination of the uterine and UA Doppler indices may offer prognostic insight into the hypertensive complication of pregnancy. However, the efficacy of uterine arterial Doppler in improving perinatal outcome remains to be shown.

Doppler Velocimetry and Management of High-Risk Pregnancy

Principles of managing a high-risk pregnancy utilizing UA Doppler velocimetry in conjunction with other fetal surveillance test findings are described in this section. Abnormal elevation of the umbilical arterial Doppler indices usually precedes ominous changes in other tests. Thus a high or increasing S:D ratio warrants more intense fetal surveillance, which consists of weekly or biweekly umbilical Doppler, NST, and BPP. If these tests are reassuring, fetal surveillance should continue unless intervention is indicated because of other complications. On the other hand, if these tests indicate fetal compromise, delivery should be planned, which may be accomplished either by induction or by cesarean

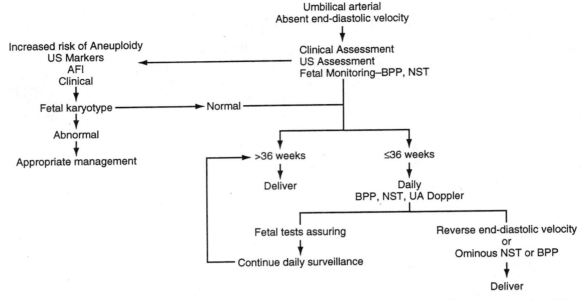

Figure 2. Algorithm for managing absent end-diastolic velocity in the umbilical artery. US, ultrasonography; AFI, amniotic fluid index; BPP, biophysical profile; NST, non-stress test; UA, umbilical arterial.

section depending on other obstetric factors and according to the current standards of practice.

In contrast to an elevated S:D ratio, the development of AEDV indicates more urgent action, as it is associated with an unusually adverse perinatal outcome. Other obstetric factors are considered in planning the optimal course of intervention for an individual patient. These include the gestational age, acuity of fetal compromise, and the presence of fetal aneuploidy and malformations. The plan of management is outlined in the algorithm in Figure 2 and is discussed here.

AEDV and Near-Term Pregnancy. The development of AEDV should prompt consideration of delivery when fetal lung maturity is anticipated or proven. Although the prudence of emergency delivery for this complication has been questioned, randomized clinical trials and their meta-analyses have shown improved outcome from obstetric interventions based on UA Doppler velocimetry. Obstetric intervention is, therefore, recommended when this complication develops at or near term (>36 weeks) when continuation of the pregnancy presents a greater threat to fetal safety and well-being.

The mode of delivery is determined by assessing relevant obstetric factors, including cervical status, fetal presentation, and the severity of fetal compromise. If reversed end-diastolic velocity develops in the umbilical arteries, the probability of impending fetal death is very high;

therefore, it may be more prudent to deliver the infant promptly by cesarean section rather than to test its tolerance to the rigors of labor induction. This management approach, however, is not applicable if lethal aneuploidy or malformation is present (see later).

AEDV and Preterm Pregnancy. In a preterm pregnancy (≤36 weeks) when significant risk of fetal pulmonic immaturity is present, the management is conservative and further assurance of fetal well-being is sought by daily surveillance with UA Doppler, NST, and BPP. Delivery is indicated when a single test or a combination of these tests indicate imminent fetal danger. The ominous signs include the reversal of end-diastolic component of the UA Doppler waveform, nonreactive NST, poor fetal heart rate baseline variability, persistent late decelerations, oligohydramnios, and BPP score less than 4. The optimal mode of delivery should be decided by assessing relevant obstetric factors as stated previously in relation to the term pregnancy.

An alternative, more aggressive approach proposes obstetric intervention at 34 completed weeks of gestation when many consider the fetal risk from a hostile intrauterine environment to be greater than that from pulmonic immaturity. A further modification of this approach involves confirmation of fetal pulmonic maturity in preterm pregnancies between 34 and 36 weeks by lecithin/sphingomyelin and phosphatidyl glycerol determination; delivery is recommended if the test results are assuring.

AEDV with Fetal Malformation or Aneuploidy. When absent or reversed end-diastolic velocity develops early in the third trimester, especially in the absence of any pregnancy complications associated with AEDV, the fetus should be assessed to rule out any malformations or aneuploidy. Fetal anatomic integrity is evaluated using targeted ultrasonography. Fetal karyotype should be determined if an increased risk of aneuploidy is suggested by clinical or ultrasonographic information. The latter includes the presence of multiple anomalies, other sonographic markers of chromosomal aberrations, and normal amniotic fluid volume (suggesting the absence of chronic fetal deprivation and stress). Contrary to the conventional wisdom, there is no preponderance of symmetrical growth compromise, although fetuses with abnormal chromosomes tend to be growth restricted. If lethal aneuploidy (trisomy 13 or 18) or malformations are identified, an appropriate management plan should be instituted.

It should be noted that these recommendations do not provide a solution for every contingency that may develop in the course of a high-risk pregnancy. The physician must individualize the care in light of the myriad of variations in the clinical situation. The information presented in this chapter should be used as a pragmatic guideline that integrates the new modality with the existing standards of fetal surveillance. As new evidence accumulates and experience grows, evidence-based integration of the various methods of fetal monitoring in appropriate sequence and frequency will add further refinement to this plan of management.

Fetal Death Syndrome

Perry A. Henderson, MD

Fetal loss may occur at any time during pregnancy. Losses that occur late in pregnancy are most distressing. When a fetal death occurs before 20 weeks of gestation and the fetal products are retained, it is termed an abortion or missed abortion. After 20 weeks' gestation, it is referred to as an intrauterine death or intrauterine fetal demise. Diagnosis, complications, and appropriate management present significant challenges and vary according to the age of the fetus. In addition, the physician must be sensitive to the potential emotional impact this may have for the parents. The development of ultrasonography as a diagnostic technique and newer modes of treatment have greatly facilitated the management of fetal death.

Rarely is the exact cause of fetal death known, such as with a cord prolapse. More often it is associated with a maternal condition with a known increased risk for fetal loss but for which the causal mechanism is obscure (eg, hypertensive diseases of pregnancy or diabetes mellitus). There are also patients who have a normal prenatal course until late in pregnancy, when the fetus dies unexpectedly and without any demonstrable explanation.

Diagnoses

The presence of fetal cardiac activity whether detected as heart tones by direct auscultation, Doppler ultrasonography or by real-time ultrasonography, is the easiest and most reliable sign of fetal life. Conversely, its absence is diagnostic of fetal death. Recent improvements in resolution of real-time ultrasonographic equipment and the increased accessibility of this equipment make it a definitive tool for the diagnosis of fetal death. The presence of fetal heart tones should be verified at each prenatal visit by either direct auscultation or Doppler ultrasonography. If fetal heart tones are not heard, a fetal ultrasonographic examination is indicated as soon as possible to evaluate the condition of the fetus.

Late in pregnancy the lack of fetal movement is most often the heralding event noted by the mother that prompts the obstetrician's evaluation for fetal death. Early in pregnancy, however, when this cannot be depended upon, the failure to detect fetal heart tones by auscultation or Doppler ultrasonography should prompt further evaluation of the fetus. With the use of real-time ultrasonography, fetal cardiac activity can be reliably visualized at 8 to 10 weeks' gestation. Failure to observe cardiac activity in a fetus before 8 to 10 weeks is not unusual, and subsequent examinations may be necessary to demonstrate fetal viability. In addition, after 12 to 16 weeks of gestation, the absence or loss of fetal limb motion, aortic pulsations, fetal breathing, or normal posturing are additional real-time ultrasonographic findings indicative of injury or fetal death. If the fetus has been dead for a significant period of time, the uterus usually fails to grow or even decreases in size, and this may be an additional clue indicating fetal death.

Traditionally, radiographic signs indicative of fetal death include overriding of fetal cranial skull bones (Spalding's sign) or gas in the fetal heart or great vessels (Robert's sign). These signs may not appear until several days to several weeks after fetal death. They are not as reliable as ultrasonographic findings and are now primarily of historical interest.

The natural history varies with the timing and cause of fetal death. Overall, three fourths of patients labor spontaneously within 2 weeks, and 90% within 3 weeks of the event. The interval, however, tends to vary inversely with the length of gestation.

Complications

Intrauterine fetal death often has strong emotional and psychological ramifications for the mother. This is especially true with a fetal death late in pregnancy. However, it may occur earlier in pregnancy and may be associated with a spontaneous abortion. This is clearly apparent with infertility patients who suffer a fetal loss of a pregnancy accomplished sometimes only after heroic attempts. There may be evidence of anger, depression, and/or guilt with or without an associated sense of shame and failure.

Other maternal morbidity is usually secondary to either infection or coagulopathy. Rupture of the membranes with retention of the necrotic fetal products increases the risk of infection. Vigorous treatment with antibiotics should be initiated when a diagnosis of infection is made. However, the definitive treatment is evacuation of the uterus, which may be accomplished by either medical or surgical means.

The most serious complication of fetal death is a consumptive coagulopathy arising from thromboplastin liberated from the dead products of conception and released into the maternal vascular system. This condition develops relatively late after fetal death, and its course is typically gradual. Some laboratory evidence of coagulopathy can be found in 25% of patients who retain a dead fetus for as long as 4 weeks. The initial changes in the coagulation system are hypofibrinogenemia and increase in fibrin degradation products. The platelet count may also be reduced, although severe thrombocytopenia is uncommon. Elevation of the prothrombin time and partial thromboplastin time may also occur. Clinical manifestations such as life-threatening hemorrhage usually do not occur until the serum fibrinogen level has reached 100 to 150 mg/dL or less. The hematologic alterations are reversed by the administration of heparin, confirming that the underlying cause is disseminated intravascular coagulation (DIC).

Therapeutic Options

Among the therapeutic options available in documented fetal death are expectant management, suction curettage, dilatation and evacuation, amnioinfusion, intravenous oxytocin, and vaginal prostaglandin E_2.

Expectant Management

Treatment of suspected intrauterine death should be expectant until the diagnosis is firmly established. Since the majority of women deliver within 2 weeks of fetal death, delivery may be delayed for this length of time if there are no other complications. However, the decision to proceed with termination often is made because of the mother's emotional or psychological inability to continue the pregnancy. The mother's desire for intervention may be a legitimate reason for termination but must be carefully weighed against the medical situation. If expectant management is chosen, serial weekly levels of fibrinogen, fibrin degradation products, and platelet determinations should be monitored. Intervention should be instituted if the fetus is retained for 4 weeks. If during expectant management intrauterine infection occurs, antibiotic therapy should be instituted and the uterine contents evacuated immediately by the most appropriate means.

Suction Curettage

Dilation of the cervix and vacuum aspiration of the uterine contents are safe as long as the pregnancy is not too far advanced, assuming the surgeon is skilled in this technique. When the uterus is no larger than that of a 14-week gestation, suction curettage is usually the method of choice. With more advanced gestations, the risk of uterine perforation and other complications increases and because of the size of the fetus may more appropriately be termed dilatation and evacuation.

Suction curettage following fetal death is associated with greater risk than for the same operation for the interruption of normal pregnancy. The likelihood of hemorrhage is increased, and technical difficulties of dilating the cervix and removing the products of conception are more likely. Therefore, the procedure should be done in an operating room, with appropriate anesthesia and intravenous infusion established for medications and/or possible blood transfusions. Laminaria may be inserted in the cervical os the evening before dilatation and curettage or 8 to 12 hours prior to the procedure. This greatly softens the cervix and facilitates cervical dilatation.

Dilatation and Evacuation

Fetal death in pregnancies of 14 to 18 weeks' gestation is particularly problematic. Because of the relatively early gestation, the uterus responds poorly to oxytocics and prostaglandin E_2 suppositories. In addition, with fetal death there is usually a resorption of the normal amount of amniotic fluid, making amniocentesis and subsequent infusion of hypertonic saline or urea and prostaglandin relatively difficult. For those surgeons skilled in the technique, dilatation and evacuation may be a reasonable alternative. Insertion of laminaria into the cervical canal 12 hours or so prior to the procedure may aid in subsequently dilating the cervix. The cervix should be maximally dilated to allow total extraction of the fetal parts, especially the fetal head. Following dilatation of the cervix, the amniotic fluid and whatever tissue can be obtained are aspirated with a large suction curette. Then, utilizing ovum forceps or ring forceps, the fetus and placenta are extracted. It is imperative that all of the major parts of the fetus be identified following removal and that the surgeon is assured at the end of the procedure that the uterine cavity is empty by performing a sharp curettage with a large curette. Pelvic ultrasonography may be used to confirm that all fetal parts have been removed from the uterus. There should be an intravenous line open and oxytocics may be administered to aid the uterus in contracting and to decrease the amount of blood loss. Should the etiology of the fetal death be obscure, bear in mind that following the procedure an intact fetus will not be available for clinical evaluation.

Amnioinfusion

Intra-amniotic injections of medications have been used to terminate second-trimester pregnancies complicated by intrauterine fetal death. Hypertonic saline has been used in the past, but intra-amniotic urea and prostaglandin $F_{2\alpha}$

are being used more commonly today. A serious disadvantage of the hypertonic saline is the risk of inadvertent intravascular injection. This complication is more likely with a dead fetus with its tendency toward oligohydramnios than with a normal pregnancy. There is also the increased risk of disseminated intravascular coagulation with hypertonic saline amnioinfusion. On the other hand, the amnioinfusion of 80 g of urea with 5 mg of prostaglandin $F_{2\alpha}$, although not without risk, is somewhat safer. Extreme care in technique is essential. A needle is placed in the intra-amniotic cavity under ultrasound guidance. As much amniotic fluid as possible is withdrawn and the urea and prostaglandin $F_{2\alpha}$ are injected. Care should be taken to inject the fluid into the amniotic cavity and avoid an inadvertent intravascular infusion. Some physicians prefer the medications to be infused by gravity and not by injection. Either way, the system should be checked for return of amniotic fluid repeatedly during the amnioinfusion. Following this, the patient usually experiences intermittent uterine contractions associated with progressive cervical dilatation and ultimately expulsion of the products of conception. On occasion, augmentation with oxytocin infusion may be necessary.

Vaginal Prostaglandin E_2

The vaginal insertion of prostaglandin E_2 suppositories is probably the most frequent method used to evacuate the uterus when fetal death occurs after 16 to 18 weeks. The technique is simple, rapid, effective, and useful in second-trimester or early third-trimester pregnancies. It can be used when the uterus is too large for suction curettage or oligohydramnios is present so that an amnioinfusion technique cannot be used. Prostaglandins carry a high incidence of undesirable side effects such as fever, gastrointestinal symptoms (nausea, vomiting, and diarrhea), and cardiovascular/respiratory effects (tachycardia, hypotension, and bronchospasm). More serious complications such as uterine rupture and myocardial infarction have been reported following the use of vaginal prostaglandin E_2. Also, this should not be used concomitantly with intravenous oxytocin because of the increased risk for uterine rupture or cervical laceration.

A factor of some significance is that the United States Food and Drug Administration has given limited approval for use of prostaglandin E_2 vaginal suppositories in fetal death to pregnancies of 28 weeks' gestation or less. Thus, although the agents are undoubtedly used in fetal deaths after 28 weeks, there are medical/legal implications should any complications occur if used after this stage of pregnancy. Suppositories contain 20 mg of prostaglandin E_2, and the usual dose is one suppository every 4 hours until labor is well established. Typically three or four doses are needed. In instances in which a reduced dosage seems desirable (eg, relatively late in pregnancy or in a patient with an irritable uterus), the suppositories may be cut in half.

Several commercial products are now available that contain small doses of prostaglandin E_2. When placed in the posterior vaginal fornix or in the cervix, these may ripen the cervix and allow for an easier induction of labor. It should be noted that smaller doses are used for intracervical application than when placed in the posterior vaginal fornix.

Intravenous Oxytocin

Oxytocin is a familiar and relatively safe drug. Unfortunately, the uterus is often insensitive to oxytocin, particularly prior to term, and the failure rate in cases of fetal death is high. Moreover, oxytocin in doses of 40 mU/min or higher has an antidiuretic effect and therefore carries a risk of water intoxication. Oxytocin should be given as a relatively concentrated solution in an electrolyte-containing medium (eg, 50 units in 1000 mL of lactated Ringer's solution). Administration should be by constant infusion pump with an initial rate of 0.5 to 1.0 mU/min and increased stepwise to an amount causing contractions of the appropriate interval, duration, and intensity.

Occasionally oxytocin induction of labor, even at term, is unsuccessful. After an adequate trial of labor, it is appropriate to discontinue the oxytocin infusion and repeat it at a later date as long as the membranes remain intact and the patient's condition remains stable. Artificial amniotomy with subsequent oxytocin infusion may be considered if the patient's cervix is ripe. However, once amniotomy has occurred, delivery must be effected within a reasonable time to avoid infectious complications.

Suggestions for Management
Uncomplicated Cases

In fetal death during the *first trimester* or later in cases in which the uterus recedes to no larger

than 14 weeks' gestational size, suction curettage is clearly the safest and simplest method of termination. The conditions and precautions outlined earlier should be observed.

During the *second trimester*, vaginal prostaglandin E_2 represents the preferred method, with an amnioinfusion of urea and prostaglandin $F_{2\alpha}$ the second choice.

Third-trimester fetal death presents a dilemma. Vaginal prostaglandin E_2, as 20 mg suppositories, has been used and appears to be reasonably safe, but the fact remains that it is not specifically approved for use during this trimester. With this in mind, the safest course is probably amnioinfusion of urea and prostaglandin early in the third trimester and intravenous oxytocin (with or without amniotomy) when fetal death occurs near term. Traditional contraindications to induction of labor by any method should be considered. These include prior classic cesarean birth, complete placenta previa, maternal cardiac failure, and invasive carcinoma of the cervix.

Complicated Cases

Certain maternal diseases represent relative contraindications to one or another technique of termination. Prostaglandins should be avoided in patients with cardiovascular disease, asthma, or other respiratory diseases. Urea should be used with caution in patients with renal disease. If such complications are present, the proper therapeutic approach may be that of expectant management and awaiting spontaneous labor and delivery. DIC caused by prolonged retention of a dead fetus may occasionally occur. However, this is usually only after retaining the dead fetus for 4 weeks or longer. Monitoring plasma fibrinogen weekly should be adequate to detect a problem before serious coagulopathy develops. If DIC should occur, proper management would include heparinization with intravenous heparin, 1000 to 2000 units per hour by intravenous pump for 24 to 48 hours. This should reverse the hematologic changes, after which the uterus can be evacuated by means appropriate to the circumstances. Heparin should be used only with an intact vascular system, and in no instances should it be used in the presence of overt bleeding.

Special Diagnostic Tests

A number of diagnostic tests may be helpful in identifying the cause of an apparently unexplained fetal death. Laboratory indices of potential value in this regard include serologic tests for syphilis, Rh, and other antibody titers, glucose tolerance testing, and renal function studies. Recently, both lupus anticoagulant and anticardiolipin antibodies have been associated with fetal losses. These antibodies are found frequently in patients with lupus erythematosus and other autoimmune diseases but they may also occur without apparent disease. The association between lupus anticoagulant and pregnancy loss appears to be stronger; however, more studies are needed to further elucidate the relationship between antiphospholipid antibodies and the etiology of fetal death.

Autopsy of all stillbirths should be done. Unfortunately, unless done by an individual experienced in perinatal pathology, the results typically reported—"macerated stillborn"—are not often helpful. In stillbirths near term, clinical or physical examination of the fetus may be independently rewarding. The assistance of a clinical geneticist in this examination is often useful. Photographs and radiographs may also be helpful in identifying an otherwise unrecognizable syndrome.

Karyotyping of fetal tissues should be considered. Instances of chromosomal abnormalities as high as 5% have been reported in large series of stillbirths. Unfortunately, the substantial cost of karyotyping represents a deterrent to widespread use. Among conditions that seem to be particularly associated with chromosomal anomalies and therefore increase the yield of karyotyping are anomalies other than those involving the nervous system, fetal growth retardation, and a previous history of fetal wastage.

Fetomaternal hemorrhage has recently been recognized as a relatively common finding in otherwise unexplained fetal death, with spontaneous fetal exsanguination accounting for approximately 10% of cases. Therefore, every woman carrying a dead fetus should be tested, preferably before delivery, by Kleihauer-Betke staining of a peripheral blood smear.

Emotional Support and Care

Fetal death, particularly when it occurs unexpectedly, is an emotionally wringing experience for the prospective parents and the physician. It is normal to encounter denial, anxiety, guilt, hostility, and depression in either or both parents. This must be acknowledged and faced squarely. It is the physician's role to be available and to resist the temptation to avoid the patient, to be reassuring in allaying any guilt feelings, to explain the grieving process, and to answer questions. Although the cause of the fetal death may be unexplained, invariably parents have many other questions that can be easily answered.

Formerly, patients with a dead fetus were sedated heavily during labor, not permitted to see the stillborn infant, and housed postpartum in an area other than the maternity ward. Current opinion holds that this approach is generally erroneous. Couples sustaining a fetal death usually need assistance in facing the reality of the event. Therefore seeing, touching, and/or photographing the infant should be encouraged if the parents desire. This is true even if the infant is macerated or malformed. Frequently, the fears and anxieties of the couple about how the baby will look greatly exceed the actuality of the appearance of the stillborn infant. Other questions such as naming the infant or holding memorial services need to be explored gently and nonjudgementally.

The loss of an unborn baby is a painful experience, and parents who suffer through this usually have an overpowering grief. Although many people are exposed to death in our society, how we respond to a fetal loss has several unusual characteristics. These include a sense of nonreality of the event, a perceived loss of control by the parents, and the inappropriate reactions of an uninformed society. Patients suffering a fetal death may be viewed as passing through three phases following an acute crisis. They seem to be in a period of shock for several days to weeks. This is followed by a longer period of suffering or disorganization in which they suffer tremendous emotional turmoil. Finally, usually after months, they begin to recuperate during a third period of recovery or reorganization. The final goal of accepting a fetal death may be reached only after as long as 18 to 24 months. This is dependent upon the degree of bonding that has occurred with the pregnancy.

During this prolonged period of adjustment, patients undergo a number of emotional responses over which they have no control and which are accordingly designated "involuntary coping mechanisms." Examples of these include denial, anxiety, anger or hostility, guilt, bargaining, depression, withdrawal, and shame. It is important to acknowledge these emotions and assure the patient that these are normal responses.

In addition to these involuntary coping mechanisms, there are other specific acts that grieving couples perform or are encouraged to perform which seem to help them cope with a fetal death. These have been characterized as "voluntary coping strategies," examples of which include verbalizations (discussing the loss), holding, seeing, and touching the baby, mementos (eg, baby's bracelet, cap, pictures), autopsy, funeral or memorial service, and burial or cremation. These are conscious efforts of patients which help them cope and attempt to make real this nonreal event.

The physician should continue to be available to the patient and her partner following termination of the pregnancy or delivery of the stillbirth. Some contact is advisable approximately 2 weeks following hospitalization. It is at this time, when the initial shock and denial of the event have passed, that many questions arise and the need for reassurance is great. A postoperative routine follow-up at 4 to 6 weeks is an opportunity not only to ascertain the physical status of the patient but to explore her level of adjustment to the fetal loss. Finally, a 3-month perinatal loss review conference can be very useful. It is at this time that the autopsy report can be reviewed and its implications discussed. Questions can be answered whether or not the cause of the fetal death was determined. Within the context of the discussion at this conference, when or if to pursue a subsequent pregnancy should be discussed.

The patient's perception of "loss of control" is closely linked to the related perception of the "nonreality of the event." Assisting the patient to regain control can be accomplished through a continual process of support, acknowledging the significant impact of the fetal death and repetitively answering questions that initially may seem superficial. Providing options also helps patients regain a sense of control—for example, involving the couple in the decision to have prostaglandin induction of labor in the second trimester rather than a dilatation and evacuation. Although the latter may be more expeditious, a prostaglandin-induced delivery would provide an intact fetus for postmortem evaluation as well as a baby that can be seen, touched, and held if the parents so desire.

Lastly, the patients need to be prepared to meet with nonunderstanding relatives and friends. Like the patient, they usually need to be educated as to what to expect and how to relate to couples who have experienced a fetal death. They frequently do not appreciate the duration of acute grief following a pregnancy loss and do not understand why it takes so long to resolve the grief of a fetal death. Or they offer insensitive comments such as "it was better that way" or "you can have another baby." The most difficult

reaction is no reaction at all, as friends and relatives join in a "conspiracy of silence" and avoid or do not speak to the couple with a pregnancy loss. Often the patient may have to initiate conversation or mention the subject, in effect giving permission to discuss fetal death.

Care During Subsequent Pregnancies

Care during a subsequent pregnancy should be individualized in accordance with the needs of the patient. Particular attention should be paid to emotional support and reassurance in view of the high level of anxiety certain to be present. The patient should be seen more frequently than customary, and more than the usual amount of time should be spent with her at each visit.

Some types of special tests (e.g., glucose tolerance test or midtrimester amniocentesis for genetic diagnosis) may be indicated by specific events or findings of the earlier pregnancy. Following a previous unexplained fetal death, tests should be performed to rule out syphilis, isoimmunization, diabetes, renal disease, or collagen diseases. Fetal surveillance techniques such as kick counts, antepartum heart rate testing, and/or biophysical profiles are advisable in late pregnancy if for no other reason than to provide reassurance. This reassurance is most often needed at that period of gestation in which the prior fetal death occurred.

Fetal Distress in the Intrapartum Period

David Jackson, MD

This discussion examines the clinical tools necessary to identify and manage fetal distress in labor. Almost invariably, the mischief preceding a hypoxic, acidotic, and asphyxiated fetus is recognizable in hindsight. As such, the medicolegal milieu surrounding such cases is divided into failure to anticipate, failure to diagnose, and failure to treat in a timely fashion. Practitioners from midwife to physician can no longer simply "follow" labors, they must intelligently lead labor to a successful outcome. In an age of technology and high cesarean section rates, the challenge is to develop accurate fetal surveillance and intervention that does not compromise the natural beauty and safety accompanying the majority of delivery experiences.

Relevant History

Anticipating and preventing distress relies on relevant history, appropriate auscultation (albeit electronically in many cases), and decisive intervention. Patients today are well informed regarding their upcoming labor experience. Birthing classes, advocate books, and practitioners' office materials stress an active role for mothers and partners in the labor room, but fail to educate on individual risks. As such, patients need realistic expectations regarding their risk for decreased fetal perfusion in labor. The top maternal conditions associated with distress in labor include hypertension, diabetes, third-trimester bleeding, heavy smoking or drug use, postmaturity, extreme prematurity, and prolonged preterm premature ruptured membranes. Correlative fetal conditions include intrauterine growth restriction, oligohydramnios, elevated Doppler umbilical blood flow, congenital anomalies, meconium in amniotic fluid, and abnormal antepartal monitoring results. For patients at risk, adequate time is required during prenatal visits to stress benefits, risks, and alternatives of labor augmentation (active rupture of membranes, oxytocin), surveillance tools (intermittent auscultation and electronic monitoring), resuscitation tools (positioning, hydration, oxygen), and delivery tools (episiotomy scissors, forceps, vacuum, and cesarean section). In our experience, explaining the at-risk clinical situation usually creates an expectation that the practitioner will be on site during active phases of labor. Practitioners in groups need to relay to covering partners the patient's clinical status and expectations. In simple terms, if you say you will be there throughout labor, be there. If a historical risk factor is present, be sure to be in attendance to identify distress and intervene in a timely fashion.

Surveillance and Management Tools

Monitoring of labor has become immersed in the controversy over electronic tracing versus intermittent auscultation. The controversy is ultimately irrelevant, as long as the pregnancy is monitored. Auscultation requires listening every 15 minutes from active dilation to 10 cm dilation and every 5 minutes from complete dilation to delivery. Auscultation should include timing of heart rate post-contraction. Electronic monitoring is usually continuous. Tracing interpretation and documentation should occur with at least the same frequency as auscultation. The presence of tachycardia, bradycardia, or intermittent decelerations warrants documentation and intervention. Conversely, the presence of normal heart rate baseline (120–160 bpm), presence of reactivity, presence of fetal movement, and presence of heart rate variability are all indicative of an intact fetal nervous system without depression.

Often confusion arises over the relative severity of "distress." This confusion can lead to a delay in intervention, which frequently occurs in centers with electronic monitoring. Discussion is carried out over deceleration type, presence or absence of variability, and presence or absence of reactivity. This approach has several practical pitfalls that should be avoided. The first is to review the strip away from the bedside, so that speculative conversation will not unduly worry the family. The second is to ask the simple question "Is the tracing *completely* reassuring?" Any answer other than "yes" requires management, even for periodic changes alone in the setting of normal variability and normal baseline. Since the monitor indirectly reflects the fetal environment, when the tracing is anything other than reassuring, the patient should be informed of its nature, expected etiology, strategies for reversal, and timeline for delivery. Initial approaches universally accepted for intrauterine resuscitation include hydration with bolus of intravenous fluid, positioning with right or left tilt, oxygen by mask at 6 to 10 L, and blood pressure check. Intravenous fluids correct hypovolemia, and placing the patient in the lateral recumbent position will additionally improve uterine blood flow and placental perfusion. It should be explained to the patient that the large vessels returning blood to the heart can be compressed by the gravid uterus pushing against the maternal lower spinal curvature. This decrease in cardiac preload reduces cardiac output and placental perfusion. Fluids, position, and oxygen improve cardiac output and maternal oxygen pressure. Since oxygen masks are distressful to the patient, avoid stating that "It's for the baby" without explaining that the fetus is very efficient at extracting oxygen from the maternal system, and even small improvements in maternal oxygen pressure facilitate increased fetal oxygenation. This helps alleviate the mother's worst fears that her child is lacking oxygen and will be brain damaged. It should also be explained that if the decelerations persist and are associated with excessive uterine activity, oxytocin will be discontinued. In the setting of excessive uterine activity and decelerations, we administer an agent such as terbutaline 0.25 mg subcutaneously or 0.25 mg intravenously. The patient should be forewarned of the expected tachycardia and anxious feeling associated with these medications.

For prolonged decelerations unassociated with excessive contractions, immediate vaginal examination for occult cord prolapse or rapid fetal descent is needed. At the time of examination, the practitioner should stimulate the fetal scalp and note fetal movements or acceleration of the fetal heart rate. The presence of fetal movement or heart rate accelerations does not negate the intermittent decelerations, but it does give a variable timeline (often 20 minutes or less) to effect complete resuscitation prior to delivery. Persistent variable decelerations (especially with an associated maternal risk factor for oligohydramnios such as hypertension, intrauterine growth restriction, postmaturity, or prolonged ruptured membranes) should be treated with amnioinfusion. We utilize an intrauterine pressure catheter system with a separate port for infusion. Bolus of 400 to 600 mL of warmed or at least room temperature saline over 1 hour is followed by continuous infusion at a rate of 180 mL/hour. We monitor for uterine overdistention and visually assess that fluid is returning from the vagina. For centers where continuous infusion is not desired, then bolus of 600 mL over 1 hour can be utilized and periodically repeated when fluid escapes and decelerations resume.

Intrauterine resuscitation of the fetal patient also requires correction of hypotension. If the blood pressure has not been recently recorded, it should be taken and repeated at regular intervals (every 10–15 minutes) during the efforts to resuscitate the fetus. Maternal hypotension related to epidural block requires fluid replacement and judicious ephedrine use (2.5–10 mg increments IV). If severe hypertension is noted, then appropriate agents to lower blood pressure and improve placental perfusion should be initiated.

Special Circumstances of Anemia

Rarely, maternal or fetal anemia will be severe enough to produce periodic decelerations, tachycardia, decreased variability, or all three. The maternal hemoglobin, hematocrit, and blood type should be obtained in labors at risk or with the onset of nonreassuring heart patterns. Blood replacement for severe maternal anemia may be necessary prior to operative delivery and may correct fetal decelerations. Fetal anemia from chronic sources (isoimmunization, viral illness,

fetal-maternal bleed) may manifest as sinusoidal heart tracings or be inferred from fetal hydropic changes. Acute fetal anemia from post-amniocentesis vessel compromise or eccentric umbilical cord insertion with fetal vessel rupture may be heralded by sudden bradycardia followed by tachycardia, late decelerations, or a combination of these. If fetal distress occurs in close proximity to membrane rupture and is associated with vaginal bleeding, then attempts should be made to confirm fetal or maternal origin to the bleeding. Kleihauer-Betke stain or APT testing will be helpful but often is time consuming. Since delivery by cesarean section may be imminent to save the baby's life, a clinical decision is necessary, to be followed by immediate delivery room transfusion. The pediatric staff should be prepared to transfuse non-crossmatched, universal donor blood. For centers with no blood bank capabilities, we have heard of collecting cord blood for autotransfusion. If no other source is available, blood from the mother may be necessary to reverse severe neonatal cardiovascular collapse in the setting of ruptured vasa praevia.

Second Stage Decelerations

Many times the most confusing fetal monitoring occurs in the second stage of labor. The severity of distress may be lost in the monitored patient in whom the return to baseline is never quite complete prior to a new contraction and new deceleration. In the absence of a reassuring tracing, persistent decelerations in the second stage should also be managed with position, hydration, and oxygen. Oxytocin should be discontinued and tocolytics used judiciously if the decelerations are related to excessive uterine activity. The patient may be coached to avoid excessive pushing while resuscitation is attempted. The anticipated timeline to delivery should be calculated. Clearly a multiparous patient with adequate progress and rapid fetal descent is at less risk of needing to tolerate prolonged decelerations than the woman with her first delivery and slower descent. Macrosomia, occiput posterior, and maternal pelvic outlet contraction should be documented and utilized in careful decision making. Cesarean section in a timely fashion is preferable to a difficult operative vaginal delivery with subsequent shoulder dystocia. In centers where it takes time to assemble the anesthetic and surgical teams, parallel preparation for vaginal or cesarean delivery should be occurring during the attempts to correct distress. If decelerations continue, documentation of fetal movements and appropriate scalp stimulation will allow for continued labor as long as delivery is anticipated in a short interval. Direct scalp pH may be useful if attempting to confirm the absence of acidosis with confusing tracings. Emergent delivery should be enacted if the tracing is nonreassuring, fetal decelerations persist, and fetal descent is lacking.

Timing of Delivery

A plan that delays intervention until absolute signs of fetal acidosis and central nervous system depression are in place will lead to neonatal catastrophe. Delivery by cesarean section for uncorrected decelerations, loss of variability, rising baseline, and nonreassuring tracing is individual to the maternal situation. As mentioned earlier, in centers where it takes time to assemble the anesthetic and surgical teams, parallel preparation for cesarean delivery should be occurring as you are attempting to correct distress. If decelerations continue, documentation of fetal movements and appropriate scalp stimulation will allow for continued labor as long as delivery is anticipated in a short interval. Direct scalp pH may be useful if attempting to confirm the absence of acidosis with confusing tracings. Emergent delivery should be enacted if the tracing is nonreassuring, fetal decelerations persist, and labor progress is lacking.

Pediatric Attendance, Cord pH, Placental Pathology

The postpartum management of intrapartal distress is crucial to successful obstetrics. Pediatric attendance with experience in resuscitation of a depressed neonate should be requested for all situations that are not reassuring. The pediatric resuscitation team should have been forewarned of their anticipated attendance with the onset of abnormal heart tracing or based on historical maternal risk factors, as mentioned earlier. Obtaining a cord pH is useful in understanding the impact of the labor changes on fetal and neonatal physiology. A documented low pH with a healthy neonatal response does not increase legal risk and may assist the pediatric monitoring of the neonate. We regularly send the placenta to the pathology laboratory to assist in documentation of placentally mediated syndromes such as infarction, infection, meconium, and abruption. Finally, discussion with the patient regarding the conduct that occurred during labor is essential. Even with careful monitoring and aggressive de-

livery, neonatal depression may occur. Often the timing of neurologic insult preceded labor and was unavoidable. A supportive team approach of nursing, pediatric, and obstetric staff is required to assist the family without becoming overly defensive. In those rare situations in which an extremely depressed neonate is delivered, expert support for delivery staff is also encouraged to avoid the damaging situations of guilt and adversarial defensiveness. Specialists such as perinatologists, nurse managers, and risk assessment personnel are experienced at facilitating appropriate reviews and support and should be consulted in a timely fashion.

Fetal Movement Charting

William F. Rayburn, MD

Maternal perception of gross fetal movement is the oldest and least expensive technique for monitoring fetal well-being. Recording such activity may serve as an indirect means of evaluating fetal central nervous system function and integrity, since coordination of whole body motion requires complex neurologic control similar to that of the newborn infant. A mother's perception of a loss or significant decrease in propulsive fetal activity has been traditionally regarded as a warning sign, especially when fetoplacental insufficiency is suspected. Many investigators have reported on the value of daily fetal movement charting as a means for signaling impending fetal jeopardy and possible demise. Perceived inactivity requires a reassessment of any underlying antepartum complication and a more precise evaluation of fetal well-being either by fetal heart rate (FHR) testing or by performing a biophysical profile.

Gross Fetal Movement Patterns

Recognized patterns of fetal movement correspond to different stages of development. With the use of ultrasonography, twitching of the fetus can be detected at 7 to 10 weeks' gestation, independent limb movement by 10 weeks, combined movements of limbs, head, and torso by 16 weeks, and respiratory efforts by 20 to 24 weeks. Fetal movements during the second half of pregnancy can be perceived when they last for more than 1 second. These involve an extension of the limbs or head relative to the trunk ("stretching"), displacement or rotation of the torso ("rotation"), and isolated forceful movements of the lower limbs (strong "kick").

Perceived total movements can be confirmed by ultrasonography; conversely, an average of 82% of all visualized movements of fetal limbs are perceived by the patients. A gradual decline in movement is expected as gestation advances because of refinements in motor coordination. The number of perceived or visualized fetal movements does not change significantly, however, in an otherwise healthy fetus.

A normal daily range of perceived fetal movements is difficult to predict, since the number per hour is highly variable. Fetal activity is normally perceived to range from 8 to 40 movements per hour. Fetal activity is unrelated to the time of day (except perhaps during the very early morning hours) or to a glucose challenge.

Fetal activity is related to "sleep-awake" cycles, which are independent of the maternal sleep-awake states. The "sleep" portion of the cycle may range from 20 minutes to as much as 2 hours. Discerning between this physiologic rest period and an abnormally low activity pattern is often difficult. A 1-hour counting interval is frequently adequate. Fetal inactivity of more than 1 hour may not be physiologic, however, and can be associated with a greater likelihood of fetal jeopardy.

Clinical Applications

Fetal movement charting has been accepted by many to be a useful adjunct in predicting impending fetal compromise. Periods of fetal activity as noted by maternal perception, Doppler monitoring, or ultrasonographic imaging are reassuring findings. Perceived fetal inactivity should be evaluated by more objective fetal monitoring techniques and by reassessing any underlying complication (eg, hypertension, diabetes, intrauterine infection, fetal growth disparity, oligohydramnios).

We encourage movement charting to be used by any woman reporting decreased fetal activity on routine prenatal questioning. Applying fetal movement recording to all low-risk patients is appealing, since approximately one half of all stillbirths occur without obvious cause. In one study, this application was found to have a positive effect on decreasing the fetal mortality rate while increasing the total amount of antepartum testing by only 13%.

Most investigators would agree that fewer than 10 fetal movements per hour for 2 consecutive hours constitutes evidence of fetal inactivity. Inactivity is present at some time in 2.5% to 15% of all high-risk pregnancies during the last trimester. Depending on the clinical definitions and patient population, 46% to 81% of inactive fetuses will have an unfavorable perinatal outcome (nonreassuring heart rate pattern during labor, low Apgar scores, umbilical artery acidosis, intensive care nursery admission, perinatal death).

Fetal movement charting is especially helpful in a pregnancy predisposed to uteroplacental insufficiency or fetal heart failure. Such conditions include maternal acute or chronic hypertension, Rh isoimmunization, fetal anemia, maternal diabetes, severe fetal growth retardation, oligohydramnios, preterm ruptured membranes, arrested premature labor, and postdate pregnancies. Not all stillbirths can be avoided by using fetal movement charting. Unfavorable outcomes despite prior documented fetal activity often relate to acute changes such as a placental abruption or an umbilical cord complication.

Fetuses suspected of being growth retarded are more likely to have reduced activity, especially if the delay is severe. Under these circumstances, an underlying vascular, structural, genetic, or chronic inflammatory process is more likely to be present. Postmaturity, another form of growth retardation, is occasionally accompanied by fetal inactivity. Postnatal complications that would account for increased perinatal morbidity are frequently attributable to postnatal metabolic or respiratory complications, which cannot be fully anticipated by antenatal testing in general and by fetal movement charting in particular.

Fetal growth disparity or heart failure is more common in multifetal gestations. Differentiating between twin fetuses from day to day by movement charting is difficult and often impossible. "Boxing matches" occur often. The mother's observation that her fetuses are quite active is reassuring, but it is common for a mother to report one fetus to be less active than the other. More objective techniques are required to assess fetal growth and to better evaluate biophysical wellbeing.

Most infants with major malformations are active in utero, with gross body movements usually being indistinguishable from those of normal fetuses. If the spinal cord remains intact, sufficient preservation of the iliopsoas and quadriceps muscles should allow for spastic lower limb motion and positioning. Those perceived to be inactive usually have an abnormality in central ner-

To know more about your baby, we ask you to count how many minutes it takes for you to feel ten distinct movements (kicks, stretches, or roll-overs—not hiccoughs). Do this any time while lying on your side.

Circle the letter corresponding to the number of minutes.

A=0–15 minutes   C=31–45 minutes
B=16–30 minutes   D=46–60 minutes

WEEK	SUNDAY	MONDAY	TUESDAY	WEDNESDAY	THURSDAY	FRIDAY	SATURDAY
	ABCD	ABCD	ABCD	ABCD	ABCD	ABCD	ABCD
	ABCD	ABCD	ABCD	ABCD	ABCD	ABCD	ABCD
	ABCD	ABCD	ABCD	ABCD	ABCD	ABCD	ABCD
	ABCD	ABCD	ABCD	ABCD	ABCD	ABCD	ABCD

Contact us if more than one hour is needed. Otherwise, please bring this chart with you at your next visit.

Figure 1. An example of a fetal movement chart: the "count to 10" chart.

vous system pathways, muscular dysfunction, space-occupying masses, extreme dwarfism, or excessively increased or decreased amniotic fluid volumes. Unlike polyhydramnios, reduced amniotic fluid after rupture of the membranes does not usually impair perception of fetal activity and its predictability.

Role in Antenatal Fetal Surveillance

Many methods have been described for fetal movement charting. The "count to 10" technique is perhaps most attractive, because it presents the least time restrictions (10 movements are often perceived in less than 20 minutes). Maternal compliance is more likely when the counting scheme requires 1 hour or less. Other described methods of fetal movement charting require counting for 1 to 12 hours daily. Figure 1 shows an example of our "count to 10" fetal movement chart. Using this chart, our patients "grade" their fetus' activity as being an "A," "B," "C," or "D." A lack of 10 movements in 1 hour warrants notification of the clinic or physician by the patient.

Regardless of technique, the mother should be instructed to lie on her side, preferably in a quiet room, and to concentrate on fetal activity. Recordings may be done at any time, although the evening hours are usually most convenient. Gross fetal body movement is unaffected by a recent meal, making a glucose challenge unnecessary before testing.

The patient should be given a clear description about how to keep a movement chart. The importance of recognizing and acting promptly on a perceived reduction of movement must be emphasized. The chart should be reviewed by the practitioner at each prenatal visit. Patients complaining of decreased fetal movement warrant further evaluation in the labor and delivery unit or clinic. A reactive nonstress test or a biophysical profile score of at least 6 is reassuring. Use of ultrasonography to demonstrate fetal movements and muscle tone should relieve maternal apprehension and may improve the patient's accuracy if she is having perception difficulties. Continued fetal movement charting should be encouraged after discharge.

A decision to deliver should not be based on fetal movement patterns alone. Documented fetal inactivity in either low- or high-risk pregnancies requires at least antenatal FHR testing (primarily nonstress testing) or real-time ultrasonographic visualization. Observed propulsive movements (at least three discrete body/limb movements in 30 minutes) with an adequate amniotic fluid volume or a reactive FHR pattern is a reassuring finding and does not necessitate further evaluation. A nonreactive pattern, despite vibroacoustic stimulation or any fetal inactivity observed for more than 40 minutes, requires additional observation that same day or serious consideration for delivery.

Patient compliance with this protocol has generally been favorable. She should understand charting instructions, be seen primarily by the same physician, and understand treatments necessary for any underlying antepartum complications.

In summary, daily fetal movement charting is an inexpensive screening tool for fetal assessment outside the office setting. Evidence of an active fetus is reassuring of an intact central nervous system, whereas perceived inactivity requires further evaluation. Patient cooperation is necessary and may require repeated encouragement. With proper utilization of the described technique, a decrease in stillbirth rate is possible and the cost of fetal surveillance may be reduced.

Fetal Scalp Stimulation

Frank C. Miller, MD

The accurate diagnosis of fetal distress remains a major goal of obstetric management. Traditionally, fetal heart rate (FHR), fetal blood gas analysis, and the color and volume of the amniotic fluid have been utilized to diagnose fetal hypoxia and asphyxia. Periodic FHR decelerations with normal baseline variability and fetal respiratory acidosis reflect acute changes in the fetal status. Repetitive late decelerations with a smooth or changing baseline rate, metabolic acidosis, and reduced amniotic fluid volume reflect varying degrees of more prolonged asphyxia. Vintzileos and colleagues proposed a gradual hypoxia concept: The biophysical activities that appear first in fetal development are relatively more resistant to hypoxia than activities controlled by central nervous system (CNS) areas, which mature later and require more oxygen for growth. According to this concept, severe fetal asphyxia is associated with cessation of all biophysical activities, whereas milder hypoxia initially results in the loss of FHR reactivity and fetal breathing movements (Table 1).

Changes in FHR, such as late decelerations and loss of baseline variability and reactivity, are the earliest signs of fetal hypoxia. Murata and colleagues demonstrated that late decelerations appear before accelerations disappear (pH 7.23 versus pH 7.21) in a rhesus monkey model. Yet accelerations of the FHR with movement or response to a direct tactile stimulus are the basis for the non-stress test, indicating the presence of an intact autonomic nervous system and a healthy fetus. A reactive non-stress test is predictive of fetal well-being at the time of the test and has been associated with fetal survival for 1 week in 99% of cases.

Accelerations of FHR of at least 15 beats per minute that last at least 15 seconds during labor are also reassuring and are associated with normal fetal scalp blood pH values. FHR accelera-

tion in response to a tactile stimulus, even in the presence of FHR patterns suggesting acidosis, appears to be an excellent indication of fetal well-being. Clark and colleagues reported that no fetus with acidosis (pH < 7.20) had an acceleration of FHR in response to digital stimulus or scalp blood sampling. All fetuses who did respond had pH levels of 7.20 or greater. These findings suggest that the presence of FHR accelerations in response to scalp stimulation may be a better tool than fetal blood pH for diagnosing fetal distress because it provides a biophysical measure of autonomic function of the fetus rather than a biochemical measure. Thus, this noninvasive technique can reduce the need for fetal scalp blood sampling and provide information regarding the metabolic state of the fetus during labor. It may be of special value during early labor, when fetal scalp blood sampling would be technically difficult, or in clinical settings where scalp blood pH monitors are not available. The sporadic use of fetal blood sampling in an attempt to diagnose fetal distress is an idealistic goal, but it is unrealistic in most clinical settings. In one study, an adequate fetal blood sample could not be obtained in 17% of all cases of suspected fetal distress.

The technique for fetal scalp stimulation is quite simple. With the patient in the dorsal lithotomy or lateral Sims' position, a vaginal examination is performed. Pressure is applied by the examining finger directly to the fetal presenting part. Fundal pressure may be necessary in some cases to prevent disengaging the presenting part in early labor. Occasionally, sweeping the examining finger in a circular motion (much like stripping membranes) is necessary to evoke a fetal response. FHR acceleration may or may not be immediate. A persistent increase in baseline FHR or accelerations that are delayed (occurring within 10 minutes of the stimulus) are as predictive of fetal well-being as are immediate accelerations (Fig. 1).

We do not routinely pinch the fetal scalp with an Ellis clamp, as was reported in an initial study. However, during the process of preparing to take

TABLE 1. Fetal Central Nervous System Centers

Fetal tone	Cortex (subcortical area?)		↑
Fetal movements	Cortex nuclei	Embryogenesis	Hypoxia
Fetal breathing movements	Ventral surface of fourth ventricle	↓	
Non-stress test	Posterior hypothalamus, medulla		

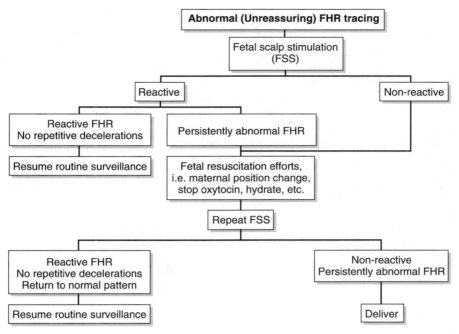

Figure 1. Algorithm for utilization of scalp stimulation to diagnose fetal distress.

a fetal scalp blood sample, inserting the viewing cone frequently stimulates FHR accelerations. These accelerations are as predictive of a nonacidotic fetus as any other stimuli, and thus the scalp puncture is not necessary. On rare occasions, one may resort to pinching the fetal scalp for 5 seconds with a long, loose Ellis clamp when the fetus does not respond to either digital pressure or the pressure from the viewing cone against the presenting part.

Fetal Surgical Management of Congenital Hydronephrosis

Michael R. Foley, MD

Since the early 1960s, prenatal diagnosis has become increasingly sophisticated, leading to an expanded knowledge of the pathophysiology and natural history of many structural fetal anomalies. As a natural consequence to this evolution in diagnostic capabilities, advances in fetal thera-

peutic modalities have also progressed. Until the early 1980s, however, little was known about the natural history of congenital fetal hydronephrosis. During the last decade, a better understanding of the natural history and pathophysiology of fetal obstructive uropathy has been elucidated using experimental animal models. These models have established rationales for the current concept of urinary decompression in an attempt to preserve fetal renal and pulmonary development. The purpose of this chapter is to review current prenatal diagnosis, prognostic indicators, and fetal surgical intervention for congenital fetal hydronephrosis.

Prenatal Diagnosis

Technologic improvements in ultrasonographic image quality have led to earlier detection of fetal urinary tract abnormalities. Current diagnostic capabilities allow for detection of urinary tract abnormalities in fetuses as early as 12 to 14 weeks' gestation. The goals of the diagnostician are to distinguish normal physiologic urinary pelvic distention from pathologic hydronephrosis that may potentially benefit from serial ultrasonographic assessments or invasive fetal surgery, or both. Figure 1 presents the initial diagnostic ap-

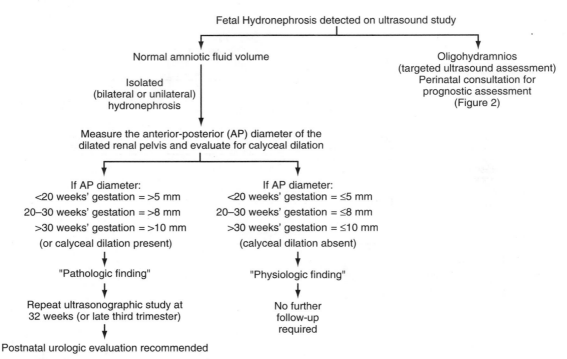

Figure 1. Algorithm for the initial assessment and management of congenital fetal hydronephrosis.

proach to the fetus with hydronephrosis. Once the fetus with pathologic hydronephrosis has been identified, the etiology for the abnormality should be investigated. Table 1 lists the various etiologies for congenital fetal hydronephrosis.

Prognostic Evaluation

After careful ultrasonographic assessment of the fetal urinary tract and karyotype evaluation, attention should be directed toward investigating the impact the abnormality has had on fetal structure and development. The two areas of primary concern for the clinician are the extent of fetal renal injury and the adverse developmental consequences from the resultant oligohydramnios. In humans, oligohydramnios adversely affects pulmonary development and, depending on the embryologic phase in which oligohydramnios occurs, may result in life-threatening pulmonary hypoplasia. Table 2 reviews the important phases of embryologic pulmonary development. The mechanism by which oligohydramnios causes pulmonary hypoplasia is uncertain. Several possible theories have been entertained, in-

TABLE 1. Etiologies of Congenital Hydronephrosis

Bilateral Hydronephrosis	Unilateral Hydronephrosis
Obstruction above the bladder	Ureteropelvic junction obstruction
Bilateral ureteropelvic junction obstruction	Ureterovesical junction obstruction
Bilateral ureterovesical junction obstruction	Congenital megaureter
Obstruction below the bladder	Renal duplication
Urethral atresia	
Posterior urethral valves	
Obstructing urethrocele	
Other	
Prune belly syndrome	
Vesicourethral reflux	
Megacystis-megaureter complex	

TABLE 2. Embryologic Phases of Fetal Lung Development

Period		Development
Pseudoglandular period (5th–17th week)	⟶	Conductive airways formed
Canalicular period (17th–24th week)	⟶	Respiratory bronchioles formed; pulmonary vasculature expanded
Terminal sac period (24th week–term)	⟶	Primitive alveoli formed, surfactant produced from Type II pneumocytes
Alveolar period (term–8 years)	⟶	Mature alveoli formed

cluding decreased lung fluid, extrinsic thoracic compression, and limited fetal breathing movement. Uncorrected oligohydramnios has been associated with a neonatal mortality rate approaching 100%, whereas if the amniotic fluid volume is restored to near normal levels, the survival rate has been reported to be approximately 94%. Intrauterine fetal renal failure may occur as a consequence of the imposing urinary pathologic process. Even if adequate amniotic fluid has been present to allow for uncompromised fetal pulmonary development, survival for a neonate with renal failure is extremely unlikely. The goal for the clinician, therefore, is to identify the intrauterine problem early enough in the course of the disease to potentially favorably influence the outcome of the fetus. The practical circumstances surrounding the detection and referral of the fetus with urinary tract abnormalities prior to significant fetal compromise, however, make this goal difficult to attain. The clinician is often placed in a position of being unable to determine whether irreversible fetal injury has already occurred. Prognostic indicators in the form of abnormally appearing fetal kidneys and abnormal fetal urinary electrolyte levels (measured by serial fetal vesicocenteses) have been successfully employed to assist the clinician in identifying those fetuses that may benefit from invasive fetal surgical decompression (Fig. 2). Table 3 lists the sonographic and urine biochemi-

cal criteria that are considered to indicate "favorable prognosis" for fetal decompression.

In Utero Vesicoamniotic Shunt Placement

As the results of the prognostic evaluation become apparent, patients with a "favorable" prognostic assessment should be counseled regarding the risks and benefits of in utero urinary decompression. In our institution, the primary method for urinary decompression is ultrasonographically guided fetal vesicoamniotic shunt placement. The risks of this procedure include the following:

1. Procedure-related mortality of approximately 4% to 5%
2. Chorioamnionitis up to 14%
3. Catheter obstruction or dislodgement
4. Fetal injury during placement
5. Potential iatrogenic gastroschisis
6. Potentially inadequate urinary decompression

The use of the KCH catheter (Rocket USA, Inc, Branford, CT) has minimized morbid complications in our institution (Fig. 3). The severity of renal dysplasia and pulmonary hypoplasia at birth clearly depends on the timing and severity of the urinary obstruction prior to birth. The proper selection of the fetus with a "favorable"

TABLE 3. Sonographic and Urine Biochemical Criteria to Be Considered "Favorable Prognosis" for Fetal Decompression*

Chromosomal Evaluation	Sonographic Criteria	Urine Biochemistry
Normal karyotype	Absent fetal renal cortical cysts Normal low renal echogenicity	Sodium <100 MEq/L Chloride <90 MEq/L Osmolarity <210 mOsm/L Calcium <2 mmol/L Phosphate <2 mmol/L B-2 microglobulin <2 mg/L

*"Poor prognosis" is implied if values or descriptions are not consistent with the criteria for "favorable prognosis."

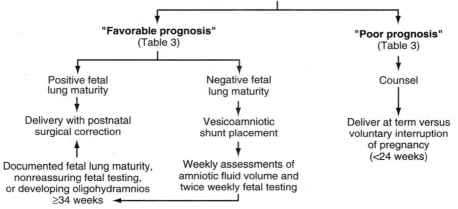

Figure 2. Fetal prognostic assessment.

prognostic assessment for in utero decompression improves the reported success of this procedure but does not guarantee a favorable outcome. It appears that the best outcomes follow decompression during the most active period of nephrogenesis (20–30 weeks' gestation), allowing for early normalization of amniotic fluid volume and minimizing continued renal injury. Patients and families should acknowledge a clear understanding of the indications for the procedure, the risks of the procedure, and the potential success (without guarantee) before intrauterine therapy is initiated.

Fetal Surgical Procedure

Under direct ultrasonographic guidance, in a sterile operating suite, the trochar with sheath

(see Fig. 3A) is introduced into the amniotic cavity above the anterior lateral aspect of the fetal bladder. Warmed normal saline is infused to create an amniotic fluid pocket outside of the fetus in which to leave the proximal pigtail catheter coil. The trochar with sheath is then advanced into the fetal bladder. The trochar is removed and the KCH catheter is uncoiled and threaded into the sheath. The short obturator (see Fig. 3A) is then used to push the distal pigtail coil into the bladder. The sheath is then pulled back slowly until it is free from the fetal anterior abdominal wall within the amniotic cavity. The long obturator (see Fig. 3A) is then placed, pushing the proximal pigtail coil into the amniotic cavity. The bladder will be seen to decompress, allowing fetal urine to egress into the amniotic space. Figure 4 illustrates how ultrasonographic

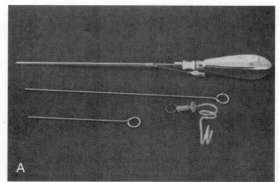

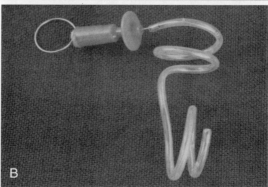

Figure 3. A, The trochar and sheath used for the KCH catheter. Below are the long and short obturators. The KCH catheter is to the right for scale. **B,** A close-up view of the KCH catheter with the pigtail ends at 90 degrees to each other. (From Crombleholme TM: Invasive fetal therapy: Current status and further directions. Semin Perinatol 1994;18[4]:389.)

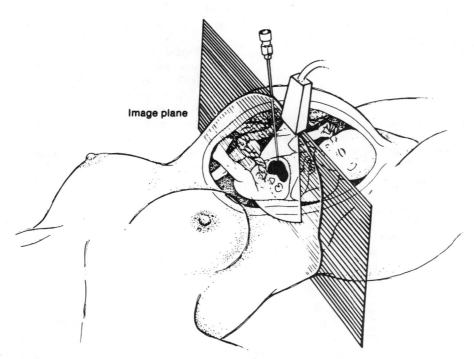

Figure 4. Illustrative representation of ultrasound-guided access to the fetal bladder. (From Finberg HJ, Clewell WH: Ultrasound-guided interventions in pregnancy. Ultrasound Q 1990;8[3]:197–226.)

assistance helps obtain access to the fetal bladder.

Summary

The prenatal diagnosis and management of fetal congenital hydronephrosis is a challenging process. Recent advances in the quality of our ultrasonographic equipment and improvements in the understanding of the pathophysiology and natural history of this disease have, through more careful selection of appropriate candidates for intervention, led to increased fetal survival and lessened overall morbidity. Fetal surgical intervention is a highly specialized procedure that, in appropriately selected and counseled patients, may be offered as a valuable therapeutic option.

Glucose Metabolism, Hypocalcemia, and Hypomagnesemia in the Newborn

Leandro Cordero, MD

Hypoglycemia

At birth, umbilical cord glucose levels correlate with maternal values; on the average they are higher in infants born following cesarean delivery (105 mg/dL) than those born vaginally (80 mg/dL). Blood glucose levels decrease during the first 2 hours of life to about 50 mg/dL and following the surge of counter-regulatory hormones (epinephrine and glucagon) rise slowly and stabilize. During this transitional period, it is not unusual to observe single instances of borderline or low blood glucose value. The diagnosis of hypoglycemia is usually based on two consecutively low values on samples taken 30 minutes apart. Hypoglycemia in full-term and premature infants is defined by a true blood glucose of 35 mg/dL (1.7 mM/L) or less during the first 3 hours of life, less than 40 mg/dL (2.2 mM/L) during the remainder of the first day, and 45 mg/dL (2.5 mM/L) or less thereafter. Following birth, preterm infants also experience a fall in blood glucose but, unlike full-term infants, are less able to mount an effective counter-regulatory response; some investigations, therefore, are challenging the old notion that premature infants can tolerate lower blood glucose levels. We no longer define hypoglycemia in the premature infant at lower levels than those of the full-term infant.

Over the last 20 years, the biochemical definition of neonatal hypoglycemia has changed slightly, and yet, surprisingly, the overall incidence of this condition remains undetermined. Transient hypoglycemia affects 0.5% to 4% of apparently healthy full-term neonates; other well-defined clinical entities place certain infants at much higher risk. Premature infants whose birth weights are below 2000 g (33 to 34 weeks of gestation) seldom experience hypoglycemia because they are usually admitted to newborn intensive care units (NICUs) where they receive continuous intravenous infusions of dextrose. On the other hand, larger premature infants (34 weeks to 37 weeks of gestation), who usually receive the traditional care reserved for full-term infants, experience hypoglycemia about 30% of the time. In nondiabetic pregnancies, 8% of large for gestational age (LGA) and 15% of small for gestational age (SGA) infants become hypoglycemic at an average age of 3 and 6 hours, respectively. SGA infants are at extreme risk for hypoglycemia due to their minimal fat and glycogen reserves. Neonatal hypoglycemia among infants born to diabetic mothers (IDMs) tends to be less common and milder in the infant whose mother's condition is well controlled throughout pregnancy and who remains euglycemic during labor and delivery. In clinical practice, screening for low blood glucose is done with a chromogen strip test (Chemstrip). The results of this simple and rapid test should be interpreted cautiously. Comparative studies have shown that Chemstrip readings will underestimate 10% of hypoglycemic values (false negatives) and will overdiagnose hypoglycemia in up to 20% of borderline cases (false positives). In addition, samples with hematocrit over 70% will produce falsely low blood glucose readings about 50% of the time. In spite of these statistics, chromogen strip tests are valuable, especially when they are promptly followed by "true" (serum or plasma) blood glucose determinations.

In 1993 the American Academy of Pediatrics (AAP) discouraged universal screening for hypoglycemia while strongly advocating it for infants at risk (eg, LGA or SGA infants, IDMs, meconium-stained infants, infants with perinatal distress or congenital malformations, premature infants). A recent clinical study shows that 72%

of 236 infants with such risk factors developed hypoglycemia. Since the incidence of hypoglycemia varies with the type of obstetric population and clinical practice, the AAP condones universal screening in institutions with large numbers of infants at risk for hypoglycemia.

The clinical diagnosis of hypoglycemia is difficult since the majority (60–70%) of infants remain asymptomatic. These signs are lethargy, hypotonia, jitteriness, poor feeding, tachypnea, apnea, diaphoresis, shrill cry, and seizures. Symptomatic infants usually present with a combination of these signs.

Nursing and medical management of newborns strongly influences the incidence of transient hypoglycemia. Short delivery room stay, careful control of environmental and body temperature, establishment of early feedings, and aggressive blood glucose screening undoubtedly minimize the occurrence of neonatal hypoglycemia. The use of intravenous dextrose in the nondiabetic mother during labor increases the incidence of neonatal hypoglycemia, especially when β-adrenergic agonists (some tocolytic agents) are added since they increase fetal insulin release. Forty percent of infants of appropriate size for gestational age born by cesarean section to nondiabetic mothers and 37% of those born vaginally were reported to have blood glucose levels of 40 mg/dL (2.2 mM/L) or less at 2 hours of life. This transient hypoglycemia has been linked to the high incidence of the use of regional anesthesia in that obstetric population.

In our institution, the average healthy full-term infant leaves the delivery room 20 to 45 minutes after birth. Transport to the well-baby nursery usually takes 5 minutes and is conducted in a battery-operated incubator. If, on arrival to the nursery, the skin temperature is 96°F or less, the newborn is considered to be hypothermic and at risk for hypoglycemia and a stat Chemstrip test is performed. Readings in the abnormal range are promptly followed by a true serum blood glucose test and an oral feeding. Although the incidence of hypoglycemia associated with hypothermia is undetermined, we believe it to be common. Other infants at risk for hypoglycemia are those who experienced any form of perinatal distress (eg, low Apgar scores, meconium-stained fluid, maternal hypertension, Rh incompatibility). Neonatal hypoglycemia is often transient (as in the cases described earlier) but on rare occasions can be persistent and refractory to treatment. Such is the case with hereditary defects in amino acid and carbohydrate metabolism, single or multiple hormonal deficiencies, or hyperinsulinemic conditions (eg, nesidioblastosis, Beckwith-Wiedemann syndrome).

Infants at Risk for Hypoglycemia

Upon the infant's arrival at the triage nursery, a Chemstrip test is done and oral feedings (breast milk, D10W, or formula) are started. We prefer formula or breast milk because they provide more energy per milliliter than D10W, supply important nonglucose fuels, and promote ketogenesis and gut maturation. The energy content of formula is 2750 kJ/L while that of D10W is 1600 kJ/L. For infants with poor sucking, gavage feedings are provided. Chemstrip values that are borderline or definitely low (<40 mg/dL) are confirmed with serum glucose determination (turnaround time from sampling to report is about 20 minutes). Failure to measure blood glucose concentrations promptly after sampling allows blood cell glucose oxidation resulting in falsely low plasma values. The Chemstrip test and serum glucose levels are repeated ½ hour apart until the next feeding and as needed thereafter. If, after the initial oral feeding, glucose levels remain abnormally low or if the infant is symptomatic (regardless of glucose levels), transfer to the NICU is considered urgent and mandatory. On admission, a peripheral venous access is immediately obtained but if this proves to be difficult or if the symptoms are severe, we advise the temporary placement of an umbilical venous catheter. Once this is done, we administer a slow (2-minute) intravenous infusion of 2 mL/kg D10W to be followed by 100 mL/kg/24 hours of D10W (equivalent to 8 mg/kg/minute of glucose).

We continue to monitor blood glucose hourly until the symptoms have disappeared and the serum glucose values have returned to normal. If, in spite of these measures, serum glucose levels remain abnormal or if the symptoms have not abated, we increase the continuous infusion 2 mg/kg/minute at the time to a maximum of 12 mg/kg/minute of glucose infusion (using D10W, that represents an intravenous fluid infusion of about 180 mL/kg/day). We do not favor administration of higher concentrations of glucose in water (hypertonic glucose boluses) since they inhibit glucagon secretion, decrease the threshold for insulin release ("positive feedback loop"), and depress hepatic glucose release.

After serum glucose control has been obtained with the intravenous regimen and if the infant's condition so allows, oral feedings (gavage if necessary) are restarted. During the next 24 to 48 hours, the intravenous glucose load is tapered while the oral intake is increased.

Symptomatic Infants

Whether high risk or not, infants who present with signs compatible with hypoglycemia should be treated expeditiously. In our nurseries, apnea, cyanosis, and seizures mandate immediate admissions to the NICU. Increased respiratory rate, temperature instability, poor feeding, hypotonia, and sweating, if not relieved by one or two feedings, also lead to an NICU admission. Many clinical signs of hypoglycemia may be due to other underlying pathology such as sepsis or pneumonia. Thus, treatment of hypoglycemia often requires a thorough clinical, radiologic, and laboratory differential diagnosis.

Infants of Diabetic Mothers

It is well established that IDMs are at risk for problems other than hypoglycemia. Delayed pulmonary maturation, a high incidence of congenital malformations, polycythemia, hyperbilirubinemia, hypocalcemia, and hypomagnesemia are some of the multiple challenges affecting these infants. We recommend that on admission of an LGA or SGA infant born to an insulin-dependent or gestational diabetic mother to the triage nursery, a hematocrit and hemoglobin and a capillary (or arterial) blood gas be obtained. A deliberate effort should be made to prevent cold injury by postponing baths or prolonging the time these infants spend under radiant warmers. Considering that IDMs are deficient in peripheral catecholamines, do not have normal glucagon surges in the first hours of life, and have an inadequate hepatic glucose production, some investigators advocate simultaneous use of glucose infusions and glucagon administration (200 µg/kg intravenous bolus). In our institution, approximately 8% of the 3800 newborns delivered every year are IDMs (one third insulin-dependent and two thirds gestational diabetic). Since our goal is to prevent hypoglycemia, we initiate intravenous dextrose infusions in about 80% of insulin-dependent and 20% of gestational diabetic infants (Table 1). The selection of the patients is based on coexisting risk factors for hypoglycemia. Since we do not administer intravenous fluids to patients in the well-baby nurseries, this procedure requires direct admission to the NICU. Among infants who do not receive immediate intravenous dextrose infusions, 25% of insulin-dependent and 10% of gestational diabetic infants develop hypoglycemia and require delayed admission to the NICU.

TABLE 1. Admissions to the Neonatal Intensive Care Unit Among Infants Born to Diabetic Mothers°

State at Birth	Infants Born to Insulin-Dependent Mothers (n[%])	Infants Born to Gestational-Diabetic Mothers (n[%])
Premature	21 (100)	42 (74)
LGA	55 (73)	48 (13)
AGA	40 (63)	117 (5)
SGA	14 (78)	15 (20)
Total	130 (82%)	222 (21%)

°Total n = 352 born at the Ohio State University Medical Center, 1994–1995.
  AGA, average for gestational age; LGA, large for gestational age; SGA, small for gestational age.

Hyperglycemia

A serum glucose level higher than 150 mg/dL (6.9 mM/L) biochemically defines hyperglycemia during the neonatal period. Due to the placental transfer of glucose, maternal hyperglycemia corresponds to transient neonatal hyperglycemia. This increase in serum glucose level produces an insulinemic response that eventually could result in "rebound" hypoglycemia. Similar responses are also triggered by therapeutic infusions of glucose at high concentrations (D15W to D50W). Furthermore, high concentration solutions are highly osmolar and quite damaging to vessels and soft tissues.

Hyperglycemia occurs in about 5% of NICU admissions, especially in very low birth weight infants. In an effort to prevent this, we advocate the use of D5W infusions for infants with birth weights less than 1000 g. It has been shown that low tolerance to glucose infusion is related to birth weight, dosage, and the infusion of lipids. Associations of hyperglycemia and other pathologic conditions are still unclear. It is known that hyperglycemia results in increases in serum osmolarity (a 180 mg glucose infusion is accompanied by an increase of 10 mOsm/dL). Experimental work with kittens provided linkage between serum osmolarity shifts and intracranial hemorrhages. Very low birth weight infants who receive excessive infusions of glucose (10–16 mg/kg/minute) often experience glucosuria and occasionally may develop hypovolemia.

In the majority of cases of hyperglycemia, strict control of the glucose intake suffices to correct the problem. Occasionally in very small premature infants, slow infusion of regular insulin (0.05–0.1 unit/kg/hour) may be required.

Hypocalcemia and Hypomagnesemia

Approximately one half of premature infants of diabetic mothers develop early transient hypocalcemia. Although the cause for the high incidence of this complication is unclear, it is well recognized that it relates to the severity of maternal diabetes, perinatal distress, and prematurity. Often, hypocalcemic infants display low serum magnesium values. In poorly controlled maternal diabetes, serum, amniotic fluid, and fetal and neonatal magnesium levels are low. Neonatal hypomagnesemia seems to impair parathyroid hormone secretion and also blunts end-organ response, all of which leads to hypocalcemia. Irritability, jitteriness, tongue thrusting, lip smacking, apnea, and, occasionally, seizures can be the presenting signs. The majority of infants, however, may be clinically unrecognizable. In the newborn period, hypocalcemia is defined as total serum calcium values lower than 6 mg/dL (3 mEq/L) or ionized calcium levels below 4 mg/dL (2 mEq/L). Ionized calcium levels, although more physiologically accurate, require a heparinized larger blood sample.

Infants who remain symptomatic after correction of hypoglycemia or who have low serum calcium values are treated with a slow infusion of 10% calcium gluconate (100 mg/kg). For premature infants or those with refractory hypocalcemia, a 400 mg/kg/day intravenous infusion is established. In the rare case of newborns who, in spite of this treatment, remain symptomatic or who present with magnesium levels below 1.5 mg/dL (0.7 mM/L), a single intramuscular injection (0.1–0.3 mL/kg) of 50% magnesium sulfate solution should be considered.

Hydrocephalus: Diagnosis and Treatment

James A. O'Leary, MD
James L. O'Leary II, JD

In recent years, the diagnosis and evaluation of fetal hydrocephalus and its ethical implications have become a greater challenge as well as an exercise in meticulous differential diagnosis. Unfortunately, the outlook remains very poor, with a high perinatal death rate and a high incidence of mental retardation in survivors.

Hydrocephalus is not a rare disorder; its incidence is between 0.5 and 1.8 per 1000 live births. It is usually sporadic in its occurrence and there is rarely a positive family history. In most cases the etiology is unknown. In our experience, this disorder poses difficult practical and ethical problems for the family, since they are often faced with a very poor prognosis for normal intellectual development, as well as the potential for long-term care of a completely dependent person.

Hydrocephalus is the most common major anatomic abnormality seen in neonatal brain. This abnormality may result from aqueductal stenosis or may be associated with a spinal diastrophism. Other developmental anomalies such as holoprosencephaly or hydranencephaly may also be identified. It is important to note that many significant congenital anomalies, such as heterotopias, cannot be identified radiologically. The newest imaging modality applied in the neonatal period is magnetic resonance imaging scanning. This technique is especially valuable for examining white matter changes and delineating the anatomy of the posterior fossa. Delayed myelination has been observed in neonates with complicated perinatal courses.

Pathophysiology and Associated Anomalies

We categorize enlargement of the cerebral ventricles into two main groups: ventriculomegaly due to obstruction of the flow of fluid through and out of the ventricular system with subsequent elevation of intraventricular pressure and dilatation of the ventricles, or primary destruction of brain tissue with excess accumulation of cerebrospinal fluid without elevated pressure.

Hydrocephaly dilating the ventricles compresses the developing cortex and eventually destroys neurologic function. Early damage is mainly to the white matter, which thins out, while gray matter is untouched. The increased pressure causes periventricular edema, flattening and disruption of the ependymal lining, and nerve fiber destruction in the subependymal white matter and the corpus callosum. As edema subsides, periventricular gliosis ensues with or without reconstitution of the ependyma.

Obstruction of the fluid outflow is the usual cause of increased intraventricular pressure. Reduced absorption or increased production by a papilloma of the choroid plexus is much more rare. Obstruction is very often not an entity by itself but rather a manifestation of cytomegalovirus, rubella, syphilis, toxoplasmosis, and chromosomal anomalies (especially trisomy 13 and 18).

Hydrocephalus is commonly associated with other congenital anomalies (37%). They include hypoplasia of the corpus callosum, cephalocele, arteriovenous malformation, and arachnoid cyst. Extracranial anomalies are present in 63% of cases and include meningomyelocele, renal anomalies (bilateral or unilateral renal agenesis, dysplastic kidneys), cardiac anomalies (ventricular septal defect, tetralogy of Fallot), gastrointestinal anomalies (colon and anal agenesis, malrotation of the bowel), cleft lip and palate, Meckel's syndrome, gonadal dysgenesis, sirenomelia, arthrogryposis, and dysplastic phalanges.

Etiology and Prenatal Diagnosis

Conditions causing obstruction include aqueductal stenosis in about 40% of cases; blockage of the subarachnoid pathway, referred to as communicating hydrocephalus or extraventricular hydrocephalus in about 40%; Dandy-Walker syndrome in about 10%; and other types of anatomic abnormalities in about 10%. The majority of cases are multifactorial in origin.

Observation of a normal cerebellum effectively rules out Arnold-Chiari and Dandy-Walker malformations. The presence of the corpus callosum should be noted on coronal views of the head.

The anatomic features of various abnormal karyotypes are inconstant and may be relatively subtle on ultrasonogram. Congenital heart disease, especially endocardial cushion defects, are relatively common in Down syndrome. The inability to obtain a normal four-chamber view of the fetal heart should suggest the possibility that the fetal karyotype may be abnormal. The finding of cysts in the liver or kidney should suggest the possibility of Meckel's syndrome, which has a

very poor prognosis regardless of the degree of ventricular enlargement. Even minor details may be critically important to making an etiologic diagnosis. The finding of multiple anomalies makes an abnormal karyotype highly likely.

Viral infections as a cause of fetal hydrocephalus carry an extremely bad prognosis. They cause both obstruction to the drainage of cerebrospinal fluid and direct destruction of brain tissue. One can suspect this etiology if certain telltale features are seen. Nonimmune hydrops fetalis may occur and may be transient. Cerebral calcifications may be seen, but more commonly one sees subtle abnormalities of brain texture on ultrasonogram. While none of these features are completely diagnostic of congenital viral infections, they are suggestive enough to warrant viral cultures.

We offer every affected family fetal karyotype and viral cultures. These must be interpreted with caution because amniotic fluid viral cultures may not be positive with fetal infection. Furthermore, viral culture techniques are highly specific and one can only culture for relatively common organisms such as cytomegalovirus. It seems likely that other organisms can also cause congenital infections with hydrocephalus. Culture of amniotic fluid cells for karyotype is highly reliable and almost always reflects the fetal karyotype. While amniocentesis is usually sufficient, there will be occasions when the finding is suspect or a more rapid analysis must be obtained. In these cases, we recommend fetal umbilical blood sampling.

Prognosis

Unfortunately, in a great number of cases the etiology is imprecise, which makes prediction of the outcome very difficult. The natural history depends more on the underlying process than on the extent of ventriculomegaly or width of the cerebral mantle. Although a cortical width of less than 10 mm seems to be associated with a grim outcome, this correlation is imperfect, and excellent neurologic outcomes have been observed after early shunting with mantle thicknesses of less than 10 mm. This parameter should not be used as the sole criterion for obstetric management.

Earlier studies indicated a high infant mortality rate; however, the advent of prenatal diagnosis, judicious obstetric practices, and expert neonatal and surgical care has resulted in a marked improvement in prognosis. About 80% of infants with spina bifida have hydrocephalus as well;

possibly as a consequence of this association, a perinatal mortality rate of about 75% has been reported.

The most important prognostic consideration is the presence and nature of the associated anomalies, and a fetal period of more than 2 months after the diagnosis of hydrocephalus. When the hydrocephalic state develops early in utero, the outcome is usually considerably poorer, with only a 15% survival rate after an average follow-up period of 13 months. Most of these cases have several etiologic causes and frequently are associated with other anomalies. Poor signs in the early hydrocephalic fetus include multiple extracranial anomalies.

Congenital hydrocephalus has an overall recurrence risk of 1.4%. Since hydrocephalus is often the final common pathway of a number of etiologic agents, it is difficult to assess individual prevalences by agent.

Treatment

Several options are available when fetal hydrocephalus is diagnosed: termination of pregnancy, withholding therapy, and fetal surgery.

At late gestations, delivery and neonatal treatment are clearly the best option. With enlargement of the fetal head, vaginal delivery may not be a viable option. We recommend that delivery be carried out in a hospital with a special care nursery and the availability of a pediatric neurologist and neurosurgeon. Prior consultation with the specialists to be involved in the care of the baby increases the family's confidence in the specialists and reduces their stress level.

Termination of pregnancy is recommended if legally permissible, if the diagnosis is made sufficiently early, with indications of worsening of the ventriculomegaly, and if there are no religious or moral objections.

In midpregnancy, delivery is not usually a reasonable option. Owing to the relatively large size of the ventricles in early pregnancy, the diagnosis usually cannot be made with confidence prior to about 20 weeks' gestation. Once ventriculomegaly is suspected, the next step is confirmation of the finding and determination of the rate of progression. There is usually about a 2-week wait for the viral cultures and karyotype to be reported.

We feel that management options depend on the severity of the ventriculomegaly at the time of diagnosis and on the rate of progression. Mild disease may require no specific treatment in the perinatal period. In these cases, management decisions are made after delivery based on neonatal evaluation. Some infants will have extremely severe ventricular enlargement when first seen. In these situations one must provide humane care for the family and the fetus. One must avoid a natural sense of urgency and recognize that this is not an emergency and that decisions are best made after the family has dealt with the initial shock of diagnosis.

Progressive disease detected in midpregnancy poses the most distressing problem for the family and the physicians. Delivery is not an option due to extreme prematurity. While waiting for maturity there is progressive loss of brain tissue owing to elevated intraventricular pressure. The helplessness of the family and physicians is most acutely felt in those cases in which the obstructive hydrocephaly appears to be an isolated lesion. It is this group of patients that prompted the attempt to treat hydrocephalus in utero.

If the diagnosis is made too late for termination of the pregnancy, if there are objections to termination, or if severe malformation or signs of intrauterine infections make fetal therapy inappropriate, a "wait and see" policy is adopted. The decision as to when to deliver the fetus has to take into consideration the degree of enlargement of the fetal head. Similar considerations apply to deciding how the baby will be delivered, that is, vaginally versus by cesarean section, and whether cerebral decompression will be performed.

We feel there are few data to support any specific management plan. Our general recommendations include delaying delivery until fetal lung maturity is documented, avoiding cephalocentesis, and using cesarean section for obstetric indications only. Fetal lung maturity is determined by performing weekly amniocentesis beginning at 36 weeks of gestation.

Fetal Treatment

Cephalocentesis

Cephalocentesis, the transabdominal or transvaginal aspiration of cerebrospinal fluid to avoid cesarean delivery, is associated with perinatal mortality in excess of 90% and its use should be limited to those instances in which hydrocephaly is associated with anomalies carrying a dismal prognosis (eg, thanatophoric dysplasia and Meckel's syndrome). In our 35-year experience, cephalocentesis has resulted in a 100% mortality rate. This procedure should be performed under sonographic guidance. Macrocrania or overt hydrocephaly (head circumference above the 98th percentile for gestational age) in the absence of any other associated anomaly suggesting poor prognosis is not an automatic indication for cephalocentesis. Cesarean section is reserved for standard obstetric indications (eg, fetal distress, failure to progress in labor) and if the biparietal diameter is greater than 10 cm.

When a pregnancy is complicated by hydrocephalus with macrocephaly, there may be a role for cephalocentesis. Because the use of cephalocentesis carries a high rate of morbidity and mortality in a fetus shortly before birth, ethical justification is required for its use. This justification can be based on an analysis of beneficence-based and autonomy-based obligations to the pregnant woman and the fetus she is carrying.

Shunting

Intrauterine treatment consisting of the implantation of a ventriculoamniotic shunt for the relief of intracranial pressure during gestation has been attempted by others. Although experience in animal models appears encouraging, the clinical application of these procedures remains undetermined. In a group of 39 treated fetuses, the perinatal mortality rate was 18%, and 66% of the survivors were affected by moderate to severe handicaps.

The following guidelines have been proposed:

1. The hydrocephalus should be detected sufficiently early that delivery and postnatal shunting are not realistic options.
2. The hydrocephalus should appear as a simple obstructive variety without major dysmorphic brain development.
3. The hydrocephalus should not be associated with other major malformations (including positive viral cultures for the amniotic fluid or fetus).
4. Each pregnancy should be evaluated for chromosomal abnormalities and associated neural tube defects during the initial assessment.
5. The ventricular dilatation should be progressive.
6. Pretreatment evaluation should include a multidisciplinary consultation including specialists in perinatology, neonatology, ultrasonography, neurosurgery, and genetics.

A set criterion for fetal treatment was also established and supported by the Society of Fetal Medicine. Careful selection of the fetal patients is based on team opinion of those involved in antenatal treatment, natural history of the fetal defect, exclusion of severely affected fetuses who will not benefit from antenatal treatment because of pre-existing irreversible damage, and exclusion of severely affected fetuses who will benefit from postnatal treatment. Consultations are concerned with legal arrangements and family commitments for a long-term follow-up. The specific criteria are as follows:

1. Ventriculomegaly with no evidence of multiple malformations
2. Affected fetus too young for early delivery (before 30 weeks of gestation)
3. Sonographic evidence of continuous enlargement of ventricles and decreases of cortical mantle
4. A singleton pregnancy
5. The patient's understanding of the experimental treatment by the team of experts
6. The patient's commitment to long-term follow-up

In 1985, the total world experience of shunted infants was 40 cases. Thirty-four fetuses were delivered alive but 50% were severely handicapped and 8% were mildly handicapped. Of the 40, 8 died during treatment or within a short time after delivery, and in 4 (10%), intervention was probably the direct cause of death. Altogether, about 30% of shunted fetuses developed into normal babies. Comparison of these figures with published results for development of babies with congenital hydrocephalus diagnosed near term or after delivery fails to show any advantage of fetal shunt operations.

We believe there are several facts that militate against the performance of antenatal shunting:

1. Shunting did not improve the histopathologic damage of the brain.
2. Ultrasonography is incapable of distinguishing the fetus with dilated ventricles who has increased intracranial pressure, and these are obviously the only ones who are helped by a shunting procedure.
3. In shunted lambs, degenerative white matter changes and intraventricular adhesions have been observed.
4. There have been displacements, malfunctions, or occlusions of the shunts, necessitating multiple procedures with inherent increase in complications.
5. The only fetuses to benefit from the procedure and in whom it is justifiable to perform it are those with pure isolated hydrocephalus, and these cases are relatively rare. In fact most fetuses with ventriculo-

megaly do not require intervention before birth.

6. Intrauterine treatment increases the number of handicapped survivors, not the number of normal survivors.

In our opinion, the following treatment scheme is reasonable:

1. When hydrocephalus is extreme, the best solution, depending on fetal age, is either termination of pregnancy or nonintervention and eventual vaginal delivery after cephalocentesis.

2. When brain tissue exists there are three options: termination of pregnancy, withholding therapy until a further decision is made, or active treatment. If one chooses to withhold therapy, serial ultrasonographic follow-up should be performed. Thickness of under 10 mm is frequently a very poor prognostic sign.

Laparoscopic Approaches to Fetal Disease

The recent resurgence of interest in laparoscopic techniques has resulted in an explosion of new technology for laparoscopic procedures. However, the ability to perform major fetal surgery under direct vision through small puncture sites in the uterus has only recently become a realistic possibility. However, a number of modifications of current laparoscopic instrumentation and technique will be required to make fetal application possible.

Risk Management

The probability of detecting hydrocephalus prior to viability will depend on the nature of the lesion and its rate of progression. This can result in false-negative diagnoses. In contrast, incorrect diagnosis (false-positives) are also possible, since the data were generated in a general population and some normal fetuses will by definition fall outside the limits of normality. However, severe ventriculomegaly associated with macrocephaly should be identifiable. Associated anomalies are also frequently missed, including spina bifida. In addition, hydrocephalus may be mistaken for hydrencephaly, agenesis of the corpus callosum, and holoprosencephaly, and vice versa. Such an improper designation certainly does not constitute a departure from current standards of obstetric care.

We prefer to provide our patients with printed instructions. These are signed by the patient and witnessed at the next office visit.

Legal Aspects

We recommend that all reasonably available means be used to regularly monitor the size of the fetal head. The full spectrum of technology, including ultrasonography, magnetic resonance imaging (MRI), fetoscopy, and traditional methods should be used to properly evaluate the existence of hydrocephalic symptomatology. To maximize the utility and cost of performing the MRI, it would be most helpful if done at or around 20 weeks. The use of the MRI scan will help detect ventriculomegaly. A detailed history coupled with MRI will help detect the significant risk factors discussed herein. Indeed, in this day and age of increasing use of the technology for diagnostic purposes, simply failing to use the requisite technology needed to diagnosis such a condition may well be deemed negligence. Since the limits of liability traditionally have been based on what is reasonably foreseeable, once the hydrocephalus diagnosis is achieved, a significant portion of the potential liability is eliminated. If the practitioner detects any lesions or other signs of hydrocephalus in the fetus, it becomes critical to execute a detailed, thorough, and meticulous informed consent procedure to properly educate the patient of the potential devasting effects of hydrocephalus. The informed consent should thoroughly describe and explain all of the risks, benefits, and alternatives associated with hydrocephalus. The practitioner should of course aspire to deliver the often devasting and delicate news in a compassionate and sincere demeanor, as this will subjectively play a role in the patient's potential decision to seek legal recourse. Once hydrocephalus is diagnosed, it should be the practitioner's standard business practice to proceed with this detailed description of the disorder. Along with more thorough diagnostic testing, more and better documentation is critical in defending a potential claim arising out of hydrocephalus. A videotape of the informed consent may prove extremely helpful in the likely event that the patient initiates contact with legal counsel to assess the merits of a potential malpractice claim. The key is to develop systematic business procedures to standardize the process of informing the family of the hydrocephalic fetus. This ensures that this critical evidence is admissible at trial.

Conclusion

Although large clinical experiences are limited, the establishment of a more precise etiology and pathophysiologic evaluation is very important. A less invasive and more reliable decompressive technique for fetal hydrocephalus needs to be developed. Analysis of factors affecting the prognosis of intrauterine hydrocephalus in the third trimester supports the belief that the results of an ongoing hydrocephalic state may become irreversible during fetal life, especially after 60 days.

Lung Maturity Testing

Roger Lenke, MD
Edward Ashwood, MD

Respiratory distress syndrome (RDS) remains a significant cause of neonatal morbidity. Evaluation of fetal lung maturity is often used to determine the best time for delivery in either complicated pregnancies or planned deliveries. The ideal test would not only predict lung maturity 100% of the time, but would also predict actual fetal maturity without error. Conversely, an immature test would predict RDS 100% of the time. The test would have a rapid turnaround time and be easy to perform, inexpensive, and reproducible from laboratory to laboratory. The test would also be noninvasive or, as a minimum, need a small specimen size. Unfortunately, there is no such test currently available.

Neonatal Respiratory Distress

Neonatal respiratory distress is a clinical term that can have different etiologies. *Respiratory distress syndrome* is a clinical definition used when the infant has cyanosis, grunting, retractions, and progressive oxygen settings. True RDS appears to be caused by a deficiency of surfactant, which leads to atelectasis, decreased lung compliance, and increased work of breathing. Surfactant itself consists of lecithin (phosphatidylcholine), with smaller amounts of phosphatidylglycerol (PG), protein, and other lipids. Hyaline membrane disease is a pathologic definition in which there is an acidophilic membrane within the alveoli, uneven expansion of the alveoli, and variable necrosis of the pulmonary epithelium. Transient tachypnea of the newborn, infectious etiologies, and other structural anomalies (eg, diaphragmatic hernia) may often initially be confused with RDS or hyaline membrane disease.

Currently Available Tests for Predicting Fetal Lung Maturity

ACOG Criteria for Delivery at Term

ACOG guidelines state that if one of the following criteria is met, fetal maturity may be assumed and amniocentesis is not necessary:

1. Fetal heart tones documented for 20 weeks by fetoscope or 30 weeks by Doppler.
2. It has been 36 weeks since a positive serum or urine human chorionic gonadotropin pregnancy test.
3. Ultrasonographic measurement of the crown–rump length taken at 6 to 11 weeks' gestation supports a gestational age of 39 weeks or more.
4. Ultrasonographic measurements taken at 12 to 20 weeks' gestation confirm a gestational age of 39 weeks or more.

Ultrasonographic Criteria for Delivery at Term

With reasonably reliable dating criteria, the absolute biparietal diameter (BPD) also correlates well with lung maturity and the absence of RDS. In a nondiabetic population, having a BPD greater than 9.2 cm was not associated with infants that developed RDS. Before relying on the BPD, the patient should have been evaluated for diabetes and there should be no unusual discrepancies between the head measurement and other fetal measurements. Although placental grading was once thought to correlate with the presence and absence of RDS, it has not proven reliable enough to be used for the prediction of RDS.

Amniotic Fluid Evaluation

Amniocentesis Versus Vaginal Pool

Almost all other forms of evaluation for RDS risk involve some form of analysis of amniotic fluid. The most reliability and accuracy is obtained when an amniocentesis is performed under ultrasonographic guidance. The problem with studies evaluating vaginal pool samples is the inconsistency of the specimen obtained. Vaginal pool samples may be contaminated by mucus, blood, and different forms of bacteria. Differences may also arise depending on whether the vaginal pool sample was free-flowing or stagnant. When paired samples of vaginal pool specimens were compared with amniocentesis specimens from the same patient, the vaginal pool lecithin to sphingomyelin ratio (L:S) was significantly greater than that obtained at amniocentesis over 20% of the time. PG does appear to be useful in evaluating lung maturity in vaginal pool specimens, but other tests appear to be erratic.

Contamination

Even when amniocentesis is performed, there may be problems from sample contamination. If the specimen contains more than 1% fetal or maternal blood, the L:S ratio will be biased toward a value of 2 because plasma contains a high concentration of these phospholipids at that approximate ratio. PG usually remains accurate even when the sample is contaminated by blood. The presence of thick meconium makes most results not interpretable. Infections may interfere with interpretations. Even PG results have been reported as inaccurate in the presence of certain bacteria.

Lecithin to Sphingomyelin Ration

The L:S ratio is probably the most widely known test currently employed for fetal lung maturity evaluation. Unfortunately, it has many technical and clinical limitations. The procedure is extremely complicated and needs trained personnel. It is a slow, labor-intensive procedure that is difficult to standardize and reproduce from one laboratory to another. There are also many false-negative results (ie, immaturity predicted, but no RDS develops).

Phosphatidylglycerol

Although it has many proponents, evaluation for PG has limited clinical usefulness. The presence of PG may be determined by either thin layer chromatography with a methodology similar to that of the L:S ratio or by rapid slide test evaluation. The biggest problem with PG evaluation is that it is usually not present until near term. Only 56% of patients with pregnancies between 36 and 37 weeks' gestation will have positive PG. Even at 40 to 41 weeks, approximately 10% of the population will still not have detectable PG.

The currently available slide test is rapid and qualitative. Unfortunately, it has limited value because if positive there is a low incidence of RDS, and if negative there is also a low incidence of RDS. Quantitative evaluation of PG may eventually prove more useful, but at present the procedure is cumbersome and is usually performed only in a research setting.

Foam Stability Testing

Foam stability testing is based on the concept that surfactant maintains a stable bubble in the presence of ethanol after shaking. Whereas proteins, bilirubin, free fatty acids, and phospholipids produce foam, only saturated phosphatidylcholine will maintain a stable bubble in the presence of 47.5% ethanol. Although a rapid test, foam stability suffers from the same problems as PG. Thus, if positive, there is a low incidence of RDS, but if negative there is also a low incidence of RDS. Blood and meconium can also interfere with the results.

Fluorescence Polarization

Measurement of fluorescence polarization depends on the rotational diffusion of fluorescent dyes. Originally, Shinitzky hypothesized that fluorescence polarization (fpol) might reflect the lipid composition of surfactant and thus predict lung maturity. The original procedure proposed by Shinitzky was fast, precise, and simple. The accuracy was at least as good as that of the L:S ratio. Unfortunately, it required an instrument that was not commonly available and the dye used was not chemically stable when exposed to oxygen. Two other tests are currently available using the same technology and a polarimeter already available in most laboratories (Abbott TDx instrument). These two newer fpol methods actually reflect the amount of surfactant compared to the amount of albumin. The commercial version sold by Abbott Laboratories has a recommended reference range that is more conservative than that used in the other fpol methodology. The non-Abbott fpol evaluation uses a fluorescent lipid dye (NBD-PC) that is stable when exposed to oxygen. The procedure usually takes less than 30 minutes, requires a specimen of less than 1 mL, and has a coefficient of variation (CV) of only 1% to 2%. The Abbott version is reported in different units (milligram surfactant per gram albumin) and has a CV of 5%. Similar to the L:S ratio, blood and meconium can cause major interference. Values can be classified as mature, immature, and transitional. Using this technology, adjustment for the presence of diabetes does not appear necessary.

Lamellar Body Counts

This new method for assessing fetal lung maturity is promising but should not be used alone until more prospective clinical outcome studies are published. This technique uses the platelet channel of the Coulter Counter (a common clinical laboratory instrument) to count the number of surfactant particles per microliter. The technique has a CV of 10% at the maturity threshold of 60,000/μL. Blood contamination lowers the lamellar body count by up to 20%. The mucus frequently found in vaginal pools can spuriously elevate immature results into the mature range. The accuracy of the test in a diabetic population is not yet known. This novel test is slightly faster than the fpol.

Conclusions

It must always be remembered that fetal lung maturity should not be confused with fetal maturity. There are other organ systems besides the lungs that may cause problems in the nursery. One study evaluated infants delivered with a mature L:S ratio and compared outcomes with gestational age. Of babies with a "mature" L:S ratio and gestational age of less than 33 weeks, 47% still developed RDS and 7% developed necrotizing enterocolitis. Before planned delivery, the clinical situation should always be evaluated and the risks and benefits determined. For the patient at term, it is acceptable to use the dating criteria as outlined by ACOG. If the ACOG criteria cannot be used, then consider using ultrasonographic evaluation of the biparietal diameter but make sure that diabetes is first ruled out. If ultrasonographic criteria cannot be used, or if the BPD is not in the mature range, then look for a mature fpol evaluation. If vaginal pool specimens are used, there may be problems with reliability.

Multifetal Pregnancy Reduction

Lauren Lynch, MD

The incidence of multifetal pregnancies has increased dramatically in industrialized countries throughout the world. This increase is mainly because of the widespread use of ovulation induction agents and assisted reproduction techniques. In the United States from 1972 to 1974 and from 1985 to 1989, the rate of multifetal births defined as three or more live births increased by 113% among white mothers and by 22% among African-American mothers. The increase was particularly large in white women aged 30 to 39 years. The rate of triplet live births increased by 156%, quadruplets by 356%, and quintuplets and higher-order births by 182% between 1972 and 1989.

Natural History of Multifetal Pregnancies

Despite modern perinatal management, the rate of prematurity in multifetal pregnancies has not changed since the 1960s. However, the perinatal mortality rates have had a significant decline, probably because of improved neonatal care. The mean gestational age at delivery of triplet pregnancies is 33 weeks. Ninety percent deliver before 37 weeks, 25% before 32 weeks, and 8% before 28 weeks. The average triplet birth weight is 1797 g. The perinatal mortality in most recent series has been relatively low (22 to 59 per 1000 births); however, there is very little information regarding long-term follow-up of the survivors. Therefore, accurate statistics regarding the incidence of permanent sequelae of prematurity are virtually nonexistent.

The mean gestational age at delivery of quadruplet pregnancies is 31 weeks. Ninety-seven percent deliver at less than 37 weeks, 45% at less than 32 weeks, and 12% at less than 28 weeks. The perinatal mortality rate in the largest series was 67 per 1000 births. Here again, the data on long-term follow-up of the survivors are extremely limited. One small study showed that after 2 years of follow-up, 30% of quadruplet survivors had evidence of neurodevelopmental abnormalities.

As stated, the data on long-term morbidity and mortality of survivors of multifetal pregnancies are very limited; however, it seems safe to assume that the larger the number of fetuses, the greater the risk of prematurity and long-term sequelae. One study using a multiple-birth registry found that the risk of producing at least one child with cerebral palsy was 1.5%, 8%, and 43% for twin, triplet, and quadruplet pregnancies, respectively.

Multifetal Pregnancy Reduction: Technical Aspects

Most institutions performing multifetal pregnancy reduction procedures utilize one of two methods: transabdominal or transvaginal intrathoracic injection of potassium chloride. The procedures are generally performed at 10 to 12 weeks of gestation. Most operators recommend reducing to twins; however, most will reduce to triplets and some to a singleton if the patient so desires.

The transabdominal approach utilizes a 22-gauge spinal needle directed into the fetal thorax under ultrasonographic guidance. Generally 2 to 5 mEq of potassium chloride is required to achieve asystole. This procedure is then repeated for each fetus to be terminated. The most important factor in selecting the fetus or fetuses to be terminated is accessibility, which usually signifies those fetuses closest to the uterine fundus. At 10 to 12 weeks, detailed examination of the anatomy of each fetus is not possible, but if an obvious abnormality is observed or if one fetus is significantly smaller than the others, that fetus should be selected for termination.

The transvaginal approach utilizes endovaginal ultrasonographic guidance and insertion of a needle into the fetal thorax via the vaginal fornix and injection of potassium chloride.

At this time, there is no consensus regarding the advisability of performing prenatal diagnosis before the reduction in women with indications such as advanced maternal age, the concern being subjecting the pregnancy to another invasive procedure in a relatively short period. Some argue that prenatal diagnosis is best performed in the survivor via amniocentesis at a later date. In my opinion, women whose fetuses are at a significant risk of mendelian disorders or aneuploidies should be offered chorionic villus sampling before the reduction procedure, whereas those with a smaller risk can be offered amniocentesis after being fully counseled regarding the risks and benefits of both procedures. If chorionic villus sampling is elected, it should be done only on the placentas of those fetuses that are not intended to be terminated, rather than on all

of the fetuses, to minimize the number of needle and catheter insertions.

Pregnancy Outcome After Multifetal Pregnancy Reduction

In our experience with 400 cases of multifetal pregnancy reductions, most of which were reductions to twin pregnancies, the average gestational age at delivery was 35.4 weeks, and 88% delivered at or after 32 weeks. There were 32 pregnancy losses (8%), but only 4 (1%) of these occurred within 4 weeks of the procedure; thus it is impossible to know how many of the remainder were caused by the procedure itself because some of the losses occurred many weeks later. Among the losses were 2 (0.5%) cases of chorioamnionitis secondary to the procedure, and they were successfully treated with uterine evacuation and intravenous antibiotics. No other serious maternal complications were encountered. Some of the patients experienced leakage of amniotic fluid shortly after the procedure, but it was always from the sac of one of the terminated fetuses. These cases were managed with bedrest at home as long as ultrasonographic examinations revealed normal amniotic fluid volume in the sacs of the living fetuses. Fluid leakage always ceased within days and the pregnancies continued uneventfully.

Prenatal Care After Multifetal Pregnancy Reduction

In general, prenatal care after a multifetal pregnancy reduction to twins should be the same as for any twin pregnancy, with two exceptions:

1. Maternal serum alpha-fetoprotein is always elevated in patients who have undergone a reduction, even if tested many weeks later. This elevation is caused by the presence of the dead fetus and not by fetal or placental abnormalities. Therefore, maternal serum alpha-fetoprotein screening for neural tube defects and aneuploidies is useless in these patients and should be replaced by a detailed anatomic ultrasonographic examination and amniocentesis if karyotyping is indicated.
2. Although intrauterine growth retardation is more common in twins than in singleton pregnancies, it appears that it is even more common in twins after a reduction compared to nonreduced dichorionic twin

pregnancies. Therefore, patients with this type of pregnancy should be followed with serial ultrasonographic examinations at least every 4 weeks for fetal growth estimation. Although many practitioners would follow this regimen in any twin pregnancy, in reduced twin pregnancies it is essential.

Who Should Be Offered Multifetal Pregnancy Reduction?

It is clear that multifetal pregnancy reduction is effective in improving the perinatal outcome of pregnancies with four or more fetuses. The improvement in gestational age at delivery is so dramatic that it must lead to an improvement in survival and long-term outcome (ie, intact survival). The benefits of reducing triplet pregnancies are less obvious. However, all couples with a triplet pregnancy should be offered the procedure for the following reasons:

1. Triplets that are reduced to twins deliver an average of 3 weeks later than nonreduced triplets. More importantly, the risk of delivering before 32 weeks is reduced from 25% to 8%. Furthermore, studies comparing twins after a reduction from triplets to nonreduced triplets have shown a prolongation in the mean gestational age at delivery, larger birth weights, a decrease in the perinatal mortality rate, and a decrease in the incidence of neonatal respiratory complications and intraventricular hemorrhage. Although these studies did not compare long-term outcome of the survivors, it is likely that the improvement in perinatal outcome leads to a better long-term prognosis.

2. Reducing a triplet pregnancy to twins may in fact decrease the risk of spontaneous abortion. The reason for this is that the spontaneous abortion rate is related to the number of fetuses within the uterus. For example, one recent report of 140 triplet pregnancies, all of whom were determined to be alive by ultrasonographic examination before 9 weeks of gestation, found that of the 106 women who continued their triplet pregnancies, 21% spontaneously aborted the entire pregnancy before 24 weeks of

gestation. The 34 patients who underwent a multifetal pregnancy reduction to twins experienced only a 9% spontaneous abortion rate. Therefore, it appears that the risk of spontaneous abortion related to the larger number of fetuses is greater than the risk of undergoing a multifetal pregnancy reduction.

3. The social and financial concerns of raising three children, especially if one or more has a disability, may be enough reason for some couples to elect reducing their triplet pregnancy to a smaller number of fetuses.

What Is the Ideal Number of Fetuses in Reduction?

In most cases, the ideal number of fetuses to reduce to is twins. Some patients will elect to reduce from a larger number to triplets, but because of the reasons mentioned, this is not the optimal number if the goal is to deliver infants at or close to term. However, if the couple understands the risks and benefits of this decision, the pregnancy should be reduced to triplets. On the other hand, some patients will request a reduction to a singleton rather than to twins, although the improvement in perinatal outcome in singletons as compared to twins is marginal at best. The disadvantage of reducing to a singleton is that if, after the reduction, the fetus is found to have a structural or karyotypic abnormality, the couple will be left with no normal fetus. In these cases, one should strongly consider performing a chorionic villus sampling in the fetus one intends to retain before the reduction instead of an amniocentesis at a later date if there is an indication for prenatal diagnosis. Some patients will have medical indications for having the pregnancy reduced to a singleton, such as previous very early preterm delivery, uterine anomalies, or maternal medical conditions that would make a twin pregnancy too risky. These patients should be counseled to reduce to a singleton. However, some couples will request an elective reduction of their multifetal pregnancy to a singleton pregnancy. Although some operators are reluctant to do this, I believe that if the couple is fully aware of the risks and benefits, they should be offered the procedure.

Nonimmune Hydrops

Vern L. Katz, MD

Hydrops fetalis was originally described in conjunction with Rh isoimmunization, and, until recently, the great majority of hydrops cases were due to immunologic erythroblastosis. With the advent of routine maternal antibody screening and the use of Rh immune globulin, the etiologies have changed. Eighty-five to 90% of hydrops is now from nonimmune causes. The incidence of nonimmune hydrops is approximately 1 in 1500 to 1 in 3500 deliveries. Thus, most obstetricians will encounter hydrops not uncommonly.

Nonimmune hydrops fetalis (NIHF) is a confusing diagnosis in that it represents an end-stage fetal or neonatal condition rather than a specific disease entity. Hydrops refers to abnormal fluid collections in the baby. It may be thought of as circulatory collapse, although it is not always cardiogenic. By convention, two or more fetal compartments must have excess fluid to fit the criteria for hydrops fetalis. These body cavities or compartments include generalized skin edema greater than 5 mm, pleural effusion, pericardial effusion, ascites, and placental edema with thickness greater than 6 cm. Dilatation of fetal organs such as hydrocephalus, hydronephrosis, or cardiomegaly is not considered hydrops. However, these conditions often coexist with NIHF. Once the descriptive ultrasonographic diagnosis is made, the next step is determination of a specific etiology. NIHF has multiple etiologies. Management and prognosis are dependent on the particular etiology. A definite etiology may be found in 80% to 85% of NIHF cases. Unfortunately, this is often found only after fetal or neonatal death.

The presentation of NIHF may be as an asymptomatic finding on ultrasonography, or it may present symptomatically. Symptomatic presentations are usually in the late second and third trimester. Symptoms may be decreased fetal movement as the fetus becomes sick, increasing abdominal girth in the mother with the development of polyhydramnios, or development of symptoms of pre-eclampsia in what has been described as "mirror syndrome," with both mother and fetus being edematous.

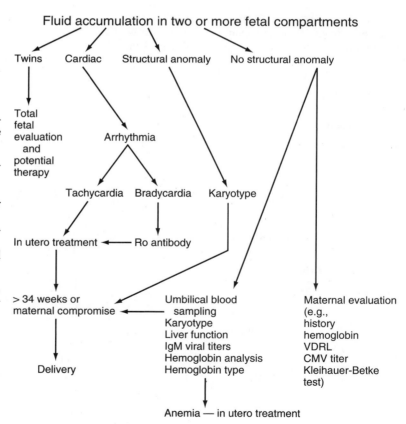

Figure 1. Algorithm for fetal evaluation of suspected nonimmune hydrops:

1. Ultrasonographic examination
2. Maternal antibody screen
3. Maternal evaluation for pre-eclampsia
4. If >24 weeks, glucocorticoid therapy
5. Amniocentesis or umbilical vein sampling

CMV, cytomegalovirus; VDRL, Venereal Disease Research Laboratory.

Etiology

NIHF is an end-stage condition of circulatory failure that may develop from over 100 individual diseases. These etiologies may be divided into broad categories, as shown in Table 1. The categories include cardiovascular etiologies, which constitute approximately 20% to 40% of NIHF cases; chromosomal anomalies, constituting approximately 15% to 20%; twin-twin transfusion syndrome, constituting approximately 5% to 10%; infection, constituting approximately 10% to 15%; syndromic, such as metabolic diseases, constituting approximately 10%; structural lesions, constituting approximately 15% to 20%; and idiopathic, constituting approximately 15% to 20%. Certain etiologies are found more commonly in specific populations; for example, alpha thalassemia may account for more than 50% of NIHF cases in Southeast Asian populations.

Pathophysiology

The various etiologies and diseases of NIHF may produce a hydropic state in the fetus through several varied mechanisms. Abnormal lymphatic damage, for example Turner's syndrome, may lead to hydrops by steady accumulation of extravascular fluid. Obstruction of venous return from thoracic cystic adenomatoid malformations may lead to cardiac failure. Myocardial disease, for example, may lead to venous congestion, ascites, effusions, and cardiac failure. Fetal supraventricular tachyrhythmia may lead directly to cardiac failure. High output cardiac failure may arise from vascular lesions such as a chorioangioma of the placenta. Decreased oncotic pressure from fetal hepatitis secondary to infection may lead to generalized edema. Increased capillary permeability from endovascular damage from infection will also lead to generalized edema. In most instances, more than one pathophysiologic mechanism contributes to the development of hydrops. For example, an infection may lead to myocardial damage, endovascular damage, and hepatitis. As is obvious, the reversal of a disease process in utero is extremely difficult, and thus there is a very poor prognosis of most cases of NIHF. NIHF carries a mortality rate of more than 80%.

Diagnosis

Once the diagnosis of NIHF is made, particular attention must be given to several aspects of the fetus and the fetal condition. The following questions should be evaluated:

1. Gestational age. NIHF prior to 24 weeks' gestation has a very poor prognosis. A much greater proportion of these fetuses have chromosomal lesions. Additionally, very few of the cases that develop early are amenable to therapy. The overall prognosis

TABLE 1. Categories and Examples of Etiologies of Nonimmune Hydrops Fetalis

Category	Example
Cardiovascular, 20–40%	Arrhythmias Structural malformations Myocarditis
Chromosomal, 15–20%	45,XO Trisomies
Twin-twin transfusion, 5–10%	
Infections, 10–15%	Parvovirus (anemia) Cytomegalovirus Syphilis
Structural malformations, 15–20%	Cystic adenomatoid malformation Skeletal dysplasias Fetal teratomas
Syndromic, 10%	Thalassemia Gaucher's disease Myotonic dystrophy
Idiopathic, 15–20%	

of NIHF at this gestational age is more than 95% fatal. If the fetus is older than 34 to 35 weeks' gestation, delivery should be considered because extrauterine therapy is more efficient in the great majority of cases.

2. Growth and measurements, skeletal integrity. If fetal long bone size is appropriate for dates, this is a better prognostic sign. Intrauterine growth retardation in the presence of hydrops carries a worse prognosis. Additionally, the skeletal dysplasias are associated with NIHF, so rib cage shape and size should be examined.

3. The sonographic cardiac characteristics. The largest single category of NIHF etiologies is cardiovascular causes. Cardiac rate, rhythm, and chamber size need to be closely evaluated. The tachyarrhythmias greater than 200 beats per minute in many cases may be treated successfully in utero, often with reversal of NIHF. In utero therapy has included maternal digitalis administration, quinidine, propranolol, and verapamil. Fetal therapy via umbilical venous injection has also been performed.

   Bradyarrhythmias are associated with structural malformations up to 50% of the time. Bradyarrhythmias without structural malformations may be associated with a maternal immunoglobulin G antibody, the Ro antibody that accompanies systemic lupus, or Sjögren's syndrome.

   Bradyarrhythmias have also been treated in utero, although less successfully than tachyarrhythmias. A careful analysis of fetal cardiac anatomy including chamber size and myocardial contractility should be made. Intracardiac tumors and rhabdomyomas may cause NIHF. Tuberous sclerosis is associated with rhabdomyomas. This disease is autosomal dominant, although many cases are sporadic mutations. Measurements of the fetal cardiac biventricular outer diameter may be helpful in assigning prognosis and in following disease progression.

4. Chest anatomy. The presence of space-occupying lesions, either abdominal viscera from diaphragmatic hernia or the common cystic adenomatoid malformations, is a common cause of NIHF. Congenital chylothorax is also a common cause of NIHF. It may present initially as an isolated pleural effusion, which may progress into generalized hydrops.

5. Fetal anatomy. A complete generalized fe-tal survey, including face, cranium, intercranial anatomy, and abdomen, should be undertaken to identify any structural lesions. The presence of multiloculated fluid cavities in the skin suggests lymphatic lesions such as lymphangiomas or Turner's syndrome. Teratomas most commonly found in the sacral-coccygeal areas may lead to high output failure. Arteriovenous malformations in other areas of the body have also been associated with NIHF. If ascites is present, a good view of the fetal liver is often possible. A large liver or dilated umbilical vein at the entrance to the liver (0.9 mm) is suggestive of secondary erythropoiesis with venous congestion.

6. Extrafetal evaluation. Obviously, twin-twin transfusion will be apparent on the initial ultrasonographic overview. However tempting it may be to assign this etiology, however, many cases of suspected twin-twin transfusion have turned out to be anatomic lesions in one twin, or even infection causing the hydrops. Therefore, careful fetal evaluation should be made of both infants before assigning this diagnosis. NIHF may occur in the donor or the recipient twin in twin-twin transfusion. The twin-acardiac twin sequence is also associated with NIHF. Twin-twin transfusion may be treated in utero or temporized with serial amniocentesis. There is often but not always a growth discordance between the fetuses.

Umbilical cord lesions, including thrombosis and torsion, are rare causes of NIHF. Placental tumors and chorioangiomas may cause NIHF through high output failure similar to arteriovenous malformations. These are large echolucent, complex masses most commonly found at the cord insertion.

Laboratory Testing

At the time of ultrasonographic examination, consideration should be given to invasive fetal assessment. For gestations over 24 weeks, umbilical blood sampling is preferable because of the rapid turnaround of results and the ability to assess fetal chemistries and hematologic indices, as well as fetal chromosomes. Table 2 lists helpful fetal tests that may be obtained at the time of invasive examinations. The results of the ultrasonogram help guide which tests to order. Fetal chromosomes are important in almost all cases of NIHF, however.

TABLE 2. Laboratory Tests in the Diagnosis of Nonimmune Hydrops*

Tests on Fetal Samples	Tests on Maternal Samples
Umbilical blood samples	Antibody screen (indirect Coombs') and titer
Chromosomes	Kleihauer-Betke
IgM—parvovirus, CMV, toxoplasmosis	Maternal IgM and IgG—titers for parvovirus, CMV,
Total IgG, total IgM	toxoplasmosis
SGOT, SGPT, alkaline phosphatase	VDRL (or other syphilis tests)
Fetal hemoglobin type	Maternal hemoglobin analysis
Complete blood count	Ro antibody
Amniocentesis	Thyroid-stimulating antibody
CMV culture	
Chromosomes	
PCR—adenovirus, parvovirus	

*Which laboratory tests are ordered will vary, depending on the history and ultrasonographic findings. CMV, cytomegalovirus; Ig, immunoglobulin; PCR, polymerase chain reaction; SGOT, serum glutamic-oxaloacetic transaminase; SGPT, serum glutamate pyruvate transaminase; VDRL, Venereal Disease Research Laboratory.

Maternal testing is extremely valuable in elucidating an etiology. Several conditions in the parents should be evaluated. The laboratory evaluation on the parents is derived from the history.

1. A maternal history should be taken for the presence of genetic diseases in the family such as storage diseases, tuberosclerosis, and previously affected children or other relatives. A history of medication ingestion should be obtained, particularly ingestion of over-the-counter medications such as aspirin, ibuprofen, nonsteroidal anti-inflammatory agents, or aspirin-containing medicines that may cause premature closure of the ductus.
2. Antibody screen–indirect Coombs' test. Even in mothers who are Rh positive or have had negative antibody screens earlier in pregnancy, this treatable cause of hydrops should be reassessed.
3. Hemoglobin electrophoresis: racial/ethnic origin. Women of Mediterranean and Southeast Asian descent should be evaluated for hemoglobinopathy.
4. Maternal-fetal hemorrhage may cause NIHF. Even without a history of trauma, a Kleihauer-Betke test should be ordered to evaluate for the presence of fetal cells in the maternal circulation.
5. Anti-thyroid antibodies may induce a tachyarrhythmia even though the mother may have had her thyroid removed. Ro antibody should be ordered if there is a bradyarrhythmia. A history of thyroid disease and autoimmune disease should be sought in conditions of fetal cardiac arrhythmias.
6. Maternal infections may cause NIHF; most of these may be asymptomatic. Parvovirus and cytomegalovirus are often asymptomatic or so slightly symptomatic as to be confused with general pregnancy symptoms. Occupational history of teachers and daycare workers may suggest such etiologies. Thus titers for cytomegalovirus, parvovirus, toxoplasmosis, and syphilis testing are valuable laboratory tests. Maternal laboratory studies are listed in Table 2.

Management

Management is dependent on etiology and fetal condition (see Fig. 1). At gestational ages beyond 34 to 35 weeks, treatment is usually more effective ex utero. At gestational ages less than 35 weeks, diseases amenable to in utero therapy include anemias by fetal transfusions, tachyarrhythmias by maternal antiarrhythmia medications, and some infections such as syphilis and cytomegalovirus treated by maternal medications. Twin-twin transfusion has been treated with in utero surgery and more commonly with serial amniocentesis. We believe that glucocorticoid therapy to help induce fetal lung maturity is appropriate in all gestations over 24 weeks. We use 12 mg intramuscular betamethasone in two doses 24 hours apart.

Obstetric management is based on etiology and fetal condition. Fetal thoracentesis prior to delivery for large pleural effusions should be considered, since postdelivery oxygenation may be impossible with collapsed lungs. Cesarean delivery is usually the indicated mode of delivery because the cardiac failure and placental congestion usually produce fetal distress in labor.

Many cases of fetal NIHF are complicated by poor placental separation, and the frequency of polyhydramnios often leads to postpartum hemorrhage. Appropriate obstetric preparations for postpartum hemorrhage should be undertaken prior to delivery. This includes type and cross-matching of blood. The placenta should be sent for pathologic examination. Histologic stains should be made for viral inclusions. If necessary, placenta and membranes may be used for chromosomal analysis. Intrapartum management should also include delivery with neonatologists present. Hydropic infants have extremely difficult transitions to the extrauterine environment.

Another issue of management is maternal status. The excessive fluid accumulations within the uterus and the increased placental growth lead to a pre-eclampsia-like syndrome termed *mirror syndrome*. This condition should be managed like pre-eclampsia, and its presence is an indication for delivery. Mirror syndrome pre-eclampsia may be severe. HELLP (*h*emolysis, *e*levated *l*iver functions, and *l*ow *p*latelets) syndrome and eclampsia have been seen with NIHF. This syndrome may lead to maternal morbidity and mortality and should not be taken lightly even though its origin is understood.

Prognosis

The prognosis for NIHF is in general poor. It is particularly poor for early hydrops in a fetus of less than 24 to 28 weeks' gestation. If oligohydramnios or intrauterine growth retardation is present, then the fetal condition may actually be worse than expected and the prognosis grave. Fortunately, the recurrence of most etiologies is usually low. Since prognosis is poor, avoidance of maternal complications should be an important factor in counseling and management.

Percutaneous Umbilical Blood Sampling

Lisa J. Farkouh, MD
John C. Hobbins, MD

Since the fetal circulation provides extremely useful diagnostic information, it is no wonder that the technique of percutaneous umbilical blood sampling (PUBS), also referred to as cordocentesis, has generated so much attention over the last 15 years. Until recently, only a few centers in the United States performed this diagnostic technique, but now there are few prenatal diagnostic programs that do not offer this option.

Background

It became clear in the early 1970s that amniotic fluid was insufficient to diagnose fetal hemoglobinopathies such as beta-thalassemia and sickle cell disease. A technique was developed to obtain fetal blood through the intrauterine insertion of an endoscope (fetoscopy). Fetal blood was aspirated from a punctured vessel on the chorionic plate through a needle housed in a side channel adjacent to the endoscope.

The fact that it was impossible to sample directly from the tiny placental vessels without introducing some amniotic fluid limited the diagnostic potential of the technique. This stimulated investigators to take the brave step of approaching the umbilical cord. After demonstrating that it was possible to obtain pure samples of fetal blood from the umbilical cord with modest rates of fetal mortality, the centers involved in direct fetal sampling adopted this approach. By the mid-1970s, conditions with predictable inheritance patterns such as beta-thalassemia, sickle cell disease, and hemophilia and very rare conditions such as chorionic granulomatous disease could be reliably diagnosed through acquisition of fetal blood. Since reported fetal mortality rates were between 1.5% and 5%, the technique was attempted only in those at high risk for the condition in question.

Frustrated by an inability to obtain the very thin endoscope required to perform the fetal blood sampling by the current standard method, Daffos decided in 1983 to utilize a technique that required guiding a 20-gauge needle into the umbilical cord with the use of ultrasonography alone. He demonstrated in 600 cases that fetal blood could be consistently obtained with fewer procedure-related fetal losses than with fetoscopy. Since then, others have reported similar results.

Methods

The technique can be accomplished with linear arrays, sector scanners, or curvilinear transducers. Most operators are now using 22-gauge needles, which are small enough to limit morbidity yet stiff enough to be redirected once they are through the maternal abdominal wall.

Some operators advocate using a needle aspiration guide that is attached to a sector or curvilinear transducer. Most, however, use a "freehand" technique, which is a modification of a standard method of real time–directed amniocentesis. The operator chooses a sampling site on the umbilical cord that is approximately 1 cm from its insertion on the placenta. Here the cord is essentially "fixed" and will move little when entered by the needle. An entry site is chosen on the maternal abdomen that allows direct access to the umbilical cord. If the procedure lasts more than a few minutes (as in an intrauterine transfusion), then local anesthesia is used in the abdominal insertion site. Depending on the needle's position with respect to the transducer, the tip appears as a bright echo or the entire needle is visualized. The needle is then advanced by ultrasonographic guidance to the umbilical cord.

Although most operators choose umbilical vein blood for sampling, one investigator preferentially chose the fetal heart as a sampling site. Protocols vary between institutions regarding use of maternal and fetal sedation and paralysis of the fetus.

The degree of difficulty of the procedure seems to depend most on the size of the target, which is dependent on gestational age. For example, the umbilical vein varies in size from about 3 to 4 mm at 18 weeks of gestation to about 10 mm at 33 weeks. Since the side-to-side (azimuthal) resolution of most transducers is 2 to 3 mm, one can understand how much more difficult it is to place the needle tip into an 18-week umbilical vein than to approach the umbilical vein in the third trimester.

When approaching a viable fetus, we suggest that the procedure be performed either near or in a cesarean section room in case an intractable bradycardia develops. Postoperative monitoring need not be extensive and, in most cases, the patient can leave the hospital shortly after the procedure is completed. We do keep a patient overnight whose fetus has had an intrauterine transfusion. The use of antibiotics following PUBS is optional.

Uses

1. *Cytogenetics.* Rapid karyotyping is the most common indication for PUBS in the second trimester, usually when fetal anomalies are sonographically detected. Fluorescent *in situ* hybridization (FISH) techniques applied to amniotic fluid samples or placental biopsy are replacing PUBS as a technique for rapid karyotyping.
2. *Thrombocytopenia.* Until several years ago, PUBS was commonly performed in patients with *idiopathic thrombocytopenic purpura* at term to determine whether the fetus was affected. Some recent studies, however, suggest that the incidence of severe neonatal thrombocytopenia and intracranial hemorrhage may be too small to warrant an invasive procedure such as PUBS. Although the management of idiopathic thrombocytopenic purpura remains controversial, PUBS still offers precise determination of the fetal platelet count if desired. *Neonatal alloimmune thrombocytopenia* poses a threat to the fetus, and early assessment of the fetal platelet count is recommended.
3. *Fetal anemia.* PUBS provides the most accurate measurement of the fetal hematocrit, which is important in conditions such as Rh isoimmunization, Kell sensitization, parvovirus B19 infection, or fetomaternal bleeding. Intrauterine transfusions can be performed in the event of severe fetal anemia or hydrops.
4. *Intrauterine infection.* In cases of maternal infection with cytomegalovirus, *Toxoplasma gondii*, or parvovirus B19, PUBS may be helpful in determining the presence of fetal infection. Blood can be analyzed for white blood cell count, immunoglobulin G and M, or culture, although this method has recently been supplanted by amniotic fluid studies.

Risk

Although PUBS provides invaluable information in select clinical situations, it is not an entirely innocuous procedure. The risk of fetal loss varies from 0.8% to 4% when performed by experienced operators. Alternatives to PUBS include the following:

1. *Placental biopsy.* Analogous to transabdominal chorionic villus sampling, this procedure is gaining popularity in Europe as an alternative to midtrimester cordocentesis. It is especially useful if PUBS is technically difficult and an anterior or fundal placenta permits easy access for biopsy. The risk has been reported to be similar to that of second trimester amniocentesis.

2. *Doppler indices.* Fetal acid-base status can easily be determined by PUBS. Recently, two studies have shown an indirect correlation between fetal Doppler indices and acid-base status, possibly obviating the need for invasive techniques.

3. *Amniotic fluid culture and polymerase chain reaction.* Amniocentesis provides substrate for the most sensitive tests of prenatal cytomegalovirus and toxoplasmosis infection.

4. *Amniotic fluid for fetal Rh status.* Prenatal fetal Rh typing can be reliably accomplished by polymerase chain reaction with amniocytes. The finding of an Rh-negative fetus in an Rh-sensitized pregnancy would eliminate the need for further invasive measures.

Rh and Other Blood Group Immunizations

John T. Queenan, MD

Isoimmunization, due to Rh and other blood group antigens, can cause erythroblastosis fetalis (EBF), which is responsible for a significant portion of perinatal mortality and morbidity. Isoimmunizations due to the Rho(D) antigen occur less frequently today because of the prophylactic use of Rh immune globulin. Rh immunizations still occasionally occur because of transplantal hemorrhages, inadequate doses of Rh immune globulin, or failure to administer Rh prophylaxis altogether.

Rh Incompatibility

Pregnant Rh-negative women constitute a unique group of high-risk patients. This risk

group may be defined by Rh typing. Screening by the indirect antiglobulin (Coombs') test for Rh antibodies will determine those at risk for EBF. This screening should be done at the initial prenatal visit for all women and at 28 weeks for the Rh-negative woman. Rh immune prophylaxis is administered at 28 weeks, provided the mother is not already immunized. If the program is followed carefully, clinically significant disease will not go undetected. If there are no Rh antibodies, there can be no EBF caused by Rh incompatibility (Rh-EBF).

When a new antibody is detected, it is important to perform a titer. The titer determines the strength of the antibody. A critical antibody titer is the level at which an intrauterine or neonatal death may occur. In laboratories in which a low volume of titers is performed, the accuracy of these tests may be questioned. The laboratories should freeze all serum specimens so that they may be used to run subsequent titers in duplicate.

Today, the Rh-immunized pregnancy can be managed by five complementary modalities:

1. Antibody titers
2. Amniotic fluid deviation in optical density at 450 nm (AF ΔOD_{450}).
3. AF DNA Rh typing
4. Cordocentesis
5. Sonographic evaluation

When the antibody titer is very low (e.g., 1:4) the outcome is generally favorable because the disease is mild. Following serial antibody titers is all that is necessary to evaluate the pregnancy in mild disease. In situations in which the titer is higher, the outcome is not as predictable, and the AF ΔOD_{450} and sonography are used to determine the fetal condition. AF DNA Rh typing is performed on amniocytes at the time of the initial amniocentesis. If the fetus is determined to be Rh-negative, then no further testing is necessary and the fetus is delivered at term. If the fetus is found to be Rh-positive, then additional AF ΔOD_{450} tests are necessary. When very severe Rh-EBF is suspected, then the operator performs a cordocentesis to proceed with a fetal transfusion if the anemia is severe.

Antibody Titers

Antibody titers are most helpful clinically with mild immunizations. Allen, Diamond, and Jones showed that patients with low indirect antiglobulin (Coombs') titers had favorable pregnancy outcomes. In 174 patients with titers of 1:32 or lower and no history of stillbirth or hydrops fetalis, 167 (96%) of the fetuses were alive at 37 weeks' gestation. In a first immunized pregnancy, if the antibody does not reach a critical level, the pregnancy can be managed without amniocentesis. Once the titers reach critical level, then amniocentesis with AF ΔOD_{450} and AF DNA Rh typing must be done.

Amniotic Fluid ΔOD_{450}

AF ΔOD_{450} analysis is a valuable clinical tool that recently was made even more accurate by the addition of DNA Rh typing of the amniocytes. Many methods of AF analysis have been proposed. The Liley method has been a standard. It is applicable from 27 weeks to term and is based on prediction of fetal anemia. In 1993, a four-zone method (Queenan and colleagues) was proposed that is based on analysis of 789 single and serial AF ΔOD_{450} measurements. An advantage of this method is that it is efficacious in both the second and third trimesters. In addition, it integrates the complementary modalities of AF ΔOD_{450}, amniocyte Rh typing and sonographic monitoring (Fig. 1).

In the Rh-negative (unaffected) pregnancies, the AF ΔOD_{450} values rise until 24 weeks, then fall until term. In Rh-positive fetuses at risk of dying in utero, the values are higher and the trends of AF ΔOD_{450} values rise. There are four zones of increasing severity: Rh-negative (unaffected), Rh-positive (affected), indeterminate, and intrauterine death risk. Establishing which zone an amniotic fluid falls in determines a management scheme for that fetus. By following this protocol, the Rh-negative fetuses have the least intervention and the fetuses at risk of dying in

utero are recognized early enough for fetal transfusions.

If the AF ΔOD_{450} value falls in the Rh-negative zone, most likely the fetus is Rh-negative. The AF is sent for DNA Rh typing. If the fetus is Rh-negative, deliver at term and no further testing is necessary. If the fetus is Rh-positive, then repeat the AF ΔOD_{450} every 2 to 4 weeks, depending on the clinical situation.

If the value falls in the indeterminate zone, an AF DNA Rh typing is done. This zone contains fetuses that are both Rh-positive and Rh-negative. If the fetus is Rh-negative, deliver at term and no further testing is necessary. If the fetus is Rh-positive, then repeat the AF ΔOD_{450} every 1 to 2 weeks depending on the clinical situation.

If the value falls in the Rh-positive zone, follow the AF ΔOD_{450} values to determine the safety of keeping the fetus in utero and gaining valuable maturity, or to determine the timing of fetal transfusion for the fetus in jeopardy of dying. Decreasing values generally mean that the fetus has mild or moderate EBF. Rising trends indicate severe disease and even death if the fetus is not delivered or transfused, depending on the gestational age. Incipient hydrops may give lower values due to dilution.

If the value falls in the intrauterine death risk zone, or the trend of values will cross over into this zone, the fetus is in jeopardy of dying in utero. Cordocentesis should be performed to determine the fetal condition, and when indicated, to provide access for intrauterine transfusion.

Amniotic Fluid DNA Rh Typing

AF DNA Rh typing is very accurate and can clearly differentiate between an Rh-negative (no disease) and an Rh-positive (affected) fetus. The test should be done at the initial amniocentesis because when the values fall in the two lowest zones it is difficult to differentiate between the Rh-negative and the Rh-positive fetus. Adding this modality solves that problem. It also has value in the occasional Rh-negative fetus whose values fall in the Rh-positive zone, since an Rh-negative fetus can rarely have a value that high.

Cordocentesis

Cordocentesis is performed when AF ΔOD_{450} values fall in the intrauterine death risk zone or if they fall in the Rh-positive zone with an upward trend of values such that they would enter

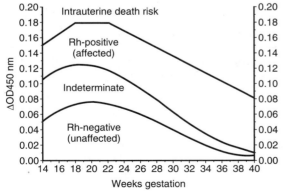

Figure 1. Amniotic fluid ΔOD_{450} management zones.

the intrauterine death risk zone. It provides the ability to directly evaluate the fetal hemoglobin and hematocrit and thus measure degree of hemolytic anemia. Cordocentesis is not a substitute for the AF ΔOD_{450} because it is a more complex procedure and has a higher mortality rate than the amniocentesis. It can cause further maternal immunization and should not be used unless severe disease is suspected.

Sonography

Sonography is a very valuable in detecting signs of fetal deterioration in moderate to severe disease. Signs such as cardiomegaly, pericardial effusion, polyhydramnios, and ascites usually indicate that the fetus is rapidly deteriorating due to heart failure or hypoproteinemia. However, significant EBF can occur without detectable sonographic signs. This modality is not capable of distinguishing normal (no EBF) from mild disease. Sonographic evaluation serves as an excellent safety net because it is accurate and noninvasive and almost always reveals when a fetus is undergoing serious deterioration due to EBF. Therefore, it is commonly used with antibody titers or AF ΔOD_{450} to rule out any undetected fetal deterioration.

Intrauterine Transfusion

When it is determined that a premature fetus is a very anemic, an intrauterine transfusion can be life-saving. The original technique as described by Liley involved instillation of blood directly into the fetal peritoneal cavity. The blood cells were absorbed directly into the fetal circulation over a period of 6 days. Whereas this technique corrected the fetal anemia and often saved the life of the fetus, it was not effective against hydrops fetalis.

Today, intrauterine transfusion is performed by cordocentesis, which has certain advantages. This technique provides immediate correction of anemia and a sampling of fetal blood for hematocrit, uses a smaller needle, and is effective for fetuses at 18 to 23 weeks and even for hydropic fetuses. Transfusions are generally done with group O, Rh-negative, cytomegalovirus-negative blood that has been irradiated to destroy donor white blood cells. If the transfusion is being done to a hydropic fetus, whole blood is preferable because the fetus is usually acutely deficient in serum proteins as well as red cells. Usually the hydrops does not disappear until after the second transfusion.

Although the cordocentesis is the usual technique employed today, occasionally a combined procedure is done with direct transfusion into the umbilical vein and then blood is also instilled into the fetal peritoneal cavity. This has the advantage of providing prolonged absorption of blood, permitting longer intervals between transfusions.

Rh Immune Prophylaxis

Individuals who lack the Rh antigen in the surface of their red cells are called Rh-negative. Exposure to as little as 0.25 mL of Rh-positive red cells may cause an individual to be immunized. A woman can become immunized by a spontaneous abortion, induced abortion, ectopic pregnancy, chorionic villus sampling, amniocentesis, transplacental hemorrhage, and, rarely, through a mismatched blood transfusion.

Today, the possibility of preventing Rh immunization has been increased markedly by the administration of concentrated Rh antibody in the form of Rh immune globulin. Rh immune prophylaxis should be given whenever the patient is exposed to Rh-positive red cells. This will prevent Rh immunization. One ampule of Rh immune globulin contains 300 μg of antibody and will protect against 30 mL of Rh-positive blood. Generally, one ampule of Rh immune globulin is administered at 28 weeks' gestation to protect against transplacental hemorrhage. An indirect antiglobulin (Coombs') test should be done to assure that the mother is not already immunized. She is then protected until the time of delivery. During the first 72 hours postpartum, the sooner the better, another 300 μg of Rh immune globulin is administered to the Rh-negative patient delivering a Rh-positive infant.

Most Rh-negative women who deliver Rh-positive babies receive Rh immune globulin at 28 weeks and postpartum. If they are in other situations that could cause exposure to Rh-positive blood such as amniocentesis or abdominal trauma causing a transplacental hemorrhage, then additional Rh immune globulin should be administered.

Other Blood Group Immunizations

The Rh-negative and the Rh-positive patient may become immunized to other blood group antigens. Antigens such as Kell, Duffy, Kidd, c, e, C, and E may cause significant EBF. Indeed, they may cause intrauterine death. Therefore, the work-up and management should be similar to that for Rh immunization.

Blood group antigens such as Lewis antigens Le[a] and Le[b] generally cause immunoglobulin M antibodies that are large molecules and do not cross the placenta. Even if the immunization contains a component of immunoglobulin G antibodies that cross the placenta, there is no risk of significant EBF because the Lewis antigens are not yet attached to the fetal red blood cells. They circulate in the plasma and will attach to the fetal red cells after birth. Therefore, a Lewis immunization does not require amniocentesis or preterm delivery.

It should be remembered that all obstetric patients are potential recipients of blood transfusions. In the setting of a blood group immunization, even though EBF may not be anticipated, the blood bank should be alerted, because promptly getting compatible blood for an emergency cesarean section or postpartum hemorrhage could be difficult.

ABO Incompatibility

In Rh-EBF, 40% of EBF caused by ABO incompatibility (ABO-EBF) occurs in the first pregnancy. Although by far the most common cause of EBF, it may go undetected because the disease is often mild.

The direct antiglobulin (Coombs') test is usually positive; however, the reaction may be very weak. The disease most commonly occurs in Group O mothers with Group A or B infants, because these mothers produce an immunoglobulin G type of antibody. The ABO-EBF is usually very mild and rarely needs to be treated by exchange transfusion. The problem can be managed adequately with phototherapy because the neonatal bilirubin levels generally do not become markedly elevated. With the trend toward early discharge from the hospital, the clinician should be alert to detect ABO-EBF by doing a direct antiglobulin (Coombs') test on the cord blood. One should observe the neonate for early signs of jaundice, because, if undetected, the disease could cause kernicterus.

Fetuses do not die in utero because of ABO incompatibility. Therefore, amniocentesis and AF analysis are not indicated in this disease. There are no antibody studies that are useful clinically. This clinical entity is a pediatric rather than an obstetric problem. Although preterm delivery is not indicated, a scheduled, prepared delivery at term is appropriate management.

Seizures in the Neonatal Period

Leandro Cordero, MD
Randy Miller, MD

Overt forms of seizure activity occurring during the neonatal period have been recognized for many years. Recently, however, attention has been given to more subtle forms such as lip-smacking, chewing, pedaling, and staring. Clinical presentation of seizures is different in premature infants than it is in full-term newborns and older infants. These differences are related to neuroanatomic characteristics of the particular developmental stage. Although by about the 24th week of gestation the human cortex has the full complement of neurons, it is not until a year later that the so-called organizational period is completed. It is during this developmental phase that layering, alignment, and orientation of cortical neurons and axonal and dendritic ramifications take place. The absence of cortical organization and the paucity of dendritic connections characteristic of the newborn prevent, or at least modify, the propagation of a generalized seizure and explain the rarity of typical grand mal, tonic-clonic attacks. In contrast, during the last weeks of intrauterine life, there is a relatively advanced cortical maturation of limbic structures and their connections to the diencephalon and the brain stem. This anatomic characteristic explains the predominance of oral-buccal-lingual and oculomotor movements as expressions of seizure activity.

The basic pathophysiologic event leading to rapid synchronous firing of cortical neurons is a sudden depolarization, often due to failure of the sodium-potassium pump, alterations of membrane potential, or imbalance of excitatory and inhibitory neurotransmitters.

Clinical Presentation

The most common presentation of neonatal seizures is the subtle form. Lip-smacking, chewing, tongue-thrusting, twitching, bicycling, pedaling, and staring are some examples of this type of seizure activity. Abrupt changes in heart and respiratory rate and blood pressure may also be subtle manifestations of seizures. Diagnosis of subtle forms can be difficult, since they must be differentiated from normal physical behavior such as startle, clonus, tremors, grimacing, and non-nutritive sucking. It should be noted that movements during the newborn period relate to the state of sleep or wakefulness. Therefore, familiarity with the different states of sleep and their behaviors facilitates recognition of seizures. By far the most common form of clonic activity seen during the neonatal period is tremor (jitteriness). These rhythmic high-frequency movements of the limbs can be present in normal infants but are more frequently found in pathologic conditions such as hypoglycemia, perinatal asphyxia, and drug withdrawal. Unlike true seizures, tremors can be started by exogenous stimuli and can be stopped by holding the limbs. These tremors are alternating movements of equal rate and intensity and they do not have the jerky fast and slow components of a true clonic seizure. When seizure activity presents as apnea, it is usually accompanied by other subtle forms and, unlike primary apnea of the newborn, is not usually associated with bradycardia.

Generalized tonic seizures can be observed more often in premature than in full-term infants. They are characterized by stiffening of the entire body and extremities with or without flexion of the upper limbs. They are also accompanied by other subtle manifestations of seizures. Multifocal clonic seizures are commonly seen in asphyxiated full-term infants. Focal clonic episodes used to be common in the past, when they were thought to be associated with obstetric trauma. Myoclonic convulsions (single muscular jerks) are even less common. The advent of video electroencephalographic (EEG) recordings has made it possible to establish behavioral and electrographic correlates with important physiopathologic and diagnostic implications. Thus, seizures can be classified into clinical (normal EEG recording), electroclinical (behavioral and EEG manifestations), and electrographic (clinically asymptomatic with EEG abnormalities). Focal/multifocal clonic, focal tonic, and generalized myoclonic seizures belong in the electroclinical category. Electrographic confirmation is usually absent in generalized tonic, focal, or myoclonic seizures (clinical). Asymptomatic seizures detectable only by EEG scan (electrographic) are surprisingly common and carry a prognosis as severe as that of the electroclinical type.

Incidence

The incidence of neonatal seizures is very difficult to estimate, since in about half of the cases it will be subclinical, while only 70% of clinically suspected episodes will be confirmed by EEG recordings.

In light of the diagnostic difficulties, especially with the subtle forms, it is not surprising that the reported incidence of neonatal seizures varies so greatly. Between January, 1983 and December, 1987, approximately 3000 infants were admitted to the neonatal intensive care unit of the Columbus Children's Hospital. During that 5-year period, 256 neonates presented with or developed seizures during the neonatal period. In 1994 and 1995, 116 newborns were admitted with similar complaints. Like other authors, we have observed a decline over the years in the number of full-term infants presenting with seizures. On the other hand, as the number of smaller premature infants who survive continues to increase, the incidence of convulsions among them remains constant.

Etiology

The most common pathologic conditions associated with seizures in the neonatal period encountered in our experience are presented in Table 1. In decreasing order of frequency, these diagnoses are perinatal asphyxia, intracranial bleeding, congenital malformations, bacterial and viral infections (sepsis/meningitis), metabolic disorders, trauma, apnea, and miscellaneous. This group includes a few infants experiencing drug (opiates) withdrawal and a sizable number of neonates who present with poorly documented isolated convulsions.

Perinatal Asphyxia

Perinatal asphyxia has remained the single most common cause of neonatal seizures, especially in

TABLE 1. Patients with Neonatal Seizures Admitted to Columbus Children's Hospital

Associated Pathology	Patients (*n* [%])	
	1983–1987	1995–1996
Perinatal asphyxia (full term)	72(28)	25(22)
Intracranial bleeding	57(22)	20(17)
Congenital anomalies°	42(16)	20(17)
Sepsis/meningitis (viral/ bacterial)	35(14)	16(14)
Apnea	10(4)	6(5)
Birth trauma	6(2)	4(3)
Seizure of unknown origin	34(14)	25(22)
Total	256	116

°Includes inborn errors of metabolism.

full-term infants. Approximately 30% of asphyxiated infants develop convulsions that usually start between 6 and 12 hours of age. Hypoxic ischemic encephalopathy is a well-defined syndrome that occurs often in severely asphyxiated neonates. Aggressive, modern obstetric and neonatal management has somewhat reduced the mortality and, to some extent, the severity of neurologic sequelae. Serial EEG monitoring is important because seizures with EEG correlates carry a more severe prognosis.

Intracranial Bleeding

Until recently, clinical diagnosis of intracranial bleeding was made in the presence of a falling hematocrit, a bulging fontanelle, a deteriorating condition, and the occurrence of posturing or seizures, or both. The development of ultrasonography now allows the detection of otherwise unsuspected brain hemorrhages. Furthermore, the location and severity of the hemorrhage can be ascertained with ease. When the more severe forms of hemorrhage produce neonatal seizures, the mortality increases significantly and the possibility of intact survival is almost nonexistent. The incidence of severe intracranial bleeding is inversely related to gestational age. The majority of these seizures start anywhere from the first to the fifth day of life.

Perinatal Infections

A variety of intrauterine infections have been associated with neonatal seizures. Toxoplasmosis, cytomegalic inclusion disease, and herpes have been the most common of the TORCH complex (*toxoplasmosis, rubella, cytomegalovirus,* and *herpes* simplex) to be incriminated. *Escherichia coli,* group B *Streptococcus,* and *Listeria monocytogenes* are the bacteria most commonly associated with meningitis. In recent years, we have observed an increased number of enteroviral central nervous system (CNS) infections, resulting in seizures, some very refractory to treatment. Convulsions in this category may start as early as the first hour of life (e.g., disseminated cytomegalovirus infection) or as late as several weeks (e.g., late-onset group B streptococcemia).

Congenital Anomalies

In our series, approximately one half of the patients with congenital anomalies (see Table 1) presented with malformations involving the CNS (e.g., encephalocele, hydrocephalus, Arnold-Chiari and arteriovenous malformation). Chromosomal disorders (eg, trisomies 13 and 18) and nonchromosomal malformations were found in one third of the patients. The remaining patients included those with inborn errors of metabolism.

Metabolic Problems

Hypoglycemia is a common problem that affects infants of diabetic mothers, premature infants, small-for-gestational-age infants, postmature infants, and asphyxiated infants. Even when blood glucose is not detectable these newborns may remain asymptomatic or present with only jitteriness. Early blood glucose monitoring and prompt intravenous glucose administration should be ordered for all newborns in the high-risk group.

Hypocalcemia (serum level below 7 mg/dL) occurs in small premature infants, in offspring of diabetic mothers, and in asphyxiated infants. Subtle signs such as irritability, jitteriness, chewing, and lip-smacking may be present but overt seizures are not uncommon. Hypomagnesemia may coexist with hypocalcemia and occasionally produce neonatal convulsions. A rare though treatable cause of neonatal seizure is pyridoxine (vitamin B_6) dependency. Every infant who has a refractory neonatal seizure of unclear origin should receive a trial of pyridoxine (50–100 mg IV) during EEG recording.

Drug Side Effects

Benzodiazepines are commonly prescribed for infants and children as a sedative, anticonvulsant, antiemetic, or amnesic agent. Lorazepam is commonly used as a sedative in newborns undergoing mechanical ventilation and as an anticonvulsant. Recently, myoclonic multifocal seizure-like activities have been observed within minutes of lorazepam administration in premature as well as full-term infants. Although this side effect is rare, we have observed it in 1% of the lorazepam-treated infants but not when the drug was administered in a 20-minute infusion. The onset of these myoclonic seizures may be related to the time of the entry of lorazepam into the cerebrospinal fluid. The relatively low plasma protein binding, the low volume of distribution for lorazepam, and its delayed clearance in newborns may contribute to relatively high concentration of the drug in the cerebrospinal fluid. Free unbound lorazepam across the blood-brain barrier may paradoxically stimulate neural synapsis because of interactions with already low levels of γ-aminobutyric acid. Although this myoclonic seizure-like activity is self-limited and not associated with neurologic sequelae, further sedative dosage should be restricted in affected newborns.

Treatment

Untreated or uncontrollable seizures during the neonatal period should be considered a true emergency, since they may aggravate the neurologic damage already present. Depletion of brain glucose, increased oxygen consumption, accumulation of lactate, and changes in cerebral blood flow are some of the disturbances encountered during convulsions. Neuronal death may also result from the release of endogenous neurotoxic compounds that act on subtypes of glutamate receptors, resulting in an increased influx of calcium ions to cells. Uncontrollable seizure activity may indirectly compromise the patient, as in the case of persistent fetal circulation, where poor gas exchange (i.e., hypoxia) could further increase pulmonary vascular resistance and decrease pulmonary blood flow. Apnea may also lead to hypoxia, hypercarbia, and hypotension. In the small premature infant with fragile periventricular vessels, the hypertension observed during seizures could initiate or increase intraventricular bleeding. In treating neonatal seizures, one must stabilize the patient (e.g., establish an airway), correct the underlying cause (e.g., hypoglycemia), and start anticonvulsant therapy.

Owing to its effectiveness and low toxicity, phenobarbital remains the single most valuable therapeutic agent (Table 2). An intravenous loading dose of 20 mg/kg should control seizures in about 80% of cases. If this is not effective within 10 minutes, we repeat another dose of 10 to 20 mg/kg. Maximizing therapy with phenobarbital to achieve a serum concentration of 20 to 40 µg/mL is recommended before adding a second agent. In our experience, only 5% of patients

continue to have seizure activity and require the addition of phenytoin. Owing to its high osmolarity (15,570 mOsm/L), phenobarbital should be administered through a vein to avoid the occluding endarteritis that may affect small vessels.

The pharmacokinetics of phenobarbital in neonates differs from that in adults in its absorption, distribution, and elimination. The volume of distribution is substantially larger in neonates, which explains the necessity of higher loading doses. Changes in blood pH can also affect the volume of distribution of phenobarbital, since its dissociation constant (pK) is very close to physiologic pH. Plasma protein binding is less in newborns than in adults. The primary metabolic pathway for phenobarbital is by parahydroxylation and subsequent glucuronide conjugation, a pathway that is not mature in the preterm infant. Renal excretion may account for up to 60% of the eliminated drug during the first week of life. Infants with impaired renal function should be monitored for phenobarbital accumulation. The half-life of phenobarbital is approximately 100 hours during the first week of life and decreases to 70 hours during the second to third week of life. Therefore, the maintenance dose of phenobarbital for infants less than 7 days old is 3 mg/kg/day, and it is increased to 5 mg/kg/day for infants greater than 1 week of age. The dosing interval has traditionally been every 12 hours, but daily dosing has been shown to be safe and equally effective owing to the drug's long half-life. Serum concentrations should be monitored to maintain therapeutic levels of 20 to 40 µg/mL. Symptoms of toxic levels (greater than 50 to 60 µg/mL) include poor feeding, hypotonicity, unresponsiveness, and respiratory depression. Oral liquid phenobarbital is available only in the elixir form, which contains 13.5% alcohol. Bioavailability is approximately 80% for oral preparations.

Phenytoin is generally considered a second choice in neonates owing to difficulties in drug administration, dosing, and interpretation of se-

TABLE 2. Treatment of Neonatal Seizures

Drug	Loading Dose	Maintenance	Serum Level
Phenobarbital	20 mg/kg IV	3–5 mg/kg/day q12h IV	20–40 µg/mL
Phenytoin	15–20 mg/kg IV	5 mg/kg/day q12h IV only	10–20 µg/mL
Lorazepam	0.05–0.1 mg/kg IV	N/A	N/A
Dextrose (D$_{10}$W)	200–400 mg/kg IV	6–10 mg/kg/min	N/A
Calcium gluconate (10%)	200 mg/kg IV	N/A	N/A
Magnesium sulfate (50%)	50–100 mg/kg IV	N/A	N/A

N/A, not applicable.

rum concentrations. The loading dose of phenytoin is 15 to 20 mg/kg given by slow intravenous push (0.5 mg/kg/min) to avoid bradycardia and cardiovascular collapse. Phenytoin is metabolized in a manner similar to that of phenobarbital. However, a reliable half-life cannot be ascertained, since the clearance of phenytoin decreases as the serum concentration increases owing to nonlinear metabolism. Maintenance doses of phenytoin are 5 mg/kg/day administered every 12 hours. A suspension is available for oral use, but bioavailability is a problem, particularly when it is administered with or near enteral feedings. Another consequence of nonlinear kinetics is that the higher the maintenance dose, the longer it takes to reach steady state, causing slow unsuspected drug accumulation and possible toxicity. Serum levels of phenytoin are very difficult to interpret in neonates because of variable protein binding. Total phenytoin serum concentrations of 10 to 20 μg/mL are considered therapeutic in adults, but this may not be applicable to neonates. Protein binding has been shown to be less than 70% in preterm infants, making the free fraction more than three times greater than that of an adult. Phenytoin toxicity may be more dangerous than that of phenobarbital, since high levels can induce seizures. Lethargy and nystagmus are also symptoms of phenytoin toxicity. In light of the above, we prefer to discontinue phenytoin after 2 weeks of treatment.

In cases of neonatal seizures refractory to treatment with phenobarbital and phenytoin, benzodiazepines could be given. Diazepam, although effective in slow infusion, may produce apnea and hypotension in the presence of phenobarbital. Lorazepam, which is longer acting, given at a dosage of 0.05 to 0.1 mg/kg intravenously over a 20-minute infusion, is commonly used in our institution (see earlier discussion).

Duration of anticonvulsant treatment for acute cases is still a matter of controversy. A recent survey of neonatologists revealed that 40% will discontinue the medication prior to discharge and only 10% will maintain it for over a year. Patients with status epilepticus or uncontrollable seizures should remain on medication for at least 4 months. Those with malformations of the CNS and those with abnormal EEG tracings should remain on medication longer. In all other cases, we let the patient "outgrow" the dose before discharge from the hospital. Considering that 8% to 15% of infants who experienced neonatal seizures will have recurrence, close clinical surveillance of this population should be maintained.

Successful treatment of seizures depends not only on anticonvulsants but also on recognition and treatment of the underlying cause. In our experience, diagnosis of seizures is mainly clinical, since it is logistically difficult to obtain EEG and video recordings during the acute phases. In patients receiving pancuronium bromide, muscular paralysis may mask seizure activity; therefore it may be prudent to delay anticonvulsant therapy until EEG recordings are obtained. Whenever a metabolic abnormality like hypoglycemia or hypocalcemia is suspected, its correction should precede any specific anticonvulsant medications.

Prognosis

The majority of neonatal seizures are self-limited events that do not lead to epilepsy. The morbidity and mortality resulting from neonatal convulsions depend more on the underlying cause than on the seizure itself. In our experience, 12% of full-term infants with perinatal asphyxia and 30% of premature infants with intracranial bleeding who experienced seizures do not survive.

The longer the lack of response to anticonvulsants, the greater the chance of death and disability. EEG recordings, especially during the interictal period, are valuable outcome predictors. Approximately 80% of the infants with convulsions who have an abnormal EEG recording at the time of discharge continue to experience seizures and suffer significant neurologic sequelae. On the other hand, those with normal EEG recordings are unlikely to develop convulsions later on. Unfortunately, EEG recordings, especially in premature infants, are difficult to interpret. Convulsions complicating bacterial and viral meningitis and perinatal asphyxia may lead to severe neurologic sequelae in as many as 50% of the patients. No more than 20% of premature infants experiencing intracranial bleeding and seizures should be expected to be normal. Generalized tonic, myoclonic, and subtle seizures reflect diffuse CNS involvement and have worse prognosis than clonic manifestations. The prognosis for patients experiencing true hypoglycemic seizures may be as severe as that of asphyxiated infants. Unprovoked recurrent seizures (epilepsy) have been observed among 15% of preterm and 30% of full-term survivors whose neonatal seizures were diagnosed only by clinical criteria. It has been reported that this incidence is higher among infants or children who had electrographically confirmed neonatal (electroclinical) seizures.

Primary Care

Acne Vulgaris

Marina Ball, MD
Gerald D. Weinstein, MD

Acne vulgaris is a skin condition with a variety of typical lesions on the face, neck, and upper trunk and is the classic dermatologic sign of puberty. For many young adults, it is only a passing disturbance of minor significance. In some, however, it has varying amounts of short- and long-term morbidity, with even psychological difficulties. Fortunately for most of these affected individuals, there are effective therapeutic approaches that minimize the impact of the disease until it spontaneously runs its course. The primary lesion of acne stems from the comedo (blackhead) or hair follicle impaction. The impaction is due both to retention and to increased production of squamous epithelial cells. Impactions form in the superficial portion of the hair follicle (comedones) and may eventually rupture into the dermis, resulting in inflammatory lesions (papules, pustules, nodules). Even though these morphogenetic events are widely accepted, the precise primary pathogenetic event eludes us. Heredity, androgens, 5-alpha-reductase, sebum, free fatty acids, microorganisms (especially *Propionibacterium acnes*) and their enzymes, and intercellular cements all have ill-defined and controversial roles. Although questions remain and research continues, we have been fortunate in developing or finding effective forms of therapy.

Treatment of acne is not difficult in most patients, especially if a regimen can be appropriately individualized. Implicit in this statement is the concept that both the disease and the patient vary considerably. As a result, acne is usually treated with more than one active agent and a number of adjunctive measures (Fig. 1).

A vital aspect of the successful management of acne is the first office visit. It is during this critical, formative interchange that the bonds of mutual trust and understanding are formed. Adequate time should be allotted during this first visit to sit quietly and discuss, in simple terms and with the help of a drawing, the basic anatomy of the obstructive and inflammatory lesions of acne. Explanations of the chronicity of acne, its waxing and waning course, and, most importantly, the fact that amelioration and control

rather than cure are the only realistic goals with currently available therapy will prevent later disappointment over expectations of cure. This interview then serves as a basis for the greater acceptance of therapies, which all require cooperation of the patient over many months or years.

Patients with numerous open and closed comedones (blackheads and whiteheads) without inflammatory papules require "unplugging" of the occluded follicles. Such unplugging (keratolytic) agents include topical retinoic acid and topical benzoyl peroxide.

Retinoic acid is available in several strengths—cream base, 0.025%, 0.05%, and 0.1%, and gel base, 0.01% and 0.025%. Retinoic acid can cause mild irritation and dryness of the face initially. This is usually due to one or more of the following: (1) application of too much medicine—it should be applied in a very thin film, gently smoothed in, and used in strength and frequency that just begin to produce erythema and peeling; (2) pooling in natural crevices—care should be taken to avoid the crevices of the mouth, eyes, nasal-facial junction, and nasolabial fold; (3) application too soon after washing the face—since retinoic acid penetrates hydrated skin more readily, the patient should

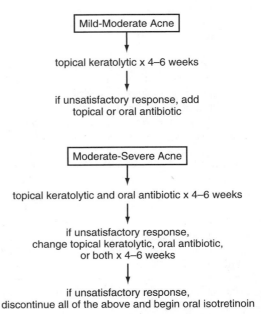

Figure 1. Algorithm for the management of common acne.

wait at least 20 minutes after washing before applying the medication; (4) additive effects of other irritants—these include various over-the-counter peeling agents containing sulfur and/or salicylic acid and/or resorcinol, α-hydroxy acid lotions, abrasive cleansers, excessively frequent washing with soap and water, and frequent use of astringents; (5) injudicious sun exposure—retinoic acid increases the sensitivity of the skin to sunburn; retinoic acid should be applied only at night, and use of a sunscreen with an SPF (sun protection factor) of 15 or greater is recommended.

Since we cannot be certain about percutaneous absorption of topical tretinoin or its metabolites and the possibility of teratogenicity, we ask patients to stop using topical tretinoin if they are, or are attempting to become, pregnant. At least two new second-generation topical retinoid preparations will soon be available with potential advantages—Avita Cream and Differin—with the former having less irritation than the original preparation.

Benzoyl peroxide has keratolytic properties as well as being antibacterial and reducing the surface free fatty acid level. It also can hasten the involution of some existing lesions. This product is available by both prescription and over-the-counter sale. Benzoyl peroxide is marketed as a gel or cream in several strengths—2.5%, 5%, and 10%. It is best to start with the lowest concentration to avoid excessive irritation until the skin begins to "harden" (not to be confused with resistance, which does not occur). The incidence of allergic contact dermatitis due to benzoyl peroxide is quite low, about 1% to 2%. With the exception of enhanced sensitivity to sun exposure, the same usage patterns that tend to produce problems with retinoic acid–induced irritation should be looked for with benzoyl peroxide. Additional benefit can usually be achieved by using benzoyl peroxide in combination with retinoic acid, e.g., benzoyl peroxide in the morning and retinoic acid at night. One may find that pretreating for 1 week with benzoyl peroxide alone may decrease the irritancy of the retinoic acid used subsequently. Topical benzoyl peroxide is considered nonteratogenic, since no cases of birth defects have been reported in women using this medication during pregnancy.

A mild soap is recommended initially so that the patient will not experience further dryness of the face from normal cleansing. Expression of comedones with a comedone extractor (acne surgery) can be beneficial in comedonal acne. Often it is best to use the comedone extractor after therapy with an unplugging agent has already

been used for 2 to 4 weeks. By this time, an early "softening" of the lesions occurs and their mechanical removal is facilitated. If too heavy a hand is used, the possibility exists of creating deeper, more inflammatory lesions by rupturing the comedones.

When the acne patient presents with comedones as well as inflammatory papules or pinhead-sized pustules, therapy is initiated with an antibiotic along with either retinoic acid or benzoyl peroxide. Antibiotics for acne can now, of course, be given by either the oral or topical route. The most common topical antibiotics for acne include clindamycin phosphate, 1% (Cleocin T), and erythromycin in cream, gel, and lotion preparations. Oral antibiotics most often used are tetracycline, erythromycin, and minocycline.

The most common cause of apparent failure with topical antibiotics is the expectation that these medications will clear up existing lesions. Their role is prophylactic, preventing or decreasing the formation of new inflammatory lesions. Therefore, little or no effect can be seen before about 4 to 8 weeks, a similar time period as for retinoic acid and benzoyl peroxide. Adding topical antibiotics for mild to moderate inflammatory acne ordinarily is more effective if combined in a regimen including retinoic acid or benzoyl peroxide, e.g., topical antibiotics applied in the morning and afternoon, with retinoic acid or benzoyl peroxide applied at night.

There are no adequate and well-controlled studies of any of the topical antibiotics in pregnant women. Nevertheless, a recent preliminary controlled human study on the in vivo percutaneous absorption of several anti-acne drugs has shown that each of the three topical antibiotics—clindamycin phosphate, erythromycin, and tetracycline—was absorbed less than 1% through the skin and less than 0.1 mg of each was detected in the urine. There has been one case of pseudomembranous colitis directly attributable to topical clindamycin reported in the literature. Patients should be instructed to stop any antibiotic, topical or oral, if diarrhea occurs and to call a physician if it persists. The treatment of pseudomembranous colitis is vancomycin.

A new topical prescription acne medication, azelaic acid, 20%, has just been released for use in acne. It is chemically different from other topical agents. Neither of us has had a chance to evaluate it in our practices.

If, in the opinion of the physician, pitted scarring may develop from the active acne lesions, oral antibiotics are preferred initially, along with an unplugging agent. When prescribing oral antibiotics, it is important to check for drug allergies and to make sure the female patient is not pregnant and is not considering pregnancy in the near future. Tetracycline is usually prescribed in a divided dosage of 1 g/day to be taken on an empty stomach (1 hour before a meal or 2 hours after a meal). Side effects include nausea, diarrhea, phototoxicity, and onycholysis. The drug is contraindicated in pregnancy and in children less than 12 years of age because of permanent staining of teeth. Oral tetracycline does pose a threat to the pregnant woman herself. During the third trimester there is a risk of developing hepatic failure from acute fatty liver in patients taking tetracycline. It is also contraindicated in patients with liver or kidney disease. Erythromycin, both oral and topical, is generally thought to be a safe drug during pregnancy. In general we try to refrain from using any oral medication for acne during pregnancy, but in a pregnant woman whose acne is severe and cannot be controlled with topical therapy, oral erythromycin may be used for a period of time not to exceed 6 weeks. Erythromycin is usually prescribed in a divided dosage of 0.5 to 1.0 g/day, not necessarily on an empty stomach. Epigastric distress is a common side effect. Minocycline is a potent tetracycline that does not need to be taken on an empty stomach and is prescribed in a divided dosage of 100 to 200 mg/day. It carries the same contraindications in pregnancy and in children as tetracycline. In addition, dizziness and cutaneous pigmentation are dose-related side effects.

Breakthrough bleeding and, rarely, pregnancy have been reported in women who were taking oral contraceptives and antibiotics concurrently. Such interactions have been reported for rifampin, ampicillin, and tetracycline. The antibiotics induce microsomal enzymes in the liver that presumably accelerate the metabolism of estrogen. In some cases, this apparently has resulted in subtherapeutic blood levels of the estrogen component of the oral contraceptive. Oral contraceptive therapy is not considered a contraindication to antibiotic therapy, but the physician and patient should be aware of the potential interaction. The problem would be expected to occur more frequently with the low-estrogen preparations. With concurrent, long-term antibiotic therapy and oral contraceptive use, mechanical contraception could be used near mid-cycle as a precaution, if desired. Breakthrough bleeding first occurring with oral contraceptives after initiating antibiotic therapy suggests that re-evaluation of the contraceptive preparation used by the patient would be appropriate.

With all of the above-mentioned oral antibiotics used to treat acne over a long period of time, candidal vaginitis is a frequent side effect. More rarely, a gram-negative folliculitis superinfection may result.

Cystic acne can be most difficult to treat. Initially, therapy with oral antibiotics is begun (tetracycline, 1 g/day up to 2 g/day, in divided doses on an empty stomach, or minocycline, 100 mg bid). The topical treatment depends on various factors, including the severity of the cystic acne, the degree of skin oiliness, and the presence of comedones, inflammatory papules, or nodules. Therefore, either retinoic acid, benzoyl peroxide, or soaks may be suggested. Triamcinolone suspension in a concentration of 2.5 to 5 mg/mL is often beneficial when injected directly into the cyst with a 30-gauge needle. Because of potential skin atrophy, injections of this nature should not be performed into the same cyst more often than once every 3 weeks. Incision and draining of the cyst is not recommended because of its scarring potential.

Despite strict adherence to the therapeutic principles outlined here, a small group of patients seem truly refractory to treatment. In these patients, careful evaluation is required to rule out additional aggravating factors. These include hormonal imbalance, overgrowth of resistant organisms (gram-negative folliculitis), emotional stress, and a variety of external factors such as abusive cleansing, friction, and cosmetics.

Hormonal imbalance may be suggested by scalp hair loss, hirsutism, and menstrual irregularity, as well as by aggravation of acne, and requires evaluation for adrenal 11- and/or 21-hydroxylase deficiency as well as other causes of increased androgen secretion or Cushing's syndrome.

One should also verify whether the patient is taking an "androgen-dominant" oral contraceptive such as those containing the progestational agent norgestrel or very low estrogen–containing drugs with the progestational agent norethindrone.

Crops of recurrent pustules on the chin and perinasal area as well as indolent nodulocystic lesions in the same location should lead one to suspect overgrowth of gram-negative organisms resistant to the antibiotic being administered. These can readily be identified by culture and appropriate therapy instituted according to the sensitivity of the organism cultured. One should also look for the source of the organism—not infrequently the nares or the external auditory canal (otitis externa).

Emotional stress can frequently aggravate existing acne and can, at times, be explosive in its onset. While one can attempt to assist the patient with this emotional stress, brief courses of treatment with prednisone (20 to 40 mg/day) may be required. The drug should be tapered rapidly over a period of usually not more than 3 weeks.

A variety of external factors have been implicated in either the initiation or the aggravation of acne. Occupational exposure to halogenated hydrocarbons has long been known to be acnegenic. More recently, it has been demonstrated that hair pomades and occlusive, oily cosmetics also may induce or aggravate acne. In addition, inflammatory acne is aggravated by the use of abrasive cleansers or devices, and all forms of acne can be aggravated by heat, humidity, and friction such as may occur under athletic equipment or when the patient constantly rests her chin in the palm of the hand. These are easily treated by advising the patient of their nature and avoidance. Many patients develop a habit of "picking" at their lesions, producing small ulcerations. This habit can cause the greatest long-term damage, because it produces residual scarring of the face.

Isotretinoin (Accutane) remains the most dramatically useful and effective drug for severe acne. This drug, given orally in doses of 0.5 to 1.0 mg/kg/day, decreases sebaceous gland activity up to 90%. Remission of up to 30 months or longer following 20 weeks of therapy occurs in over 60% of cases of severe cystic acne. Clinical toxicity, which is dose-dependent and reversible, is limited principally to the skin and mucous membranes (cheilitis, xerosis, dry nasal mucosa, conjunctivitis). A transient, dose-dependent elevation of serum triglycerides occurs in about 25% of patients, the greatest risk being in those with elevated levels prior to therapy or with predisposing medical conditions (diabetes, obesity, increased alcohol intake). Pseudotumor cerebri has been reported infrequently and occasionally when tetracycline is taken simultaneously with Accutane. Even though the half-life of 13-*cis*-retinoic acid is relatively short (about 1 day), there is now no doubt that isotretinoin is teratogenic in humans. The teratogenic effects do not appear to be dose-related and can occur within the first 3 weeks of gestation. Exposure to the drug is associated with an unusually high relative risk for a group of characteristic major malformations involving one or more of the following systems: central nervous system, cardiac, thymus, and craniofacial. In addition, a number of patients exposed to isotretinoin have spontaneous abortions. Despite this knowledge and warnings by the Food and Drug Administration and the manufacturer, inadvertent use of isotretinoin

during pregnancy continues to cause birth defects. Exposure during pregnancy is preventable if physicians strictly adhere to the following established guidelines for use of isotretinoin in women of childbearing age:

1. Isotretinoin should be used only for the approved indication (severe, recalcitrant, nodular, or cystic acne that is nonresponsive to conventional therapy).
2. The physician must be certain that the woman is not pregnant when therapy is initiated. Two acceptable forms of contraception should be in use before, during, and for 1 month after treatment. The initial dose should be postponed until the second day of her next menstrual period.
3. The patient's informed consent is absolutely critical (physician counseling to inform the patient about the teratogenic potential of the drug, necessity of using adequate contraception). If the physician feels the patient is, for any reason, unlikely to comply with advice about contraceptives, isotretinoin should not be prescribed.

A standardized procedure kit has been made available by Roche Laboratories for physicians prescribing Accutane. The kit is helpful for both patients and physicians, providing information for patients in a detailed and clear manner to minimize the risks of accidental exposure to the drug by a pregnant woman.

Refer to Figure 1 for an algorithm of common acne management.

AIDS and HIV Infection

David A. Wininger, MD

Epidemiology

Since the early 1980s, when the acquired immunodeficiency syndrome (AIDS) was initially recognized in homosexual and bisexual men, attention to AIDS in women has been steadily increasing. Of American adult and adolescent AIDS cases in 1995, 19% involved women, of whom 38% acquired HIV via injected drug use and 38% via sexual contact with an at-risk male. The death rate from AIDS among white men in the United States had plateaued by 1994, while in women and black men it was continuing to rise. The AIDS-related death rate in black women (age 25–44 years) exceeded that of white men of the same ages, and AIDS was the third leading cause of death among all women in that age group.

Pathogenesis

Infection by the human immunodeficiency viruses (HIV-1 worldwide and HIV-2 primarily in western Africa) culminates in immune system destruction, which predisposes patients to the opportunistic infections and malignancies that characterize AIDS. HIV enters the body primarily via direct introduction into the bloodstream or through sexual contact and targets CD4+ T lymphocytes as well as the monocyte/macrophage system. The retrovirus integrates into the patient's DNA and rapidly replicates, achieving peak serum viral levels prior to the development of the primary immune response. During this period of primary infection, an associated "mononucleosis-like" syndrome (which can include fever, rash, pharyngitis, lymphadenopathy, arthralgias, headache, aseptic meningitis, and other constitutional symptoms) occurs in an ill-defined proportion of patients.

The immune system responds to the expanding viral load with heightened production of antibodies and cytotoxic T lymphocytes, resulting in a suppressed serum viral burden. The body also attempts to replenish CD4 lymphocytes destroyed by virus. Over time, relentless viral replication occurs in reservoirs of infections, primarily the lymph nodes. The body's capacity to sustain this battle is overwhelmed, and serum viral burden rises as the immune system fails. Selection of viral strains that have increased virulence may add to this dynamic process. The decline in the CD4 lymphocyte count correlates with suppression of cell-mediated immunity and a concomitant increased risk for bacterial, fungal, viral, and protozoal infections. Infection by HIV can directly contribute to chronic fatigue, wasting, diarrhea and dementia.

Case Definition

The Centers for Disease Control and Prevention's (CDC) case definition of AIDS is met in HIV-infected patients who develop any one of a long list of opportunistic infections, a specifically defined wasting syndrome, HIV encephalopathy, or certain malignancies such as Kaposi's sarcoma, primary central nervous system lymphoma, or non-Hodgkin's lymphoma. Some diseases are so distinctive of AIDS (e.g., *Pneumocystis carinii*

pneumonia [PCP]) that they can define a case in the absence of confirmed HIV infection as long as no other cause of immunodeficiency is present. The definition was expanded in 1993 to include patients with established HIV infection who had CD4 lymphocyte counts less than 200 cells/μL or had pulmonary tuberculosis, recurrent bacterial pneumonias, or invasive cervical carcinoma.

Progression of Disease

Although AIDS was initially observed to be rapidly fatal, patient survival from primary HIV infection until the first AIDS-defining condition currently averages 10 years. After meeting the case definition of AIDS, average life expectancy is 2 to 3 years, although some patients surpass that despite CD4 lymphocyte counts near 0 cells/μL. Less than 10% of patients are noted to be asymptomatic with stable, relatively high CD4 counts more than 13 years after infection, and the viral, immunologic, and environmental factors responsible for "long-term nonprogression" are being actively pursued by researchers.

The CD4 lymphocyte count has been a reasonable surrogate marker of disease progression, with certain opportunistic conditions tending to manifest when this count falls within certain ranges. Although the lower limits of normal are loosely defined, most HIV-uninfected patients with normal immune systems have CD4 lymphocyte counts ranging from 600 to 1900 cell/μL. During the early years of HIV infection, generalized lymphadenopathy, cutaneous manifestations such as tinea pedis, folliculitis, and localized herpes zoster can be noted. As counts approximate 500 cells/μL, recurrent sinusitis, vaginal candidiasis, and oral thrush may manifest. With additional decline, recurrent bacterial pneumonias, especially with *Streptococcus pneumoniae*, are more common. *Pneumocystis carinii* pneumonia can be observed as CD4 lymphocytes fall below 200 cells/μL, while cytomegaloviral retinitis or gastrointestinal disease and disseminated *Mycobacteria avium* complex disease are generally not seen until counts have dropped below 50 to 100 cells/μL.

Testing for HIV Infection

Analyses for HIV by enzyme-linked immunosorbent assay (ELISA) with confirmatory Western blot tests provide sensitivities and specificities greater than 99%. Infection by the virus can usually be detected serologically within 3 months, although repeat testing 6 months after the last high-risk exposure can further exclude the possibility of a false-negative result occurring during the window period of seroconversion.

To whom should HIV testing be offered? Testing clearly cannot be limited to the highest risk populations, such as injected drug users or men who have sex with men. Testing during pregnancy is advised, given the substantial potential for reducing vertical transmission with the use of peripartum zidovudine. Diagnosis of another sexually transmitted disease warrants a recommendation for HIV testing. Manifestations of possible HIV infection (such as recurrent oral or vaginal candidiasis, profound weight loss, prolonged fever, herpes zoster infection, and generalized lymphadenopathy) without a reasonable alternative explanation should also prompt testing for HIV.

Caring for a Newly Diagnosed Patient

During the initial assessment of a newly diagnosed HIV-infected patient, many issues can compete for the caretaker's attention. The history and physical examination should suggest the extent of disease and can uncover active opportunistic infections, which require acute management. Patients require education about the nature of HIV/AIDS and transmission prevention. Sexual or needle-sharing partners and state health departments may need to be notified.

Baseline laboratory studies should be obtained for future reference. The CD4 lymphocyte count has been the primary marker of disease stage, but recently sensitive measures of viral RNA in serum have been demonstrated to be a superior indicator of long-term prognosis. Blood cell counts, liver enzymes, and blood urea nitrogen and creatinine can screen for abnormalities attributable to HIV, opportunistic conditions, and medications. Screening for prior or latent infections should include a rapid plasma reagin test, toxoplasma IgG, cytomegalovirus IgG (so that negative patients can be designated to receive only leukocyte-filtered blood products), purified protein derivative test (followed by a chest radiograph if positive), and hepatitis A and B serologies (if vaccinations for these viruses are being considered).

Even though immunizations have been shown to have an acute negative effect on HIV load, most authorities continue to advise the use of annual influenza vaccines and the multivalent pneumococcal vaccine (every 5 years) in all HIV-infected patients. Hepatitis A and B vaccines should be offered to high-risk patients who lack serologic evidence of prior exposure.

Gynecologic Primary Care

According to the CDC, all newly diagnosed HIV-infected women should have a Pap smear, and if it is normal, it should be repeated in 6 months. After the second normal examination, annual Pap smears are recommended. Colposcopic examination is recommended for squamous intra-epithelial lesions and atypical squamous cells. The Pap smear should be repeated in 3 months if there is severe inflammation with reactive squamous cellular changes. In addition to the increased frequency and aggressiveness of cervical neoplasia in HIV-infected women, these patients have a high incidence of condyloma from human papillomavirus infection. Effective treatment for ulcerative genital infections in the patient and her partners has heightened importance, since the associated lesions can serve as a cofactor in HIV transmission.

Prophylaxis for Opportunistic Infections

Prophylaxis for certain opportunistic processes are initiated based on the patient's CD4 lymphocyte count and history of opportunistic infections. Patients with a prior history of PCP, oral thrush, or a CD4 lymphocyte count less than 200 cells/μL should be placed on prophylaxis for PCP indefinitely. Trimethoprim/sulfamethoxazole (TMP/SMX) (generally one double strength tablet daily) is the optimal prophylactic regimen, with dapsone (100 mg PO every day) the preferred second choice (outside of pregnancy). While previously popular, inhaled pentamidine can fail to adequately penetrate certain segments of the lung and provides no protection from extrapulmonary pneumocystosis. TMP/SMX is a more reasonable choice after the first trimester of pregnancy because of its superior efficacy.

For toxoplasma IgG–positive patients, TMP/SMX (or dapsone plus pyramethamine) provides the added benefit of prophylaxis against toxoplasmosis reactivation in addition to PCP; it is recommended by the CDC for patients with CD4 lymphocyte counts less than 100 cells/μL. Toxoplasma IgG–negative patients should avoid contact with cat litter and the eating of undercooked meat to prevent acute primary toxoplasmosis, especially if pregnant.

Patients positive for PPD with no evidence of

active tuberculosis should receive isoniazid and pyridoxine for 12 months if they have not previously done so.

The CDC recommends that prophylaxis for disseminated *Mycobacterium avium* complex (MAC) disease be considered for patients with less than 75 cells/μL, weighing several factors.

1. Prophylaxis can delay the onset of mycobacteremia and associated fever and anemia but does not prolong survival.
2. Active infection with *M. tuberculosis* and MAC must be ruled out prior to initiation of prophylaxis.
3. Prophylaxis may promote the development of antimicrobial resistance.
4. Significant drug-drug interactions and intolerance are associated with prophylactic medications. Rifabutin was the original agent approved for MAC prophylaxis, but more recent data support consideration of clarithromycin and azithromycin.

The use of prophylaxis for cytomegaloviral retinitis in patients with extremely low CD4 lymphocyte counts is controversial. Although approved by the Food and Drug Administration (FDA), not all studies support the use of high-dose oral ganciclovir in this setting. Expense and potential hematologic side effects have caused many clinicians to rely on regular (e.g., every 6 months) screening to enhance early detection of retinitis rather than employing primary prophylaxis.

Primary prophylaxis for fungal infections is not generally recommended. Frequent recurrent candidiasis can respond to intermittent or chronic therapy with topical antifungals or oral triazoles, although resistance to these agents is a growing concern. Lifelong secondary prophylaxis following primary infection with histoplasmosis, cryptococcosis, or coccidiodomycosis is always indicated, owing to the substantial risk for relapse in HIV-infected patients.

Patients with frequent recurrences of anogenital herpes simplex virus infection may benefit from suppressive acyclovir or possibly one of the newer prodrugs, famciclovir or valacyclovir. Acyclovir-resistant herpes simplex virus may respond to more intensive acyclovir dosing, but alternatives such as foscarnet or topical trifluridine are sometimes required.

Antiretroviral Therapy

Options for directly attacking HIV have greatly expanded since zidovudine (AZT, ZDV, Retrovir) was introduced. The initial class of antiretrovirals are the inhibitors of reverse transcriptase (RT), the enzyme necessary for deriving HIV DNA from RNA for incorporation into the host cell genome. Zidovudine, didanosine (DDI, Videx), zalcitabine (DDC, Hivid), stavudine (D4T, Zerit), and lamivudine (3TC, Epivir) are all nucleoside RT inhibitors approved for use by the FDA. RT inhibitors that are non-nucleoside analogues (e.g., delavirdine and nevirapine) are being studied in ongoing clinical trials.

Early trials of zidovudine monotherapy demonstrated a survival advantage, and there was a delay in progression to AIDS-defining illnesses in patients who started zidovudine "early" (200–500 cells/μL) compared with patients who waited until CD4 lymphocyte counts were lower (<200 cells/μL). In subsequent studies, the lack of a survival advantage in patients given early zidovudine compared with delayed treatment was attributed in part to the development of zidovudine-resistant virus.

More recent studies have focused on combination therapies and the introduction of the newer RT inhibitors. Combinations such as zidovudine with didanosine and zidovudine with zalcitabine as well as didanosine monotherapy are superior to zidovudine monotherapy even in zidovudine-naive patients. Recent data suggest that zidovudine with lamuvidine may be another superior RT-inhibitor combination.

Protease inhibitors are the newest class of antiretroviral agents and provide the theoretical advantage of attacking the virus at an alternative site in its life cycle, closer to final viral particle assembly. Of the three FDA-approved agents, ritonavir (Norvir) and indinavir (Crixivan) appear more efficacious in clinical trials than saquinavir (Invirase), possibly due to differences in bioavailability. Data from short-term clinical trials of these agents in combination with zidovudine in patients with advanced-stage disease demonstrated dramatically improved viral burdens and CD4 lymphocyte counts compared with zidovudine monotherapy. Correlation with long-term clinical outcome is pending.

Patients need to be monitored both for response to therapy (general well-being, weight gain, CD4 lymphocyte counts, probable viral burden) and side effects (neurosensory examination, blood cell counts, liver enzymes, amylase, etc). Drug intolerance or evidence of progressive disease are the most common indications for altering the antiviral regimen. Nausea, vomiting, headache, and skin changes are side effects common to several of the agents. Zidovudine and lamivudine can suppress the bone marrow, whereas neuropathy and pancreatitis are more commonly associated with didanosine, zalcitabine, and stavudine. The protease inhibitors can cause nausea and diarrhea and alter levels of hepatically metabolized medications, and indinavir is associated with nephrolithiasis. Pre-existing conditions such as neuropathy or pancytopenia often preclude the use of certain agents and help to focus treatment options.

Formal clinical guidelines for the use of antiretroviral therapy rapidly become obsolete as new data and new agents become available. The timing of initiation of therapy is controversial. There is growing enthusiasm for earlier therapy to attempt to minimize viral burden before the immune system reserves are exhausted. A less optimistic approach involves delaying treatment to avoid early selection of resistant viral strains. The appropriate timing of changes in antiretroviral medications to minimize the impact of viral resistance remains elusive, is often determined by changes in the patient's CD4 lymphocyte count and general sense of well-being, and likely will be guided by measures of viral RNA burden in the future.

Annual Examination

Vicki C. Darrow, MD

The annual examination is undoubtedly one of the most important mechanisms that obstetricians and gynecologists have to prevent disease and promote health. Traditionally, obstetricians and gynecologists have been at the forefront of prevention of diseases, as exemplified by the decrease in the incidence of cervical cancer through the recommendation of the annual Pap smear and the early identification of pre-eclampsia with the advent of prenatal care. It is imperative that, as the field of Obstetrics and Gynecology continues to evolve, prevention of disease and health promotion continue to be a priority. The opportunity to perform evaluations on an annual basis allows obstetricians and gynecologists to continue as primary health care providers for the prevention of disease in women (Fig. 1).

Prevention Focus

One of the primary goals of the annual examination is to prevent acute and chronic disability

TABLE 1. Leading Causes of Death in Women

Age (years)	Cause of Death
13–18	Motor vehicle accidents, homicide, suicide, leukemia
19–39	Motor vehicle accidents, cardiovascular disease, homicide, AIDS, breast cancer, coronary artery disease, cerebrovascular disease, uterine cancer
40–64	Cardiovascular disease, coronary artery disease, breast cancer, lung cancer, cerebrovascular disease, colorectal cancer, obstructive pulmonary disease, ovarian cancer
Over 65	Cardiovascular disease, coronary artery disease, cerebrovascular disease, pneumonia/influenza, obstructive lung disease, colorectal cancer, breast cancer, lung cancer, accidents

and premature death. If this goal is to be met, it is important that the physician be aware of the leading causes of morbidity and mortality in women. Table 1 lists the age-related leading causes of death, and Table 2 lists the age-related leading causes of morbidity in women.

Components of the Annual Examination
Patient/Physician Relationship

It is helpful to interview the patient fully dressed in a comfortable and private setting, then to move to the examination room for the physical examination. Some physicians provide a women's

TABLE 2. Leading Causes of Morbidity in Women

Age (years)	Cause of Morbidity
13–39	Upper respiratory tract infections and ear infections Viral, bacterial, parasitic infections Sexual abuse Injuries, acute urinary conditions
40 and older	Upper respiratory infections Hypertension Heart disease Orthopedic back pain, injuries Osteoporosis, arthritis Urinary incontinence Hearing and vision impairments

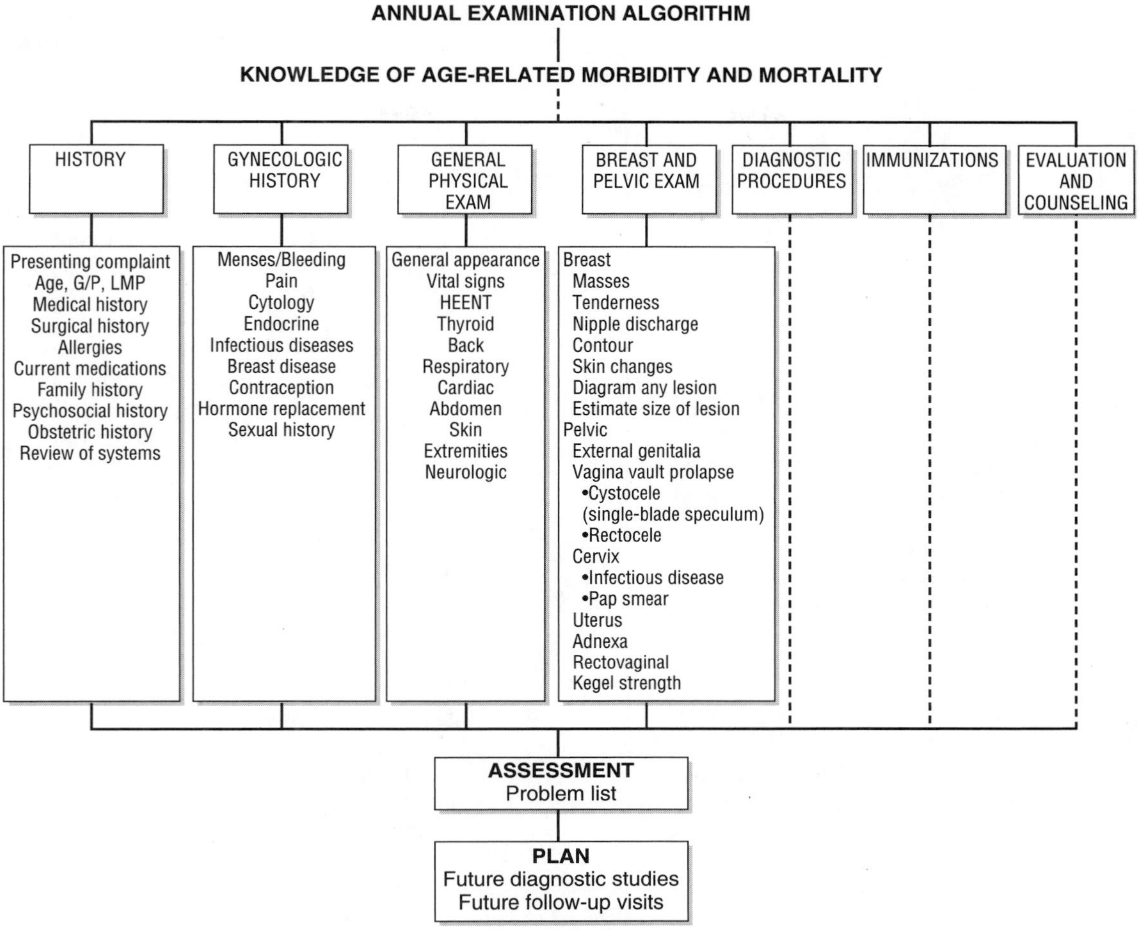

ANNUAL EXAMINATION ALGORITHM

KNOWLEDGE OF AGE-RELATED MORBIDITY AND MORTALITY

HISTORY	GYNECOLOGIC HISTORY	GENERAL PHYSICAL EXAM	BREAST AND PELVIC EXAM	DIAGNOSTIC PROCEDURES	IMMUNIZATIONS	EVALUATION AND COUNSELING

Presenting complaint Age, G/P, LMP Medical history Surgical history Allergies Current medications Family history Psychosocial history Obstetric history Review of systems	Menses/Bleeding Pain Cytology Endocrine Infectious diseases Breast disease Contraception Hormone replacement Sexual history	General appearance Vital signs HEENT Thyroid Back Respiratory Cardiac Abdomen Skin Extremities Neurologic	Breast 　Masses 　Tenderness 　Nipple discharge 　Contour 　Skin changes 　Diagram any lesion 　Estimate size of lesion Pelvic 　External genitalia 　Vagina vault prolapse 　　•Cystocele 　　(single-blade speculum) 　　•Rectocele 　Cervix 　　•Infectious disease 　　•Pap smear 　Uterus 　Adnexa 　Rectovaginal 　Kegel strength			

ASSESSMENT
Problem list

PLAN
Future diagnostic studies
Future follow-up visits

Figure 1. Algorithm for the annual examination. G/P, gravida/para; HEENT, head, ears, eyes, nose, and throat; LMP, last menstrual period.

health questionnaire to the patient prior to her office visit so that she can answer questions completely and confidentially. These questionnaires are often helpful when addressing topics with the patient that she might not have felt comfortable bringing up on her own.

Patient's History

The following aspects of the patient's history should be explored:

1. Presenting issue or complaint. The physician should ask the patient to thoroughly describe her presenting complaint. This includes the nature of the complaint, the duration, the severity, any previous treatments, and any concerns she may have regarding this complaint.
2. Age, gravida, para, last menstrual period.

3. History of any major medical illnesses:
   Diabetes
   Respiratory illnesses
   Cardiovascular disease
   Childhood illnesses
   Liver and gall bladder disease
   Cancer
   Infectious diseases, eg hepatitis and tuberculosis
   Hypertension
   Renal disease
   Urinary tract infections
   Embolic disease
   Thyroid disease
   Neurologic disorders
   Migraines
4. Previous surgery or trauma, history of blood transfusion.
5. Allergies to medications, medications currently in use.
6. Family history:

Diabetes
Breast cancer
Colon cancer
Any congenital anomalies
Any inherited diseases, eg sickle cell, cystic fibrosis, thalassemia, Tay-Sachs
Hypertension
Any gynecologic cancer
Other cancer
Cardiovascular disease
Twins

7. Psychosocial history:
Marital status
Number of children
Substance abuse, including alcohol, tobacco, illicit drugs
Significant psychosocial stressors, including a history of child abuse, sexual abuse, or domestic violence
Support system
Exercise
Nutrition/vitamin supplements
Symptoms of depression
Occupation

8. Obstetric history:
Numbers of pregnancies
Pregnancy outcomes, including year of pregnancy, mode of delivery, weight of baby, weeks of gestation, condition of child at the time of the examination
Pregnancy complications
Number of pregnancies resulting in ectopic pregnancies, elective abortions, molar pregnancies, spontaneous abortions, or still births

9. Review of systems. Any standard review of physiologic systems is appropriate.

10. Gynecologic history (including breast diseases)
a. Menses/beeding:
Last menstrual period
Age at menarche
If menopausal, when did menses cease
Interval and duration of menses
History of dysmenorrhea or menorrhagia
Any irregular vaginal bleeding (between menses, postcoital)
b. Pain:
Symptoms of pelvic pressure
History of dyspareunia
History of pelvic pain any time during the cycle
c. Cytology:
Any history of DES exposure
Date of last Pap smear
Any history of abnormal Pap smears and treatment

d. Endocrine:
History of virilization: change of voice, change in facial or body hair
Any symptoms of premenstrual syndrome
Menopausal symptoms (hot flashes, mood swings, vaginal dryness, age at menopause, any vaginal bleeding)
Any history of treatments for infertility
e. Any previous gynecologic infectious diseases:
Vaginal infections: bacterial vaginosis, trichomonas, yeast infections
Cervical infections: gonorrhea, chlamydia
Perineal: herpes, human papillomavirus
Any history of pelvic inflammatory disease
Any history of any other sexually transmitted diseases, including hepatitis, syphilis, and human immunodeficiency virus (HIV)
f. Breast disease:
Any history of fibrocystic breast changes
Any history of a previous breast biopsy
Any abnormal findings during breast-self examination
Any nipple discharge
Date of the last mammogram
g. Current therapeutic regimens (where applicable):
Contraception
Hormone replacement therapy
Antibiotic suppression for urinary tract infections or herpes
h. Other:
Symptoms of urinary incontinence
Sexual history
Any previous gynecologic surgeries
Current method of contraception, past methods, duration of use

Physical Examination

The intent of the physical examination performed at the time of the annual examination is that it be complete. This is as true for young women who present for contraceptive counseling requesting only an annual Pap smear as it is for post-menopausal women requesting gynecologic care for hormone replacement. The following examinations should be made:

General appearance
Vital signs
Head, ears, eyes, nose, oral cavity, throat, and neck, including the thyroid
Back
Breast (discussed in detail later)
Respiratory and cardiovascular

Abdominal

Skin–note any signs of hirsutism (reinforce the importance of protection from the sun)

Extremities, including observation for edema, varicosities, and pulses

Basic neurologic

Breast and Pelvic Examinations

Breast

It is crucial for the obstetrician/gynecologist to perform a complete breast examination (Fig. 2). Initially, the patient should be sitting in the upright position, and both breasts should be inspected visually for any abnormalities in contour or skin retraction. It is sometimes helpful to have the patient place her hands on her hips and compress so that any changes in the contour of the breasts are evident. After this inspection, the patient is asked to lie on the examination table in the supine position. She should be draped appropriately, so that each breast is examined individually while the other breast is covered. It is often easier to examine the breast with the patient's arm above her head. The key to an adequate breast examination is to thoroughly palpate all of the breast tissue in all quadrants, including the axillary tail. Fifty percent of all breast cancers are found in the upper outer quadrant of the breast, which includes the tail. There are many different specific methods for examining the breast, all of which are acceptable. One commonly used method is to move the finger tips in a circular motion throughout all of the breast tissue and then to palpate the nipples, noting any discharge. In addition, the patient's axillary, supraclavicular, and suprasternal lymph nodes should be palpated. During this examination, it is important to reinforce the monthly breast self-examination. Eighty-five percent of breast cancers are found by the patient.

Pelvis

External Genitalia. The physician should visually inspect the entire area of the external genitalia, including the vulva, labia majora and minora, clitoris, urethral meatus, and fourchette, noting evidence of lesions. Palpation should be performed along the gland areas, including Bartholin's and Skene's glands.

Figure 2. (1) Examination of breasts begins with inspection. The patient is disrobed to the waist and comfortably seated facing the examiner. Asymmetry, prominent veins, and skin changes may be signs of disease. (2) The patient raises her arms above her head, thereby altering the position of the breasts. Immobility or abnormal cutaneous attachments may become evident. (3) Inward pressure on the hips tenses the pectoralis major muscle. Abnormal attachments to its overlying fascia and skin can produce retraction or dimpling of the skin. (4) Palpatory examination of the supraclavicular lymph nodes. (5) The deltopectoral triangle is palpated for evidence of infraclavicular nodal enlargement. (6) Each axilla is examined for nodal enlargement. Proper placement of the examiner's hands and of the patient's arm is important. (7) Thorough palpatory examination of entire breast for masses is performed with patient in supine position. A fine rotational movement of the hands is useful to appreciate the consistency of the underlying tissues. (8) The nipple is compressed to elicit discharge. (From Scott JR, Disaia PJ, Hammond CB, et al: Danforth's Handbook of Obstetrics and Gynecology. Philadelphia: Lippincott-Raven, 1996.)

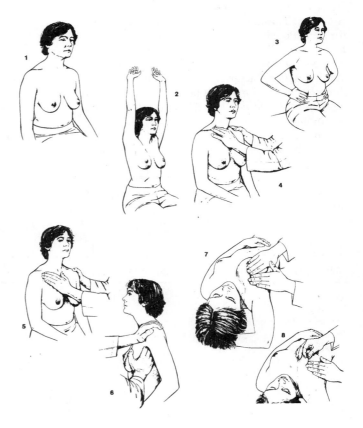

Vagina. The physician should observe the appearance of the vagina, inspecting for masses or lesions. Any hypoestrogenic effects should be noted, such as atrophy, erosions, or the presence or absence of a vaginal discharge. If the patient has any signs of vaginal vault prolapse, it is important to have her perform a Valsalva maneuver at this point to evaluate for rectocele, enterocele, and cystocele. A warm speculum is then inserted gently into the vagina. It is perfectly acceptable to lubricate the speculum with water or a small amount of lubricant. The walls of the vagina are inspected as the speculum is inserted and then the cervix is viewed.

Cervix. The physician should visually inspect the cervix for state of parity and any abnormalities, including lesions, polyps, discharge, or bleeding.

Infectious Disease Screening. If the patient has any concerns about a vaginal discharge or any sexually transmitted disease or pelvic pain, it is important to perform a wet mount and cultures at this point.

In screening for bacterial vaginosis, trichomonas, or vaginal yeast infection, these entities are best diagnosed by wet mount rather than by culture. For a wet mount, a cotton tip applicator is placed inside the vagina and some discharge is removed. The material on the cotton tip applicator is then applied to two glass sides, one of them with saline and the other with KOH. KOH is used for two indications, (1) to perform the Whiff test for bacterial vaginosis, and (2) to examine under the microscope for the presence or absence of *Candida*. Table 3 delineates diagnostic findings seen on wet mounts.

Culture samples for chlamydia and gonorrhea should be taken from the endocervical area. Since chlamydia is an obligate intracellular organism, it is imperative to obtain endocervical cells for diagnosis by placing a dacron-tipped applicator inside the endocervix.

Since 50% of women diagnosed with chla-mydia are assymptomatic, it is important to have a high index of suspicion and to screen frequently. Prevalence of chlamydia does vary according to populations; routine screening should be considered in areas with high prevalence.

Pap Smear. The ectocervical area, which includes the entire portio and transformation zone, is sampled with a spatula in a 360-degree fashion. The cytobrush is then gently inserted into the endocervix, rotated 360 degrees, and then removed and wiped on a cytology slide. It is important to spray the slide immediately with a fixative to reduce the incidence of drying artifact. The speculum is gently removed.

If there has been any evidence of prolapse or any history of urinary incontinence, it is important to perform the single-blade speculum examination.

Single-Blade Speculum Examination. The speculum is split in half and the single blade of the speculum is then replaced into the vagina. Initially it is placed in the posterior area of the vagina and the patient is asked to perform the Valsalva maneuver; the degree of prolapse is noted. The single blade is moved circumferentially around the vagina, and any prolapse after the Valsalva maneuver is noted. In addition, it is appropriate to ask the patient to cough to see if there is any demonstration of stress incontinence. In addition to this examination in the supine position, it is important to repeat the single-blade speculum examination in the upright position to further delineate the degree of prolapse noted and any further evidence of incontinence.

Bimanual Examination. Place a small amount of lubricant on your examination fingers and gently place your fingers inside the patient's vaginal vault, moving very slowly and gently to the cervix. Evaluation of the cervix is important. It is important to note the consistency, size, and mobility. Place your other hand on the patient's abdo-

TABLE 3. Diagnostic Findings on Vaginal Wet Mounts

Diagnosis	Discharge	pH	Microscopic	Reaction to KOH
Bacterial vaginosis	Copious, milky, homogeneous, gray	5–6	Clue cells	Amine odor
Trichomoniasis	Frothy, gray or yellow-green	6–7	Motile trichomonads, many white blood cells	Mildly positive amine odor
Candida	White, curdy	4–5	Pseudohyphae	No odor
Normal	Slate gray to white	3.8–4.5	Free-floating bacilli	No odor

men to palpate the uterus and adnexal structures. It is important to note the size, shape, consistency, position, and mobility of the uterus and the presence or absence of tenderness. Examination should include palpation of the uterosacral ligaments and posterior cul-de-sac. When examining the adnexa, note the size, position, and mobility of the ovaries and the presence or absence of masses and tenderness. It is important to confirm your bimanual examination with a rectovaginal examination. In addition, for women over the age of 40, a sample should be obtained for a fecal occult blood test.

Kegel Exercise. It is important to instruct all women in the proper use of Kegel exercises. These exercises build pelvic floor support, which prevents or improves symptoms of urinary incontinence.

At the conclusion of the bimanual examination, prior to the rectovaginal examination, the physician places one or two fingers in the patient's vagina. She is asked to tighten her vagina around the physician's fingers. These exercises are most effective when the pubococcygeus muscle is contracted in isolation from other surrounding muscles, so the abdominal and gluteal muscles should remain relaxed. Symmetry of the contraction, strength, and duration should be noted. A woman with good perineal strength can usually hold the contraction for 6 seconds or more.

The patient should be instructed to perform these exercises by squeezing for 3 to 10 seconds, then relaxing for 3 to 10 seconds, in sets of six to 10, four or five times per day. She should not do a larger number of sets at one time because this may cause muscle fiber fatigue.

In addition, the patient should be instructed not to perform Kegel exercises while urinating. During micturition, the detrusor muscle of the bladder is contracting while the urethra is relaxing. If one overrides this process by repetitively contracting the muscles to stop urine, this may cause long-term nerve damage to the system.

Health Promotion Screening and Review

- Diet
  Folate supplementation for women age 13–46: prevention of neural tube defect; 1000–1500 mg calcium supplementation; 400–800 IU vitamin D supplementation
- Weight
- Exercise
  Weight-bearing exercise, 20 minutes, three times per week

- Substance abuse screening and counseling
- Sexually transmitted disease and HIV prevention counseling (including hepatitis, syphilis, gonorrhea, and chlamydia)
- Pregnancy prevention counseling
- Community violence/firearms
- Domestic violence: Do you feel safe at home?
- Seat belts and bicycle/motorcycle helmets
- Smoking cessation
- Suicide, depression
- Sun exposure and skin cancer prevention
- Monthly breast self-examination
- Additional areas for the older woman:
  Hormone replacement therapy
  Visual actuity/glaucoma/hearing
  Environmental control: prevention of falls
  Durable power of attorney/living will/advanced directives

Diagnostic Procedures

Diagnostic procedures should be geared toward the age-related risk and any high-risk circumstances that pertain to a particular patient (Table 4). Screening tests are intended to reduce morbidity and mortality in a group at a reasonable cost. Criteria for appropriate screening tests include: (1) the disease is significant in terms of prevalence, morbidity, and mortality; (2) screening, and thus early detection, can reduce the morbidity or mortality; and (3) the screening test is safe, reasonably priced, sensitive, and specific.

Frequency of Pap Smears

1. Annual Pap smears when the patient is sexually active or at least 18 years old.

TABLE 4. Age-Related Diagnostic Procedures

Age (years)	Procedure
13–18	Pap smear yearly when sexually active or at age 18
19–39	Pap smear yearly; cholesterol every 5 years
40–64	Pap smear yearly; cholesterol every 5 years; mammogram every 1–2 years until 50, then yearly; fecal occult blood yearly; sigmoidoscopy every 5–10 years after age 50
Over 65	Pap smear yearly; cholesterol every 3–5 years; mammogram yearly; fecal occult blood yearly; sigmoidoscopy every 5–10 years urinalysis yearly; thyroid-stimulating hormone test every 3–5 years

2. After a patient has had three or more consecutive, satisfactory, normal annual Pap smears and is low risk, the time interval between Pap smears may be extended to 3 years.
3. Risk factors that necessitate annual Pap smears include the following:
   History of human papillomavirus or other sexually transmitted diseases
   Cigarette smoking habit
   HIV-positive status
   History of multiple sexual partners

Other Screening Tests

Many risk factors serve as indications for various screening tests (Table 5). These recommendations are for screening tests only. If the patient presents with pertinent history and physical findings that indicate the need for diagnostic studies, the physician should proceed as clinically indicated.

For all diagnostic procedures that are ordered, it is imperative that appropriate follow-up be obtained so that any abnormalities in the diagnostic tests will be acted upon in an expeditious manner.

Immunizations

Immunizations are one of the key ways to prevent major life-threatening illnesses. Research advances continue to bring new immunizations to the forefront; therefore, physicians should remain vigilant about new immunization recommendations.

The current recommended schedule and indications for immunizations are given in Table 6.

TABLE 5. Risk Factors as Indications for Screening Tests

Test	Risk Factor
Varicella and rubella titer	Women of childbearing age lacking evidence of immunity
TB skin test	Close contact with a person with TB
	HIV infected
	Health care workers
	Resided in country or institution of high prevalence
Lipid profile	Elevated cholesterol
	History of parent or sibling with high cholesterol or premature coronary artery disease
	Diabetes mellitus or smoking
Mammogram	35 years or older, family history of premenopausally diagnosed breast cancer in a first-degree relative (or 10 years prior to the age at diagnosis of family member's breast cancer)
Fasting glucose every 3–5 yrs	Family history of diabetes, history of gestational diabetes
	Obese
Thyroid-stimulating hormone	Family history of thyroid disease
	Other autoimmune disease
Colonoscopy	History of inflammatory bowel disease or polyps
	Family history of polyps, colorectal cancer
Bacteriuria testing	Persons with diabetes mellitus
HIV and hepatitis B and C testing	STDs, IVDA
	Multiple sexual partners
	Reside in area of high prevalence
	Blood transfusion 1978–1985
	Abnormal cervical cytology
	Pregnancy
STD testing	Multiple sexual partners
	Partner with multiple contacts
	History of repeated episodes
Hemoglobin	Persons of Caribbean, Latin American, Asian, Mediterranean or African descent
	Excessive menstrual flow

HIV, human immunodeficiency virus; IVDA, intravenous drug abuse; STD, sexually transmitted disease; TB, tuberculosis.

TABLE 6. Schedule and Indications for Immunizations

Immunization	Frequency/Indication
Mumps, measles, rubella	Once if nonimmune
Tetanus-diphtheria booster	Once between the ages of 14 and 16 Every 10 years thereafter
Influenza vaccine	Annual for women age 65 or older, residents of chronic care facilities, persons with chronic diseases (e.g., HIV positive)
Pneumococcal vaccine	Once for women age 65 or older and patients with medical conditions (e.g., HIV positive) that increase the risk of pneumococcal infection
Varicella vaccine	Once if nonimmune and considering pregnancy (this vaccine should not be administered during pregnancy), patients who are immune compromised (e.g., HIV positive)
Hepatitis A vaccine	Patients who live in or travel to endemic areas, HIV positive, hepatitis C positive
Hepatitis B vaccine	IVDA, blood product recipients, HIV positive, hepatitis C positive Health care workers Multiple sexual partners, adolescents, household contacts of hepatitis B carriers

HIV, human immunodeficency virus; IVDA, intravenous drug abuse.

Conclusion of the Annual Examination

At the conclusion of the annual examination, it is important that the physician discuss the findings, normal and abnormal, with the patient. The patient may have further questions provoked by the history and physical examination process, and these should be answered. Finally, the physician should discuss recommendations for continued prevention of disease and health promotion and recommendations for follow-up. It is often helpful to develop a problem list on which are listed current problems, any past problems of significance to current status, further diagnostic work-up planned for each problem, treatment planned, date of identification and resolution for each problem, medications, drug allergies, and plans for health maintenance (eg, date of next Pap smear, mammogram, tuberculosis test).

Documentation

It is imperative to carefully document the complete annual examination in the patient's medical record. The medical record is the only permanent way of confirming that the physician did, in fact, a take a complete history on the patient, perform a complete physical examination, counsel her appropriately for all the indicated diagnostic procedures and immunizations, and discuss any lifestyle changes and plans for future follow-up. In addition, if an abnormality is found on physical examination, it is helpful to diagram the lesion and to estimate the size.

In addition to documenting what was done, it is equally important to document what was not done. In fact, if the physician made a recommendation to a patient and she declined that recommendation, it is important to document her declining.

Atelectasis in the Postoperative Period

Russell P. Woda, DO

Thomas E. Reilley, DO

Atelectasis is a pulmonary complication that threatens every bedridden patient. It is the most common postoperative complication and with an associated pneumonia is the leading cause of postoperative morbidity and death. Pre-existing risk factors include cardiopulmonary disease, smoking, obesity, and advanced age. The risk is also increased in emergency surgical procedures. Obstetric surgical patients have gestational factors that may predispose to this condition. Atelectasis is a physical collapse of the geometric lung unit of the alveolus, usually in adjacent segments, which then removes that portion of the alveolar capillary membrane from participation in respiratory gas exchange and probably affects the nonrespiratory functions of that lung unit as a metabolic organ, that is, clearance of vasoactive agents, lymph flow, and release of prostaglandins.

Complete obstruction of subsegmental bronchi resulting from absorption of alveolar gases is thought to be the most common cause of atelectasis; however, other factors are probably more important. The development of discoid atelectasis can be demonstrated within 15 minutes in normal volunteers who are anesthetized and paralyzed in the prone position without operation. Cephalad displacement of the dorsal portion of a lax diaphragm in a supine anesthetized patient occurs from the weight of the abdominal contents themselves, resulting in an altered ventilation-perfusion ($\dot{V}/\dot{Q}$) ratio. It has also been demonstrated that anesthesia decreases the functional residual capacity by affecting the function of the rib cage itself. These effects may be lessened by regional anesthesia and laparoscopic surgical techniques. In addition to physical collapse of basilar alveoli, the change in $\dot{V}/\dot{Q}$ is worsened by the addition of positive-pressure ventilation to a patient paralyzed with neuromuscular blocking agents. Clinically, the anesthesiologist recognizes a decrease in the expected partial pressure of arterial oxygen (PaO_2) for a given fraction of inspired oxygen (FIO_2) during an otherwise uneventful operative procedure. The increased abdominal pressure of the gravid uterus has been shown to diminish functional residual capacity (FRC) through a decrease in both residual volume and expiratory reserve volume. Since other intra-abdominal operative procedures can decrease FRC by as much as 75%, the addition of pregnancy to the factors of diaphragmatic $\dot{V}/\dot{Q}$ alteration during anesthesia as explained earlier are significant in the development of atelectasis during operative procedures. The collapsed atelectatic alveolus may not produce surfactant because of loss of its geometric form, thus promoting continuance of atelectasis as a result of the loss of surface tension–reducing properties of surfactant.

Three other factors are poorly appreciated in their role in producing or promoting atelectasis. They are mucociliary clearance, oxygen administration, and excessive and improper suctioning.

Mucociliary clearance, by which the normal tracheobronchial tree clears itself of secretion, is greatly inhibited by both dry anesthetic gases and the presence of an endotracheal tube itself. In addition, overstimulation of mucus production may occur, and the mucus is then undercleared. Prolonged administration of increased FIO_2 can decrease tracheal ciliary action as well as cause further absorption atelectasis when the splinting effect of alveolar nitrogen is replaced by absorbable oxygen. Although mechanical suctioning of the airway and tracheobronchial tree is a common hospital procedure, it has many complications and may cause atelectasis itself when improperly applied. Endotracheal suctioning should be performed only when there are retained secretions and should be limited in duration, preceded by adequate oxygenation, and followed by careful hyperinflation to re-expand atelectactic areas that may have been created by the suction catheter itself.

The diagnosis of atelectasis becomes apparent as a reduction in oxygenation by arterial blood gases or pulse oximetry, elevated temperature, and other physical and radiologic signs within 24 hours of surgery. Tachypnea may occur with significant hypoxemia, and chest auscultation reveals decreased breath sounds and moist rales with occasional wheezes; however, except for increased temperature these physical signs may be completely absent.

The therapy of atelectasis is in using minimally adequate sedation or narcotics while encouraging deep spontaneous ventilation in the upright position. Even if the patient is bedridden, the upright position allows the lung bases to expand their basilar segments. Humidified supplemental oxygen should be provided to ensure adequate hemoglobin saturation. Incentive spirometry is effective when ordered every 1 to 2 hours while the patient is awake. Patients should be ambulated or sat at the side of the bed as soon as possible. When comparing cough and deep-breathing with incentive spirometry and postural drainage, the frequency and adequate supervision of respiratory therapy are more important than the type of therapy used. More severe forms of atelectasis require the judicious application of continuous positive airway pressure (CPAP) therapy. CPAP therapy by mask can be employed up to 15 cm H_2O if these specific masks are available. Few commercially available masks fit well with proper tension, and caution must be used to avoid nasal skin necrosis from mask pressure. A functioning nasogastric tube should be in place to prevent gastric distention above 15 cm H_2O CPAP therapy, and the patient should be alert enough to protect the airway. An endotracheal tube is generally required if CPAP therapy is used beyond 15 to 20 cm H_2O.

Battered Woman

Julianne S. Toohey, MD

During the last decade, increased attention has been given to the complex crime of domestic violence. It is disturbing, however, that most practitioners continue to be unaware of the magnitude and terrible consequences of spousal abuse and are unclear on how to diagnose and respond. **Domestic violence is the number one cause of injury to women in the United States.** One in five women has been or will be abused in an intimate relationship and 4000 will die each year in this country as a result. Ninety-five percent of domestic violence victims are women, so while the problem is one of intergenerational family violence between both genders, it continues to be valid to talk about "the battered woman." This chapter provides assistance with identification of and appropriate intervention for domestic violence in the clinical setting.

Diagnosis

Management cannot proceed without correct diagnosis (Fig. 1). Prevalence estimates find that 22% to 35% of injured women presenting to the emergency room have been abused by their partners, but only 1 in 25 is correctly identified. Approximately 20% to 25% of women presenting to family practice clinics and 17% of obstetric patients are in violent relationships. These num-

bers differ greatly from the numbers identified by physicians.

Health care providers fail to diagnose most women suffering from abuse because of various barriers. Battered women feel great shame and fear for their safety if they confide in anyone. Some women have been abused so long they no longer see this behavior as abnormal and may even believe they deserve the abuse. Most of them are filled with despair and have no hope for their future or confidence in the response of the system.

Physicians also erect barriers to correct diagnosis. They are uneducated about the frequency of abusive relationships and they are filled with prejudices about what women could be at risk. It is vital for health care providers to know that battered women come from all socioeconomic, racial, religious, and educational backgrounds and that violence is seen in both homosexual and heterosexual relationships and in all ages. Physicians are also afraid of offending their patients, have limited time during patient visits, and do not know how to appropriately respond. In spite of all these factors, the number one reason physicians fail to diagnose most cases of domestic violence is that they do not ask the right questions.

Routine assessment of all women is the key to improving diagnostic efforts. It removes the specter of prejudice and is a form of education in itself. Certainly all women presenting to the emergency room, for prenatal and postpartum care, and for routine doctor's visits should be screened. It is appropriate to begin with "Unfor-

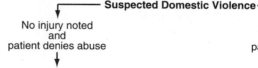

Figure 1. Algorithm for the management of domestic abuse.

Note: Screen ALL women for abuse, whether suspected or not, especially during prenatal care and postpartum. Always inquire about child abuse.

Suspected Domestic Violence

No injury noted
and
patient denies abuse

1. Teach the cycle of violence.
2. Give referrals to shelters and local domestic violence organizations.
3. Reappoint frequently.
4. Don't give up!

Suspicious injury
and/or
patient reports abuse

1. Use patient's own words.
2. Document injury carefully; include photos, body chart.
3. Treat injuries and hospitalize if necessary.
4. Teach the cycle of violence.
5. Make safety assessment and plan.
6. Refer to social services, local shelters, and domestic violence organizations.
7. Report to the local police department with the patient's knowledge. Refer to own state laws.

tunately, violence in relationships is a common problem for many women. Are you or have you ever been in a relationship where you were frightened or hurt?" Always assess your patient in private without her partner or other family member or friend. Private time with your patient is essential for many issues and she deserves this attention and respect.

Every battered woman is a unique individual with a unique situation. However, there are certain characteristics that many of these women share. Typically, a battered woman is isolated from friends and even family. She rarely joins groups or social functions without her spouse. She may use clothing or glasses that cover her injuries and often does not carry money, credit cards, or checks. She presents to the physician's office or emergency department with multiple somatic complaints or is noncompliant with her visits and delays treatment for injuries. It is important to call patients when they miss scheduled visits and to reschedule as soon as possible. A battered woman may miss work frequently because she is too sore or she does not want her coworkers to notice her bruises. Her spouse often calls at work or appears suddenly to ensure she is where she should be. Women most at risk for domestic violence are those with increased dependence on their spouses or boyfriends, for example, teenagers, pregnant women, those with disabilities or language barriers, and those isolated geographically in rural areas or who are unable to drive.

Domestic violence is about abuse of power and control. The batterer, almost universally a victim of abuse as well, has such low self-esteem that he desperately tries to control as many aspects of his life as possible. His attempts to control his wife or girlfriend often includes making all family and financial decisions, controlling her time and her use of the car, dictating her career, and when or whether she will be pregnant. He accomplishes this by threats, intimidation, and physical abuse.

These couples are typically caught in a cyclic pattern of behavior, described as the cycle of violence, which includes three phases. Phase one is the tension building phase, when the batterer is increasingly angry and irritable. Phase two is the actual battering incident that may include anything from verbal and emotional abuse, a slap, or push to repeated beatings, rape, and even death. Phase three has been called the Honeymoon Phase. During this time, the batterer is repentant, tells his victim he loves her and will never hurt her again. This phase gives her hope and may therefore be the most dangerous phase of all. Studies have shown that with time the Honeymoon Phase gets shorter and shorter and the abusive incidents escalate.

If your patient denies abuse but she is a high-risk individual or you are suspicious, it is appropriate to teach the cycle of violence and its escalation. Schedule frequent appointments. If she has a suspicious injury, it may be more effective to ask, "In my experience, when a woman has a bruise like this, someone has hurt her. Did this happen to you? Are you safe at home?" Do not expect your patient to immediately trust and confide in you. She is overcoming years of conditioning and fear and she does not need to fulfill your timetable. Because of frustration, a physician may become inappropriately controlling. The health care provider needs to offer education, support, and referrals. It is always the woman's choice to reveal or deny the abuse and badgering her is not helpful. Remember that she knows her situation best and she deserves autonomy and decision-making opportunities. It is obvious, however, that many women need help and counseling to be able to make good decisions. Tell her that you are concerned, that you are available to talk, and that if she is in an abusive relationship her life is in danger. Always provide information about domestic violence in the women's restroom, where the patient may find referral or hotline numbers in privacy. If she denies abuse but you are concerned, document your worries and your educational and referral efforts and schedule frequent appointments.

Pregnancy provides a unique opportunity for obstetricians to respond to domestic violence. It is clear that abuse increases in severity and frequency during a women's pregnancy and probably also during the postpartum period. One in six neonates will go home to a woman who was battered during her pregnancy. During prenatal visits, the health care provider has the advantage of seeing the patient on a regular basis and may therefore more easily establish trust and rapport. Family dynamics may become more apparent with the increased involvement of spouses in the birthing process. This fact, however, may also make private assessment of each patient more difficult. It is imperative that physicians be open to changing their office routine to ensure private time with each new patient. Remember to ask each patient if the pregnancy is wanted and of her options. Battered women have an increased incidence of unwanted pregnancies, low birth weight infants, and stillbirth. Battery is also most likely implicated in some cases of premature rupture of membranes, preterm labor, preterm delivery, and abruptio placenta. In addition to routinely screening all pregnant women, these cases deserve careful scrutiny.

While violence is more common during pregnancy, it is also known that a woman is more likely to seek help during this time. The postpartum period is also an excellent time for a physician or nurse to spend private, quiet time with a patient and help ensure that the future of this new family is not in jeopardy. Provide frequent educational efforts to staff and nursing and include domestic violence information in the postpartum packets given to all new mothers. Informational videos are also helpful in our hospital during the postpartum stay.

The association between battery and teen pregnancy is frequently overlooked. Dating violence has reached epidemic proportions and a great many of our teenagers are pregnant as a result of rape. Many girls fear that if they "say no" to intercourse or take contraceptives, they will be beaten by their boyfriends. All teenagers in your practice deserve extra time and attention for violence screening whether they are pregnant or not.

Management

Once a patient has confided in you that she is a victim of domestic violence, make immediate adjustments to spend more time with her. Call social services or a domestic violence intervention team if available. Review when the violent behavior began, and how often and how severely she has been or is injured. Inquire about child abuse in her home. In over 50% of cases of domestic violence, the children are also injured.

If the patient is currently injured, have her describe when and how the injury occurred. A careful and complete physical examination should be performed, documenting all current bruises, cuts, scars, and the state of the patient's clothing. Pay special attention to the head and inside of the mouth. Remember that bruises may not show up until later. Any neck swelling or discomfort should be carefully assessed for evidence of attempted strangulation. Injuries should be measured and described and all foreign material, for example, carpet fibers, glass, or splinters, removed from wounds should be documented. A body chart or photographs are very helpful in court.

Always ask about rape. This form of abuse is common in cases of domestic violence and it is especially hurtful and humiliating. If a rape has occurred, proceed with the appropriate forensic collection of evidence with the kit provided by the sheriff-coroner and a careful pelvic examination with a colposcope to help document injuries. Offer emergency birth control if the assault occurred within 72 hours (Ovral 50 mg, two tablets immediately and again in 12 hours) and screening for sexually transmitted diseases.

It is possible the patient may be helped by psychiatric assessment. In addition to frequent problems with depression and suicide attempts, many battered women are dependent on alcohol or drugs to cope or as part of their abuse. It has been noted that many physicians discriminate against patients who are under the influence and often do not prescribe sufficient or appropriate pain medication. Remember that it is never the physician's role to make judgments and that an acute situation is not the time to begin drug rehabilitation.

Once a patient is more calm and her injuries have been treated, a safety plan must be formulated. If she is to be hospitalized, ensure that the staff knows not to give out information regarding her presence and condition. Do not have patient's names on boards or charts that are in clear view.

If she does not require in-house care, ask her what she feels is best in her situation. Remind her that violence escalates and that her life and the lives of her children may be in danger, in spite of the fact that her partner may now be repentant. Besides the frequency and severity of the beatings, there are specific signs that point to a very dangerous situation: recent escalation of violence, a gun in the house, signs of depression, threats of suicide or homicide from the batterer, and kidnapping of the children. Does she have a safe place to go? Can she be admitted to a shelter for battered women? As much as possible, encourage this route. Shelters have provided a safe haven for many women, including counselors and support groups. Shelter personnel may also help plan for the patient's safety regardless of whether she stays there or not. I strongly advise physicians to be familiar with their local shelters and to call them for guidance.

It is frustrating for the physician if the patient chooses to return to her partner. However, the reality is that this will occur more often than not. It is important not to allow this frustration to keep you from providing the best care possible. Sit down with her and suggest an emergency kit containing extra keys, money, medicines, diapers, phone numbers, custody papers and other important documents. She should keep this kit at a neighbor's house or where her partner would not find it. Also review some basic safety tips:

1. It may sometimes be appropriate to give the batterer what he wants to ensure your safety.
2. If an argument begins, stay away from areas of the house where there is a gun or other weapons. For example, the kitchen is a very dangerous room because of the knives kept there.
3. Plan ahead of time all possible exits from your home.
4. Devise a code word you can use with your children or friends that means you need the police immediately.
5. Tell a neighbor about your situation.
6. Talk to others. Breaking the isolation is the first step to breaking the cycle of violence.
7. Carefully plan when you will leave. Never threaten to leave, as this will only enrage him. **Remember that the most dangerous time for you is the time of separation.**

Many states have mandatory reporting laws in cases of domestic violence. Make sure you are familiar with your state's requirements. For example, in California, a physician or other health care provider must report immediately to the police if a patient presents for treatment of an injury that is or most likely is the result of domestic violence. A physician must report the incident to the local police immediately and file a written report within 2 working days even if the woman does not wish to press charges. Failure to report may result in 6 months jail time and/or a $1000 fine. When the police are called on a case, document the officer's name, the case number, and the action that was taken.

Experts in the field of domestic violence disagree on whether mandatory reporting by the medical community is advisable, primarily because of concern for the woman's safety. While there is room for continued discussion on this controversy, I believe that mandatory reporting is essential to improve not only the physician response but the response of the entire system. It clearly identifies spousal abuse as a crime that should be punishable to the full extent of the law. However, it is vital that health care providers understand that reporting to the police alone does not ensure their patient's safety and that this is obviously their primary responsibility.

The physician's role in combating domestic violence should reach beyond universal screening, diagnosis, and appropriate, compassionate

intervention. Former Surgeon General C. Everett Koop and the American College of Obstetricians and Gynecologists have clearly identified domestic violence as a medical and public health issue. The physician must involve himself or herself in community efforts to improve the response of the police, the courts, and shelters to make it truly possible for the battered woman to successfully leave her dangerous situation and lead the life she deserves.

Breast Cancer: Principles of Therapy

Dirk Kiebeck, MD

Fritz K. Beller, MD

Only a minority of gynecologists in the United States manage patients with malignancies of the breast. But patients with breast cancer frequently consult with gynecologists regarding hormonal manipulation as part of an adjuvant therapeutic regimen, for advice on hormone replacement therapy after treatment, or as the physician who initially recommended the screening. Breast cancer is the most common malignant tumor in women in the Western cultures. This translates into more than 145,000 new cases per year and more than 54,000 annual deaths in the United States. Because the gynecologist is the primary care provider for many women at the time breast cancer is diagnosed, it is imperative that he or she understands the principles affecting the management of breast cancer.

Risk Factors

The importance of identifying risk factors associated with the development of breast cancer is spurred by the knowledge that 1 in 10 women will develop breast cancer in their lifetimes. Of many risk factors identified (early menarche, late menopause more than two biopsies performed even for benign lesions, proven atypical fibrocystic disease or carcinoma in situ, and many others), a positive family history has the greatest influence on directing surveillance strategies and in some cases definive treatment. When a first-degree relative is known to have had a breast malignancy, the risk for the patient increases two to three times.

Recently, the breast and ovarian cancer genes *BrCa1* and *BrCa2* were identified; these are frequently present in high-risk families. Social and ethical issues of genetic testing are very complex, and testing cannot be recommended on a routine basis. Preliminary results of the first controlled intervention trials show a risk reduction in the 90% range for women who undergo bilateral mastectomy after positive genetic testing, but this is obviously not a choice for all patients at risk. For the much more common nonfamilial breast cancer, there is evidence of the presence of a mutated progesterone receptor gene as a possible genetic risk factor, increasing the breast cancer risk twofold. As an isolated finding this would not prompt surgical intervention at the time of discovery; conclusive data are pending.

Biology

Most tumors come to the attention of the physician as a result of patient breast self-examination. At the time cancers first become palpable, tumor size is approximately 2 cm, and the tumor has probably been growing for 6 to 8 years. Over this period of time, a tumor has had ample time to metastasize. Surgical interventions alone, encompassing a spectrum from wide local excision to radical mastectomy, seem to have little influence on survival if adjuvant therapy is not considered. Although a rate of lymph node metastasis of up to 16% has been described even in tumors under 0.5 cm in diameter, our own investigations in a large series have not found nodal metastasis from tumors under 0.6 cm. This group of small tumors is therefore most amenable to curative surgical intervention. It must be taken into account that carcinogenesis is often a bilateral event. In surgical biopsies of the contralateral breast at the time of initial surgery, 10% of tumors of 0.5 cm appeared with a simultanous malignancy of similar size in the contralateral breast at the time of diagnosis.

Diagnosis
Imaging

In addition to monthly self-examinations, biannual mammograms in patients between the ages of 40 and 50 years and annual mammograms after 50 years of age are recommended by the American Cancer Society. A baseline mammogram should be obtained around age 35. It has been shown that a population of women under-going routine mammographic screening has an increased overall life expectancy. The high diagnostic value of mammographic imaging is due to the fact that women in the age group with the highest incidence of breast cancer usually have fatty involution of the breasts, which renders the tissues very transparent on radiographic examination. In the absence of a delineated mass, atypically configured microcalcifications are important indicators of early malignant disease; this is the most important target of all diagnostic efforts. Sixty percent of intraductal carcinomata show microcalcifications. The radiographically dense breasts of younger women, however, or the presence of pronounced fibrocystic disease presents a problem for mammographic evaluation. Originally used mainly for the distinction of cystic versus solid lesions, breast sonography has been shown to be able to diagnose small malignant tumors in this group of patients. The use of Doppler ultrasonography with analysis of the perfusion pattern of a suspected lesion appears to further increase diagnostic accuracy. Ultrasound imaging provides superior differentiation between benign and malignant solid lesions in dense breast tissue but is less valuable in fatty involution and cannot screen for microcalcifications. Therefore at the present time it is not a suitable tool in population screening for breast cancer.

Cytology

There are two methods of needle biopsy of a breast mass: cyst aspiration and fine-needle aspiration for the cytologic examination of a solid lesion. In young patients a perimenstrual cystic mass can often be drained easily with or without ultrasonographic guidance. Given the current medical-legal climate, the aspirated fluid is sent for cytologic evaluation even though intracystic carcinoma is very rare. It should be suspected if cysts show protrusions into the lumen or there are irregularities of the cyst wall. In these cases, cystography with air filling of the cystic cavity and a subsequent repeat mammogram can be helpful. In the majority of these patients, histologic evaluation by biopsy is performed. For a solid lesion, fine-needle aspiration and cytology or immediate excisional biopsy may be indicated, depending on clinical suspicion. Considering the high false-negative rate of aspiration cytology, only positive results should lead to a final therapeutic decision.

Fine-needle aspiration and cytologic examination in combination with mammography and ultrasonography performed by trained personnel are valuable tools to decrease the number of unnecessary surgical biopsies. Furthermore, stereotactically targeted needle biopsies performed under ultrasonographic or mammographic guidance are now available and can further improve the results obtained by reducing the number of surgical biopsies carried out under anesthesia.

Excisional Biopsy

There are two schools of thought regarding the presence of a breast mass. One group observes and follows the patient if triple diagnostics (mammography, ultrasonography, and fine-needle aspiration) are negative for cancer. The other group proceeds to excisional biopsy regardless of the results of the above-mentioned studies. Excisional biopsy may be diagnostic, therapeutic, or both. The complete excision of a suspicious breast lesion enables a definite histologic diagnosis, and in cases in which the histologic findings are benign, such as in fibrocystic disease of fibroadenoma, further therapeutic intervention may not be needed. It is generally accepted that incisional biopsy does not spread disease provided that definitive therapy is undertaken within 10 days of the initial biopsy. However, it remains an important surgical dictum to approach excisional biopsy with the intent of obtaining a wide healthy margin, thereby obviating any doubt about final diagnosis and therapy. Stereotactically guided removal of small benign-appearing lesions or clustered microcalcifications by excision of a tissue cylinder under local anesthesia has helped to obtain a histologic diagnosis with optimal cosmetic results and minimal trauma (i.e., advanced breast biopsy instrumentation, ABBI).

Staging

There are two staging systems for breast cancer, one clinical and one based on the surgical specimen and its histologic evaluation.

The clinical staging is based on palpation of the tumor and axillary nodes as well as so-called "staging exams" to screen for metastasis. A clinical stage 1 tumor is a tumor of up to 2 cm with no palpable nodes and no metastasis; a stage 2 lesion is a tumor of 2 cm to 5 cm with or without palpable nodes or a tumor more than 5 cm in diameter with no palpable nodes. Stage 3 refers to a large tumor with palpable nodes, and a stage 4 tumor constitutes any tumor with distant metastasis. The tumor-node-metastasis (TNM) system differentiates T1 (0–2 cm), T2 (2–5 cm), T3 (> 5 cm), and T4 lesions (any size tumor involving the skin or fixed to the chest wall). N0 stands for histologically negative axillary nodes, N1 is histologically positive nodes, N2 represents histologically positive numerous or large and conglomerated nodes, and N3 is used for histologically positive nodes close to the collar bone. Because the rate of false-negative nodal diagnosis on clinical examination is in the 30% range, surgical sampling of axillary nodes is so far regarded as mandatory for prognostically and therapeutically correct staging. Staging examinations for metastasis include x-ray of the lungs, bone scan, and liver ultrasonography, as well as pelvic ultrasonography.

Intraoperatively, identification of the first lymph node draining the tumor area can be improved by using the so-called "sentinel lymph node technique." In this method, radioactively labeled colloid is injected subcutaneously close to the tumor and is enriched in the first draining lymph node. Using a Geiger counter, this node can be located intraoperatively, removed, and examined in detail, detecting an additional 11% of nodal metastasis that would be missed by conventional histologic techniques.

Pathology

Benign breast disease is not considered a precursor to breast cancer. The relative risk is increased only if there is proliferation or atypical proliferation (Table 1). Two histologic diagnoses are considered to be in situ lesions: lobular carcinoma in situ (LCIS) and ductal carcinoma in situ (DCIS). LCIS is associated with a two- to fourfold increased risk of invasive disease over a 20-year period. This increased risk causes some to view LCIS as a marker of future malignancy rather than as a true premalignant lesion. However, prophylactic surgery or radiotherapy is generally not indicated. DCIS, however, is associated with a risk of invasive disease 30 to 40 times greater than that seen in the general population. When a positive family history is superimposed, this increased risk can approach 100%. These data are responsible for the controversies surrounding the management of this entity. Unfortunately, current data are inadequate and do not enable the physician to objectively counsel a patient; there are no prospectively controlled randomized trials.

Three general approaches to management are often considered: (1) frequent follow-up, (2) prophylactic mastectomy, and (3) prophylactic radiation. Currently, radiation therapy or mastectomy

TABLE 1. Relative Risk for Invasive Breast Carcinoma Based on Pathologic Examination of Benign Breast Tissue

No increased risk
  Adenosis, sclerosing, or florid
  Apocrine metaplasia
  Macro or micro cyst lesions
  Duct ectasia
  Fibroadenoma
  Fibrosis
  Hyperplasia (mild, two to four epithelial cells in
    depth)
  Mastitis (inflammation)
  Periductal mastitis
  Squamous metaplasia
Slightly increased risk (1.5 to 2 times)
  Proliferation, moderate or florid, solid or papillary
  Papilloma with a fibrovascular core
Moderately increased risk (5 times)
  Atypical hyperplasia
  Ductal
  Lobular
Insufficient data to assign a risk
  Solitary papilloma of lactiferous sinus
  Radial scar lesion

with immediate reconstruction seems to be favored, although it is important to keep in mind that the data regarding the effectiveness of this approach are still limited.

The most frequent histologic type of breast cancer is the infiltrating ductal carcinoma (about 70% of all cases), followed by invasive lobular carcinoma (about 10%). Medullary and inflammatory cancers have a poorer prognosis than other types. Nuclear grading on histologic examination provides further information about the aggressiveness of the individual cancer. Lymph–vascular space involvement, perifocal carcinoma in situ, or multicentricity points to a poor prognosis.

Prognostic Factors

Tumor size, cell differentiation, nodal involvement, lymph–vascular space involvement, and multicentricity as well as estrogen and progesterone receptor expression are the most important predictors of prognosis. Prognostically, nodal involvement and the absence of estrogen/progesterone receptor expression are equally ominous. Long-term survival is around 95% for small T1 N0 estrogen receptor–positive tumors and drops rapidly to the 50 to 70% range with increasing tumor size, nodal involvement, absence of estro-

gen receptor expression, and other risk factors. Because small tumors (< 1 cm in diameter) usually correspond to negative nodal status, the value of early detection cannot be overemphasized. An increasing number of prognostic factors have become available from recent research in addition to the traditional stratification by tumor size, lymph node involvement, receptor expression, and menopausal status. These new prognostic markers include the following:

1. Expression of the *HER-2/neu* oncogen with adverse outlook for *HER-2/neu*–positive tumors.
2. Mutations in the tumor suppressor gene *p53*. Tumors with a mutated and thereby inactivated *p53* gene exhibit a more aggressive clinical pattern.
3. Cathepsin D production in the tumor, with adverse prognosis correlating with high levels.
4. Urokinase contents of the breast cancer correlates with more malignant behavior, probably because this protein facilitates tumor invasion.
5. *BrCa1*, the genetic risk factor detectable in healthy women with familial or heritable breast cancer, can also be detected within the tumor of otherwise genetically normal individuals. There is some evidence that these nonfamilial malignancies with *BrCa1* expression grow more aggressively.

The prognostic significance of the progesterone receptor status is on average one order of magnitude higher than the prediction on the basis of estrogen receptor expression alone, but it is less important as a therapeutic discriminator. With the current immunocytochemistry techniques, only the presence or absence but not the function of the receptor is evaluated. In this respect, the traditional hormone-binding assay, although impaired by the possibility of healthy tissue contamination, offers the advantage of testing the functioning of the present receptor by testing actual hormone binding. Estrogen receptor mutations and variants have been described in breast cancer, possibly explaining treatment failures in immunocytochemically receptor–positive patients. The expression of significant progesterone receptor levels is induced only by an intact and functional estrogen receptor protein. Therefore, the value of the progesterone receptor assay lies in the assurance that this autoregulatory loop is intact within the tumor, making antiestrogen therapy a promising treatment approach.

Tumor DNA aneuploidy, S-phase fraction, and thymidine-labeling index are also used to characterize the individual cancer. The tumor markers CA 15-3, CA 12-5, and CEA are tested not in the tumor but in the patient's blood. They are used as markers for distant metastasis and treatment evaluation in follow-up.

Surgical Treatment

For a long time modified radical mastectomy was the standard of care for the treatment of a malignant breast lesion. Today, lumpectomy or quadrantectomy with a wide surgical margin is a treatment option that can be offered to the majority of patients.

Initially, breast-conserving surgery was limited to tumors up to 2 cm in diameter. At present the size limit depends more on the ability of the surgeon to resect the tumor with a satisfactory margin of healthy tissue, on the cosmetic aspect of breast size in relation to tumor size, and on the decision of the patient.

After breast-conserving surgery, radiotherapy to the operated breast with a dose of 45 to 50 Gy is indicated. Some centers give an additional boost of radiation to the tumor bed. Multicentric lesions, inflammatory carcinoma, and tumors with skin involvement are excluded from the breast-conserving surgical approach. Mastectomy with the option of immediate reconstruction by rotational or free musculocutaneous flaps from latissimus dorsi, rectus, or transverse abdominal muscles can be offered to the patient with locally more advanced disease or to patients who prefer mastectomy to breast-conserving surgery plus irradiation.

Axillary lymph node dissection is regarded as standard because nodal status is required for staging and adjuvant therapeutic decisions. In the future, this approach may be modified by the sentinel lymph node technique. This technique involves the injection of a technetium-marked colloid suspension into the subcutaneous area at the axillary margin of the lesion. This colloid is then transported by the lymphatics toward the first lymph node, where it is trapped. The one to two lymph nodes that accumulated the radioactive colloid are detected intraoperatively with a modified Geiger counter and removed. Very thorough evaluation of these lymph nodes is performed, including the use of immunohistochemical stains to detect single tumor cell involvement. According to the data available so far, an additional 11% of positive lymph nodes are found in this way. Preliminary data indicate that the sensitivity of the sentinel lymph node technique compared with a formal axillary lymph node dis-

section is 98%, with only a 2% skip metastasis. The fact that a defined sentinel lymph node can be found in approximately 89% of the patients makes it likely that in the future the number of lymph nodes needed for diagnostic and prognostic information can be considerably reduced. In summary, the trend toward an individually tailored surgical approach prevails, resulting in increasingly reduced morbidity and better cosmetic results without sacrificing prognosis.

Adjuvant Therapy
Chemotherapy

Adjuvant chemotherapy has been shown to improve survival for many breast cancer patients. It is considered standard for patients with lymph node metastasis and negative estrogen receptor status as well as for premenopausal women. Most frequently used are combination regimens like cyclophosphamide, methotrexate, and 5-fluorouracil (CMF) or doxorubicin and cyclophosphamide (AC) (Table 2). Adjuvant chemotherapy also has been able to prolong the disease-free interval of all patients regardless of menopausal status or receptor expression. For postmenopausal patients with positive estrogen-progesterone receptor status, treatment with antiestrogens remains favored. The latest evaluations of the largest and best controlled breast cancer trial ever undertaken, the National Surgical Adjuvant Breast Project (NSABP) trial, show very clearly that every subgroup of patients, regardless of additional risk markers or their absence, profits from adjuvant chemotherapy with or without ad-

TABLE 2. Frequently Used Drugs for Chemotherapy

Single agents	Abbreviation	Abbreviation use in combination regimens
Doxorubicin (Adriamycin)	DOX	A
Cyclophosphamide	CTX	C
Methotrexate	MTX	M
5-Fluorouracil	5-FU	F
Paclitaxel	TAX	T
Mitoxantrone	DHAD	N
Vinblastine	VLB	V
Thiotepa	TSPA	T
Prednisone	PRED	P
Combinations:		
CAF, CMF, CMFP, CNF, AC, FAC, MF, MFT, MV, VAC, VATH		

ditional antiestrogen therapy. Increased disease-free survival, reduced risk of local recurrence or regional and distant recurrence, and better long-term survival were observed in every subgroup. However, the improvement of prognosis was most pronounced in patients age 49 years or younger. It was also shown that in elderly women, less aggressive chemotherapy regimens (MF or MFT; see Table 2) can be used safely, omitting the cyclophosphamide, which accounts for most of the side effects of the CMF regimen. For tumors with high-risk nodal involvement and other ominous signs, high-dose chemotherapy with stem cell rescue is widely used; conclusive data are pending. For metastatic disease, a variety of drug combinations are used, with response rates between 15 and 25%.

In general, the use of adjuvant chemotherapy has been the only measure by which survival time of breast cancer patients could be improved in the past decades; the more limited surgical approach that is now standard has greatly improved quality of life for the individual patient.

Endocrine Therapy

Surgical or radiologic oophorectomy has given way to pharmacologic manipulation. Adjuvant endocrine therapy prolongs disease-free intervals and survival in postmenopausal women but probably does not in premenopausal women. At present it is being tested in the latter group as a possible prophylactic agent for healthy high-risk individuals in a large prospective randomized trial. Tamoxifen is the most widely used compound; it is a nonsteroidal agent structurally similar to clomiphene. Tamoxifen binds to estrogen receptors in the area of the hormone-binding domain, sharing one binding site with estrogen and binding to another site at a tamoxifen-specific site. It acts as a weak estrogen receptor agonist, with the desired antiestrogenic effect becoming apparent after only 6 weeks of treatment. Originally used mainly for advanced-stage breast disease, the main indication for use of this agent has become the adjuvant treatment of postmenopausal women with receptor-positive tumors. It was originally recommended for a 2-year course of therapy, but there is a widespread trend toward prolonging the administration in

relapse-free women. It was agreed recently, however, that exceeding a 5-year period does not improve results.

Patients receiving tamoxifen should undergo yearly endometrial biopsy or vaginal ultrasonography, as the unopposed weak estrogenic effect of tamoxifen may lead to endometrial carcinoma. An endometrial thickness of greater than 5 mm may indicate abnormal stimulation of the endometrium and should be histologically evaluated. Although they are rare, tamoxifen-induced endometrial cancers are usually poorly differentiated. Routine monitoring of the uterine cavity prevents these tumors from adversely affecting breast cancer patients' prognosis. Recently, so-called pure antiestrogens have become available (droloxifene/raloxifene); they promise to be effective more rapidly and without the agonistic side effects of tamoxifen. For treatment of metastasis, endocrine therapy (e.g., antiestrogens, progestins, aromatase inhibitors, and GnRh-agonists) is used on a highly individualized basis.

Contraception

The preferred method of contraception in patients with a history of breast cancer is the intrauterine device or, when this is not feasible, the barrier methods and finally tubal ligation. Most physicians feel that steroid hormones are contraindicated, although some studies argue that progestins may have beneficial effects. Conclusive studies are lacking.

Treatment of Menopausal Symptoms

According to recent studies, hormonal replacement therapy does not adversely affect the risk of recurrence or death in breast cancer patients after treatment. Some centers recommend estrogen replacement therapy for breast cancer patients with estrogen receptor–negative tumors. Widespread controversy, including the so-called alternative therapies, exists, and data from controlled studies are needed. As standard recommendations cannot be given, the treatment approach should depend on the severity of symptoms of the postmenopausal patient as well as on the prognostic markers of the patient's tumor.

Breast Mass and Nipple Discharge

Douglas J. Marchant, MD

The American Board of Obstetrics and Gynecology has recognized the special role of the obstetrician/gynecologist in the diagnosis and treatment of breast disease, and a knowledge of breast disease is now required in its certification process. The American College of Obstetricians and Gynecologists also has increased its efforts to more clearly define the role of the obstetrician/gynecologist in the diagnosis and treatment of breast disease. Several postgraduate courses address these issues, and the College has provided guidelines for screening and two technical bulletins, one dealing with benign breast disease and the other with breast cancer. In this article, the contemporary management of the breast mass and nipple discharge is discussed. Recently, the Council on Residency Education in Obstetrics and Gynecology announced the availability of "mini" fellowships in selected breast centers.

Breast Mass

Evaluation

It is important to emphasize that the physical findings on breast examination present a judgment call. The patient often presents or is referred with the diagnosis of a "lump." This may or may not be confirmed by careful examination. The usual finding is a vague thickening, particularly in the upper outer quadrant. In the mature female, most of the breast tissue is located in this area and beneath the nipple areolar complex, and it is not surprising that most of the benign changes and cancers are found there. In addition, the physical findings may vary depending on the amount of adipose tissue. In a woman who has recently lost considerable weight, particularly in the breast, the breasts feel lumpy. The cushion of fatty tissue is absent and palpation reveals breast tissue. This has a feeling similar to that of tapioca pudding, with small spherical aggregates and a rather indistinct outline.

The evaluation of a breast mass begins with a careful history and a thorough examination of the breast. The breasts are first examined in the sitting or standing position. Contour, symmetry, and skin changes are noted. The vascular pattern is observed and the condition of the areola and nipple recorded. These changes may be exaggerated by asking the patient to elevate the arms or by asking her to place the hands on the hips, thus contracting the pectoralis major muscles and exaggerating any small changes noted on routine examination. Standard textbooks usually discuss obvious signs of malignancy such as a mass, erythema, edema, retraction, and ulceration. These represent late signs of malignancy for which current treatment modalities are equally ineffective. One must look for subtle changes. Is there slight flattening in the inframammary fold? Is one nipple slightly elevated? The search for these changes requires considerable time.

While the patient is in the sitting or standing position, palpate the axilla, being careful to support the arm with the opposite hand. This relaxes the pectoral muscles and permits careful examination of the axilla. Even if well performed, this examination is inaccurate. It has been reported that 40% of patients carefully examined and thought to have a negative axilla will at the time of axillary dissection be found to have involved nodes. On the other hand, it is important to detect clinically evident metastasis prior to recommended treatment.

Following these maneuvers, the patient is placed in the supine position. The breast is palpated in a systematic manner with the flat of the hand. The use of pHisoHex or talcum powder permits the identification of even minor alterations. (Approximately 80% of women discover their own lesions, often while taking a shower. The use of this so-called "wet technique" permits the identification of very subtle changes in breast texture.) Following the careful examination of all quadrants, the areola and nipple should be carefully examined and the nipple gently squeezed. Any discharge is evaluated for location and color.

The physician must carefully evaluate the chief complaint and then on the basis of a thorough examination decide whether the findings represent a mass or an exaggeration of normal breast tissue associated with fibrocystic changes. In the very obese patient with very large breasts it is unlikely that anything but the most obvious lesion will be discovered by routine breast examination. The large breast is an indication for mammography to augment what is, in most cases, an inadequate physical examination.

Diagnosis

Once a lesion has been described as a mass or a lump or is measured or drawn, it must be resolved. The palpated mass may be cystic, solid, benign, or malignant. There are no obviously benign masses, with the exception of the fibroadenoma in the teenager. This neoplasm appears predominantly in young women and presents as a firm, painless, mobile mass. The lesions tend to be multiple but are bilateral in only 10% to 20% of cases. They are usually discovered accidentally. They may not increase in size; however, occasionally they may grow rapidly during adolescence, pregnancy, or menopause with exogenous estrogen stimulation. If the size of the mass increases dramatically, one must consider the possibility of a cystosarcoma phyllodes or a sarcoma. In my opinion, there are three reasons for recommending removal of these lesions.

1. They will not disappear, and, once discovered by the patient, they produce anxiety and are eventually removed.
2. They do not increase dramatically in size, but over a period of years they may grow, making their removal more difficult and less cosmetic.
3. We live in a mobile society and patients diagnosed in one city may move. If this patient becomes pregnant and a mass is noted, can we believe the patient when she states that "it has been present for many years?"

When multiple fibroadenomata are palpated, I perform an ultrasonographic examination to determine exactly how many lesions are present in each breast. Once the number of lesions has been stabilized, the decision can be made concerning elective removal. Nonpalpable lesions should not be removed, at least in the young patient. They can be considered "asymmetric densities" and followed by mammography to assess stability. Lesions that are obvious and symptomatic should be removed through cosmetic incisions as noted earlier. Judgment and tact are required for these young patients with multiple lesions.

Aspiration

An attempt should be made to aspirate any dominant mass with a fine gauge needle. Local anesthesia is not required. The mass is immobilized with the fingers, the needle is inserted, and the fluid is withdrawn. If the fluid is clear or cloudy and no residual mass is palpated immediately following the aspiration, follow-up examination in 1 month with reassurance and reinforcement of monthly breast self-examination are recommended. If the mass remains immediately following the aspiration, if the fluid is bloody, or if there is a residual mass on the first follow-up visit in 1 month, open biopsy is recommended. It cannot be overemphasized that the mass must

completely disappear at the time of the initial aspiration and should not return on follow-up evaluation in 1 month.

It is not necessary to deliberately aspirate multiple macrocysts noted by breast examination or other diagnostic aids such as mammography and ultrasonography. Macrocysts are common, particularly in the late reproductive years. The etiology of this condition is unknown, but most are asymptomatic. If a patient known to have macrocysts is seen because of a tender mass, an attempt should be made to empty this cyst. If, however, the patient is totally asymptomatic and a number of macrocysts have been confirmed by ultrasonography, one should not attempt to aspirate each and every one of these either by ultrasonographic guidance or repeated attempts with an open biopsy.

Cytologic evaluation of cyst fluid is seldom rewarding. Most reports indicate "foam cells" with slight atypia and they do not aid in establishing a differential diagnosis. A positive cytologic examination of cyst fluid in the absence of other indications for biopsy is exceedingly rare, and routine cytology cannot be recommended.

Fine Needle Aspiration

If the mass is solid, fine needle aspiration or open biopsy is recommended. Fine needle aspiration requires an understanding of the technique involved and a cytopathologist capable of interpreting the smear. A standard disposable syringe can be used with a 23- to 25-gauge needle. A large needle should be avoided. Local anesthesia is helpful because several "passes" may be required to obtain an adequate sample. The technique in essence provides an evaluation of "tissue juice." It is therefore important that sufficient material be withdrawn and placed on the slide for appropriate evaluation. The material should not enter the syringe and is placed directly on the slide. In some instances, the fluid is diluted for Millipore filter evaluation. The result should be available within a few minutes. This technique is most useful for the obvious mass with signs suggesting carcinoma either by physical examination or by mammographic findings. A positive fine needle aspiration permits immediate treatment planning and discussion of alternative treatments with the therapeutic team. Except in rare instances, this finding is confirmed by open biopsy at the time of definitive treatment.

There is considerable controversy concerning a negative fine needle aspiration. It is quite clear from the literature that in expert hands, fine needle aspiration is accurate and few false-negative results are obtained. On the other hand, it has been my experience that physicians, particularly primary care physicians who perform the technique infrequently or who rely on a cytopathologist not adequately trained in the evaluation of these cells, too often rely on a negative aspiration only to discover an invasive cancer at a later date. Recently, I was referred a patient at the Breast Health Center who had had a fine needle aspiration 1 year previously. She was in her middle 30s, the aspiration was negative, and her case was followed up by the physician. A year later, the mass had increased in size, mammography revealed obvious cancer, and biopsy confirmed an invasive ductal cancer. The recommendation that the primary care physician, particularly the obstetrician/gynecologist, rely on physical examination, fine needle aspiration, and mammography is appropriate in theory and in expert hands. However, it does not represent reality in usual office practice. Few, if any, breast surgeons recommend reliance on the negative fine needle aspiration; indeed, the most recent article in the *New England Journal of Medicine* discussing the management of the breast mass advises against it.

Mammography and Ultrasonography

Other diagnostic studies include mammography and ultrasonography. Ultrasonography is useful to clarify the diagnosis of an asymmetric density noted on the mammogram but, in my opinion, should not be performed routinely to confirm the presence or absence of a cyst when this lesion is palpable. Simple aspiration is adequate and is certainly more cost effective.

Mammography is performed as a screening examination or to clarify the diagnosis following the discovery of a palpable lesion. Recently there has been considerable controversy concerning screening in the younger patient, that is, those aged 40 to 49 years. With the availability of new data, the National Cancer Institute and other organizations are now suggesting that the original guidelines—screening beginning at age 40 and continuing every year or every other year—are appropriate. Obviously, risk factors such as family history may suggest screening beginning as early as age 30. While there may still be some questions concerning the advisability of *annual* screening in women aged 40 to 49 years, there is no question that all organizations recommend annual screening beginning at age 50 and probably continuing until at least age 75 or 80. There is some debate about the wisdom of continuing annual screening in the very elderly patient.

In most institutions, screening mammography in patients under the age of 30 is discouraged, and in my own institution, it is impossible to obtain a mammogram in a patient under 30 years of age for any reason unless the indications are personally discussed with the radiologist. Too often we see young patients in their mid-20s referred for another opinion and "with their mammogram."

Finally, a word must be said about the negative mammogram associated with a palpable mass. In the best of screening clinics, a false-negative rate of 10% is seen. This may be the result of the dense breast parenchyma or the fact that the lesion cannot be technically imaged because of its location. A negative mammogram in the presence of a palpable mass should never preclude the recommendation for open biopsy.

Nipple Discharge
Evaluation

Nipple discharge may be spontaneous or provoked. The patient should be questioned concerning the nature of the discharge. Is it bilateral or unilateral, clear, yellow, greenish, watery, sticky, serosanguineous, or bloody? Spontaneous discharge may be associated with ovulation, the use of drugs such as tranquilizers, and oral contraceptives. Most physiologic discharges are white or greenish in color. Occasionally, the discharge may be clear or yellow. Unilateral spontaneous discharge raises the possibility of an underlying malignancy, and a serosanguineous or bloody discharge must be investigated.

The initial approach to the diagnosis and treatment of nipple discharge begins with an accurate history. The most common cause of spontaneous nipple discharge is galactorrhea; in this case a prolactin level is obtained, and, if it is elevated, the patient should be referred to the reproductive endocrinologist for further evaluation.

Patients should be questioned carefully on when the discharge is noted. Does it appear on the bra or nightgown, or does it occur in the shower, with sexual stimulation, or during breast self-examination? In addition, patients who jog several miles a day, particularly when they do not use a support bra, and the occasional patient using the Nautilus machine with weight lifting may have physiologic discharge. These activities stimulate the pectoral muscles, producing spontaneous or occasionally provoked nipple discharge.

The most common cause for physiologic discharge, other than that related to medications and physical activity, is duct ectasia. Typically, the discharge is greenish and appears from multiple ducts. The patient often confuses this with "bloody" discharge. The true diagnosis is easily obtained by placing a gauze over the nipple and noting that the discharge is black or green rather than serosanguineous or bloody. Usually this is bilateral but occasionally it is unilateral. No specific treatment is required.

Unilateral spontaneous discharge raises the possibility of an underlying malignancy, and a serosanguineous or bloody discharge must be investigated. The most common lesion is a benign intraductal papilloma. However, breast cancer occurs in 5% to 15% of the cases. The diagnosis therefore must be confirmed by histologic evaluation. Usually, the involved quadrant of the breast can be located by firm pressure. Occasionally, if this is not possible, I use Hemoccult paper pressed on the nipple. This may show the involved duct and permit surgical excision. Occasionally, the patient will report bloody discharge, but neither the physician nor the patient can produce this at the time of examination. In this instance, I send the patient home with a small piece of gauze and ask her to bring it in following the next episode of discharge. If bloody discharge is confirmed, exploration is indicated. It is also possible to confirm bloody discharge by utilizing a Pap smear. If the smear, in fact, shows a significant bloody background, this confirms the nature of the discharge and again, exploration is indicated. This usually is performed on a day-surgery basis under local anesthesia.

In summary, discharge from a nonlactating nipple is seen in approximately 5% of women. It is most frequent in premenopausal women, and galactorrhea is the most common cause. Reported rates of malignancy in cases of serosanguineous or frankly bloody discharge range from 5% to 15%. The risk increases with the association of a palpable mass. Cytologic study of the discharge may be helpful, but false-negative results often are obtained.

Summary

The opinions and recommendations in this section are the result of a considerable experience dealing exclusively with breast disease. For many years at our Breast Health Center we have seen approximately 100 patients a week with various forms of breast problems. There is no mass that is obviously benign with the single exception of

that in the teenager. Hormonal or other forms of medical management are not recommended for nipple discharge except for galactorrhea associated with high levels of prolactin. Most of the lesions discussed in this section require diagnosis and, when indicated, prompt surgical intervention.

Bulimia Nervosa

Michael P. Levine, PhD

Bulimia nervosa (BN) occurs in 1% to 3% of females aged 14 to 35 years, although inclusion of subthreshold variants pushes this figure to 5%. BN is unusually prevalent among women seeking treatment for infertility or substance abuse and in subcultures emphasizing slenderness, competition, and perfection (eg, dance and gymnastics). Gynecologists can play an important role in detection, referral, and collaborative management of this serious and potentially chronic eating disorder.

Characteristics

Clinical Features

Eating Binges ("Bulimia")

Binge-eating refers to consumption of unusually large amounts of food during a discrete period of time, accompanied by a frightening experience of loss of control over eating. Typically, "episodes" take place in secret and involve fattening foods ordinarily excluded as part of a restrictive diet. Frequency varies from once or twice a week to several times daily.

Purging

Binge-eating is precipitated by a build-up of negative feelings. Gorging temporarily relieves dysphoria but eventually produces physical discomfort and acute anxiety about weight gain. In most cases these consequences motivate self-induced vomiting followed by a guilty determination to re-establish "control" over eating and weight by restrictive dieting and rigorous exercise. Misuse of stimulant-type laxatives, diuretics, and fasting is also common. As BN worsens, purging rationalizes and counteracts future losses of control over eating.

Pathogenic Attitudes About Weight and Shape ("Nervosa")

The "nervosa" in BN is very similar to that in anorexia nervosa (AN): a morbid fear of becoming fat, a strong drive for thinness, body image distortion, low self-esteem, difficulties in identifying and expressing internal states, and preoccupation with both eating and dietary restraint. Most patients also struggle with depression and anxiety disorders and control.

Weight Status

Although 70% to 80% of females with BN are at a statistically normal body weight for height and the disorder may occur at any weight status, many patients with BN have a genetic and personal history of overweight. Thus, a significant percentage of those at a statistically normative weight are well below their personal set-point. This semi-starvation state in a person of ostensibly "normal weight" is marked by irritability, a tendency to binge-eat, serum elevations of beta-hydroxy butyric acid and free fatty acid, and abnormal fasting hypoglycemia. Whatever their current weight status, BN patients have a history of significant weight fluctuation, which probably contributes to their risk for amenorrhea and oligomenorrhea.

Clinical Signs

Bulimia nervosa is hard to diagnose. Clinical signs are subtle and there are no definitive laboratory tests. Moreover, patients are usually ambivalent about giving up a reliable and presumably discreet, albeit destructive, means of tension control. Secretiveness is fueled by shame, hopelessness, and a self-conscious desire to appear "perfect."

Table 1 presents some warning signs of BN. Suspicion should not be mitigated by weight status.

Excessive Weight and Shape Concerns

Women in our society, whether or not they are pregnant, tend to be concerned about weight and shape. The effects of pregnancy on such concerns is highly variable and poorly understood, but it appears that while they are pregnant many women become *more* accepting of body shape and size, make fewer attempts to control weight, and are more likely to eat a balanced

TABLE 1. Warning Signs of Bulimia Nervosa

Excessive weight and shape concern
Intractable menstrual difficulties
Electrolyte disturbances
Hyperemesis gravidarum that is protracted and responds poorly to standard interventions
Maceration or hyperpigmentation of the fingers or knuckles (caused by finger-initiated vomiting)
Bilateral hypertrophy of the parotid or submandibular salivary glands
Dental erosion (perimolysis) causing complicated and unusual dental procedures
Perioral irritation (caused by regurgitated stomach acid)
Dehydration and elevated blood urea nitrogen levels (caused by vomiting, abuse of laxatives, or diuretics)
Frequent weight fluctuations in both directions of ≥10 pounds
Idiopathic edema ("puffiness" or "bloating") of the face, stomach, or extremities
Pancreatitis (signaled by acute abdominal pain, vomiting, elevated serum amylase levels)
Gastrointestinal complaints (eg., heartburn, esophagitis, stomach cramps, hematemesis)

diet. A study of 100 primagravid women found that during pregnancy they reported few uncontrollable eating binges and no mean change in a tendency to overeat. Thus, persistent, anxious, or "odd" statements or questions about binge-eating, weight, shape, calories, water retention (diuretics), laxatives, vomiting, or eating disorders should arouse concern.

Intense anxiety about weight gain or loss of control over eating during pregnancy is not normal or harmless. Particular attention should be paid to women who (1) express panic and humiliation in response to weigh-ins, (2) adhere rigidly to a "magical" weight goal, (3) indicate that their weight determines their value as a person, or (4) are eating but failing to gain weight appropriately.

Menstrual Difficulties

Half of patients with BN will be amenorrheic or oligomenorrheic, while another 40% will have luteal dysfunction or problems with follicular development. Two gynecologic problems—persistent infertility in women (and especially those who are slightly underweight) with anovulatory cycles or short luteal phase, and polycystic ovary syndrome—are often attributable to unhealthy weight control practices, including BN. Schweiger, Pirke, and colleagues at the Max

Planck Institute in Germany found that about half of 30 BN patients had inadequate follicular development as judged from consistently low estradiol levels. Patients in this group also had lower body weights, as well as lower mean values and low peak sizes of luteinizing hormone. The remaining subgroup manifested a regression to an early postpubertal pattern: estradiol levels during follicle development and the preovulatory period were normal, but luteal phase was short in conjunction with low levels of estradiol and progesterone. In both groups, 24-hour pulsatile gonadotropin secretion and luteinizing hormone response to estradiol are reduced (data on follicle-stimulating hormone response are inconclusive). The relative contributions of erratic eating patterns, weight fluctuations, poor nutrition, and purging and other weight control behavior to menstrual disturbances in patients with BN are unknown.

Electrolyte Disturbances

Approximately one half of patients with BN—probably those who purge frequently—have hypokalemia, hypochloremia, and hyponatremia. An elevated serum phosphorus level appears to be a sensitive and specific sign, and metabolic acidosis in a young woman strongly suggests laxative abuse associated with BN.

Diagnosis and Referral

Diagnosis

It is appalling how often pregnant women tell their gynecologist directly about an eating disorder, only to be dismissed with either an empty admonition to "forget than nonsense and eat right" or outright reinforcement for their unhealthy desire to be thin. If self-report or warning signs point to BN, an attitude that is concerned and insistent but nonjudgmental and nonaccusatory will be most effective in referring for expert assessment and for supporting ongoing psychological therapy.

It is also distressing that 50% to 70% of pregnant women who have had or currently have an eating disorder never spontaneously mention it to their gynecologist. An even higher percentage of infertile women undergo costly, complicated endocrinologic examinations but *are never asked about eating problems*. Thus, for all patients a careful menstrual history should be supplemented with information about weight history, weight management practices, type and fre-

---

TABLE 2. A Quick Screen for Eating Disorders

Does gaining weight mean you are out of control?
Is the thought of gaining 20–40 pounds during pregnancy very upsetting?
If you know that a nurse is going to weigh you, do you feel anxious to the point of wanting to starve yourself or exercise intensely to lose weight?
Do you have a lot of shame or anxieties about food, eating, and weight, but keep them to yourself?
Do you ever eat in secret?
Do you go on uncontrollable eating binges to the point where you feel sick and make yourself vomit?

---

quency of exercise, use of cigarettes and other appetite suppressants, and past and current episodes of AN or BN. Screening laboratory tests should include a complete blood count, liver function tests, serum electrolytes, blood urea nitrogen, creatinine, serum glucose, and determination of uric acid, phosphorous, magnesium, and calcium.

At a minimum, all pregnant patients and all women seeking help for infertility should be asked the questions in Table 2. A written questionnaire may yield the fullest information.

Referral

Early detection plays a major role in effective treatment. If possible, referrals should be made to experienced professionals who use a multidisciplinary framework that acknowledges biomedical, nutritional, and psychosocial factors in etiology and therapy. The best programs try to (1) eliminate binge-eating, purging, and unhealthy dieting; (2) reform pathogenic attitudes about weight, shape, and self; (3) strengthen interpersonal skills and coping strategies; (4) encourage pleasurable, self-nurturing activities; and (5) mobilize the support of family and friends. Normalization of eating patterns and restoration of a weight that is "normal" for the individual are important for eliminating binge-eating, for maintaining menstruation and fertility, and for maximizing the chances of a healthy pregnancy.

General Management Issues

Menstrual Difficulties

The ideal outcome is a spontaneous return of consistent menstrual cycles and fertility with elimination of binge-purge behavior, reduction in chronic distress, and achievement of body fat in the minimal range of 17% to 22%. Encourage BN patients to think of health in these terms, as opposed to a weight goal or the cultural ideal of slenderness. Patients should be forewarned that, for unknown reasons, menstruation and fertility may be delayed for up to a year following attainment of physical and psychological health.

Misuse of Diuretics and Laxatives

Since marked alkalosis or hypokalemia is cause for considerable concern about cardiac dysfunction, hospitalization should be considered. Regardless, patients who misuse diuretics or laxatives should be withdrawn from these substances. Gynecologists should not prescribe diuretics and laxatives to patients who show unusual interest in them or who are unwilling to discuss use.

Management of Pregnancy

Effects of Pregnancy on Bulimia Nervosa

Patients suffering from both AN and BN at the time of pregnancy are at significant risk for a worsening of symptoms during and after pregnancy, for pregnancy and birth complications, and for smaller babies with lower 5-minute Apgar scores. These patients are well advised to postpone pregnancy until their disorders are in remission.

The effects of pregnancy on BN have not been studied extensively or rigorously. It appears that, upon discovering they are pregnant, most bulimic women become determined to improve their eating habits to ensure the health of their fetus. Indeed, most do significantly reduce or eliminate bulimic symptoms by the third trimester, although perhaps one in six will experience a worsening of symptoms. Unfortunately, at least half of those who improve will relapse during the puerperium, and a significant minority of these will binge and purge more frequently postpartum than pre-pregnancy.

Gynecologists should reinforce the improvements that are likely to occur during a bulimic woman's pregnancy. However, they should not assume that symptom reduction means sustained recovery and a lessened need for treatment. Self-acceptance of a heavier shape as "natural" and a resolve to be healthier constitute an excellent opportunity for referral to (and support of) treatment programs. Gynecologists also need to be aware that off-hand comments or jokes about fat,

as well as reprimands about weight gain during pregnancy, may well contribute to a worsening of the disorder—most bulimic women, despite sincere concern for their baby, still have the potential to translate weight and shape concerns into binge-eating and purging during pregnancy and after.

Effects of Bulimia Nervosa on Pregnancy

Studies that do not distinguish between AN and BN find an increased risk of low birth weight babies, spontaneous abortions, premature birth, perinatal mortality, and various pregnancy and birth complications in women with a "history of eating disorders." The few investigations of BN yield a confusing and incomplete picture. One study found that, compared with age-matched control subjects, normal-weight women who were actively bulimic during pregnancy had a higher miscarriage rate (39% vs. 17%) but were not statistically different in weight gain during pregnancy, duration of gestation, neonatal birth weight, and pregnancy outcome. Another uncontrolled study of 20 untreated normal-weight bulimic women found that 9 became hypertensive (including two with pre-eclampsia), 8 had breech deliveries, and 2 had babies born with a cleft palate or cleft lip, not attributable to prenatal benzodiazepine use.

Gynecologists should treat BN as a (high) risk factor for pregnancy and birth complications. Pregnant women who are currently bulimic or recently recovered should be informed matter-of-factly about its potential negative consequences for mother and fetus (eg, deficits in certain vitamins and trace elements) and for mother and infant (eg, failure of the baby to thrive due to the mother's irrational concerns about weight and shape). An excellent resource in this regard is Mitchell JE et al: Medical complications and medical management of bulimia. Annals of Internal Medicine, 1987;107:71–77. Some experts recommend hospitalization of pregnant women with frank BN in order to facilitate fetal assessment, nutritional rehabilitation, and psychotherapeutic consultation.

Conclusion

With respect to all patients, gynecologists need to be aware of the nature of BN, its warning signs, and the role they can play in effective referral, collaborative treatment, and support. Until eating behavior is carefully assessed and clearly stabilized, infertility specialists are well advised to refrain from inducing ovulation in those women with secondary menstrual problems who are suspected of an eating disorder or who present with low body weight. Such women are at risk for spontaneous abortion and low birth weight babies.

With respect to women with BN who are now pregnant, gynecologists can contribute to healthy development of mother and fetus in the following ways. First, encourage even "silly questions" and otherwise support the mother's desire to improve the quality of her life and that of her child. Second, help bulimic women find or remain in professional, multidisciplinary treatment. Third, discuss the viability of continuing certain psychotropic medications (eg, fluoxetine) while reinforcing the need to discontinue, as possible teratogens, vomiting, laxatives, diuretics, excessive exercising, and cigarette smoking. Fourth, educate about (1) the healthy *range* of weight they can expect to gain during pregnancy, and (2) the relationship between proper prenatal nutrition and healthy weight gain. Fifth, advise them to eat their meals on two plates, one for themselves and one for the developing fetus. Finally, be sensitive to anxieties about weight gain and body image. Emphasize the naturalness and beauty of a pregnant shape. In addition, give all your patients, including those with BN, the choice of being weighed facing outward from the scale so that they can receive assurances that their pregnancy is proceeding normally while remaining ignorant of their weight.

It is strongly recommended that this combination of sensitivity, monitoring, support, and education be continued postpartum. Several studies have shown that the fairly high percentage of mothers with BN who relapse during the puerperium are likely to provide restrictive, insufficient diets for their infants and to be neglectful and inadequate parents in other ways, too.

Headache

George Paulson, MD

Headache is one of the most ubiquitous problems of humankind, and over 20% of Americans treat themselves for headache at least once every 2 weeks. Most headaches are innocuous, many are brief, but all can cause distress to patients. A few types of headache offer major concern for physicians. Headaches are generally considered to be more common in females, with hormonal factors perhaps instrumental. A new headache in pregnancy is particularly alarming, and pregnancy is a time when some analgesics, all ergots, and most other medicines commonly used for headache are used reluctantly, if at all. Classification of headache, with constant awareness of any potential "worst-case scenario," is the cornerstone of appropriate intervention.

The clinician must be attuned to potentially serious underlying problems, although migraine and tension-type headache are far more common. A general physical examination with a focused neurologic examination is mandatory for all patients with headache. Occasionally, mental status examination is similarly important, since depression or psychic unrest is often linked to chronic headache. Aside from general observation, observing the gait, and watching the patient to assess distress, examination of the eyes is probably the most important part of the examination. All patients with headache do deserve an adequate evaluation of the eyegrounds and a look for swelling of the optic nerve disc or chronic inflammation, as well as a quick check for visual fields. If venous pulsations are present, then increased intracranial pressure is unlikely. Visual field examination by gross confrontation is highly desirable and can be done quickly; indeed, a quite adequate screening ophthalmologic examination can be done almost within the time it took to read the above sentences. After examination of the eyes and other cranial nerves, a check of the motor system and sensory function is usually appropriate, with return once again to the history. It is almost always the case that the history elucidates the problem. With an adequate history and a normal screening examination it is usually possible to avoid radiographic techniques in pregnant women. Recent data from the American Academy of Neurology have confirmed that there is absolutely no proof that computed tomography or magnetic resonance imaging is of any value in assessing classic migraine or tension-type headache. These techniques may be used to rule out something worse, but neuroimaging is no help with the 90% of patients with headache who have either migraine or tension-type headache.

Migraine and Tension-Type Headache

Migraine and tension-type headache are far more common than neoplasm, subarachnoid hemorrhage, stroke, infection, or eclampsia. The International Headache Classification is altogether too detailed for general use, with criteria that tend to be restrictive and cumbersome and that are changed almost every decade. The best criteria to distinguish migraine from tension headache are the pattern of the pain, aggravation by routine physical activity such as climbing stairs (troublesome for patients with migraine), and associated symptoms. Some experts feel that migraine and tension-type headache not only merge into one another but also represent related pathophysiologic processes, with both mediated through serotonin receptors in the brain as well as via trigeminovascular pathways (Table 1).

Migraine tends to be familial, may be unilateral, and is more common before the age of 40. Although the occurrence of migraine in childhood may be similar for boys and girls, migraine is more common in adult females than it is in males. The pain of migraine may vary but can be severe and is sometimes described as throbbing or pulsating. A typical episode lasts from a few hours to several days and can include associated symptoms such as scintillating scotoma, gastrointestinal distress, photophobia, and phonophobia. For some patients, sleep eases the symptoms; for the young, nausea, vomiting, and sleep may terminate the headache.

Migraine can be precipitated in vulnerable persons by specific environmental factors, including red wine, tobacco, hunger, chocolate, aged cheese, loss of sleep, and so on. Some are more vulnerable at "let down" times, such as the first day of vacation. Some women are more vulnerable during menstrual periods, and a few have severe pain only during menstruation, so-called catamenial migraine. Although menopause can trigger episodes of migraine, menopause is usually associated with amelioration in the frequency and severity of attacks. Oral contraceptives can be instrumental in causing headache, as can estrogen-type compounds in the later years of life. In most patients with headache who are taking oral contraceptives, the headache is not primarily due to the oral contraceptives, but there is no way to be sure without months off of the medication.

As a rule migraine tends to improve during pregnancy, but as many as 15% of females with migraine will experience their first attack during pregnancy. New onset of migraine in pregnancy can be isolated or can signal the onset of a recurrent problem. Migraine attacks are said to be most common in the first trimester, and the migraine of pregnancy even in the first trimester is often associated with an aura or with visual phenomena. Headache is common in postpartum women with previous migraine and is most frequently noted on postnatal days 3 to 6. Normal offspring are born as commonly to patients with migraine during pregnancy as to those without.

Complicated Migraine

Complicated migraine is the variant of migraine that is associated with focal neurologic deficit, and this clearly can occur during pregnancy and can begin in pregnancy. Deficits may include hemisensory deficits or hemiparetic episodes and tend to be transient. Transient amnesia or visual symptoms also occur, and a few patients have

TABLE 1. Common Headache Syndromes

	Duration	Location	Frequency	Associated Symptoms	Aura	Age and Gender Prevalence
Tension-type headache	Variable	Generalized	Very frequent	Rare nausea, occasional dizziness Stress-related in some	None	Any Female prevalence, 5:4
Migraine	12–24 hrs	Often unilateral, temporal	Every 1–5 months	Nausea, photophobia	Common	Childhood, young adult Tends to diminish with age Female prevalence, 3:1
Cluster headache	0.5–3 hrs	Retro-orbital	Clusters, nocturnal	Nasal congestion	None	4th–6th decade Male prevalence, 16:1

ophthalmoplegia, hemianopia, or persistent scotomata. Aphasia and dysarthria are less common; confusion and somnolence are rare but can occur. Complicated migraine can occur without the headache at all, but this phenomenon is rare and always raises the fear of stroke or hemorrhage. Motor and sensory phenomena may last hours rather than the 20 minutes typical of visual aura, and such lasting symptoms logically lead to neuroimaging.

Tension-Type Headache

Tension-type headache has also been referred to as muscle contraction headache and is probably the most common headache of pregnancy. Tension-type headache usually persists during pregnancy in women who have it prior to becoming pregnant and may become more frequent with the added pressures of pregnancy. Tension-type headache tends to be less severe than migraine and is usually bilateral. It is noted in the frontal and occipital regions. There may be a diffuse cranial pain or pressure encircling the head, and the pain may or may not be incapacitating but is often chronic. The pain in tension-type headache is usually not exacerbated by routine physical activity. Tension-type headache can be seen with depressive syndromes or with fibromyalgic pain in the shoulders. Tension-type headache can occur for the first time associated with postpartum depression. Depression by itself can lead to a generalized and diffuse headache. Some patients with tension-type headache develop chronic daily headache, never an easy problem to treat.

Treatment of Migraine and Tension-Type Headache

It is appropriate to consider migraine and tension-type headache together, since the headaches do often overlap. The patient may discover self-help measures, including better health habits, balanced diet, exercise, and so on. Occasionally, psychological counseling and physical therapy are of value, but it is rare that biofeedback, hypnosis, formal stress management, or relaxation techniques will be required. Psychological therapies can be especially helpful in treating pregnant women when pharmacotherapy must be minimized. Physical therapy can teach various stretching or aerobic exercises and encourage massage and good posture. Patients can be instructed on the use of hot and cold packs. Ultrasound or electrical stimulation therapies are

TABLE 2. Pharmacologic Treatment of Acute Migraine

Serotoninergic agents (ergot derivatives, sumatriptan)
Isometheptene, etc (Midrin, etc)
Analgesics; all standard ones can be tried for prophylaxis also
Prescription nonsteroidal agents (naproxen, Indocin, etc)
Higher potency analgesics (propoxyphene, codeine, etc; use with caution)
Antiemetics
Sedatives
Neuroleptics

rarely of benefit, and I do not commonly use trigger point injections. Some patients have tight muscles around the scalp and neck and selective local injections with analgesics or steroids may be helpful for them. Physical therapy has also been reported to help prevent tension-type headache.

Combination pharmacotherapy with symptomatic or abortive medications—abortive for the headache—and scheduling a prophylactic drug are crucial approaches after self-help measures have failed (Table 2). Headaches that are persistent or chronic, or that occur as more than three episodes per month, suggest the need for prophylactic therapy. The goal of abortive measures is to treat the headache and reduce or eliminate the associated symptoms. Early intervention is prudent for the chronic headache patient, in an effort to attenuate exacerbations. Over-the-counter analgesics including aspirin, acetaminophen, and ibuprofen have been utilized. There are dozens of medicines for headache, proof that we do not have a curative medicine. For prophylaxis, I favor a trial of several agents, including cyproheptadine hydrochloride (Periactin), long-acting propranolol (Inderal LA), amitriptyline (Elavil), divalproex sodium (Depakote), or one of the many nonsteroidal drugs (Table 3). Adding caffeine to an analgesic seems to enhance the effects. Aspirin and acetaminophen are available with caffeine, or one can use medications such as lorazepam (Ativan) or butalbital (Fiorinal) to promote relaxation and to alleviate anxiety. Isometheptene (a mild vasoconstrictor) and dichloralphenazone (a mild sedative) are available in combination with acetaminophen as Midrin or Isocom. Midrin is a favored first-line combination therapy in migraine, dosed as two capsules at the onset of symptoms and with one capsule repeated every 1 hour up to a total of five within a 12-hour period. Some people also use this

TABLE 3. Prophylactic Drugs

β-Adrenergic agents
Calcium channel blockers
Tricyclic antidepressants
Nonsteroidal anti-inflammatories
Monoamine oxidase inhibitors
Valproic acid
Methysergide
Steroids
Lithium

medication for tension-type headache, dosed one to two capsules every 4 hours up to eight capsules per day. We rarely use the latter regimen and prefer to reserve this medication for migraine. Ergots (often as Cafergot suppositories) are another class of medications used with success to abort migraine, but ergots should probably be avoided during pregnancy. Sumatriptan (Imitrex) is a useful new compound that can be used either intramuscularly or orally but again should probably not be used in pregnancy. Another abortive therapy commonly chosen as first-line medication for prophylaxis of migraine or tension-type headache is the group of nonsteroidal anti-inflammatory drugs such as ibuprofen, ketoprofen, or naproxen. The physician can try various compounds because the response to nonsteroidal anti-inflammatory drugs seems almost specific for each individual. For both migraine and tension-type headache, the tricyclic antidepressants such as amitriptyline (Elavil) and nortriptyline (Pamelor) are mainstays for prophylaxis, used in low dosages. When these measures fail, calcium channel blockers and anticonvulsants have occasionally been used as prophylactic agents for patients with either migraine or tension-type headache.

It is best to reserve narcotics for special cases and to try to avoid narcotics for all headache problems. Nevertheless, careful use of narcotics may be required in pregnancy, since other pharmacologic choices are more limited at this time. All the medicines that function to avoid headache can tend to lead, when used daily, to a persistence of the headaches or to rebound headache; this is particularly true of the ergots. Dependency and rebound headaches can be seen with either the prophylactic or the abortive measures.

Other vascular headache types include cluster headache, which is considerably more common in men than women. This vascular variant is often sharply localized around the eye. The management is very similar to that for migraine, with the possible exception that steroids can be useful for prophylaxis.

Headache Associated with Other Conditions

Benign intracranial hypertension (BIH) or pseudotumor cerebri is characterized by papilledema, headache, and increased intracranial pressure without other central nervous system abnormalities. Patients tend to be young and obese. Pregnancy can be associated with BIH, as can menarche and menopause. Headaches are the most common symptom in BIH, but blindness due to papilledema is the serious consequence. When there is no visual threat, pain can be managed with analgesics. Blindness is to be particularly feared if papilledema is severe or if the patient begins to develop intermittent obscuration or transient blind episodes. Treatment strategies should concentrate on lowering intracranial pressure and on weight loss. Acetazolamide (Diamox), 250 mg once or twice a day, may be used in an attempt to decrease cerebrospinal fluid volume, and lumbar punctures can help confirm diagnosis and relieve pain.

Post-lumbar puncture headache can occur following either lumbar puncture (LP) or spinal anesthesia. The pain is characteristic, occurs in the upright position, and resolves upon returning to recumbency. Onset of symptoms often lags behind the LP by 24 hours. Therapy includes analgesics and hydration. The course is usually self-limited, with resolution within 3 to 10 days. In more difficult cases, some have used caffeine infusions with success. Refractory cases can be treated with infusion of 5 mL of the patient's blood (ie, blood patch) into the epidural space. The etiology of post-LP headaches remains unknown, but they can occur whenever the subarachnoid space has been opened and are present in 5% to 15% of all patients whose subarachnoid space has been opened. They are not caused by emotional factors.

Benign sexual headache, also called orgasmic cephalgia or coital headache, is characterized by acute pain related to sexual activity. The onset is often precisely related to the time of orgasm. Neurologic examination, computed tomographic scan of the brain, and cerebrospinal fluid analysis are normal. Evaluation is designed to rule out a subarachnoid hemorrhage. If the symptoms are similar to those of migraine, then propranolol can be tried. When symptoms mimic those of tension-type headache, then indomethacin has been reported to be the best therapeutic option.

There are, of course, major disorders that can present with or be associated with headache. In addition to all the problems such as tumor or meningitis found in males, women can have additional rare problems, including venous thrombosis or intracranial hemorrhage related to pregnancy. Most of the time, fortunately, disorders such as subarachnoid hemorrhage present as an obvious problem, and appropriate therapy follows. Examination and history always remain crucial, but imaging will be needed in almost all such patients. Management will need to be individualized, and neurologic or neurosurgical consultation is commonly required.

Most of the numerous patients with headache can be helped by analgesics, prophylaxis, or attention to factors in life style that are contributory. Fortunately, most headaches are benign, those that are not are usually obvious, and almost all patients are grateful to the doctor who tries to help.

Hemorrhoids and Anal Fissure

William E. Wise, Jr, MD
E. Christopher Ellison, MD

Every patient is susceptible to the potential problems associated with hemorrhoids and anal fissures. Although such problems are centuries old, their precise etiology and treatment are controversial. In the practice of obstetrics and gynecology, skin tags, hemorrhoids, and occasionally rectal bleeding may be encountered during pregnancy as well as post partum. These may also occur as the patient ages. An obstetrician/gynecologist is frequently asked to recommend appropriate therapy for hemorrhoids and anal fissures. Therefore, it is important to understand current thinking on the pathogenesis, diagnosis, and treatment of these lesions.

Hemorrhoids

Hemorrhoids are one of the most common afflictions of western civilization; women are particularly susceptible to the development of hemorrhoidal symptoms during pregnancy as well as the perinatal period. The increased abdominal pressure associated with pregnancy, and espe-

cially vaginal delivery, can frequently exacerbate relatively minor hemorrhoidal problems. Proper counseling of patients as well as timely intervention depends on an adequate understanding of the anatomy and pathophysiology of the anorectum.

Anatomy

Hemorrhoids are normal anatomic structures. Internal hemorrhoids exist above the dentate line, are covered with rectal mucosa, and usually occur in the left lateral, right anterior, and right posterior quadrants. These "anal cushions" dilate with increased abdominal pressure, descend with straining, and restore to normal anorectal anatomy after the act of defecation. External hemorrhoids occur distal to the dentate line, are covered by anoderm, and tend to be more circumferential in distribution.

Pathophysiology

The anal cushions become lax with conditions that predispose to increased intra-abdominal pressure. Constipation, with its attendant need to strain at stool, and pregnancy and delivery, with increased intra-abdominal pressure, both tend to contribute to the development of the clinical syndrome known as hemorrhoids. Progressive and prolonged pressure leads to downward stretch of the anal cushions and may lead to failure of the cushions to resume their normal position above the dentate line. In addition to these physical factors, increasing evidence in recent years has linked dietary factors (specifically decreased dietary fiber) to the development of constipation and hemorrhoids.

Classification

Hemorrhoids are classified into internal and external forms. External hemorrhoids occur below the pectinate line and are covered with anoderm. Internal hemorrhoids occur cephalad to the dentate line and can further be classified as first-, second-, third-, or fourth-degree hemorrhoids.

First Degree

The patient complains of painless, bright-red rectal bleeding associated with defecation. These hemorrhoids can be visualized anoscopically as projections into the lumen of the anal canal, but they do not prolapse below the dentate line.

Second Degree

Hemorrhoids prolapse below the dentate line during defecation or straining but spontaneously reduce.

Third Degree

Hemorrhoids prolapse below the dentate line with straining or defecation and require manual reduction.

Fourth Degree

These chronically prolapsed hemorrhoids cannot be manually reduced and are therefore always below the dentate line.

Signs and Symptoms

Hemorrhoids commonly present with painless rectal bleeding. The bleeding is characterized by the appearance of bright-red blood on the toilet paper, on the surface of the stool, or in the toilet bowl. Bleeding is caused by the passage of a hard stool that tears the rectal mucosa overlying the venous plexus. Patients may also complain of the presence of a lump or fullness in the perianal skin associated with straining. This prolapsed hemorrhoid may or may not be reducible into the anal canal. Internal hemorrhoids can become so engorged that they can prolapse, fail to reduce, and become gangrenous.

Itching, burning, and perianal irritation are also common complaints in women with hemorrhoids.

Diagnosis

Digital rectal examination and subsequent anoscopic evaluation are essential for the diagnosis. Further evaluation, including sigmoidoscopy, colonoscopy, or barium enema, should be undertaken to exclude inflammatory bowel disease or potential neoplastic sources of persistent rectal bleeding. All patients over 40 years of age should have a flexible sigmoidoscopic examination even if an obvious source of rectal bleeding is seen on anoscopy.

Treatment

Hemorrhoids usually respond well to nonsurgical forms of treatment. These include dietary manipulation, the addition of a fiber supplement, and the use of topical ointments and sitz baths. Ninety percent of patients will respond well and avoid surgery; the remainder may require surgical intervention to alleviate their symptoms.

Dietary Manipulation

Early, intermittent hemorrhoidal symptoms can usually be managed by dietary manipulation and bulk-forming agents. The patient should be instructed to maintain a high-fiber diet (bran and other cereals) and to supplement the diet with bulk agents such as psyllium-containing compounds. Metamucil, Perdiem fiber, and Citrucel are such agents, and each contains approximately 3.4 g of fiber per dose. Konsyl contains the highest amount of fiber as a supplement, with 6 g of dietary fiber. The fiber products come in a variety of forms, from wafers to powder to pills, and the brand chosen should be based on patient tolerance and compliance. Stool softeners are occasionally used (Colace, Surfak); laxatives and mineral oil have no role in the treatment of hemorrhoids. First- and second-degree hemorrhoids often require no other treatment.

Local Treatment

Spreading creams and lotion on the perianal skin is rarely beneficial in the treatment of an exacerbation of hemorrhoidal disease. Some patients require local treatment to reduce the swelling and inflammation often seen with first- and second-degree disease. Anusol suppositories (preparation of bismuth, benzyl benzoate, and Peruvian balsam) provide a soothing lubricant action on the rectal mucosa and may provide symptomatic relief. The addition of hydrocortisone provides an anti-inflammatory, antipruritic, and vasoconstrictive action. Over-the-counter hemorrhoidal preparations may be used, but in our experience they are not as efficacious. A response to these conservative measures is usually seen within a few days, although complete cessation of bleeding and prolapse may not occur for 2 to 4 weeks.

Surgical Therapy—Office

Symptomatic hemorrhoids that fail to respond to conservative measures can often be managed using one or more simple out-patient surgical techniques.

Band ligation may be used to treat internal hemorrhoids that fail to respond to medical therapy. This technique is particularly useful for first-, second-, or third-degree internal hemorrhoids and is contraindicated in patients with external hemorrhoids. The instrumentation is relatively inexpensive and ligation can be performed in the office with no anesthesia. The technique involves grasping the protruding hemorrhoid and slipping a rubber band around the base. The band should be placed cephalad to the dentate line to avoid the somatic innervation of the anoderm. One to two hemorrhoids can be banded at each setting, and the procedure can be repeated at monthly intervals until the patient achieves symptomatic relief or all of the hemorrhoids have been ligated. The patient should be warned that she will pass the rubber band with her stool about 10 days following ligation. Patients should be treated with bulk fiber supplements during this time period.

Fourth-degree internal hemorrhoids can also occasionally be managed with rubber band ligation after reduction of the hemorrhoidal complex. Local anesthesia with 0.25% bupivacaine and 1:200,000 epinephrine with the addition of 150 U of hyaluronidase (Wydase) can be used to create a perianal block. The hemorrhoidal complex can then be reduced and rubber bands applied to the largest of the internal hemorrhoids. This technique can often convert a severe hemorrhoidal deformity from one that requires surgical hemorrhoidectomy into one that can be managed by serial rubber band ligation.

The potential complications of band ligation include pain (if the band is placed below the dentate line), hemorrhage (usually 7 to 10 days following banding when the ligature erodes through the venous plexus), and perineal sepsis. The incidence of sepsis is very small but the consequences can be quite devastating. Sepsis is heralded by perineal pain, fever, erythema, and urinary retention and should be managed in a hospital setting with intravenous antibiotics. Failure of prompt relief mandates surgical excision of the quadrant involved.

Surgical Hemorrhoidectomy

Surgical hemorrhoidectomy should be reserved for those patients in whom vigorous attempts at nonoperative and out-patient management fail. This includes patients with large bleeding hemorrhoids that are nonreducible and may be associated with severe distortion of anorectal archi-

tecture. Multiple thrombosed or extremely painful hemorrhoids may be difficult to manage with more conservative measures and may require operative intervention. Hemorrhoidectomy may also be necessary in women with known grade 1, 2, or 3 hemorrhoids that prolapse during pregnancy or at the time of labor and delivery and are nonreducible. A discussion of techniques for surgical hemorrhoidectomy is beyond the scope of this chapter.

Thrombosed Hemorrhoids

Thrombosed external hemorrhoids present as an acute painful and hard perianal mass. The mass is tender to palpation, is usually round, and has a bluish appearance. This type of hemorrhoid arises below the pectinate line and is covered by a pale squamous epithelium. If the symptoms are severe or fail to resolve promptly with medical therapy, the thrombosed vessel should be excised under a local anesthesia. Prolapsed thrombosed internal hemorrhoids can be differentiated from external hemorrhoids by the fact that the internal hemorrhoid is covered by red rectal mucosa. This is the usual type that develops in the postpartum period. In these cases, medical therapy with cold compresses, analgesics, stool softeners, sitz baths, and bedrest usually helps. If these measures do not result in resolution of the symptoms within 24 hours, then reduction of the prolapsed hemorrhoids can be achieved with injection of a mixture of local anesthetic and hyaluronidase. In some cases of thrombosed external hemorrhoids, hemorrhoidectomy may be the only way to adequately relieve the symptoms.

Anal Fissure

Anal fissure is a common anorectal disorder. It is often seen in pregnancy and the postpartum period owing to associated constipation. The majority of fissures are the result of poor bowel habits (diarrhea or constipation). Multiple fissures or fissures in a lateral location suggest the possibility of Crohn's disease, infection, or anal carcinoma.

Etiology

The development of an acute fissure-in-ano results from the passage of a large, hard bolus of stool. The anoderm is torn, and pain and bleeding ensue.

The vast majority of fissures occur in the midline posteriorly owing to the relative lack of support of the anoderm by underlying external sphincter muscle. Women have a higher incidence of anterior fissures than men (21% versus 1%), once again owing to a relative weakness of the muscle in the anterior midline. While the vast majority of fissures heal spontaneously, continued trauma due to constipation may result in the development of a chronic fissure-in-ano.

Signs and Symptoms

Anal fissure classically presents with the acute onset of painful rectal bleeding. The pain can be quite severe and is often described as "knifelike." The pain is worsened by defecation and tends to resolve over the 2 to 3 hours following a bowel movement. Blood can often be seen as thin streaks on the toilet paper in patients with acute fissure-in-ano. Chronic fissures usually have an associated hypertrophied anal papilla and a large external skin tag.

Diagnostic Evaluation

Rectal examination is often painful or impossible in patients with an acute anal fissure. Gentle retraction of the perianal skin allows the examiner to visualize the acute fissure in the midline without significant discomfort. A topical anesthetic applied directly to the fissure may be a useful adjunct in the physical examination. As with hemorrhoids, proctosigmoidoscopy should be undertaken prior to any surgical intervention to exclude the presence of inflammatory bowel disease involving the anorectum. General anesthesia may be required to perform an adequate evaluation.

Medical Treatment

Nonoperative therapy should be attempted prior to surgical intervention. A stool softener, a high-

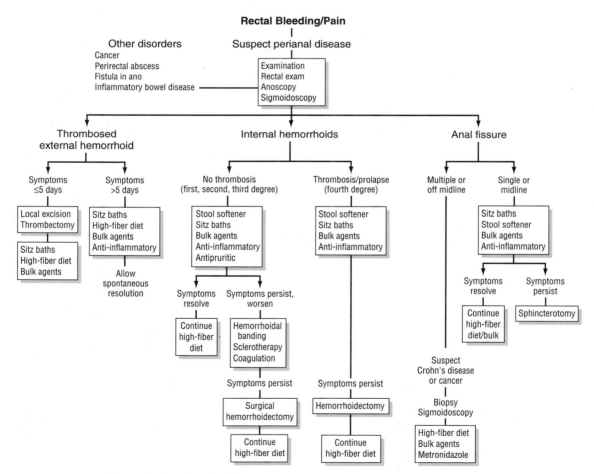

Figure 1. Algorithm for the management of hemorrhoids and fissure-in-ano.

fiber diet, and sitz baths may all provide symptomatic relief for the patient with an acute anal fissure. Topical anesthetics may be helpful in transiently relieving the symptoms; however, they may be irritating to the underlying mucosa and delay healing. Patients who complain of associated pruritus should be instructed to keep the perianal skin clean and dry, to avoid vigorous cleansing with soap and water, and to avoid coffee, cola, alcohol, and spicy foods, all of which have been implicated in symptoms of pruritus ani. These measures should result in relief of symptoms in 80% of patients and promote healing of the fissure within 4 to 6 weeks. Recurrence or persistence of symptoms should prompt a search for a systemic cause of the fissure-in-ano.

Surgical Management

Operative management depends on the physical findings as well as the duration of symptoms. Acute anal fissures respond readily to internal sphincterotomy, whereas chronic fissures often require surgical excision of the fissures combined with internal anal sphincterotomy. Lateral internal sphincterotomy can be performed on an outpatient basis under local anesthesia. Complication rates are low, and the procedure is almost uniformly successful in relieving the symptoms of acute anal fissure and preventing the development of a chronic fissure. Fissurectomy with sphincterotomy remains the treatment of choice for chronic anal fissures. Postoperative measures include only sitz baths and adherence to a high-fiber diet.

Complications

Perianal abscess, hemorrhage, and ecchymosis are all rare complications of internal sphincterotomy. Fecal soiling and incontinence for flatus should occur in less than 2% of patients. Fecal incontinence should not occur. Recurrence of anal fissure should be rare, and virtually all fissures should be healed within 2 to 3 weeks, although occasionally the healing process can be prolonged.

Summary

In summary, hemorrhoids and fissure-in-ano are commonly seen in the practice of obstetrics and gynecology. An algorithm for diagnosis and treatment is presented in Figure 1. Diagnosis needs to be confirmed in each case by digital rectal examination and anoscopy. Sigmoidoscopy is warranted in patients in whom Crohn's disease or ulcerative colitis is suspected and in patients over 40 who are at high risk for colorectal cancer. Biopsies of anal fissures may be warranted if they are located in an unexpected area. Fortunately, conservative medical management of hemorrhoids yields symptomatic relief in the majority of these cases. Minor procedures such as hemorrhoidal banding and sclerotherapy have virtually negated the necessity for closed hemorrhoidectomy except in cases in which there is extreme rectal prolapse or thrombosis. In a similar fashion, most anal fissures can be managed medically. Surgical management should consist of lateral internal sphincterotomy. Once treated, problems with hemorrhoids and fissure-in-ano may occur on a chronic basis. Prevention of hard stool and constipation is the best method to avoid symptomatic recurrence with either condition. Therefore, once treated, patients should use bulk agents and a high-fiber diet indefinitely.

Hypertension in the Nonpregnant Patient

Donald G. Vidt, MD

Based on current definitions—systolic blood pressure (SBP) 140 mm Hg or higher and/or diastolic blood pressure (DBP) 90 mm Hg or higher and/or the taking of antihypertensive medication—approximately 50 million Americans have elevated blood pressure. The prevalence of hypertension increases with advancing age and is higher in blacks than in whites. During the first half of adult life, hypertension is slightly less common among women than among men, but after menopause, prevalence among women increases to a level higher than that among men. The reason for this postmenopausal increase is not clear. Much lower rates of cardiovascular events in middle-aged women make it difficult to distinguish the degree of benefit from treatments between men and women. Recent clinical trials with older individuals support a similar approach to the management of hypertension in both men and women.

There is a scarcity of data regarding many important aspects of hypertension in women. Data that do exist, however, suggest that gender, race, and age can significantly influence both the natural history of hypertension and the response to treatment. Treatment for black women is clearly beneficial, suggesting that aggressive outreach, screening, and case finding could be important public health measures for this group. Even in this group, however, it is not known whether there are gender-related adverse effects of current therapies. Thus, black women may not be receiving maximal benefit from their antihypertensive treatment. The same discrepancies in the database exist for possible differences among specific therapies for white women as well. There is almost complete absence of data regarding two important side effects of antihypertensive medications in women: alterations in lipid profiles and sexual dysfunction. Available data from several clinical trials suggest that differences exist between men and women in terms of cigarette smoking and its effects on blood pressure, cholesterol values at baseline, and event rates during follow-up. While a considerable beneficial effect of treatment on the incidence of fatal and nonfatal stroke was clearly evident among both men and women, a significant beneficial effect of treatment on levels of total mortality could be detected only among men. The most striking difference between men and women in various aspects of their participation in hypertension trials has been the very low event rate among women, particularly for coronary heart disease.

Causes of Hypertension

Essential hypertension is the overwhelmingly prevalent type of hypertension in our society and is usually accompanied by a family history of high blood pressure and progressive cardiovascular disease. There are, however, several forms of hypertension peculiar to women that deserve mention.

Oral Contraceptives

Most women taking oral contraceptives experience a small but detectable increase in both systolic and diastolic blood pressure, usually within the normal range. Significant hypertension occurs in only a small percentage of women taking these preparations, although the risk appears to increase with age, with duration of use, and perhaps with increased body mass. In a large British study, hypertension was noted in 5% of women taking oral contraceptives for 5 years, an incidence two to three times higher than that

occurring among nonusers. It is probable that only genetically susceptible individuals develop significant hypertension with oral contraceptives; in the majority, the observed rise in blood pressure does not reach hypertensive levels.

In addition, other changes that occur with oral contraceptives that may increase cardiovascular risk include an increase in blood lipids, increased blood coagulability, and impairment of glucose tolerance. Women over the age of 35 years who smoke cigarettes should be discouraged from using oral contraceptives, since most of the cardiovascular deaths attributable to oral contraceptives have been observed in such women. Since lower doses of both estrogen and progesterone are presently in use, the current incidence of oral contraceptive–induced hypertension is probably less than reported earlier. However, accelerated or malignant hypertension has been observed in association with oral contraceptive–induced hypertension.

The mechanism by which oral contraceptives induce hypertension is imperfectly understood. Potential mechanisms are suggested by the following observations: increases in plasma volume and cardiac output associated with weight gain in users, a sodium-retaining effect of the estrogenic component of oral contraceptives, increased hepatic synthesis of renin substrate, and increased circulating levels of angiotensin II. If hypertension develops in a woman taking oral contraceptives, the pills should be stopped, after which blood pressures will usually normalize within 1 to 3 months.

Renovascular Hypertension

Renovascular hypertension, particularly in association with one of the fibromuscular hyperplasias, is much more common in younger white women than in men of all races. Fibromuscular hyperplasias account for as many as 75% of cases of renovascular hypertension observed in younger women. Although atherosclerotic renovascular disease is more common overall, it occurs in a much older age group and predominates in men.

In younger women, hemodynamically significant renovascular hypertension due to fibromuscular hyperplasia is usually amenable to therapy with percutaneous transluminal renal angioplasty. Cure rates with this procedure are very high, complication rates are lower in younger women with fibromuscular lesions of the renal arteries, and the risk of late restenosis is quite low. These results are in contrast to those observed in older women with atherosclerotic lesions of the renal arteries, in whom technical success rates with percutaneous transluminal renal angioplasty are lower, and complication and restenosis rates are higher.

Estrogen Replacement Therapy

Chronic hypertension is not a deterrent to the use of postmenopausal estrogen replacement therapy, which may in fact have a beneficial effect on cardiovascular risk. A small percentage of women will experience a rise in blood pressure attributable to estrogen therapy, and it is recommended that all women treated with hormonal replacement have blood pressures monitored periodically. The effects of transdermal estrogen on blood pressure in postmenopausal women have not been well studied.

Evaluation and Confirmation of Hypertension

The National High Blood Pressure Education Program, in its periodic reports, has recommended a practical approach to confirmation and subsequent evaluation of the hypertensive patient. Average DBP readings of 90 mm Hg or greater or SBP readings of 140 mm Hg or greater are required for diagnosis, and initial elevated readings should be confirmed on at least two subsequent visits. The current classification of hypertension in adults is listed in Table 1. The presence or absence of target organ damage or other risk factors, such as smoking, dyslipidemia, and diabetes mellitus, independently modify the risk for subsequent cardiovascular disease and hypertension. The presence or absence of major risk factors or target organ damage, or both, is determined during a routine evaluation of patients with hypertension. While obesity and physical inactivity are also predictors of cardiovascular risk, through interaction with other risk factors, they have less significance in the selection of antihypertensive drugs.

This approach enables us to focus on the total cardiovascular risk for each hypertensive patient at the time of initial evaluation, an approach that is mandatory if we wish to optimize risk reduction. Risk stratification can now be utilized for treatment decisions in each new hypertensive patient (Table 2). It is notable that patients with high normal blood pressure (130–139/85–89 mm Hg) have now been included in the risk stratification process for treatment decisions, particularly those patients with high normal blood pres-

TABLE 1. Classification of Blood Pressure for Adults Aged 18 Years And Older°

Category	Systolic (mm Hg)		Diastolic (mm Hg)
Optimal†	<120	and	<80
Normal	<130	and	<85
High-normal	130–139	or	85–89
Hypertension			
Stage 1‡	140–159	or	90–99
Stage 2‡	160–179	or	100–109
Stage 3‡	≥180	or	≥110

°Not taking antihypertensive drugs and not acutely ill. When systolic and diastolic blood pressures fall into different categories, the higher category should be selected to classify the individual's blood pressure status. For example, 160/92 mm Hg should be classified as Stage 2 hypertension, and 174/120 mm Hg should be classified as Stage 3 hypertension. Isolated systolic hypertension is defined as SBP ≥140 mm Hg and DBP <90 mm Hg and staged appropriately (eg, 170/82 mm Hg is defined as Stage 2 isolated systolic hypertension). In addition to classifying stages of hypertension on the basis of average blood pressure levels, clinicians should specify presence or absence of target organ disease and additional risk factors. This specificity is important for risk classification and treatment.

†Optimal blood pressure with respect to cardiovascular risk is <120/80 mm Hg. However, unusually low readings should be evaluated for clinical significance.

‡Based on the average of two or more readings taken at each of two or more visits after initial screening.

From the Joint National Committee on the Detection, Evaluation, and Treatment of High Blood Pressure: The sixth report (JNC-VI). Arch Intern Med 1997; 157:2413–2446.

sure in risk group C, in whom target organ damage, clinical cardiovascular disease such as heart failure, or renal insufficiency may be present, and those patients with diabetes mellitus with or without other risk factors. For patients with Stage 1 hypertension, aggressive lifestyle modification for periods of 6 to 12 months may be appropriate before consideration of drug therapy for risk groups A and B. On the other hand, patients with Stage 1 hypertension in risk group C will benefit from aggressive drug therapy. Drug therapy is recommended for all patients with Stages 2 and 3 hypertension, regardless of risk group. This classification, utilizing blood pressure stages and risk groupings, should provide practicing physicians with a simple method of identifying patients most likely to benefit from aggressive drug therapy.

In selected patients with labile blood pressure or suspected office hypertension, ambulatory blood pressure monitoring may be appropriate. A number of automatic and semiautomatic blood pressure monitors that use acoustic or oscillometric methods are currently available and acceptable for home use.

A thorough history and physical examination,

TABLE 2. Risk Stratification and Treatment of High Blood Pressure°

Stratification

Risk Group	Criteria
A	No risk factors No TOD/CDD
B	At least one risk factor, not including diabetes mellitus No TOD/CDD
C	TOD/CDD and/or diabetes with or without other risk factors

Treatment

Blood Pressure Stage (mm Hg)	Risk Group A	Risk Group B	Risk Group C
High-normal (130–139/85–89)	Lifestyle modification	Lifestyle modification	Drug therapy†
Stage 1 (140–159/90–99)	Lifestyle modification (up to 12 months)	Lifestyle modification‡ (up to 6 months)	Drug therapy
Stage 2 (≥160/≥100)	Drug therapy	Drug therapy	Drug therapy

CCD, clinical cardiovascular disease; TOD, target organ disease.
    For example: A patient with diabetes and a BP of 142/94 mm Hg plus left ventricular hypertrophy should be classified as having Stage 1
        hypertension with TOD (LVH) and with another major risk factor (diabetes). This patient would be categorized as Stage 1,
        Risk Group C, and recommended for immediate initiation of pharmacologic treatment.
  °Lifestyle modification should be adjunctive therapy for all patients recommended for pharmacologic therapy.
  †For those with heart failure or renal disease or those with diabetes mellitus.
  ‡For patients with multiple risk factors, clinicians should consider drugs as initial therapy plus lifestyle modifications.
    Adapted from the Joint National Committee on the Detection, Evaluation, and Treatment of High Blood Pressure: The sixth report (JNC-VI). Arch Intern Med 1997;157:2413–2446.

blood count, urinalysis, electrocardiogram, and automated chemistry profile provide sufficient information to determine the severity of hypertension, may help identify secondary causes, and provide baseline values for assessing biochemical effects of therapy. On occasion, when resistant hypertension is suspected, additional tests such as the measurement of urinary microalbumin, assessment of cardiac anatomy and function by echocardiography, plasma renin activity or urinary sodium excretion or both, and the measurement of cardiac output together with blood and plasma volume may be useful in assessing cardiovascular status.

Nonpharmacologic Therapy

The goal of therapy in the hypertensive patient is to achieve and maintain an arterial blood pressure below 140/90 mm Hg in an effort to prevent subsequent morbidity and mortality. The patient with Stage 1, uncomplicated hypertension should be offered a period of 6 to 12 months of aggressive nonpharmacologic treatment before the initiation of appropriate drug therapy is considered. Lifestyle modifications may represent definitive intervention in these patients and provide an adjunct to pharmacologic therapy in patients with more severe degrees of elevated blood pressure. Although nonpharmacologic therapy has not conclusively demonstrated reduced morbidity and mortality in hypertensive populations, lifestyle modifications can improve the overall cardiovascular risk profile, thus offering multiple benefits at little cost and with minimal risk to the hypertensive patient.

A clear association exists between obesity and elevated blood pressure, and all obese hypertensive patients may benefit from a weight reduction program, the goal being to achieve a weight within 15% of optimal weight. While recidivism is common and can be discouraging, the long-term goal of attenuating age-related weight gain should be kept in mind. Similarly, a high sodium intake can maintain hypertension in some patients and may limit the effectiveness of some antihypertensive agents, such as diuretics. Moderate sodium restriction (70 to 100 mEq/day) may represent definitive therapy for some patients with Stage 1 hypertension and can improve the effectiveness of these antihypertensive agents.

Excess alcohol consumption may contribute to hypertension, encouraging a recommendation that intake be limited to no more than 1 ounce of ethanol (2 ounces of 100-proof whiskey, 8 ounces of wine, or 24 ounces of beer) per day.

Although unrelated to hypertension, cigarette smoking is a major risk factor for cardiovascular disease and tobacco avoidance is essential. Use of the nicotine patch or nicotine chewing gum in conjunction with repetitive counseling has improved success rates in smoking cessation. Cigarette smoking may also blunt the beneficial risk reductions induced by selected antihypertensive agents such as beta blockers.

Regular aerobic physical activity, sufficient to achieve a moderate level of physical fitness, may prevent and treat hypertension, enhance weight loss and functional health status, and reduce the overall risk of cardiovascular disease mortality. Regular physical activity has now been demonstrated to reduce systolic blood pressure in hypertensive patients by approximately 10 mm Hg. The regimen need not be complicated for most sedentary patients; moderate activity such as 30 to 45 minutes of brisk walking, cycling, or swimming up to five times per week can be beneficial.

Because hyperlipidemia represents an independent cardiovascular risk, considerable attention has recently been focused on the cardiovascular risk benefit of a diet low in cholesterol and saturated fat. The role of stress management techniques in treating hypertensives remains uncertain, and longer, carefully controlled clinical trials are needed.

Pharmacologic Therapy

There are currently more than 100 antihypertensive drugs or drug combinations available among 10 distinct drug classes. A list of available antihypertensive drugs and their dosage recommendations is included in Table 3. A number of newer, low-dose combination agents are also available.

The clinician must possess a working knowledge of the practical clinical pharmacology of each of the available classes of antihypertensive agents if he or she is to make appropriate selections of initial and subsequent therapy for the patient with sustained hypertension. A number of issues form the current basis for empiric antihypertensive drug selection.

Efficacy

Blood pressure reduction is really not at issue in the 1990s, since the initial drug selected, regardless of class, will control blood pressure in approximately 50% of hypertensive patients and will be the only drug required. The one exception to this statement may be the vasodilators, since tolerability is poor when they are used as monotherapy, except possibly in older hypertensive patients. A review of multiple clinical trials also suggests that any two drugs in combination will control blood pressure in 80% to 90% of hypertensive patients, providing the two drugs selected are not from the same class. The importance of these statements is obvious, since therapy will usually continue for life, and the careful selection of initial and subsequent therapy is capable of providing prolonged control for the vast majority of hypertensive patients.

Controlled clinical trials over the last 25 years have demonstrated the effectiveness of blood pressure reduction in reducing stroke and cardiac and renal morbidity and mortality. A meta-analysis of 14 controlled treatment trials has demonstrated a cumulative 42% reduction in stroke but only a modest 14% reduction in coronary mortality. Clinical trials have also demonstrated that control of hypertension reduces the incidence of left ventricular hypertrophy, congestive heart failure, anginal attacks in patients with ischemic heart disease, dissecting aneurysm, and possibly symptomatic peripheral vascular disease and can preserve renal function and reduce the risk of end-stage renal disease from uncontrolled hypertension. In addition, control of Stage 1 hypertension prevents progression to more severe stages.

All of the major clinical trials that have demonstrated long-term reduction in cardiovascular morbidity and mortality have utilized oral diuretics and β-adrenergic blocking agents as basic therapy. While other classes of agents are effective in lowering blood pressure, most have not yet been subjected to well-controlled clinical trials of sufficient duration to obtain appropriate morbidity and mortality data.

The Treatment of Mild Hypertension study is a good example of the current dilemma. The study randomized 902 patients to receive placebo, diuretic, beta blocker, alpha blocker, calcium antagonist, or an angiotensin-converting enzyme (ACE) inhibitor as monotherapy. Initial monotherapy was combined with non-drug lifestyle changes in all patients. After 1 year, 83% of participants were still receiving their initially assigned medication, with good blood pressure

TABLE 3. Antihypertensive Agents

Type of Drug	Usual Dosage Range (total mg/day)*	Frequency
Initial Antihypertensive Agents		
Diuretics		
Thiazides and related sulfonamide diuretics		
Bendroflumethiazide (Naturetin)	2.5–5	Once
Benzthiazide (Exna)	12.5–50	Once
Chlorothiazide (Diuril)	125–500	Twice
Chlorthalidone (Hygroton)	12.5–25	Once
Hydrochlorothiazide (HydroDIURIL, Esidrix)	12.5–50	Once
Hydroflumethiazide (Saluron, Diucardin)	12.5–50	Once
Indapamide (Lozol)	2.5–5	Once
Methyclothiazide (Enduron)	2.5–5	Once
Metolazone (Zaroxolyn)	1.25–10	Once
Metolazone (Mykrox)	0.5–1	Once
Polythiazide (Renese)	1–4	Once
Quinethazone (Hydromox)	24–100	Once
Trichlormethiazide	1–4	Once
Loop diuretics		
Bumetanide (Bumex)	0.5–5	Twice
Ethacrynic acid (Edecrin)	25.0–100	Twice
Furosemide (Lasix)	20.0–320	Twice
Torsemide (Demadex)	5–10	Once or twice
Potassium-sparing agents		
Amiloride (Midamor)	5–10	Once or twice
Spironolactone (Aldactone)	25–100	Twice or thrice
Triamterene (Dyrenium)	50–150	Twice
Adrenergic Inhibitors		
Beta blockers		
Atenolol (Tenormin)	25–100†	Once or twice
Betaxolol (Kerlone)	5–20	Once
Bisoprolol (Zebeta)	2.5–10	Once
Metoprolol (Lopressor)	50–300	Twice
Metoprolol (long-acting) (Toprol XL)	50–300	Once
Nadolol (Corgard)	20–240†	Once
Propranolol (Inderal)	40–480	Twice
Propranolol (long-acting) (Inderal LA)	60–480	Once
Timolol maleate (Blocadren)	20–60	Once
Beta blockers with intrinsic sympathomimetic activity		
Acebutolol (Sectral)	200–1200†	Twice
Carteolol (Cartrol)	2.5–10 †	Once
Penbutolol (Levatol)	10–20†	Once
Pindolol (Visken)	10–60†	Once
Alpha-beta blocker		
Carvedilol (Coreg)	12.5–50	Twice
Labetalol (Normodyne, Trandate)	200–1200	Twice
Alpha₁-receptor blocker		
Doxazosin (Cardura)	2–16	Once
Prazosin (Minipress)	2–30	Twice or thrice
Terazosin (Hytrin)	1–20	Once

TABLE 3. Antihypertensive Agents *Continued*

Type of Drug	Usual Dosage Range (total mg/day)*	Frequency
ACE inhibitors		
Benazepril (Lotensin)	10–40†	Once or twice
Captopril (Capoten)	12.5–150†	Twice or thrice
Cilazapril	2.5–5	Once or twice
Enalapril (Vasotec)	5–40†	Once or twice
Fosinopril (Monopril)	10–40	Once or twice
Lisinopril (Prinivil, Zestril)	5–40†	Once or twice
Moexipril (Univasc)	7.5–15	Twice
Perindopril	1–16†	Once or twice
Quinapril (Accupril)	5–80†	Once or twice
Ramipril (Altace)	1.25–20†	Once or twice
Spirapril	12.5–50	Once or twice
Trandolapril (Mavik)	1–4	Once
Calcium antagonists		
Diltiazem (sustained release) (Cardizem SR)	120–360	Twice
Diltiazem (extended release) (Cardizem CD)	120–360	Once
Diltiazem (extended release) (Dilacor XR)	180–360	Once
Diltiazem (extended release) (Tiazac)	180–360	Once
Verapamil (Verelan)	120–480	Once
Verapamil (long-acting) (Calan SR, Isoptin SR)	120–480	Once or twice
Verapamil (extended release) (Covera HS)	240–480	Once
Dyhydropyridines		
Amlodipine (Norvasc)	2.5–10	Once
Felodipine (Plendil)	2.5–20	Twice
Isradipine (DynaCirc)	5–10	Twice
Nicardipine (sustained release Cardene SR)	60–120	Twice
Nifedipine (Procardia XL, Adalat CC)	30–90	Once
Nisoldipine (Sular)	20–60	Once
Angiotensin II antagonists		
Candasartan (Atacand)	8–32	Once
Irbesartan (Avapro)	150–300	Once
Losartan (Cozaar)	25–100	Once or twice
Valsartan (Diovan)	80–320	Once
Supplemental Antihypertensive Agents		
Centrally-acting alpha₂-agonists		
Clonidine (Catapres)	0.1–1.2	Twice
Clonidine TTS (Patch) (Catapres-TTS)	0.1–0.3	Once *weekly*
Guanabenz (Wytensin)	8–32	Twice
Guanfacine (Tenex)	1–3	Once
Methyldopa (Aldomet)	500–3000	Twice
Peripherally-acting adrenergic neuron antagonists		
Guanadrel (Hylorel)	10–75	Twice
Guanethidine (Ismelin)	10–150	Once
Rauwolfia alkaloids		
Reserpine (Serpasil)	0.05‡–0.25	Once
Direct vasodilators		
Hydralazine (Apresoline)	50–300	Twice to four times
Minoxidil (Loniten)	5–100	Once or twice

*The lower number is the preferred initial dose, and the higher number is the maximum daily dose. Most agents require 2 to 4 weeks for complete efficacy, and more frequent dosage adjustments are not advised except for cases of severe hypertension. The dosage range may differ slightly from the recommended dosage in the *Physician's Desk Reference* or package insert.

†Indicates drugs that are excreted by the kidney and require dosage reduction in renal impairment.

‡0.1 mg dose may be given every other day to achieve this dosage.

Adapted from the Joint National Committee on the Detection, Evaluation, and Treatment of High Blood Pressure: The sixth report (JNC-VI). Arch Intern Med 1997;157:2413–2446.

control and tolerability. Overall, blood pressure reduction was comparable in each of the five monotherapy treatment groups, and no consistent pattern in side effect differences was noted.

Age, race, and gender no longer represent characteristics that should play a major role in the empiric selection of therapy, particularly as it relates to withholding selected classes of agents from individual patients.

Safety

A primary responsibility of the Food and Drug Administration (FDA) in the drug approval process is to ascertain that agents are free from serious side effects. Generally, the FDA has met this responsibility, but it must be remembered that adverse effects may be subtle and slow to develop and may place patients at increased risk only after prolonged periods.

A host of other metabolic and clinical adverse effects associated with different agents (or classes of agents) must also be appreciated. Some classes of agents may have potentially adverse effects on lipid parameters, blood glucose, and insulin sensitivity, together with effects on potassium or magnesium concentrations. Although efforts have been made to link these drug-induced metabolic and electrolyte adverse effects with cardiovascular morbidity and mortality, incriminating data remain largely controversial. Other factors such as the effects of selected agents or classes of agents on platelet function, plasma catecholamines, uric acid concentrations, and exercise may also play a role in the physician's selection of an agent for the individual patient.

Dosage and Dosing Schedule

Historically, a leading factor in treatment failure in hypertension has been patient noncompliance, of which a notable component has been failure to correctly take medications that required multiple daily dosing. Fortunately, intermediate- to long-acting preparations are now available among all classes of antihypertensive agents to provide once- or twice-daily administration. The FDA requires peak and trough effect documentation for 12- or 24-hour duration of action for drugs to meet the claims of once- or twice-daily administration.

Dose response reactions of antihypertensives can represent an advantage or a disadvantage. As an example, the rapid dose response to short-acting nifedipine in the treatment of a hyperten-

sive urgency is a significant advantage in therapy. Conversely, that same dose response that results in a precipitous fall in blood pressure can induce cerebral ischemia in a patient with clinically significant carotid occlusive disease. The indications and cautions for short-acting as opposed to intermediate- or long-acting preparations of individual drugs must be recognized.

The FDA recently issued a warning regarding the use of short-acting nifedipine. Accumulated evidence suggests that this agent may be associated with a significant increase in coronary mortality when administered to patients at risk with underlying arteriosclerotic heart disease. The relative risk associated with nifedipine appears to be dose-related, particularly at dosages over 80 mg daily. This caution does not extend to long-acting nifedipine or other long acting calcium antagonists. Limited clinical trials with these newer, extended-release calcium antagonists have not demonstrated any increased risk from coronary mortality in patients treated with these preparations.

Longer-acting preparations have the advantage of providing potentially smoother blood pressure control. The clinician must, however, appreciate the clinical pharmacology of a given preparation. As an example, a drug with a 12- to 14-hour duration of action may be less effective when given twice a day on arising and at bedtime than when administered every 10 to 12 hours.

Twenty-four-hour monitoring of blood pressure has helped us to appreciate control problems with selected agents and in particular has focused attention on the early morning "surge" in blood pressure from the time of awakening to approximately midday. A number of events besides the rise in blood pressure and heart rate occurring during this period may potentially increase coronary risk. These factors include increased norepinephrine and epinephrine concentrations, platelet aggregation, and an increased incidence of anginal attacks, acute myocardial infarction, and sudden death. It is possible that the potential increased risk observed during this period may be alleviated by agents that effectively blunt this early morning blood pressure surge. It is also recognized that nocturnal falls in blood pressure may be accentuated by antihypertensive therapy and could add to potential risk, particularly in hypertensive patients with pre-existing ischemic coronary disease.

The first antihypertensive agent specifically designed to address the early morning surge in blood pressure was recently approved. This preparation of verapamil, called Covera-HS, is designed for bedtime administration. Design of the tablet prohibits release of any drug for the first 4 to 5 hours followed by constant drug delivery over the next 12 to 18 hours. Thus, no drug is released during sleep when blood pressure is at its lowest, and drug release first occurs before the morning surge in blood pressure. A carefully controlled clinical trial is required to determine whether this agent is effective for blood pressure control and whether the specific design of the drug will affect the occurrence of early morning cardiovascular events such as stroke and myocardial infarction.

Drug Interactions

The additive effects of antihypertensive agents, when used in combination, represent a classic example of favorable interactions among antihypertensive agents. This is particularly evident when adding an oral diuretic to a number of other classes of agents, such as the vasodilators, alpha blockers, and centrally acting α_2-agonists, which when used alone may be associated with subtle sodium and water retention. A key to optimizing additive effects is to choose agents with different mechanisms of action.

Commonly seen is the interaction between nonsteroidal anti-inflammatory drugs in blunting the effects of numerous antihypertensive agents, particularly diuretics and ACE inhibitors. The mechanism of this adverse interaction appears to be the inhibition of prostaglandin synthesis and associated sodium and water retention. Another common interaction is that observed with over-the-counter decongestant drugs, most of which contain pseudoephedrine compounds or similar agents that can increase blood pressure with repeated usage.

Interactions may be due to the direct effects of an agent on blood pressure such as that noted with oral contraceptives or may be indirectly observed through competition for the same pathway of metabolism, resulting in delayed inactivation or excretion and the enhanced possibility for drug toxicity.

Concomitant Illnesses

Antihypertensive agents may have favorable or unfavorable effects on selected coexisting or comorbid conditions. Throughout the drug development process, we have learned that selected agents should not be utilized with certain coexisting disease processes. On the other hand, sometimes predictable or at other times serendipitous

benefit has been observed in hypertensive patients in whom other complicating illnesses coexist.

Oral diuretics increase serum uric acid and may precipitate acute podagra in patients with a history of gout. Diuretic-induced hypokalemia may increase the risk of cardiac ectopy in some hypertensive patients with ischemic heart disease.

The antianginal and antiarrhythmic effects of heart rate-lowering calcium antagonists and beta blockers are well recognized benefits of using these agents in patients with hypertension and coronary artery disease. On the other hand, both classes of agents may aggravate symptoms of congestive heart failure. Both calcium antagonists and beta blockers may give specific benefit in hypertensive patients with migraine, while beta blockers would not be an agent of choice in the hypertensive patient with asthma or obstructive pulmonary disease.

Cost of Drugs

Current economic conditions and the rising cost of medical care have thrust the cost of medications into the spotlight. The cost of medications represents a major problem for a significant segment of our population: those without insurance, the underinsured, and the elderly on fixed incomes.

Generally, older, generic preparations can produce significant cost savings, but clinicians must appreciate that drug costs are market-driven, and the fact that an agent is generic or has been on the market for a long time does not necessarily translate into major cost savings. It is predictable that newer agents, particularly the ACE inhibitors and calcium antagonists, are more costly than some older preparations.

Physicians must be aware of drug cost and should take this issue into consideration in prescribing. At the same time, the cost of a drug should not be the primary consideration in drug selection.

Patient Acceptance

It has long been recognized that the key to optimal control of blood pressure is the patient's acceptance of prescribed therapy, and the leading cause of failure to control blood pressure rests with patient nonadherence. The patient's acceptance of and adherence to the treatment regimen really equates to his or her perception of overall quality of life on therapy. Quality of life is a multifaceted concept and includes the patient's perception of his or her sense of well-being, life satisfaction, physical and emotional states, cognitive function, work performance, and level of social participation.

Physician behavior and involvement is a significant factor in promoting optimal adherence to treatment. Selection of a most appropriate drug can be individualized or "tailored" according to the issues listed earlier, together with the clinician's knowledge of the practical clinical pharmacology of available agents and their potential advantages and disadvantages.

Individualized Therapy in 1999

Careful consideration of the issues discussed, together with the advantages and disadvantages of individual drug classes, should enable appropriate selection of initial drug therapy. For patients with high normal blood pressure in risk group A or B, tracking of blood pressure along with aggressive nonpharmacologic therapy remain appropriate. Because of the increased cardiovascular risks observed in patients with high normal blood pressure complicated by diabetes mellitus, target organ damage, or clinical cardiovascular disease, early aggressive drug therapy is now recommended.

Stage 1 Hypertension

Some clinicians may elect to continue careful tracking of blood pressure, without specific drug treatment, for patients with DBP in the 90 to 99 mm Hg range and SBP in the 140 to 159 mm Hg range. In those patients stratified to risk groups A or B, careful follow-up is mandatory, because blood pressures may rise to higher levels and induce target organ changes. For those patients with Stage 1 hypertension who stratify to risk group C, it is desirable to initiate aggressive drug therapy to prevent progression of target organ damage or clinical cardiovascular disease. This recommendation is also particularly relevant in patients with diabetes mellitus. Similarly, drug therapy is recommended for all patients with Stage 2 hypertension with the clear recognition that many more patients with Stage 2 hypertension will require more than one agent for optimal control of blood pressure.

Drug therapy should be started with a single drug for patients with Stage 1 or 2 hypertension. Diuretics and beta blockers are considered the preferred drugs by many clinicians, since they have been shown in carefully controlled clinical trials to reduce cardiovascular morbidity and mortality. Alternative drugs including calcium antagonists, ACE inhibitors, angiotensin II antagonists, α-receptor blockers, and the alpha-beta blocker labetalol are comparably effective in reducing blood pressure but most have not been subjected to long-term clinical trials demonstrating reductions in morbidity and mortality. The exceptions, at this time, are two dihydropyridine calcium antagonists. In the SYST-EUR trial, a long-acting nitrendipine preparation demonstrated remarkable efficacy in reducing stroke events in older patients with isolated systolic hypertension, and the recently reported Hypertension Optimal Treatment trial showed that treatment to lower goal blood pressures with felodipine, alone or in combination with other agents, reduced cardiovascular morbidity and mortality. This latter trial is of particular importance because it has shown that aggressive treatment of SBP to levels as low as 120 mm Hg and DBP to 70 mm Hg could be accomplished with relative safety. Figure 1 provides a schema that should be helpful to clinicians in the initiation of drug therapy. Therapy should be begun with a low dose of a long-acting once-daily drug, and should be up-titrated carefully. In selected patients, low-dose combinations of drugs may be appropriate.

If the patient does not respond or has troublesome side effects with the initial drug selection, a drug from another class can be substituted. On the other hand, if the response to initial treatment is inadequate, but the agent is well tolerated, it may be appropriate to add a second agent from a different class, to take advantage of additive properties. Combining drugs with different mechanisms of action usually provides an additive effect that may allow smaller doses of individual drugs to achieve control while minimizing the potential for dose-dependent adverse effects. The successive treatment steps outlined can be followed until an adequate blood pressure response is maintained. If a diuretic is not selected as the first drug, it will be particularly useful as a second agent because of an additive enhancement of drug effects.

Before proceeding to each additional step, it is important to assess possible reasons for the lack of responsiveness, which will most commonly relate to compliance, excessive sodium intake, interacting drugs, or unrecognized secondary causes of hypertension. Additional agents can be added as recommended, until blood pressure has been reduced to an initial goal below

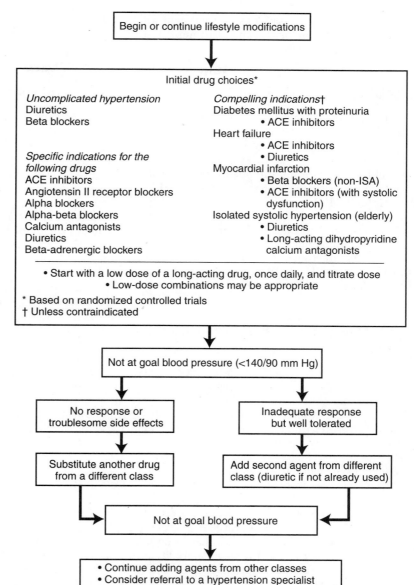

Figure 1. Algorithm for the treatment of hypertension. (Redrawn from the Joint National Committee on the Detection, Evaluation, and Treatment of High Blood Pressure: The sixth report JNC-VI. Arch Intern Med 1997; 157:2514.)

140/90 mm Hg. As noted earlier, other factors to be considered in drug selection include the metabolic and clinical adverse effects of individual agents, the potential for adverse drug-drug interactions, concomitant diseases that may derive benefit or be adversely affected by the antihypertensive agent selected, and the costs of individual drugs. The patient's perception of his or her quality of life on medication will be a major determinant for long-term adherence to therapy. Finally, the importance of controlling other cardiovascular risk factors is again noted if the ultimate goal of reduced cardiovascular morbidity and mortality from hypertension is to be achieved.

Stage 3 Hypertension

For patients with SBP of 180 mm Hg or higher, DBP of 110 mm Hg or higher, or both, modifications in the approach described may be indicated. It is often necessary to add a second or third agent after a short interval if control is not achieved. The intervals between changes in the regimen should be decreased. In selected patients, it may be necessary to start treatment with two agents concomitantly, and maximum doses of some drugs may be required.

Isolated Systolic Hypertension

Isolated systolic hypertension frequently occurs in older persons and current evidence clearly indicates the benefits of reducing SBP in older hypertensive patients. Lifestyle modifications should be used in an attempt to lower isolated systolic hypertension; however, when the SBP is consistently 160 mm Hg or higher and DBP is lower than 90 mm Hg, antihypertensive drug therapy is clearly indicated. Efforts should be made to reduce the SBP to 150 mm Hg initially, and if the treatment is well tolerated, careful further reduction of SBP to levels below 140 mm Hg is desirable.

Hypertension in the Postmenopausal Patient

The prevalence of hypertension in older women exceeds that observed in men, regardless of race. It is estimated that 83% of black women and 66% of white women over the age of 65 have blood pressures of 140/90 mm Hg or higher. These prevalence figures include those individuals with isolated systolic hypertension. Favorable reductions in cardiovascular mortality from hypertension should encourage continued aggressive management in older patients, including those over 65 years of age. Results from the Systolic Hypertension in the Elderly Program have now confirmed the benefits of treating this condition. Beneficial reductions in mortality are comparable to those observed with treatment in younger hypertensive patients. Finally, a number of prospective trials have addressed the effects of postmenopausal estrogen usage on morbidity from cardiovascular disease. Except for the Framingham trial, which reported an elevated risk of cardiovascular morbidity and a twofold increase in cerebrovascular complications with postmenopausal estrogen use, the majority of prospective studies have in fact suggested that the postmenopausal use of estrogens reduces the risk of coronary heart disease. Although the dosage of estrogens or progesterone used do not

appear to affect antihypertensive therapy adversely, use of the smallest effective doses of these agents should be encouraged.

Long-Term Follow-Up

Achievement and maintenance of goal blood pressure with the lowest possible dosage of medication requires a commitment to patient follow-up and a willingness to undertake dosage adjustment over time. Patients with Stage 1 or 2 hypertension, without significant target organ damage, should be seen within 1 to 2 months following the initiation of therapy to determine the adequacy of blood pressure control. The presence of target organ damage, associated medical problems, other major risk factors, and laboratory test abnormalities are all factors to consider in assessing the needed frequency of patient follow-up. Once blood pressure is controlled, follow-up at 3- to 6-month intervals is generally appropriate.

Remember that poor adherence to treatment, including lifestyle modifications and pharmacologic therapy, is the major reason for inadequate control of blood pressure. Therefore, patient education should be an important feature of each follow-up visit, with efforts aimed at helping patients to understand more clearly the specific therapies prescribed and the treatment goals.

Treating to Lower Blood Pressure Goals

The results of contemporary, controlled clinical studies continue to support aggressive reduction of blood pressure to lower treatment goals. A blood pressure of 140/90 mm Hg or less should now be considered an initial goal of therapy, with further blood pressure reductions encouraged if well tolerated by the patient. In particular, patients with hypertension and congestive heart failure, postmyocardial infarction, or diabetic nephropathy may benefit from reductions in blood pressure to below 130/85 mm Hg. Similarly, aggressive treatment of elevated SBP, particularly in older patients, to levels below 140 mm Hg, if well tolerated, seems advisable. Current, ongoing clinical trials continue to address not only the benefit, but also the safety of lower treatment goals for systolic and diastolic blood pressures.

Ileus

Patricia S. Choban, MD
Louis Flancbaum, MD

Ileus literally refers to any obstruction of the intestine. Clinically, the diagnosis of ileus has come to imply a "functional" obstruction of the gastrointestinal (GI) tract characterized by diminished bowel function or peristaltic activity and lack of progression of GI contents in the absence of a mechanical cause. A variety of terms have been applied to this condition, including adynamic ileus, paralytic ileus, and spastic ileus, but these designate similar entities that do not differ in etiology or treatment. While primary motility disorders and mechanical obstruction may be included in the definition of ileus, in practice significant efforts are directed toward excluding these entities before deciding on the diagnosis of ileus. The management of mechanical bowel obstructions are not addressed in this review.

Diagnosis

The diagnosis of ileus is suspected in the patient with a quiet, distended, nontender abdomen who is obstipated. The patient may complain of nausea or have vomiting. Abdominal tenderness suggests that the distention is not likely due to a simple ileus, but rather a mechanical obstruction or an intra- or retroperitoneal inflammatory process. The diagnosis of ileus is supported by radiographs demonstrating the presence of air in both the large and small intestine with variable degrees of distention in the absence of features consistent with mechanical obstruction, such as significant disproportions in the caliber of the loops of intestine, air fluid (J-loops) levels, and a lack of air in the distal GI tract. If the diagnosis is not clear on initial radiographs, serial films obtained after 6 or 8 hours are often helpful, and occasionally an upper GI study may be indicated. Once it is clear a mechanical bowel obstruction is not present, the need and urgency for intervention will vary, depending on the etiology and severity of the ileus.

Etiology

Numerous conditions are associated with the development of ileus; however, the exact mechanism by which these diverse events produce GI dysfunction is unclear. If there is an inciting condition leading to the development of ileus, it should be sought aggressively and corrected if the ileus is to resolve. These conditions may be generally categorized as anatomic, metabolic, neurogenic, vascular, and pharmacologic (Table 1).

Ileus usually occurs in the postoperative period. It is generally believed that all abdominal procedures are followed by some degree of impaired GI motility. This appears to be due to a combination of overstimulation of the sympathetic system and depression of the parasympathetic system. Return of gut function is variable

TABLE 1. Common Conditions Precipitating Ileus

Anatomic
    Postoperative or post-traumatic
    Peritonitis
    Intra-abdominal abscess
    Retroperitoneal inflammation or bleeding
    Genitourinary tract inflammation
    Thoracic inflammation
Metabolic
    Electrolyte abnormalities
        Hypokalemia
        Hypocalcemia
        Hypomagnesemia
    Uremia
    Endocrine disorders
        Hypothyroidism
        Hypoparathyroidism
        Pheochromocytoma
        Diabetic ketoacidosis
    Malnutrition
        Thiamine deficiency
        Protein calorie deficit
Neurogenic
    Parkinson's disease
    Spinal cord trauma
    Hirschsprung's disease
    Ogilvie's syndrome
Vascular
    Collagen vascular disease
    Low flow states
    Chronic ischemia
Pharmacologic
    Toxic compounds
        Heavy metal poisoning
    Drug side effects
        Narcotics
        Antidepressants
        Phenothiazines
        Antihypertensives
        Anti-parkinsonism drugs
        Antineoplastic drugs

in different segments of the GI tract. In uncomplicated postoperative ileus, small bowel motility returns within 24 hours and stomach motility by 48 hours. Colonic motility may not return for 3 to 5 days. Abdominal procedures that do not involve resection, with or without anastomosis of the GI tract, may produce only a mild ileus. This may be of no clinical consequence, and, following uncomplicated abdominal operations such as laparoscopy, appendectomy, cholecystectomy, or cesarean section, patients may often resume oral intake within 12 to 24 hours of the procedure without adverse consequences. With more major procedures, such as those involving intestinal resection or major retroperitoneal dissection, patients are often treated with nasogastric decompression and hydration for several days until signs of bowel function return. It is interesting to note, however, that if enteral access is available distal to the pylorus, most patients can absorb elemental diets even in the absence of normal motility, allowing early postoperative enteral nutrition support.

If an ileus persists past the fourth postoperative day and the etiology is unknown, an evaluation should be undertaken to identify a precipitating cause (see Table 1). In the postoperative period, this endeavor is usually first directed at excluding electrolyte abnormalities, limiting drugs that may exacerbate dysmotility, and identifying inflammatory or infectious causes. Electrolyte abnormalities are frequently the simplest abnormalities to remedy. Hypokalemia is corrected by intravenous administration of potassium chloride or potassium phosphate at a rate not exceeding 40 mEq/hr of potassium. Hypocalcemia can be corrected with calcium gluconate 1 g IV in 1L of IV fluid infused over 24 hours. Hypocalcemia may be present in the face of a low serum albumin and may not reflect a true decrease in available calcium (pseudohypocalcemia). Hyperphosphatemia should be corrected before administration of parenteral calcium. Hypomagnesemia is corrected using magnesium sulfate, 1 to 3 g in 250 mL of IV fluid over 1 to 3 hours.

Numerous drugs are known to inhibit bowel motility. The most common class of medications contributing to delayed return of bowel function in the postoperative period is narcotics. Limitation or elimination of these medications in the past has been difficult; however, the recent introduction of a parenteral nonsteroidal anti-inflammatory agent, ketorolac tromethamine (Toradol), has provided a reasonable alternative. Elimination of other medications must be directed at the underlying disease being treated, but a review of all current medications with deletion of those not absolutely necessary is often worthwhile.

Inflammatory conditions at extraperitoneal sites, such as pneumonia or urinary tract infections, should be sought and treated if present. Intra-abdominal and retroperitoneal inflammatory processes or abscesses can often be identified by computed tomography and drained percutaneously with catheters placed using computed tomographic or ultrasonographic guidance. If biliary tract disease is suspected, ultrasonography is useful in identification of cholelithiasis or dilation of biliary radicals, and radionuclide cholescintigraphy with morphine is quite sensitive and specific in identifying acute calculous or acalculous cholecystitis, even in the critically ill patient.

Management

While treatment is being directed at the underlying medical conditions identified, or if no cause is identified, supportive measures should be initiated. The GI tract is decompressed via nasogastric suction to reduce or prevent further distention by removing swallowed air, to reduce vomiting and the risk of aspiration, and to improve patient comfort. Nasoenteric or "long" tubes, such as Miller-Abbott tubes, have been advocated in the past for the treatment of severe ileus. These tubes do not appear to hasten resolution of ileus or decrease the need for operative intervention. We have found them useful in a few specific instances, which are discussed subsequently. While the gut is being decompressed, appropriate intravenous fluids, including maintenance requirements and replacement of ongoing losses, should be administered. If the patient has been without oral intake (NPO) for over 7 days or has evidence of malnutrition, nutritional assessment should be performed and the patient considered for parenteral or enteral nutrition support.

There has been interest in utilization of pharmacologic agents to increase motility or parasympathetic tone or decrease sympathetic tone or both. Prokinetic agents such as metaclopromide, cerulein, and cisapride; somatostatin; cholinergic drugs such as neostigmine or bethanechol; adrenergic-blocking drugs such as guanethidine or reserpine; and antiarrhythmics such as lidocaine have all been utilized. Results of trials have been somewhat conflicting, with some demonstrating a reduction in duration of ileus, as evidenced by passing flatus or stool, while others showed no difference between agent and placebo. Use of many of these agents is limited by systemic side effects. While intriguing, no data currently exist to suggest that these agents should be incorporated into the management of the patient with ileus.

Endoscopic decompression is the initial treatment of choice for colonic pseudo-obstruction (Ogilvie's syndrome), which may be seen with or without evidence of a diffuse ileus. This disorder requires prompt treatment if the diameter of the cecum exceeds 12 cm on abdominal radiographs. At a diameter of 12 cm or greater, there is a significant risk of ischemic necrosis and perforation of the cecum. There is no evidence that upper GI endoscopic decompression plays any role in the management of ileus at this time.

Operative intervention is generally not required in the management of ileus; in fact, unnecessary laparotomy may exacerbate the condition. Occasionally, surgery is necessary to treat an intra-abdominal catastrophe that may be causing the ileus, such as ischemic bowel or peritonitis, to drain an intra-abdominal abscess, or to exclude complete small bowel obstruction. Operative findings consistent with an ileus include dilated intestine without a transition point to decompressed bowel. If no additional pathology is identified, such as an abscess, perforation, or mechanical obstruction, there is no indication to perform other procedures. If there have been no enterotomies, one should resist the temptation to decompress the intestine via an intentional enterotomy. This does not improve the overall course of the disease and significantly increases the risk of wound infection and development of enterocutaneous fistula. The exception to this is placement of a tube cecostomy to decompress the cecum when it is dilated to greater than 12 cm, as is seen in Ogilvie's syndrome. If the intestine is dilated enough to prohibit abdominal closure, it may be possible to pass a long tube (Baker single-balloon or Baker-Nelson double-balloon) transnasally or transorally, which can then be threaded through the stomach, duodenum, and small bowel to the ileocecal valve to decompress the bowel internally and facilitate abdominal closure.

In summary, ileus is a condition that is common in the surgical patient. Its clinical course can vary from inconsequential to catastrophic. Though our ability to provide physiologic and nutritional support to these patients is increasingly sophisticated, our understanding of the basic pathophysiology is rudimentary at best. Treatment is directed at the associated precipitating conditions since, in general, these must be corrected before resolution of the ileus will occur.

Iron Deficiency

David Z. Kitay, MD

Gynecology

Chronic blood loss in gynecologic patients usually refers to abnormal (uterine) bleeding, including disorders of menstruation, in an amount sufficient to deplete iron stores and lower the hematocrit over a period of months in the absence of pregnancy. The cause of this anemia is iron deficiency, and in a number of cases iron therapy alone will suffice and may alleviate bleeding. Among women in the second or third decade, a reasonable endocrine evaluation is performed, followed by treatment of the specific disorder, nonspecific therapy to reduce blood loss (oral contraceptives, nonsteroidal anti-inflammatory drugs), and therapeutic doses of ferrous salts. Older patients should always have endometrial sampling, although liberal use of endometrial biopsy is advocated at any age.

The menstruating woman eating a nutritionally balanced diet remains in iron homeostasis each month, balancing iron intake against loss from the uterus and other organs (skin, bowel). Menstrual blood accounts for more than half of monthly iron loss. The body regulates iron metabolism at the level of intestinal absorption. There is no mechanism for excess iron excretion. Iron deficiency is a consequence of imbalance in this regulation.

Demonstration of iron deficiency is age-dependent. The teenage patient may not have heavy periods although her dietary iron intake may be compromised. The gynecologic patient may suffer anemia from blood loss due to presence of an intrauterine device (IUD), abnormal uterine bleeding, an anatomic cause of menorrhagia such as a submucous leiomyoma, endometrial hyperplasia or carcinoma, or carcinoma of extragenital organs leading to increased iron loss. Demonstration of iron deficiency in a postmenopausal woman is presumptive evidence of blood loss and demands investigation.

Subacute blood loss is defined as more immediate iron store depletion and anemia. The typical patient has a submucous myoma and has already lost tissue iron stores; the fall in hematocrit and hemoglobin may be dramatic and may occur within a few weeks. These patients require immediate therapeutic iron supplementation and diagnostic curettage or hysteroscopy, or both, over and above other specific tests to determine etiology. Hysterectomy will cure uterine blood loss, and nonsurgical therapy, such as use of gonadotropin-releasing hormone agonist to reduce bleeding, has been used. At present, both methods are expensive. Gonadotropin-releasing hormone treatment has a number of side effects and ceases to be effective when therapy is stopped. Transfusion therapy with packed red cells may be employed and is useful prior to definitive surgical therapy.

Acute blood loss in an amount sufficient to compromise oxygenation requires transfusion therapy, possible curettage, and occasional hysterectomy. Blood should be replaced as packed cells only in sufficient quantity to stabilize vital signs—no definitive hematocrit level is necessarily sought. The 1-unit transfusion is perfectly justified. Recently, erythropoietin administration to raise red cell mass among stable patients has also been successfully employed.

Hemorrhage is technically a problem in iron deficiency. After bleeding is controlled, the patient will need prolonged iron supplementation. Hemorrhage with ectopic tubal or abdominal pregnancy is also an indication for iron to replace lost stores. A woman donating a unit of blood loses as much iron as the total body stores of a term infant (approximately 250 mg). Except for reversible, occasionally annoying side effects, no harm would result from a month of iron therapy following donation. A similar course of iron administration on a yearly basis might benefit those patients wearing a copper-bearing or inert IUD.

Use of oral contraceptives may protect against iron deficiency anemia, an effect related to the 30% to 60% decrease in uterine bleeding. Both heavy menstrual bleeding and iron deficiency anemia occur with half the frequency in oral contraceptive users compared to nonusers. A similar beneficial effect occurs with Norplant. Conversely, all copper-bearing and inert intrauterine devices cause increased uterine bleeding and predispose to iron deficiency. The only hormone-containing (progestin) IUD presently on the United States market reduces menstrual blood loss by about 40%. Heavy bleeding creates the potential for reduced iron stores and iron deficiency anemia in pregnancy.

Obstetrics

Evaluation and therapy of the anemic pregnant woman must take into account preconceptional hematologic status, length of gestation when anemia is discovered, and the course of pregnancy. Pregnancy of 12 weeks may be associated with a normal initial hematocrit, which then may fall below 30% at 28 to 34 weeks. The patient with these findings may have entered pregnancy with compromised or absent iron stores. Anemia results when further iron depletion occurs with advancing gestation, since erythrocytes are the last refuge of iron storage. The fall in hemoglobin/hematocrit is the concluding event in developing iron deficiency anemia.

Iron and folic acid are essential nutrients in pregnancy, and their absence is a potential or actual cause of anemia in common obstetric practice. Prescription prenatal multivitamins should be routinely supplied. These contain 30 to 60 mg of elemental iron and more than 400 μg of folic acid. The prenatal multivitamin may be all that is necessary to maintain a normal hematocrit and assist in replacement of nutrient stores lost to the fetus.

In the otherwise healthy obstetric patient with a hematocrit of 30% and a hemoglobin of 10 g/dL, further testing for etiology may be performed unless physiologic hydremia is suspected. However, in the absence of an obvious historical or laboratory etiology, the most important step is to institute oral iron therapy and encourage ingestion of a wide variety of nutrients from various food groups. There are no substitutes for provision of oral (or parenteral) iron because no single food contains a practically sufficient amount to be therapeutically effective. For example, any normal female must absorb a minimum of 2 to 3 mg of iron daily to balance the amount normally excreted. This is the amount found in 3 ounces of steak. Assuming 10% of dietary iron is absorbed, daily ingestion of five 6-ounce steaks would be required for therapy, and approximately 10 pounds of steak for maximum remission.

Oral iron salts are the therapy of choice and should contain 60 mg of elemental iron (eg, ferrous sulfate, 320 mg tablets) administered midmorning, midafternoon, and at bedtime with water or citrus juice and without food. The iron-containing prophylactic prenatal vitamin may be substituted for the evening dose. Most prenatal vitamins have been reformulated to lower the content of magnesium and calcium because both interfere with iron absorption.

It is common practice to administer iron with meals in an attempt to minimize side effects, even though a host of foods have been shown to inhibit iron absorption. In the 15% of women who complain of nausea, diarrhea, and constipation, therapeutic iron may be given with meals, or the type, color, and shape of the iron supplement may be changed, or both strategies may be employed. Liquid iron containing 44 mg per teaspoon is available for the same dosage regimen. Only ferrous salts should be used and cost to the patient should be small. There is no evidence that any ferrous compound (sulfate, gluconate, or fumarate) is superior in therapy or in lessening side effects.

The only important complication of oral iron is acute iron poisoning, which usually occurs in children and is almost always accidental. Deliberate suicide attempts by iron overdose have been reported. Analysis of these cases places them in the broad category of attempted suicide by other means; these patients should receive appropriate consultation.

The few indications for use of parenteral iron therapy in the pregnant or gynecologic patient are (1) iron malabsorption, (2) noncompliance, (3) intolerance of oral iron, and (4) iron need greater than can be provided orally. Parenteral iron is then justified (most commonly for noncompliance) when one or more of these indications exists and there is historical or laboratory evidence of iron deficiency based on any of the following parameters:

1. Low serum iron level
2. Mean corpuscular volume of 79 or less (whether or not beta-thalassemia minor is suspected) and in the absence of a hemolytic hemoglobinopathy
3. Elevated red cell distribution width in the absence of a hemolytic hemoglobinopathy
4. Deficient serum ferritin level (below 10 µg/L, slightly higher or lower depending on laboratory norms)
5. Microcytosis, hypochromia, aniso- and poikilocytosis on peripheral smear
6. Presence of pica

Parenteral iron dextran is supplied as 50 mg/mL in 2 mL vials, although recently its manufacture seems to have rotated among various suppliers. At this writing it is American-manufactured and supplied by a single company as iron-dextran USP (InFeD) for intramuscular or intravenous administration. A dose of 0.5 mL is given intramuscularly to test for anaphylaxis, which usually develops immediately in fewer than 1% of patients. Injections are given in the buttock by the "Z-track" technique to prevent leakage. If no reaction occurs after 1 hour, the remainder of the dose may be administered. Tables and formulas are supplied to calculate the amount required for maximal response; however, a good rule of thumb is that a woman weighing more than 100 lb will need a minimum dose of 20 mL (1000 mg). One of the problems in therapy has been a manufacturer's recommendation that no more than 2 mL be given at one time and that the drug not be used in pregnancy.° Intravenous administration of 2 mL or less per day is also satisfactory, and some have given total dose infusion without problems.

In an iron-supplemented patient, when prophylaxis is begun at or before 20 weeks, the serum ferritin level should not fall below 10 µg/L. It has recently been demonstrated that an adequately supplemented patient will have a puerperal ferritin level many times this amount, indicating reasonable iron stores.

The expected response to either oral or parenteral iron in treatment of iron deficiency is essentially identical in timing and magnitude. Reticulocytosis begins after 5 to 7 days, reaches a maximum after 7 to 12 days, and then decreases. In pregnancy, especially if therapy is begun in midtrimester, normal hydremia may mask the expected rise in hematocrit. If the hematocrit remains stable or rises as pregnancy proceeds, therapy has been specific, adequate, and confirms the diagnosis. If the patient obtained oral iron by prescription or "over the counter" rather than in the clinic or office, the physician should inspect the medication to ensure that a biologically (or therapeutically) ineffective product has not been dispensed.

°The recommendation that only 2 mL be given in a single dose originally came from the experience in a single clinic in Florida with one lot number of the drug. A few pregnant women developed fever, hematuria, and arthralgias in temporal relation to intramuscular administration. The recommendation about use in pregnancy was based on animal studies and a single human stillbirth some weeks after a reaction to iron dextran.

Mastalgia and Fibrocystic Changes of the Breast

William H. Hindle, MD

Mastalgia

The innervation of the breast is from the anterior and lateral branches of the intercostal nerves originating from the T2 to T6 spinal nerve roots. Most of the pain perception in the breast is from the nerve endings in the skin from spinal nerves T3 and T4. The free nerve ending of the telodendrons follows the anatomic dermatome pattern.

All women presenting with mastalgia, most of them motivated by an underlying fear of breast cancer (chemotherapy and death), deserve a complete evaluation, which should include a breast-oriented history, complete bilateral breast examination, mammography (if over age 30), and fine-needle aspiration of any palpable dominant breast mass. If no significant abnormality is discovered, the patient can be reassured that there is no evidence of breast cancer and that her symptoms are common to many women, probably physiologic (end-organ sensitivity), analogous to physiologic dysmenorrhea, and do not increase her relative risk of breast cancer.

Most menstruating women have some diffuse breast nodularity and cyclic premenstrual breast tenderness. Forty percent of women have clinically significant cyclic mastalgia and seek medical evaluation.

About one third of women presenting with breast symptoms complain of breast pain; however, such pain is rarely a primary symptom of breast cancer. Fewer than 15% of women with breast cancer present with pain as a chief complaint. Breast cancer pain in usually localized, noncyclic, and associated with a palpable mass. Because of the pervasive fear of breast cancer, however, most anterior chest wall pain will be perceived by the patient as "breast pain."

Achalasia, angina, cervical rib, cervical radiculitis, cervical spondylosis, cholecystitis, cholelithiasis, coronary artery disease, costochrondritis, hiatal hernia, myalgia, neuritis, osteitis, pleurisy, psychological pain, rib fracture, trauma, and tuberculosis can all cause anterior chest wall pain. Mastalgia (mastodynia) is confined to the breast tissue and may be cyclic or noncyclic and diffuse or localized. The symptoms of diffuse mastalgia can often be reproduced at examination by compressing the breast tissue between the palms of the hands held parallel above and below the breast.

A few patients with severe persistent mastalgia will require pharmacologic therapy. However, more than 75% of women presenting with mastalgia, after complete breast evaluation, will be satisfied with and appropriately treated by reassurance. If further therapy is required, it should be tried in a step-wise fashion starting with the following:

1. Mechanical measures: changing to a brassiere with good support, no wires, and no pressure points; wearing a firm supporting brassiere around the clock if experiencing nocturnal mastalgia; heating pad or hot towels; massage.
2. Psychological measures: ventilation of any acute stress caused, for instance, by a change in domestic relations or exposure to breast cancer patients or information; evaluation of body image concerns; history of sexual abuse.
3. Dietary measures: weight reduction if obese, premenstrual salt restriction.
4. Over-the-counter medications: intermittent nonsteroidal analgesics.
5. Pharmacologic measures: 1/35 monophasic (or other low dose) oral contraceptive therapy; danazol for severe (incapacitating) mastalgia.

The therapeutic goal is symptomatic relief.

If danazol therapy is indicated, 100 mg should be given orally twice a day until the mastalgia is controlled. In menstruating women, danazol treatment should be begun during menstruation to avoid the possibility of pregnancy, a contraindication to danazol. If the mastalgia is not controlled on 200 mg a day, the dose can be increased incrementally up to 400 mg a day. In 80% of the women significant control of cyclic symptoms usually occurs within a month of therapy, but it may take up to 3 months to reach the maximum therapeutic effect. Noncyclic mastalgia responds to danazol therapy in about 50% of women. After the breast symptoms have been controlled for at least a month, the dose of danazol can often be reduced incrementally to as low as 50 mg a day with continued symptomatic relief. The patient should be maintained on the lowest effective dose for at least 6 months. Unfortunately, as many as 50% of women will experience return of their mastalgia within 6 months after cessation of therapy. In these cases, danazol therapy can be repeated.

Effective nonhormonal contraception should be practiced during danazol therapy. Especially at the higher dosage levels, as many as two thirds of women on danazol will have irregular menstrual patterns and variable menstrual flow. Some will experience amenorrhea. Masculinizing side effects are common on high-dose danazol therapy and may cause some women to discontinue treatment. Vigorous exercise can increase the tolerance and decrease the severity of these bothersome side effects.

Outside the United States, androgens, bromocriptine, gonadotropin-releasing hormone agonists, oil of evening primrose, progesterone, and tamoxifen have been reported to be clinically effective in the treatment of mastalgia, but they are not approved by the Food and Drug Administration for this use.

Caffeine (methylxanthine) restriction and supplementation of thyroid hormone, vitamin A, vitamin B1, vitamin C, and vitamin E have not been proved to be of statistically significant clinical benefit in prospective double-blind crossover studies.

Fibrocystic Changes

"Fibrocystic disease" is not an acceptable histologic, mammographic, or physical diagnosis. Histologic evaluation in autopsy studies has shown that as many as 75% of women have changes that used to be lumped together in this wastebasket term. In 1985, the College of American Pathologists recommended instead the use of "fibrocystic change" or, more appropriately, that the specific histologic changes be described.

In previous historical usage, both patients and insurance companies (health and life) presumed that "fibrocystic disease" was a premalignant condition, and women so designated were considered to be at higher risk of developing breast cancer. This is not true. Only atypical epithelial hyperplasia of the terminal ducts or lobules is associated with clinically significant increased relative risk of breast cancer. However, atypical epithelial hyperplasia has no characteristic mammographic signs and does not produce physical changes by examination. Thus, the diagnosis of atypical epithelial hyperplasia is usually a coincidental histologic finding in breast biopsy tissue.

The findings of fibrocystic changes of the breast by physical examination should be precisely described as, for example, tenderness, thickening, or nodularity. It is important to note the exact location of any physical findings and whether changes are localized or diffuse. Do not dignify these nonspecific physical findings with a clinical diagnosis. Such a spurious false diagnosis

is a disservice to the patient, causes undue anxiety, and confuses the clinician. A drawing or diagram of the breast in the medical record is useful in accurately recording the location of the findings. If a persistent mass is described, it must be definitely diagnosed by fine-needle aspiration cytology or open surgical biopsy.

Multiple Sclerosis

Stanley van den Noort, MD

Multiple sclerosis is an inflammatory and scarring disease of cerebral and spinal white matter that affects 1 in every 1000 adults; it favors women, usually in the third and fourth decades. The disease is notoriously difficult to recognize, and symptoms are often ascribed to psychiatric stress for many years before diagnosis. The disease begins with attacks lasting weeks or months and then gradually merges into a slowly progressive form over a half-dozen years; severity is highly variable and highly unpredictable; early symptoms are commonly impaired vision in one eye, diplopia, vertigo, facial numbness or pain, facial weakness, loss of hearing in one ear, slurred speech, choking, numbness of limbs (often painful), awkward use of hands and feet, problems with bladder control, emotional changes, cognitive difficulties, and electric shock sensations on neck flexion. A careful neurologic examination is necessary. Magnetic resonance imaging of the brain, evoked responses, and spinal fluid increases in lymphocytes, gamma globulin, and oligoclonal bands are confirmatory tests but may not be positive in earlier, mild cases. Diagnosis rests primarily on the definition of two or more lesions of the central nervous system separated in time and in anatomic space.

The treatment of multiple sclerosis is supportive and important. Patients should know the diagnosis to avoid unnecessary surgery for unusual pains or numbness; they should understand that a near majority of cases are benign or disabling in a minor way. A healthful lifestyle may be quite helpful. Exercise programs that avoid overheating, such as swimming or a Schwinn Air-Dyne stationary bicycle, are often helpful. For individual handicaps, a physical therapist and an occupational therapist are often useful. Individual symptoms require symptomatic management: fatigue, amantadine hydrochloride 100 mg qd or bid, pemoline 18.75 to 37 mg q6h prn; pain, amitriptyline 10 to 100 mg hs qd, carbamazepine 125 to 500 mg qid; vertigo, meclizine 12.5 to 25 mg tid; tremor, long-acting propranolol 60 to 120 mg bid; urgency, tolteroldine (Detrol) 2 mg q12h; retention, stop anticholinergic drugs, bethanechol may be helpful for brief intervals, terazosin (Hytrin) 1–5 mg hs qd, intermittent catheterization; constipation, combined regimens of Metamucil, Pericolase, and Dulcolax; spasticity, baclofen 10 to 30 mg qid (when baclofen, is discontinued, do it very slowly to avoid delirium).

Treatments to modify the pathology of multiple sclerosis should be undertaken with caution and with recognition that none has known long-term effectiveness. Some are high-risk drugs, and evaluating responses is usually very difficult. For severe attacks that cause a major impairment of some function such as vision or gait or cause weakness of an arm or leg or new bladder symptoms, it is usual to give 1000 to 1500 mg methylprednisolone IV over several hours IVPB qd for 4 to 5 days with or without an oral taper; or 200 mg prednisone po qid for 5 days, with or without a tapering dose. An H2 blocker (ranitidine) and a benzodiazepine for side effects are useful. Increased risk of infection, subsequent cataract, acne, brief psychosis, and transient hyperglycemia may be seen.

In patients who demonstrate frequent attacks or consistent progression that will soon lead to major levels of disability, it is now common to use immune modulation. Two forms of β-interferon, Betaseron and Avonex, are used successfully to reduce attack rate, attack severity, and MRI progression in remitting relapsing MS. Based on European studies, it is clear that these drugs also reduce progression in the secondary progressive form of MS. Glatiramer acetate (Copaxone) is a mixture of peptides with effects on disease activity similar to those of the β-interferons; this is also approved for use in relapsing-remitting MS. Interferon and glatiramer are injections that carry a cost approaching $1000 per month. All of these drugs should usually be used with contraception in women of childbearing age.

Methotrexate, 5–10 mg bid one day a week or up to 20 mg q 7d by injection, is used in an effort to slow disease progression. Another modest form of immune suppression, with fair safety, is azathioprine, 150 to 250 mg/day (adjust to keep lymphocyte count down to about 1000); I usually give 60 to 80 mg of prednisone once every third day with this regimen. In more grave circumstances, periodic treatment with intravenous cyclophosphamide or total lymphoid irradiation (sparing the spleen) may help. Both treatments may benefit from concomitant use of some prednisone once every few days. These treatments may prevent decline. They usually do not improve patients. They should be avoided in advanced cases or in relatively stable patients at this time.

Severely disabled patients require the support of a physician, physical therapist, occupational therapist, and often a social worker. Symptomatic management is often helpful.

Pregnancy has relatively little influence on the course of multiple sclerosis; in some instances there may be concern with the physical and cognitive capacity of the mother to provide optimal care for the child. During pregnancy it is common for multiple sclerosis to seem improved under the influence of autologous immune suppression. Obviously, it is desirable to eliminate or curtail most medication, although intermittent prednisone may be tolerated. No special issues surround delivery. A substantial problem with multiple sclerosis and similar dysimmune states is a relatively high risk of relapse in the first 3 postpartum months. While this risk may be immunologically mediated, it is also a time of high stress and fatigue that may be moderated by extra help in this interval.

Myasthenia Gravis

Stanley van den Noort, MD

Myasthenia gravis is an autoimmune disease that affects the neuromuscular junction, producing progressive weakness and muscle fatigue; it occurs more commonly in younger women and older men, with lesser frequency in mid-adult years. Severity varies widely but in the early phase of the illness mild may become severe rapidly and with little warning. Lability is less evident after some years of illness. It may coexist with other autoimmune diseases such as rheumatoid arthritis or thyroiditis. The muscles innervated by the cranial nerves are usually more affected than other muscles; some cases are largely limited to eye and facial movement. Failure of adequate ventilation must be a constant concern in generalized myasthenia. Diagnosis rests on history, examination, edrophonium test, electrodiagnostic tests, and measurement of acetylcholine receptor antibodies in serum; the last two of these may not be positive. The edrophonium test uses the intravenous injection of 2 mg and then 8 mg of edrophonium, with observation of dramatic changes in strength or function. Saline may be used to test for suggestibility, and atropine should be available to counteract unusual muscarinic responses. In an electrodiagnostic laboratory, repetitive stimuli at rates below 20 per second produce diminishing muscle contractions that may be reversed by edrophonium.

In 1934, Doctor Mary Walker found the first effective treatment for myasthenia gravis in neostigmine methylsulfate (Prostigmin). Today, mild and severe cases are helped by the use of a similar agent, pyridostigmine, which to some degree mimics the action of acetylcholine but primarily inhibits acetylcholinesterase. A dosage of 60 mg qid is common and usually quite safe; higher dosages up to 120 mg q2–3 hours may be required, but, at some level, this leads to conduction block or desensitization with increased weakness and risk of respiratory failure. A liquid pyridostigmine is available. For parenteral therapy it is best to use neostigmine methylsulfate 0.5 to 1.0 mg (or more) IM q2 hours. Anticholinesterases may provoke diarrhea and lead to secondary hypokalemic weakness. Anticholinergics like propantheline bromide (Pro-Banthīne) may quiet abdominal side effects without interfering with the value of pyridostigmine in voluntary muscle; these are best reserved for occasional use.

Severe grades of weakness in myasthenia are common and require more strident therapeutics. Usually this begins with prednisone in dosages of 40 to 140 mg/day with rapid conversion to a single every-other-day dosage to reduce the complications of prednisone therapy. Such treatment may of necessity begin in a hospital, since weakness may initially increase on steroids, although vigorous potassium supplements, even in the absence of hypokalemia, often prevent this. In the midst of steroid treatment, an early thymectomy should be strongly considered as offering the best chance for long-term remission. After prednisone and thymectomy (recognizing that remission after thymectomy sometimes takes a year), more vigorous forms of immunosuppressive therapy with azathioprine and other immunosuppressants may be required. Plasmapheresis several times a week is often helpful in preparing for thymectomy or getting through a crisis but has excessive costs for prolonged use. Use of cyclosporine in myasthenia is being studied experimentally. Azathioprine (2 to 3 mg/kg) in divided oral doses may serve to reduce requirements of every-other-day prednisone. A monthly pulse of 1 g or more of cyclophosphamide IV (with brisk diuresis for 6 hours after infusion) may have a similar effect. Intravenous gamma globulin, 30–36 g, over 8 hours at intervals of once a week to once a month is also helpful.

It is common for some myasthenic patients to require mechanical support of ventilation and nasogastric tube feeding at critical times. These management techniques are largely the same as in other modes of ventilation failure.

In myasthenic crises, it is generally best to provide ventilation support and to stop or greatly reduce anticholinesterase drugs. A suspension of several days may help restore sensitivity. Injections of 5 mg of edrophonium may help distinguish between over- and underdosage of anticholinesterase medication. In severe overdosage, one can inject 500 mg of pralidoxime at intervals of 10 minutes for several doses.

In nonthymectomized patients periodic computed tomography or magnetic resonance imaging of the chest to watch for thymoma is desirable. Surgical procedures in myasthenia should avoid neuromuscular blocking agents.

The influence of pregnancy on myasthenia is, like many other aspects, unpredictable. Remission with pregnancy is not uncommon, and' improvement is more likely than worsening. Careful observation of need for ventilation support is important at delivery. The newborn child may have transient myasthenia that clears after some weeks. The first several postpartum months carry some risk of exacerbation for the mother.

Nutritional Support

James W. Orr, Jr, MD, FACOG, FACS
Pamela Jo Orr, RN, OCN

The clinical outcome for any disease or treatment is adversely affected by the presence of concurrent nutritional deficits. Malnutrition is associated with an increased incidence of sepsis, prolonged hospitalization, and prolonged ventilator dependency, as well as increased risk of perioperative complications and hospital mortality. The practicing obstetrician/gynecologist often caring for young, apparently healthy women undergoing elective surgical procedures may believe that they are insulated against the potential problems associated with nutritional deficiencies. However, as many as 20% of young women are reported to have serious eating disorders. Additionally, our ever-increasing role as primary care providers necessitates that clinicians develop an increased understanding of the significance of nutritional evaluation and support. Obstetrician/gynecologists should be aware of specific risk factors and the incidence of nutritional deficits. Although primary care physicians may not be ultimately responsible for the institution and monitoring of nutritional support, they should understand predisposing factors and the importance of specific screening methods as well as the potential risks and benefits of alternative routes and methods of nutritional support. With this information appropriate consultation and nutritional support can be incorporated into the daily clinical management of women's health care.

Who Is at Risk?

Although young healthy women may appear to be nutritionally replete, it has been estimated that as many as 40% of hospitalized patients have measurable nutritional deficits. Additionally, obesity, affecting 27% of women in our society, should not be considered incompatible with nutritional deficits, as physical or biochemical evidence of nutritional deficiency occurs in as many as 50% of women with corpus cancer.

Although all patients should be considered at risk, the incidence and clinical suspicion of malnutrition should increase in subsets (Table 1) of women who have an inadequate oral intake, an altered absorptive pattern, increased nutritional losses, or increased metabolic demands from any cause. Importantly, the subtle clinical combination of multiple factors may facilitate rapid development of a significant deficit. We believe nutritional supplementation should be considered in normally nourished women whose intake is inadequate for 7 to 10 days, lowering this criterion to 3 to 5 days in women with severe measurable deficits. These criteria are clinically adjusted downward for those with serious disease or serious surgically related stress.

Metabolism

Normal Metabolism

Metabolic efficiency requires postfeeding storage of excess nutrients in a readily available form and an effective signaling mechanism to mobilize nutritional stores for metabolic support during times of fasting. Following a conventional meal, metabolic effects are predominantly regulated by the tissue-specific effects of insulin, secreted in response to hyperglycemia. In muscle, this results in increased glycogen synthesis (to provide

TABLE 1. Risk Factors for Nutritional Deficit

Inadequate oral intake
- ° Lack of access to nutritional substrate
  - ▸ Elderly
  - ▸ Poverty
  - ▸ Visual problems
  - ▸ Poor dentation

- ° Hospitalization
  - ▸ Prolonged evaluation (NPO)
  - ▸ Postoperative ileus
  - ▸ Infection

- ° Anorexia
  - ▸ Cancer
  - ▸ Drug-related
  - ▸ Psychiatric

Altered absorptive pattern

Increased losses
  - ▸ Nausea, vomiting (pregnancy, cancer, chemotherapy)
  - ▸ Diarrhea (radiation, infectious)
  - ▸ Short bowel
  - ▸ Fistulas

Increased demands
  - ▸ Cancer
  - ▸ Infection
  - ▸ Postoperative recovery
  - ▸ Pregnancy

acute fuel) and protein synthesis (for later use). In adipose tissue, insulin facilitates glucose transport, stimulates phosphorylation of glucose, and inhibits lipolysis. Associated liver effects include glycogen synthesis and inhibition of glycogenolysis and gluconeogenesis.

These effects result in the storage of 1200 carbohydrate calories (stored as glycogen in muscle and liver), approximately 140,000 fat calories, and 55,000 protein calories. Only 40% of stored protein calories are available as metabolic fuel and a 50% depletion of protein caloric stores is incompatible with life.

The metabolic process during the postabsorptive period (beginning 8 to 12 hours after last intake) is predominantly governed by the effects of glucagon, which stimulates hepatic production of glucose substrate, assists in the release of amino acids and lactate from muscle, and increases lipolysis and fat mobilization with an emphasis on fat oxidation.

Metabolic Response to Injury or Stress

Resting energy expenditure (REE) is a balance between increased metabolic needs related to catabolic influences and decreases associated with tissue depletion. Hospitalized patients may experience a 10% to 20% decrease in REE with severe malnutrition and as much as a 40% decrease with advanced cachexia. REE is rarely increased by more than 40% even in the presence of major stress. The associated hypermetabolism, muscle proteolysis, and release of amino acids (for high priority tissue use) is associated with increased urinary nitrogen excretion. During the first 3 days of non-stressed nutritional depletion, muscle and liver glycogen stores are rapidly exhausted. Internal conversion increases fat mobilization to provide metabolic fuel and minimize protein breakdown and lessen protein losses. However, protein muscle breakdown (20/24 hours) continues at a lower rate to provide for the obligate glucose requirement of the central nervous system and red blood cells. Unfortunately, specific diseases may adversely affect this protective conversion mechanism, resulting in increased protein catabolism.

Nutritional Assessment

Physician awareness undoubtedly constitutes the most important aspect of nutritional assessment. Recognizing nutritional status as a dynamic proc-ess, the alert clinician can proceed with a specific assessment (Table 2), understanding that the accuracy, sensitivity, and specificity of these techniques may differ during the evaluation of an acute or chronic nutritional deficit.

History and Physical Examination

A thorough, thoughtful history and physical examination obtained by an experienced physician remains one of the best, simplest, and most cost effective methods of nutritional assessment. Any patient who is undergoing or scheduled to be subjected to significant stress (surgical, infectious) should be evaluated for recent weight change. A recent 10% weight loss represents a critical signal for the presence of nutritional deficits and an increased risk of perioperative complications. Although the assessment may require examination and determination of actual "losses," the presence of historical clues such as recent previous therapy (radiation, chemotherapy, surgery) should also alert the physician as to the increased risk of specific nutritional deficits. In specific situations, it may be necessary to question family members or others to determine or document recent weight loss. Review of previous medical records may be more accurate than

TABLE 2. Nutritional Assessment Techniques

	Acute Serious Illness				Chronic Illness			
	Test		Predictive Value		Test		Predictive Value	
Method	Accuracy	Precision	Sensitive	Specific	Accuracy	Precision	Sensitive	Predictive
Subjective global assessment	?	?	?	?	G	G	F	F
Anthropometrics	F	P	P	P	F	F	F	G
Albumin	E	E	G	P	E	E	F	F
Transferrin	E	E	G	P	E	E	G	F
Prealbumin	G	G	G	P	G	G	G	F
Delayed hypersensitivity	F	P	G	P	F	F	G	P
Bioelectric impedance	F	F	F	P	G	G	G	G
Dual energy x-ray absorptiometry	G	G	F	F	E	E	E	E
Total body water	F	F	P	P	G	G	G	G
Neutron activation	E	E	G	E	E	E	E	E
Voluntary muscle power	F	P	G	P	F	F	G	P
Stimulated muscle power	?	?	?	?	G	G	G	F

?, Questionable benefit; E, excellent; F, fair; G, good; P, poor.

patient recall. While some believe that ideal weight is an important reference, actual weight loss appears to represent a more significant factor. Evaluation of percentage of ideal body weight may be misleading, as a significant portion of the US population may have been overweight at the beginning of their illness. Importantly, weight assessment may not be valid in an acute situation (during hospitalization), as the administration of intravenous fluids may obscure recognition of lean body weight loss.

In addition to measured weight, the patient's overall appearance (muscle wasting, decreased subcutaneous tissue) should be noted. Anthropometric measurements, which quantify and compare body habitus and body compartment to measurements in an age- and sex-matched population, may be helpful. Subcutaneous tissue constitutes 50% of the body's fat stores; therefore, a triceps skin fold measurement assists in assessment of body fat stores. Skeletal muscle constitutes 60% of total body protein and represents the major source of amino acids during stress and starvation. Mid-arm muscle circumference [(measured) − (0.341 × triceps skin fold)] represents an assessment of protein stores. Unfortunately, any single anthropometric measurement may be misleading, as the individual may have entered her illness above the normal range. Serial measurements in the same woman may be representative of nutritional status, however. Unfortunately, anthropometric measurements are of less value in the acutely critically ill patient than in the assessment of those with long-term or chronic nutritional defects.

Serum Proteins

The measurement of plasma proteins, including serum albumin, transferrin, prealbumin, and retinol binding protein, has been considered the benchmark for the evaluation of nutritional status.

Plasma albumin concentration is a valuable tool for predicting clinical outcome. Serum levels less than 3 g/dL suggest a moderate to severe nutritional deficit and an increased risk of perioperative complications. Unfortunately, albumin's long half-life (20 days) may render it an insensitive marker for acute nutritional deficits. Regardless, hypoalbuminemia in a previously nonstressed individual should prompt attention to the patient's nutritional status.

Unfortunately, the daily exchange of albumin between the intravascular and extravascular spaces is 10 times greater than its synthesis rate.

The associated increase in the acute transcapillary escape of proteins during stress (surgical, infectious) renders it a less than satisfactory marker for evaluation of postoperative nutritional status.

Plasma transferrin has a shorter half-life (8 days) and a higher sensitivity to acute changes in nutritional status. Unfortunately, while rising levels during nutritional support are a good indicator of a positive nitrogen balance, the reverse may not be true. Additionally, levels of this iron transport protein may be elevated in women with iron deficiency and lower in those receiving multiple transfusions.

Levels of prealbumin, a thyroxine carrier protein with a half-life of 2 days, are frequently reduced in those with liver disease and increased in those with renal disease. Importantly, rising levels during nutritional replenishment correlate strongly with a positive nitrogen balance.

Retinol binding protein (a serum carrier of vitamin A) has a half-life of 12 hours. Low levels are associated with hyperthyroidism, liver disease, vitamin A deficiency, and zinc deficiency. Elevated levels are common in those with renal disease.

Clinical interpretation of these serum proteins suggests that with a longer duration of nutritional deficiency, serum levels of retinal binding protein, prealbumin, transferrin, and albumin are progressively affected. In part because of its availability, it has been the authors' choice to rely heavily on the pretreatment serum albumin level as a primary biochemical assessment for the possible need for nutritional support.

Total Lymphocyte Count

The absolute lymphocyte count is a readily available marker of nutritional status, and, in the absence of infection or recent chemotherapy, levels less than 1500/mm^3 suggest malnutrition and levels less than 1000/mm^3 suggest a severe nutritional deficit. This relatively available study should be reviewed in nearly all women undergoing surgical treatment.

Creatinine

The urinary excretion of creatinine, a product of muscle metabolism, can be measured and assessed against "normal" tables. Unfortunately, this study is not reliable, as the normal creatinine clearance decreases with age and is extremely affected by the adequacy of 24-hour collection and catabolic state.

Immunocompetence

The immune response to antigen skin testing is adversely affected by severe malnutrition. Unfortunately, anergy is not uncommon in women with cancer or in those who have received recent chemotherapy. While anergy represents an adverse prognostic affect, it is of little value as a marker for nutritional status.

Measurement of Body Composition

These techniques vary in sophistication, reliability, and availability. Measurement of bioelectrical impedance reflects body water volume, which is closely related to lean tissue mass. This study is safe and easy to perform with low observer error; it is inaccurate in the presence of edema, as tissue conductivity is extremely responsive to level of hydration. Although it is of potential benefit in weight-stable patients, it is of little benefit in those with critical illness.

Dual energy x-ray absorptiometry can distinguish differences between fat and lean body tissue. Unfortunately, while reproducible, it is expensive and machine (manufacturer)-dependent and large errors may be anticipated in patients with abnormal hydration. Additionally, testing requires relative immobility, rendering it of little benefit in the critically ill.

It is assumed that potassium is present only in lean body tissue, and a whole body counter measurement of total body potassium after the administration of the emitting isotope ^{40}K allows evaluation of nutritional status. Unfortunately, lean tissue potassium concentration varies significantly with age and obesity. Additionally, the time required for testing (1 hour) renders it of little value in those patients who are critically ill.

The measurement of total body water (usually by deuterium dilution) estimates fat and fat-free mass. This technique assumes that the fat compartment is anhydrous, whereas the fat-free compartment is hydrated to a known and constant extent.

The technique of in vivo neutron activation analysis involves injection of a significant amount of radiation and offers the ability to divide the body into several compartments, which can provide information regarding elemental composition of the body. Currently, these last two techniques are available in only a few centers.

Tests of Physiologic Function

Nutritional deficits, associated with amino acid mobilization from skeletal muscle, result in increased muscle fatiguability and lessened muscle strength. Measurable deficits in muscle and respiratory function increase at 20% reduction of body protein (15% weight loss), indicate a high surgical risk, and give unequivocal evidence that nutritional support is required. Evaluation of maximal voluntary grip strength (cooperation dependent) or evaluation of contraction-relaxation response after ulnar nerve stimulation may be useful in the critically ill.

Subjective Global Assessment

Subjective global assessment incorporates important facts from the patient *history* (weight change, altered dietary intake, gastrointestinal symptoms, functional capacity, and metabolic demands) and *physical examination* (subjective loss of subcutaneous fat, muscle wasting, or the presence of edema or ascites). The reproducibility validity of the subjective global assessment when performed by an experienced physician is superb in the nonacute clinical situation.

Determining Nutritional Requirements

Although there is no single accurate determination of individual caloric, protein, lipid, carbohydrate, fluid, electrolyte, vitamin, or mineral requirements, specific guidelines can be used (Table 3). The clinician must be cognizant that any starting point can and should be altered appropriately, relating to changes in the clinical situation or specific excess or deficits.

Maintenance fluid requirements can be calculated on a kilogram, incremental kilogram, or body surface area basis. An incremental kilogram replacement administers 100 mL/kg for the first 10 kg, 50 mL/kg for the second 10 kg, and 20 mL/kg for each additional kilogram each day. Using this schema, a 50 kg woman would receive 2100 mL in 24 hours ([100 × 10] + [50 × 10] + [20 × 30] or 1000 + 500 + 600). These fluid volumes require adjustment for temperature (10 mL/kg/24 hours for each degree above 101°F), altered input, and measured and unmeasured output and extraneous losses (nasogastric suction, fistula, diarrhea, open wounds, ventilator). Daily weight determination may minimize excess fluid administration.

Caloric requirements are usually estimated us-

TABLE 3. Daily Nutrient Provisions During Total Parenteral Nutrition°

Calories	Dextrose	60–80% of requirement
	Lipid emulsion	20–40% of requirement
Protein	Crystalline amino acids	100% of requirement
Minerals	Sodium	90–120 mEq
	Potassium	90–150 mEq
	Chloride	90–150 mEq
	Calcium	12–16 mEq
	Phosphorus	20–40 mmol
	Magnesium	12–16 mEq
	Iron	10–18 mg
	Zinc	2–8 mg
	Copper	1–1.6 mg
	Chromium	10–16 μg
	Manganese	0.4–0.8 mg
	Selenium	120 μg
	Iodine	50–80 μg
	Molybdenum	20 μg
Vitamins	A	3300 IU
	D	200 IU
	E	10 IU
	B_1 (thiamin)	3.0 mg
	B_2 (riboflavin)	3.6 mg
	B_3 (pantothenic acid)	15.0 mg
	B_5 (niacin)	40.0 mg
	B_6 (pyridoxine)	4.0 mg
	B_7 (biotin)	60.0 μg
	B_9 (folic acid)	400.0 μg
	B_{12} (cobalamin)	5.0 μg
	C (ascorbic acid)	100.0 mg
	K	5 mg/wk
Essential fatty acid	Linoleic acid	4% of total calories

° Assuming absence of hepatic or renal disease.

ing the basal metabolic requirement (BMR) as calculated by the Harris-Benedict equation: BMR (Kcal/day) = 666 + (9.6 × kg weight) + (1.7 × cm height) − (4.7 × year age). Empirically, a healthy hospitalized patient needs approximately 35 Kcal/kg/day. These needs may be lessened with inactivity (−25%) or increased with severe malnutrition or stress (+20%). Overfeeding offers little benefit and a risk of other complications (Table 4).

A gram of glucose supplies 3.4 Kcal and a liter of D_5W supplies 170 Kcal. Higher concentrations of glucose (D_{20}, D_{50}) allow delivery of a significantly increased amount of carbohydrate calories using lesser volume.

One gram of protein represents 4.0 Kcal when metabolized. Routine replacement requires 1.0 to 1.5 g/kg/24 hours. Larger amounts of protein

cannot be assimilated by sick patients. While favorable clinical outcome is an important measure of adequate replacement, an alternative method requires the evaluation of nitrogen balance, which measures the balance between input and output. Nitrogen balance equals gram protein intake/6.25g − measured 24 hour urine nitrogen + 4 (extraurinary nitrogen losses). An estimation of the necessary requirement of non-protein calories requires multiplication of protein requirement by 150 and dividing by 6.25 (1 g nitrogen = 6.25 g protein).

Essential fatty acid depletion can be avoided by the weekly intravenous administration of 1 L of 10% lipids. However, 1 g of fat provides 9 Kcal, and the use of intravenous fat allows the delivery of a significant caloric intake with relatively small volume intravascular replacement. A 10% lipid infusion delivers 1.1 Kcal/mL and a 20% emulsion offers 2.0 Kcal/mL. Approximately 30% of non-protein calories are administered as lipids, although some practitioners recommend that this be 50%.

Instituting, Administering, and Discontinuing Nutritional Support

Enteral

Once the decision to offer supplement is made, the route and amount should be determined. The clinician must decide if the supplement is intended as a partial or complete replacement of

TABLE 4. Consequences of Overfeeding

Hypertriglyceridemia

Hyperglycemia
- Hyperosmolarity
- Osmotic diuresis
- Dehydration

Respiratory Complications
- Increased carbon dioxide production
- Increased minute ventilation
- Prolonged ventilator support

Hepatic Dysfunction
- Fat deposition
- Cholestasis
- Steatosis
- Hepatomegaly

Azotemia

Altered Immune Function

daily needs. With a functional intestinal tract, enteral supplementation is more physiologic, safer, and less costly than parenteral nutritional support. This assumes the absence of multiple bowel resections (short bowel), obstruction, fistulas, atrophic mucosa (ie, chronically starved), or radiation enteritis. Enteral supplementation may include effective oral supplements with protein of high natural biologic value (milk, egg, meat) or supplements via an oral or tube (gastric, small bowel) feeding. Enteral therapy maintains intestinal wall thickness, mucosal enzymes, and mucosal architectural integrity.

Numerous enteral preparations are available. Polymeric diets, composed of whole proteins, oils, and sucrose, may be blenderized whole foods, lactose-containing milk-based formulas, or lactose-free formulas. They represent a first-line source of replacement.

Defined formula or elemental diets are composed of amino acids or short chained peptides with monosaccharides or oligosaccharides. Fats are supplied with medium or long chain triglycerides. These predigested diets are easily absorbed (ideal for short bowel) but are not palatable and are usually administered by tube (nasal, gastric, jejunostomy). These hyperosmolar diets are frequently associated with diarrhea. These are instituted at full strength and in the absence of gastric retention are increased to administer adequate volume and caloric supplement over the ensuing 2 to 3 days. It is our choice to use a continuous administration via tube (preferably gastric or jejunal) to give adequate daily caloric and fluid replacement. Concurrent peripheral intravenous fluids may be necessary. Discontinuation may be relatively abrupt with little risk of involving hypoglycemia.

Peripheral

Peripheral hyperalimentation utilizing less than sclerotic concentrations of glucose ($D_{10}W$) and less concentrated solutions of amino acids is probably capable of reversing mild nutritional deficits in patients with less than severe stress. In our clinical experience, these same patients can often be supplemented enterally with equal results.

Central

Total parenteral hyperalimentation uses a high concentration of nutrients delivered via a central access catheter and is associated with a significant risk of complications (Table 5). It is appropriate to have some form of monitoring instituted to detect and minimize their severity and it should not be instituted and administered by those unfamiliar with these risks.

Central access using single lumen catheters (versus multiple lumen) is associated with a lower risk of infectious complications; however, multiple lumens offer the benefit of being placed intraoperatively and reducing the need for peripheral intravenous lines or multiple venipunctures. Permanent access provides an ideal route.

The risk of line sepsis increases in proportion

TABLE 5. Complications of Parenteral Nutrition

	More Frequent	Rare
Administration-related complications	Thrombophlebitis (peripheral vein) Infection Inappropriate tip placement Pneumothorax Central vein thrombosis	Hemothorax Air embolus Arterial laceration Brachial plexus injury Central venous catheter fragmentation and embolization
Metabolic complications	Hyperglycemia and hyperosmolarity Hypoglycemia Electrolyte disturbances BUN elevation Liver dysfunction Fatty liver Hypercapnia Cholelithiasis (long-term treatment) Hyperlipidemia from lipid emulsion	Vitamin and trace mineral deficiency Essential fatty acid deficiency Metabolic bone disease Other adverse reaction to lipid emulsion Hyperammonemia

BUN, blood urea nitrogen.

to manipulation and duration of use. We have abandoned routine line changes in most situations. When sepsis is suspected, appropriate cultures are obtained and broad-spectrum antibiotics are instituted. The decision to remove or replace the line is individually based on the source of infection, clinical response, and projected need for continued support.

After determining the safety of line placement, the contents of infused alimentation fluid should be determined. In general, a standardized form should be utilized and a standard method of follow-up should be in place. Electrolyte abnormalities and fluid volume status should be monitored regularly and corrected early. Insulin supplementation is required by 50% of patients and can be added to the solution or administered subcutaneously to minimize hyperglycemia. We typically add H_2 blockers in an attempt to minimize the gastric effects of stress.

Transient abnormalities in serum liver functions occur in 90% of patients receiving total parenteral nutrition. Although not usually clinically significant, these studies should be monitored. While any cause of hepatic dysfunction or failure may manifest itself during supplementation, the need to discontinue total parenteral nutrition is rare.

Severe hyperglycemia, osmotic diuresis, and even hyperosmolar nonketotic glycosuria may occur. Serial monitoring of glucose and ketones should confirm this diagnosis. Treatment requires the administration of insulin (and subsequent K^+ infusion), hydration, and possible discontinuation of fluids.

Monitoring for hypokalemia, hypocalcemia, hypomagnesemia, and hypophosphatemia minimizes these risks. In general, these clinical problems manifest themselves as weakness and lethargy. Anemia is treated with adequate replacement of folate, vitamin B_{12}, and iron, frequently administered parenterally.

Discontinuation of parenteral alimentation can be safely undertaken by reducing total volume by 50%. If serum glucose is 100 g/dL or greater, after 2 hours the infusion rate is again reduced by 50%. The infusion is discontinued 2 hours later.

Conclusion

Unfortunately, prospective controlled clinical trials evaluating the benefit of nutritional support have failed to provide objective support for the implementation of caloric supplementation. However, the astute clinician must recognize the adverse effects of malnutrition on specific diseases and appropriately utilize this clinical tool to assist in patient recovery when deemed necessary.

Pneumonia: Viral and Bacterial

Thomas C. Cesario, MD
Douglas A. Cesario, MD

Pneumonia is one of the most common serious infections encountered in the treatment of infectious diseases. It has been estimated that 2 to 4 million cases of community-acquired pneumonia occur each year in the United States. The overall attack rate is 10 to 12 cases per 1000 individuals per year, but increases in the incidence occur at the extremes of age, with young children and elderly adults being 5 to 25 times more prone to this disease entity. Pneumonia is the sixth leading cause of death in the United States and the leading cause of death due to infectious diseases.

Community-acquired pneumonia is differentiated from nosocomial pneumonia because the etiologies and approach to therapy are considerably different. Thus, in hospitalized patients who acquire the infection during their period of confinement, the nature of the causative organisms is such that they are considerably more resistant to antibiotics. In community-acquired pneumonia, the nature of the organism may differ depending on the population under discussion. Thus patients coming from skilled nursing facilities or debilitated patients with serious underlying diseases may acquire pneumonia with organisms more closely resembling those acquired in the hospital setting. Patients with acquired immunodeficiency syndrome (AIDS) are also prone to distinct types of pneumonia often not seen in individuals in less compromised states. Therefore, in predicting the nature of the infecting organism, it becomes important to understand the underlying nature of the patients themselves. In this review, we focus on community-acquired pneumonia in otherwise healthy individuals and not those with underlying diseases like AIDS, diabetes mellitus, or malignant disease.

Many reviews of pneumonia have focused on patients admitted to hospital, often in the setting of university referral centers. This type of review already selects for a certain type of individual and skews the type of etiology being reported. Nonetheless, in the pre-penicillin era, *Streptococcus pneumoniae* accounted for 80% of the community-acquired pneumonias reported. More recently, the incidence of these pneumonias has changed. Whether this represents a true shift or whether it merely reflects increased awareness and better diagnostic testing is not clear. In the United States today, it is estimated that *Strep. pneumoniae* accounts for 5% to 18% of cases of community-acquired pneumonia. *Haemophilus influenzae* accounts for about 10% of the cases while *Staphylococcus aureus* and enteric gram-negative rods account for 3% to 10% of the cases. *Legionella* appears to be responsible for 1% to 15% of cases of community acquired pneumonia. Other less common organisms to consider include *Moraxella, Strep. pyogenes,* and anaerobic bacteria. The role of the anaerobes is limited to cases in which aspiration occurs.

Among the nonbacterial agents known to cause community-acquired pneumonia are *Mycoplasma pneumoniae* and *Chlamydia pneumoniae* (TWAR). These two agents account for 10% to 20% of the pneumonias occurring in this setting. Finally, the true viruses such as influenza and adenovirus appear to be responsible for about 5% to 15% of the known cases. Never to be forgotten are *Mycobacterium tuberculosis* and fungal agents like *Coccidioides immitis* and *Histoplasma capsulatum,* which likely account for a small number of cases. The fungi, of course, will vary in the frequency with which they cause disease, depending on the geographic area under consideration. Of further importance is the fact that agents such as *Haemophilus* and *Legionella* usually prey on individuals with some underlying predisposition such as chronic lung disease, hypogammaglobulinemia, or alcoholism. Thus it is again worth emphasizing that the actual incidence of pneumonia caused by a given organism will vary with the individual and his or her unique features. Finally, in up to 50% of cases of community-acquired pneumonia, the specific etiology is never determined.

Since the etiologies may vary and treatments differ, it is reasonable to consider the diagnostic tests that need to be used. First is the question of documenting the pneumonia with chest radiography. It is believed this should be done in patients with respiratory symptoms who appear ill, in patients with moderately severe respiratory symptoms and underlying problems, and in patients with physical findings suggestive of pulmonary infection and systemic signs pointing to an infectious problem. Other individual considerations may be made depending on the particular case. Of major importance is establishing an etiologic diagnosis with as much confidence as possible. Recovery of a microbiologic agent from an uncontaminated specimen obtained from fluids such as blood or pleural fluid is extremely valuable and care should be taken to collect such specimens if possible. Isolation of an organism from a transthoracic lung aspiration or protected bronchoscopic brushing are also very valuable. Most physicians no longer use transtracheal aspirates because of the danger of hypoxia or bleeding. Since we either are not able or are unwilling to collect the type of diagnostic specimens mentioned, we must rely on other procedures in the less acutely ill patient or rely entirely on our clinical judgment.

Sputum collection with appropriate Gram stain and culture may be useful. One of the most important aspects of sputum collection is the care taken to obtain a specimen from the lung itself and not merely from oral secretions. Furthermore, direct observation and assessment of the quality of the sample by review of its color, character, and microscopic appearance contribute to determining the value of the specimen. Culture can only be of assistance when it is clear that the specimen reflects the flora of the infected area. Thus, it is not surprising that Gram stain may not be diagnostic in half or more of the cases, especially considering those individuals who can not produce a quality specimen. This all underlines the importance of the clinical decision-making process, not only in trying to verify an etiologic agent but also in determining empirical therapy when an adequate specimen is not available.

In addition to culture, serologies may be of value in pneumonias caused by such agents as *Mycoplasma, Chlamydia,* the true viruses, *Legionella pneumophila, Coxiella* or the fungi. Urinary antigen detection is of value with *Legionella.* Figure 1 demonstrates an algorithm for the approach to a patient with cough.

Pneumonia caused by *Streptococcus pneumoniae* is one of the most important types of pneumonia to consider. There are at least 84 different capsular types of *Strep. pneumoniae* that can cause pneumonia, although certain types are more frequently responsible for severe lower respiratory tract infection than others. The organism is a frequent inhabitant of the upper respiratory tract but has the ability to multiply rapidly in the lower tract. In most cases (75%), pneumococcal pneumonia is preceded by coryza. The onset of the pneumonia itself is usually abrupt and is usually associated with a shaking

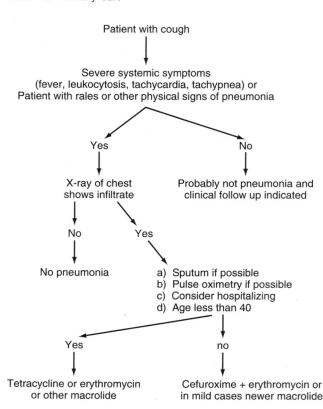

Patient with cough

Severe systemic symptoms
(fever, leukocytosis, tachycardia, tachypnea) or
Patient with rales or other physical signs of pneumonia

Yes   No

X-ray of chest   Probably not pneumonia and
shows infiltrate   clinical follow up indicated

No   Yes

No pneumonia

a) Sputum if possible
b) Pulse oximetry if possible
c) Consider hospitalizing
d) Age less than 40

Yes   no

Tetracycline or erythromycin   Cefuroxime + erythromycin or
or other macrolide   in mild cases newer macrolide

Figure 1. Algorithm for the management of a patient with cough.

chill. This is followed by fever and cough productive of blood-tinged sputum (rusty sputum). Pleuritic chest pain is very common and malaise and general prostration are frequent. The physical findings typically include tachycardia, tachypnea, and the signs of either bronchopneumonia or frank pulmonary consolidation. Abdominal findings like distension may be present.

Leukocytosis is most typical, but leukopenia often occurs in overwhelming cases. Radiographically, bronchopneumonia is more common in children and lobar more common in adults. The extent of the pneumonia depends on any delay on the part of the patient in seeking medical attention.

Many complications can occur, especially in patients who are treated late in the course of the disease. Bacteremia is seen in 25% to 30% of the cases and the usual mortality in the postantibiotic era is 5% or less. Debilitated patients are commonly afflicted by this agent and may fare worse. Other complications include empyema and pericarditis. Diagnosis is often established by appropriate stain and culture of the sputum, but culture of the blood or pleural fluid, if available and positive, is more specific.

The treatment of pneumococcal pneumonia may best be started with aftriaxone, 1 g BID.

Mild cases may respond to oral agents, but the more severe cases, especially those associated with tachypnea, hypoxia, extensive infiltration, or other underlying disease, are best treated parenterally.

Recently, penicillin-resistant pneumococci have become more frequent. Resistance is associated with an altered penicillin-binding protein in the organism. Both relative resistance (requiring higher concentrations to eradicate) and absolute resistance have been documented. Fortunately, the latter is less common. Because of these resistant strains, some believe the most severe cases of pneumococcal disease, or certainly those that either fail to respond or are associated with resistant organisms found on sensitivity tests, should be treated with third-generation cephalosporins or vancomycin until susceptibility is documented. These resistant organisms emphasize the appropriate use of the pneumococcal vaccine to prevent infection.

Haemophilus influenzae is another important bacterial cause of pneumonia. The organism is another frequent inhabitant of the upper airways. In the past, capsular type B was felt the most likely type to cause pneumonia, but recently even unencapsulated types have been reported to cause lower respiratory infections. The organism itself will most commonly cause infection in the very young or the elderly. It will also prey on the immunocompromised, especially those with chronic lung disease or agammoglobulinemia. The clinical picture resembles that of pneumonia associated with *Strep. pneumoniae,* although some believe there is a greater frequency of associated infection outside the lung, such as epiglotittis, otitis, or meningitis. This is more likely true in children. Diagnosis is again established from sputum, blood, or pleural fluid cultures.

Since almost half of the strains now produce beta-lactamase, the standard therapy of the past may well be ineffective. Therefore, currently recommended antibiotics include second-generation cephalosporins such as cefuroxime, ampicillin, and amoxicillin in combination with an inhibitor of beta-lactamase such as sulbactam or quinolones. More recently, newer macrolides such as clarithromycin or azithromycin have been found effective, especially for milder cases. The case fatality rate for pneumonia associated with *H. influenzae* is felt to be higher than that associated with *Strep. pneumoniae,* perhaps because of comorbidity due to other disease processes.

In recent years, other bacterial agents have also been found to be occasional causes of pneumonia. These include *Moraxella catarrhalis,* which produces disease under the circumstances likely associated with conditions such as chronic pulmonary disease. It responds to the same type of antibiotics used to treat *H. influenzae.*

The other common type of pneumonia associated with a bacterial agent is that attributed to *Legionella pneumophila.* This organism appears to have an affinity for water, particularly areas in air conditioning systems where water can accumulate and allow the organism to grow and disseminate. *Legionella* can become sporadic or epidemic in certain nosocomial situations. Typically patients with pneumonia due to *Legionella* are predisposed by cigarette smoking, chronic lung disease, advanced age, immunosuppression, and possibly excessive alcohol intake. The organism exists intracellularly, and, in contrast to the other forms of pneumonia discussed up to this point, cell-mediated immunity may be the body's most important defense against *Legionella.*

Clinically, *Legionella* infection may exist as a brief febrile illness called Pontiac fever or as the more typical pneumonia, Legionnaire's disease. After a brief incubation period (2 to 10 days), the patient experiences the onset of cough and chest pain. Extrapulmonary manifestations are common as they may be in any severe pneumonic process. These include diarrhea, nausea, vomiting, abdominal pain, headache, and encephalopathy.

The physical findings progress from a few rales to typical signs of consolidation. Laboratory confirmation can be made by culture of the sputum on charcoal yeast extract agar by direct fluorescent antibody stain of sputum smears, although the method is not especially sensitive. The diagnosis can also be made by measurement of serum antibody levels or detection of *Legionella*-specific antigen in urine or by use of a DNA probe.

Treatment is best accomplished with erythromycin, 2 to 4 g/day for at least 14 days. Rifampin has some activity against the agent, as do the quinolones.

Overall, the mortality from Legionnaire's disease, when appropriately treated, is under 10%.

Besides the bacterial agents, other types of organisms may produce community-acquired pneumonia. Among these is *Mycoplasma pneumoniae.* The organism is resistant to antibiotics active on the cell wall. The organism requires yeast extract and supplementary serum for growth but can be grown on artificial media.

The organism can be endemic, but distinct epidemic periods may be recognized and distinct outbreaks have been reported. Infection rates have been highest in school-aged children and young adults, and mycoplasma are known to spread extensively within the family unit. While lesser forms of respiratory illness can be seen with mycoplasma, 5% to 10% of the infections appear to result in pneumonia. Most important to the spread of the agent is the fact it may be detectable in respiratory secretions for many weeks. While immunity to the organism exists, recurrent mycoplasma infections can occur.

The incubation period for *M. pneumoniae* infections is 15 to 25 days. The disease begins with the gradual onset of constitutional symptoms, fever, and headache. Only about 10% of *Mycoplasma pneumoniae* infections actually result in pneumonia. The rest are either asymptomatic or present as pharyngitis or tracheobronchitis. The pneumonia itself is usually mild. After the period of constitutional symptoms, cough occurs, which initially is dry. Coryza, sore throat, hoarseness, and substernal pain may occur. Auscultatory findings are usually mild but include wheezes, rhonchi, and rales. Arthralgias and rash occur.

Roentgenographic findings include a subsegmental bronchopneumonia. Peripheral white blood cell count is usually normal. Gram stain should reveal polymorphonuclear cells and mononuclear cells with no bacteria or only bacteria from contamination. The best known antibody used to diagnose mycoplasma infections is the cold agglutinin. This immunoglobulin M antibody to the I antigen of red blood cells usually becomes evident at the end of the first week of illness. It is seen in about half the cases, although the sicker the patient, the more likely the antibody is to be detected. Specific mycoplasma antibody may be detected by enzyme-linked immunosorbent assay, and it is possible to culture the organism.

The clinical course of the pneumonia generally is completed in 1 to 2 weeks, although 6 weeks may be required to resolve the roentgenographic findings.

Complications of mycoplasma pneumonia include erythema multiform, erythema nodosum, sinusitis, bullous myringitis, intravascular hemolysis, meningoencephalitis, and both myocarditis and pericarditis.

The treatment of mycoplasma pneumonia is best undertaken with tetracyclines, erythromycin, and newer macrolides. It is likely that quinolones will be effective as well. Therapy should be given for 1 week and has been shown to shorten the clinical course. No vaccine is currently available.

Another recently identified cause of nonbacterial pneumonia likely seen in the community is that due to *Chlamydia pneumoniae* (also known as *Chlamydia* TWAR). This organism does not appear to have a bird or animal reservoir as does, for example, *Chlamydia psittaci*. In adults, approximately 25% to 50% of individuals have been found to have antibodies to this organism. The pathogenesis of this organism has not been well defined, but it is known to cause a variety of mild respiratory infections.

Pneumonia is perhaps the best described of the clinical illnesses associated with *Chlamydia pneumoniae*. This agent is known to cause 6% of pneumonias in one study of community-acquired pneumonias. A higher proportion has been noted in college students. The illness has many similarities to that caused by *Mycoplasma* except the cold agglutinin test can be expected to be negative. Fever, cough, and sore throat are all common features of pneumonic infections associated with *C. pneumoniae*. Infiltrates are typically modest and rales are typically present. The best treatment for *C. pneumoniae* infection is considered to be tetracycline for 10 to 14 days.

A number of true viruses are also associated with pneumonia. In children under 1 year of age, respiratory syncytial virus is probably the most common cause of this illness. Parainfluenza virus is also common as a cause of pneumonia in children. In older children and young adults, adenoviruses are an occasional cause of pneumonic infection. Typically these resemble illnesses caused by *Mycoplasma*, with the exception that the cold agglutinin test is typically negative and the course of disease is mild. No treatment or prophylaxis is generally available.

During the influenza season and during epidemic periods, the influenza virus may produce pneumonia. This is usually severe and is best known to occur in patients with mitral stenosis, although pregnancy is reported a risk factor. This is commonly a progressive illness with bilateral infiltrates and severe hypoxia. Death is common and no proven effective therapy is known, although amantadine and rimantadine are worthy of trial.

Finally, many milder cases of pneumonia in otherwise healthy individuals can be treated at home. Indications for hospitalization include (1) serious underlying disease, (2) hypoxia or tachypnea (respiratory rate greater than 25 in adults), (3) hypotension, (4) systemic toxicity, (5) patient's social circumstances that do not allow careful follow-up, and (6) extensive pulmonary infiltration.

INDEX

Note: Page numbers in *italics* refer to illustrations;
page numbers followed by (t) refer to tables.

A

Abacavir, for AIDS, 295(t)
Abdomen, examination of, in newborn, 385
  removal of IUD from, 97
  wall of, local anesthetization of, for cesarean section, 241–242
Abdominal hysterectomy. See also *Hysterectomy.*
  for fibroids, 100
  for ovarian cancer, 219
  risk of cellulitis following, in patient with vaginosis, 185
Abdominal retropubic urethropexy/ colposuspension procedure, for incontinence, 178, 179
ABO blood group incompatibility, 432
Abortion, spontaneous, 349
  recurrent, 349–354. See also *Death, fetal.*
    analyses indicated in, 226–227, 350(t)
    antiphospholipid syndrome and, 9, 351
    management of, 352–354, *354*
      allogeneic monocyte immuno-therapy in, 352, *353*
      intravenous immunoglobulin in, 352–354, *353*
  therapeutic, 358–360. See also *Selective termination.*
    in patient with PROM, 328
Abruptio placentae, 361, 363, 364
  risk of, equivocal effects of aspirin use in relation to, 302, *302*
Abscess, Bartholin's duct, 14–15
  tubo-ovarian, 130–131
Absent end-diastolic velocity (AEDV), on umbilical arterial Doppler sonography, 391
  as indicator of high-risk pregnancy, 391(t), 391–393
Absolute lymphocyte count, as marker of nutritional status, 500
Abuse, child, sexual, 156
  domestic, *453,* 453–456
  sexual, 154–156
    domestic violence and, 455
Abuser/drug addict, pregnant patient as, 269–271
AC (Adriamycin [doxorubicin]-cyclophosphamide) regimen, for breast cancer, 460
Acardiac twin, 365
Acebutolol, for hypertension, 482(t)
Acetaminophen-isometheptene-dichloralphenazone, for headache, 471–472
Acne, 437–440
  androgen excess and, 3

Acne *(Continued)*
  management of, *437,* 437–440
    during pregnancy, 439
      dangers of isotretinoin use in, 440
  oral contraceptives exacerbating, 121
ACOG (American College of Obstetricians and Gynecologists) criteria, for timing of delivery, 418
Acquired immunodeficiency syndrome (AIDS), 293–296, 440–444
  in pregnant patient, 293–296
  opportunistic infections complicating, 294
    prophylaxis against, 296(t), 442–443
  treatment of, 294, 295(t), 443–444
Actinomycin D, for trophoblastic disease, 212, 212(t)
Active management approach, to labor, 272
Actocardiography, in fetal surveillance, 373
Acute respiratory distress, after evacuation of hydatidiform mole, 216
Acute salpingitis. See *Pelvic inflammatory disease.*
Acyclovir, for herpes simplex virus infection, 71–72, 161, 162, 162(t)
  in pregnant patient, 72
Addictive drugs, effects of maternal use of, 269–271
Addisonian crisis, cortisone for, 74, 76, 76(t)
Adefovir dipivoxil, for AIDS, 295(t)
Adenocarcinoma, endometrial, 202, 207–210
  hyperplasia and, 42
  screening for, problems with, 202–203
  staging of, 209(t)
Adenoma. See also *Tumor(s).*
  adrenal, 5
    androgen-secreting, 5
  pituitary, prolactin-secreting. See *Prolactin-secreting tumor.*
    vs. lymphocytic hypophysitis, 74
  thyroid, toxic, 173
Adenomyosis, 47
Adhesiolysis, hysteroscopic, 91
  hormone therapy following, 92, 148
  pregnancy subsequent to, 92
  splinting following, with IUD, 91
Adhesions, intrauterine, 90–92, 148
  pelvic, 41, 132
Adnexa, uterine, lesions of, appearing as masses, 1
  causing dyspareunia, 42
  torsion of, 1

Adolescent patient, dysfunctional uterine bleeding in, 28
  treatment of, 29
Adrenal hyperplasia, nonclassic, 3–5
Adrenal origin, of androgen excess, 2–7
Adrenal tumors, 5
  androgen-secreting, 5
Adriamycin (doxorubicin), for breast cancer, 460
Adult morbidity/mortality, causes of, in women, 444(t)
AEDV (absent end-diastolic velocity), on umbilical arterial Doppler sonography, 391
  as indicator of high-risk pregnancy, 391(t), 391–393
Aftriaxone, for pneumococcal pneumonia, 506
Agranulocytosis, antithyroid drug use and, 174–175
  myelosuppression and, 153
  treatment of, 153
AIDS. See *Acquired immunodeficiency syndrome (AIDS).*
Albuterol, for asthma, in pregnant patient, 247
Alcohol abuse, pancreatitis due to, 314
  screening for, using TACE question-naire, 269
  teratogenic effects of, 269
Alcohol injection, for dysmenorrhea, 35
  for vulvar pruritus, 118
Alcohol-related birth defects, 269
Alendronate, for osteoporosis, in postmenopausal patient, 110
Allergen avoidance, by pregnant asthmatic patient, 245
Allogeneic monocyte immunotherapy, for recurrent spontaneous abortion, 352, *353*
Allograft, renal, pregnancy in recipient of, 341(t), 341–342
Alpha-fetoprotein, amniotic fluid, significance of, 227
Alprazolam, for premenstrual dysphoric disorder, 143
Amantadine, for fatigue, in multiple sclerosis, 495
Ambiguous genitalia, 386
Amenorrhea, 143–150. See also *Anovulation; Infertility.*
  euestrogenic, 147(t), 148
  hyperandrogenic, 147(t), 148
  hyperprolactinemic, 147, 150
  hypoestrogenic, 147, 147(t), 148
  primary, 143–146
  secondary, 146–150
    causes of, 147(t)
    evaluation of, *149*
    management of, 148, 150
      hysteroscopic adhesiolysis in, re-sults of, 92

ISBN 0-7216-7579-4